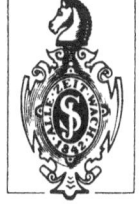

G. Baroldi F. Camerini
J. F. Goodwin (Eds.)

Advances in Cardiomyopathies

With 147 Figures and 119 Tables

Springer-Verlag Berlin Heidelberg New York
London Paris Tokyo Hong Kong

G. Baroldi, M.D.
Istituto Fisiologia Clinica CNR,
Dipartimento di Cardiologia A. De Gasperis,
Ospedale Niguarda, Ca' Granda,
Piazza Ospedale Maggiore 3, 20612 Milan, Italy

F. Camerini, M.D.
Dipartimento di Cardiologia, Ospedale Maggiore,
Piazza Ospedale 1, 34129 Trieste, Italy

J. F. Goodwin, M.D.
2 Pine Grove, Lake Road, Wimbledon,
London SW19 7HE, UK

ISBN-13:978-3-642-83762-3   e-ISBN-13:978-3-642-83760-9
DOI: 10.1007/978-3-642-83760-9

Library of Congress Cataloging-in-Publication Data
Advances in cardiomyopathies / G. Baroldi, F. Camerini,
J. F. Goodwin (eds.).
ISBN-13:978-3-642-83762-3(U.S. : alk. paper)1.Heart--Dilatation.2. Heart--
Muscle--Diseases. 3. Heart--Hypertrophy. I. Baroldi, Giorgio.
II. Camerini, F. III. Goodwin, John F. [DNLM: 1. Cardiomyopathy,
Congestive. 2. Myocardial Diseases. WG 280 A244]
RC685.D55A38 1990 616.1'24--dc20 DNLM/DLC

© Springer-Verlag Berlin Heidelberg 1990
  Softcover reprint of the hardcover 1st edition   1990

2119/3140–5 4 3 2 1 0 – Printed on acid-free paper

Preface

The international symposium organized by the Italian Study Group on Cardiomyopathies (SPIC) and planned by the organizing and scientific committees opened with a review of the history of cardiomyopathy over the last 30 years by Goodwin, London (UK) and continued with presentations on all aspects of hypertrophic and dilated cardiomyopathy by a wide spectrum of international experts.

This book includes mainly the invited contributions, but there are also many original oral presentations.

Hypertrophic cardiomyopathy is well addressed by papers on natural history, ventricular function, ischaemia and arrhythmia. Of particular interest is the note by Bonow, National Heart Lung and Blood Institute (NHLBI; USA), on the effect of beta-adrenergic stimulation with isoprenalin in increasing the rate and extent of left ventricular relaxation, beta-adrenergic blocking agents having no such effect. In contrast, verapamil improves ventricular relaxation as would be expected. These results challenge accepted belief in some ways and indicate that multiple factors – both passive and active – acting on the left ventricle, such as ischaemia, asynchrony, altered left ventricular loading and intracellular levels of calcium ions, are all operating. These aspects are the more interesting in view of the recent reports of an increase in calcium-channel receptors, but not in beta-adrenergic receptors, in hypertrophic cardiomyopathy.

The relation of arrhythmias to sudden death is outlined by McKenna, London (UK), who points out that 25% of adults with hypertrophic cardiomyopathy have nonsustained ventricular tachycardia which is an 80% marker for sudden death. Fananapazir and colleagues from the National Heart Lung and Blood Institute (USA) present electrophysiological studies in 115 patients with hypertrophic cardiomyopathy who had developed cardiac arrest, syncope, pre-syncope, palpitations or subclinical ventricular tachycardia. Programmed ventricular stimulation induces sustained arrhythmia in 45 of 115 patients. This detailed and expert work deserves close attention. The authors report no untoward effects and consider that the induction of sustained arrhythmia including polymorphic ventricular tachycardia provides an important guide to therapy. Readers may be concerned that in a larger series or in less expert hands production of a potentially lethal arrhythmia would be hazardous.

On the treatment of hypertrophic cardiomyopathy, Kaltenbach and Hopf (FRG) report that beta-blocking agents reduced outflow gradients initially but verapamil appeared more effective. Amiodarone controls arrhythmia but does not produce haemodynamic improvement. Schulte and colleagues report that septectomy (myectomy) is effective in producing significant clinical and haemodynamic improvement but comment on perioperative complications and lack of beneficial effect on prognosis. Maron and colleagues (NHLBI) report interesting data on intraoperative echocardiography used to plan the extent of septectomy and so to avoid the production of a ventricular septal defect. Wigle (Canada) reviews the well known options of medical and surgical treatment including a useful note that cardiac transplantation should be considered in endstage patients with congestive cardiac failure.

The session on hypertrophic cardiomyopathy is concluded by Epstein (NHLBI) in a paper on future research trends in which he emphasizes that the basic cellular abnormality in hypertrophic cardiomyopathy could be connected with many factors such as abnormal activity of growth factors, calcium intracellular regulation, norepinephrine kinetics or an interaction between all these various mechanisms.

The session on dilated cardiomyopathy opens with papers on the pathogenesis. Kawai's group from Japan report increased synthesis and secretion of atrial natriuretic polypeptide (ANP) in atrium and ventricle in EMC-virus myocarditis in mice. The authors suggest that increase synthesis and secretion of ANP in both chambers may have a role in the pathophysiology both of myocarditis and later cardiomyopathy. Anderson and colleagues (Salt Lake City, USA) describe work that suggests that in patients with dilated cardiomyopathy, genetically determined immune regulatory factors associated with Major Histocompatibility Complex (MHC) antigens might be involved in the causation of dilated cardiomyopathy. Maisch (FRG) notes that antimyolemmal antibodies directed against sarcolemma are diagnostic markers for both myocarditis and dilated cardiomyopathy. He concludes that antigenic mimicry operates in acute myocarditis and might be relevant to dilated heart muscle disease. Of outstanding interest is the report of Archard and colleagues (UK) who, using molecular hybridization via a specific

RNA probe, show the presence of enterovirus RNA fragments in biopsy specimens from a significant proportion of patients with myocarditis and also those with dilated cardiomyopathy. They also found probe positive results in explanted hearts from dilated cardiomyopathy patients. The RNA fragments persist until endstage disease but without eliciting a full immunological response. This, the authors consider, suggests that persistent infection results from the generation of defective virus without eliciting full immunological response. The findings help to explain the difficulty of detecting virus itself in the myocardium and absence of specific histological changes. This paper is extremely important and should be read in detail.

Billingham, Stanford (USA) describes the morphological diagnosis of myocarditis and of dilated cardiomyopathy and emphasizes the differences between dilated cardiomyopathy and anthracyclin-induced heart muscle disease, but notes that dilated cardiomyopathy could not be distinguished from alcoholic heart muscle disease or peripartum cardiomyopathy.

The section on clinical aspects of dilated cardiomyopathy includes papers on the natural history and the clinical presentation and evolution in treated and untreated myocarditis emphasizing the presence of the clinical picture of dilated cardiomyopathy in some patients with myocarditis.

Immunosuppressive treatment in active myocarditis is reviewed by O'Connell (Salt Lake City, USA) who points out that the reports of results are disparate and describes the initiation of a multicentre trial co-ordinated by the University of Utah and sponsored by the National Heart Lung and Blood Institute (USA).

Subsequent papers cover the natural history and prognosis of dilated cardiomyopathy, myocardial metabolism and perfusion and complex arrhythmias. Results of the SPIC multicentre cardiomyopathy study suggest that complex ventricular arrhythmias are not as frequent as often thought and are not related to pump dysfunction, but are a major independent determinant of sudden death.

Treatment of dilated cardiomyopathy with positive inotropic agents, vasodilators, beta-blocking agents and transplantation are dealt with in the final session. A place for digitalis but not for oral phosphodiesterase inhibitors is argued by Leier (USA). A notable contribution by J. Cohn (Minneapolis, USA) emphasizes the value of vasodilators in improving prognosis, notably a combination of oral nitrates and hydralazine (V-HeFT trial) in the United States or enalapril (CONSENSUS trial) in Europe. These trials show mortality reductions of 38% and 31% respectively. This paper deserves close study.

The rationale of beta-adrenergic treatment is well argued by Waagstein, Goteborg (Sweden). A subset of patients with dilated cardiomyopathy have auto-antibodies to beta-receptors; overstimulation of beta-1 receptors may lead to exhaustion and "down-regulation" with development of dilated cardiomyopathy. Beta-adrenergic blockade recruits more beta-receptors and the resultant 'up-regulation' improves the inotropic response to catecholamines. A small controlled study suggests that beta-blockers and ACE inhibitors together may cause an additive improvement of function.

The group from Trento (Italy) describes the use of various anti-arrhythmic drugs and concludes that amiodarone is the best choice; sotalol, propafenone and mexiletine being alternatives. The implantation of a cardioverter defibrillator might represent a bridge to cardiac transplantation in some desperately ill patients.

Cardiac transplantation is described by the group from London (Ontario) in 80 patients with dilated cardiomyopathy. Survival is 86% at 3 months, 83% at 12 months and 81% at 3 years offering a marked improvement in prognosis over medical treatment in advanced cases.

The book concludes with a report from the Mayo Clinic on dilated cardiomyopathy in children and clinical and pathological features of right ventricular dysplasia. It appears that assessing the prognosis of dilated cardiomyopathy in children is difficult because of few reports and small patient numbers in the literature. Papers from Padua by Thiene and colleagues and by Dalla-Volta give an excellent overall description of right ventricular dysplasia and its problems. They suggest a familial incidence in 75% of cases and stress that right ventricular dysplasia is a well recognised cause of familial sudden death in subjects between 5 and 30 years of age. Anti-arrhythmic treatment offers some protection.

It has not been possible for reasons of space to mention all papers in this introduction, in which we have attemped to draw attention to the most important issues raised.

G. Baroldi
F. Camerini
J. F. Goodwin

Table of Contents

II Dilated Cardiomyopathy

1 Pathogenesis of Dilated Cardiomyopathy

List of Contributors

M. Ambrosini, M. D.
Department of Cardiology and Cardiac
Surgery, University "La Sapienza", Via
Marianna Dionigi 16, 00193 Rome, Italy

J. L. Anderson, M. D.
University of Utah, Department of
Internal Medicine, Division of Cardiolo-
gy, LDS Hospital, 8th Avenue and C
Street, Salt Lake City, UT 84143, USA

E. Arbustini, M. D.
Department of Pathology, IRCCS,
Policlinico S. Matteo, Università degli
Studi di Pavia, Via Forlani 14,
27100 Pavia, Italy

L. C. Archard, M. D., Ph. D.
Department of Biochemistry, Charing
Cross and Westminster Medical School,
Fulham Palace Road, London W6 8RP,
UK

S. Berti, M. D.
Istituto di Fisiologia Clinica del CNR,
Via P. Savi 8, 56100 Pisa, Italy

R. Bettini, M. D.
Divisione di Cardiologia e Centro
Aritmologico, 38100 Trento, Italy

M. E. Billingham, M. D.
Stanford University Medical Center,
Stanford, CA 94305, USA

R. O. Bonow, M. D.
Building 10, Room 7B–15, National
Institutes of Health, Bethesda, MD
20892, USA

R. O. Cannon, III, M. D.
Cardiology Branch, National Heart, Lung
and Blood Institute, National Institutes of
Health, Bethesda, MD 20892, USA

F. Cecchi, M. D.
Cardiologia S. Luca, Ospedale di Careggi,
USL 10/E, 50100 Florence, Italy

T. Chikamori, M. D.
Department of Cardiological Sciences,
St. George's Hospital Medical School,
Cranmer Terrace, London SW17 ORE,
UK

M. Ciaccheri, M. D.
Cardiologia S. Luca, Ospedale di Careggi,
50100 Florence, Italy

J. N. Cohn, M. D.
Cardiovascular Division, University of
Minnesota, Box 488 UMHC,
420 Delaware Street SE, Minneapolis,
MN 55455, USA

C. Contini, M. D.
CNR Institute of Clinical Physiology,
University of Pisa, Via Savi 8, 56100 Pisa,
Italy

S. Dalla-Volta, M. D.
The Division of Cardiology, Dept. of In-
ternal Medicine, University of Padova
Medical School, 35121 Padova, Italy

R. De Maria, M. D.
Istituto Fisiologia Clinica CNR,
Dipartimento di Cardiologia A. De
Gasperis, Ospedale Niguarda Ca' Granda,
Piazza Ospedale Maggiore 3,
20612 Milan, Italy

G. Di Pasquale, M. D.
Divisione di Cardiologia, Ospedale
Bellaria, Via Altura 3, 40139 Bologna,
Italy

S. E. Epstein, M. D.
Chief, Cardiology Branch 10, 7B15,
NIH, Bethesda, MD 20892, USA

L. Fananapazir, M. D.
Building 10, Room 7B–15, Cardiology
Branch, National Institutes of Health,
Bethesda, MD 20892, USA

R. E. Fowles, M. D.
Salt Lake Clinic, University of Utah,
Cardiology Division, 333 South 900 East
Street, Salt Lake City, UT 84102, USA

F. Furlanello, M. D.
Divisione di Cardiologia e Centro
Aritmologico, Ospedale S. Chiara,
38100 Trento, Italy

A. Gavazzi, M. D.
Divisione di Cardiologia, Istituto di
Ricovero e Cura a Carattere Scientifico,
Policlinico S. Matteo, 27100 Pavia, Italy

E. M. Gilbert, M. D.
Division of Cardiology, 4A–100,
University of Utah School of Medicine,
50 North Medical Drive, Salt Lake City,
UT 84132, USA

J. F. Goodwin, M. D.
Royal Postgraduate Medical School,
Ducane Road, London W12, UK

E. H. Hammond, M. D.
LDS Hospital, Department of Pathology,
8th Avenue and C Street, Salt Lake City,
UT 84143, USA

M. Herzum, M. D.
Philipps-Universität Marburg, Abteilung
Innere Medizin, Kardiologie,
Baldingerstraße, 3550 Marburg, FRG

R. Hopf, M. D.
Innere Abteilung des Krankenhauses
Sachsenhausen, Schulstraße 31,
6000 Frankfurt/M. 70, FRG

W. J. Kostuk, M. D.
Cardiac Investigation Unit, University
Hospital, BOX 5339, London, Ontario,
N6A 5A5, Canada

C. V. Leier, M. D.
Division of Cardiology, The Ohio State
University College of Medicine,
666 Means Hall, 1654 Upham Drive,
Columbus, OH 43210, USA

C. J. Limas, M. D.
Department of Laboratory Medicine
and Pathology, University of Minnesota
and VA Medical Center, Minneapolis,
MN 55455, USA

B. Maisch, M. D.
Zentrum für Innere Medizin,
Schwerpunkt Kardiologie,
Klinikum Lahnberge, Baldingerstraße,
3550 Marburg, FRG

B. J. Maron, M. D.
Building 10, Room 7B–15, National
Institutes of Health, Bethesda,
MD 20892, USA

A. Matsumori, M. D.
Department of Internal Medicine,
Faculty of Medicine, Kyoto University,
54 Kawaracho Shogoin, Sakyo-ku,
Kyoto 606, Japan

W. J. McKenna, M. D.
Department of Cardiological Sciences,
St. George's Hospital Medical School,
Cranmer Terrace, London SW17 ORE,
UK

J. B. O'Connell, M. D.
Division of Cardiology, University of
Utah Medical School, 50 North Medical
Drive, Salt Lake City, UT 84132, USA

T. Richter, M. D.
Hungarian Institute of Cardiology,
P.O. Box 88, Budapest 1450, Hungary

W. Ruzyllo, M. D.
Department of General Cardiology,
National Institute of Cardiology, Alpejska
42, 04-628 Warsaw, Poland

A. Salvi, M. D.
Department of Cardiology, Ospedale
Maggiore, Piazza Ospedale 1,
34129 Trieste, Italy

H. D. Schulte, M. D.
Heinrich-Heine-Universität Düsseldorf,
Chirurgische Klinik und Poliklinik,
Abt. Thorax- und Kardiovaskularchirur-
gie, Moorenstraße 5,
4000 Düsseldorf, FRG

H. P. Schultheiss, M. D.
Heinrich-Heine-Universität Düsseldorf,
Medizinische Klinik und Poliklinik G,
Abteilung für Kardiologie, Pneumologie
und Angiologie, Moorenstraße 5,
4000 Düsseldorf, FRG

M. Sekiguchi, M. D.
Department of Internal Medicine,
Shinshu University School of Medicine,
3-1-1 Asahi, Matsumoto-City, 390 Japan

P. Spirito, M. D.
Divisione di Cardiologia, Ospedali
Galliera, Via Volta 8, Genoa, Italy

C. P. Taliercio, M. D.
Division of Cardiovascular Diseases and
Internal Medicine, Mayo Clinic,
200 First Street Southwest, Rochester,
MN 55905, USA

G. Thiene, M. D.
Istituto di Anatomia Patologica,
Via Gabelli 61, 35121 Padova,Italy

F. Waagstein, M. D.
Department of Medicine I, Sahlgren's
Hospital, University of Göteborg,
41345 Göteborg, Sweden

E. D. Wigle, M. D.
12-EN-217, Toronto General Hospital,
200 Elizabeth Street, Toronto, Ontario
M5G 2C4, Canada

Introduction: Thirty Years of Cardiomyopathy

J. F. Goodwin

Approximately 150 years ago the term myocarditis was used indiscriminately to describe virtually all disorders involving the myocardium. Lack of precision in terminology and definition hindered progress, but by the 1950s, Mattingly, Birch and Proctor Harvey in the United States were diligently collecting and studying cases of heart muscle disease. At this time, terms such as "myocardopathy" and "myocardiopathy" were often used [1]. The term "cardiomyopathy" was probably first used by Bridgen in 1957 [2] to describe conditions involving the myocardium, but not due to coronary artery disease. He described these as "non-coronary cardiomyopathies". Gradually, the cardiomyopathies came to be distinguished from myocarditis, which now is properly defined as "inflammation of the myocardium due to infection, autoimmune response, rejection, allergy or toxic agents".

In 1951 Goodwin et al. [3] defined cardiomyopathy as "a subacute or chronic disorder of heart muscle of unknown or obscure aetiology often with associated endocardial and sometimes pericardial involvement and not atherosclerotic in origin". Cardiomyopathies were then classified according to disorders of structure and function into hypertrophic, congestive, restrictive and obliterative [4]. Subsequently the definition was shortened to "cardiomyopathy, a disorder of heart muscle of unknown cause" [5]. Cardiomyopathies thus defined were separated from myocardial disorders occurring as part of a general system disease, which were described as "specific heart muscle diseases" [6]. The term "obliterative" was omitted because obliteration is a late stage of endomyocardial fibrosis (restrictive cardiomyopathy).

Following the work of Kawai [7a], I suggested in 1974 that virus infection of the heart might lead to dilated cardiomyopathy [7]. Since then, increasing evidence to support this theory has been produced [8–10], the mechanism suggested being direct destruction of myocardial cells by the virus which also sets up an autoimmune process involving suppressor T cells [11]. Recently, Coxsackie virus RNA sequences have been found in the myocardium of patients with myocarditis and others with dilated cardiomyopathy [13], further strengthening this theory, but, even so, it is improbable that more than 50% of cases of dilated cardiomyopathy can be explained on a previous virus infection.

The definition of cardiomyopathies as "heart muscle diseases of unknown cause" and the classification into hypertrophic, dilated and restrictive was endorsed by the WHO/ISFC Task Force on Definition and Classification of

Cardiomyopathies [14] and by the WHO Expert Committee on Cardiomyopathies [15].

Dilated cardiomyopathy, originally described as "congestive", was early recognised as a quite separate entity from hypertrophic and restrictive cardiomyopathies on the basis of striking differences in structure and function. The most important differences were dilatation, modest hypertrophy and severely impaired pump function in dilated cardiomyopathy as compared with massive hypertrophy, lack of ventricular dilatation and powerful pump function in hypertrophic cardiomyopathy. Fibrosis of the endomyocardium with overlying thrombosis in endomyocardial fibrosis (the commonest cause of restrictive cardiomyopathy) provided clear differentiation. It was clear also that dilated cardiomyopathy was not a single entity, but the final common path of cardiac dilatation, pump failure and congestive heart failure produced by a number of different cardiac insults. To this day, apart from the evidence suggesting a virus aetiology in some patients, no further evidence exists to implicate any other cause. Potentiating, associated or risk factors have been named such as alcohol, hypertension and pregnancy. Although deficiency diseases such as selenium produce a syndrome identical with congestive cardiomyopathy, selenium deficiency is an example of specific heart muscle disease, since the cause is known.

The term "congestive" was introduced to describe dilated cardiomyopathy at a time when patients were not diagnosed until congestive heart failure became established and no definite cause could be found. Improvement in diagnostic techniques and increasing knowledge of the natural history has permitted earlier diagnosis, so the term dilated seems more appropriate, but remains purely descriptive [14, 15].

The history of hypertrophic cardiomyopathy is more clear cut, but more complex than that of dilated cardiomyopathy and many different names have been used. Probably the first descriptions of hypertrophic cardiomyopathy were by Liouville in 1869 and Hallopeau in the same year [16, 17], followed by Schminke in 1907 [18]. The disease reappeared 50 years later when Brock in 1957 described "functional obstruction of the left ventricle" [19]. In 1958, Teare [20] reported for the first time the detailed pathology of the disease which he described as "asymmetrical hypertrophy of the heart". In 1960, Braunwald et al. [21] in the United States described it as "idiopathic hypertrophic subaortic stenosis" (IHSS), and Goodwin et al. [22], believing it to be a form of heart muscle disease, described it as "obstructive cardiomyopathy". Later the word "hypertrophic" was added, and we called it "hypertrophic obstructive cardiomyopathy" (HOCM) [23]. In 1963, Wigle et al. described the disease as "muscular subaortic stenosis" [24].

Despite recognition that diastolic faults were a more important component of the disease than outflow tract gradients, arguments have continued as to whether these gradients represent true obstruction to outflow from the left ventricle or not [25–27]. Recent research suggests that while a minority of patients have true impediment to outflow, the majority do not. (McKenna, Personal Communication 1988). The cause of hypertrophic cardiomyopathy remains uncertain, but the most likely theory is abnormal handling of catecholamines by the developing heart in utero on a familial basis [7, 28].

The commonest cause of restrictive cardiomyopathy is endomyocardial fibrosis, the history of which goes back to the early description of tropical endomyocardial fibrosis in Africa by Davies in Kampala in 1948 [29]. While originally thought to be different from the eosinophilic endomyocardial disease described by Loffler [30], it is now known that the pathology is identical in the two forms and both appear to represent the same disease in which the rogue eosinophil (which is immunologically abnormal) causes damage to the endomyocardium, initially inflammation followed by exudative fibrosis and thrombosis [30]. The cause of the eosinophilic abnormality is unknown, and may not necessarily be the same in the tropical as in the temperate climates. Both types of endomyocardial fibrosis are now known as "eosinophilic endomyocardial disease" [14].

A view of the past is incomplete without a vision of the future. This vision will include molecular biological techniques to identify cases of hypertrophic cardiomyopathy in utero. Detection of abnormal calcium channel receptors in the myocardium in hypertrophic cardiomyopathy will permit earlier effective appropriate treatment. Detection of virus material in the myocardium in myocarditis and dilated cardiomyopathy will encourage effective antiviral agents to be developed for myocarditis. Spectroscopic magnetic resonance will be used to study the biochemical pathology of the myocardium.

References

1. Goodwin JF (1979) Cardiomyopathy: an interface between fundamental and clinical cardiology. In: Hayasi S, Muraos (eds) Proceding of the VIII world congress of Cardiology. Excerpta Med. International congress series 470. Elsevier, Amsterdam, p 10
2. Brigden W (1957) Uncommon myocardial diseases – the non-coronary cardiomyopathies. Lancet 2:1179–1243
3. Goodwin JF, Hollman A, Bishop MB (1961) Clinical aspects of cardiomyopathy. Br Med J 1:69
4. Goodwin JF (1964) Cardiac function in primary myocardial disorders. Br Med J 1:1527–1595
5. Goodwin JF (1970) Congestive and hypertrophic cardiomyopathies – a decade of study. Lancet 1:731
6. Goodwin JF, Oakley CM (1972) Editorial; the cardiomyopathies. Br Heart J 34:545
7. Goodwin JF (1974) Prospects and predictions for the cardiomyopathies. Circulation 50:210
7a. Kawai C (1971) Idiopathic cardiomyopathy, a study on the infectious-immune theory as a course of the disease. Jpn Circ J 35:765
8. Cambridge G, MacArthur CGC, Waterson AP, Goodwin JF, Oakley CM (1979) Antibodies to coxsackie B virus in congestive cardiomyopathy. Br Heart J 41:693
9. Quigley PJ, Richardson PJ, Meany BT, Olsen EGJ, Monagham MJ, Jackson G, Jewitt DE (1978) Long term follow up of acute myocarditis. Correlation of ventricular function and outcome. Eur Heart J 8 (Suppl): 39
10. Abelman WH (1988) Myocarditis as a cause of dilated cardiomyopathy. In: Engelmeier RS, O'Connell JG (eds) Drug therapy in dilated cardiomyopathy and myocarditis. Dekker, New York, p 221
11. Haber E, Yasuda T, Palacios IF, Kwaw WG (1987) Scintigraphy in the diagnosis of acute myocarditis. In: Kuwaii C, Abelman W (eds) Pathogenesis of myocarditis and cardiomyopathy. University of Tokyo Press, Tokyo, p 277
12. O'Connell JB, Mason JW (1987) Scintigraphy in the diagnosis of acute myocarditis. In: Kawai C, Abelman W (eds) Pathogenesis of myocarditis and cardiomyopathy. University of Tokyo Press, Tokyo, p 281

13. Bowles NE, Richardson PJ, Olsen EGJ, Archard LC (1986) Detection of coxsackie B-virus-specific-RNA sequences in myocardial biopsy from cases of myocarditis and cardiomyopathy. Lancet 1:1120
14. Report of the WHO/ISFC Task Force on the definition and classification of cardiomyopathies (1980) Br Heart J 44:672
15. Report of WHO Expert Committee (1984) Cardiomyopathies. WHO technical report series 697. WHO, Geneva
16. Liovillie H (1869) Retrécissement cardiaque sous aortique. Gazette Med Paris 24:161
17. Hallopeau M (1869) Retrécissement ventriculo-aortique. Gazette Med Paris 24:683
18. Schminke A (1907) Über linksartige musculöse Conenstenosen. Dtsch Med Wochensch 33:2082
19. Brock R (1957) Functional obstruction of the left ventricle (acquired subvalvar aortic stenosis). Guy's Hosp Rep 106:221
20. Teare D (1958) Asymmetrical hypertrophy of the heart in young adults. Br Heart J 20:1
21. Braunwald E, Morrow AG, Cornell WP, Aygen MM, Hilbish TF (1960) Idiopathic hypertrophic subaortic stenosis. Clinical, haemodynamic, angiographic manifestations. Am J Med 29:924
22. Goodwin JF, Holman A, Clel WP, Teare D (1960) Obstructive cardiomyopathy simulating aortic stenosis. Br Heart J 22:403
23. Cohen J, Effat H, Goodwin JF, Oakley CM, Steiner RE (1964) Hypertrophic obstructive cardiomyopathy. Br Heart J 26:16
24. Wigle ED, Heimbecker RO, Gunton RW (1962) Idiopathic ventricular septal hypertrophy causing muscular subaortic stenosis. Circulation 26:325
25. Wigle ED, Henderson M, Sasson Z, Pollick C, Rakowski H (1985) Muscular subaortic stenosis (hypertrophic obstructive cardiomyopathy): the evidence for obstruction to left ventricular outflow. In: Goodwin JF (ed) Heart muscle disease. MTP Press, London, p 217
26. Criley JM, Siegel RJ (1985) A non-obstructive view of hypertrophic cardiomyopathy. In: Goodwin JF (ed) Heart muscle disease. MTP Press, London, p 157
27. Murgo JP, Miller JW (1985) Haemodynamic, angiographic and echocardiographic evidence against impeded ejection in hypertrophic cardiomyopathy. In: Goodwin JF (ed) Heart muscle disease. MTP Press, London, p 187
28. Perloff JK (1985) Pathogenesis of hypertrophic cardiomyopathy. In: Goodwin JF (ed) Heart muscle disease. MTP Press, London, p 7
29. Davies JNP (1948) Endomyocardial fibrosis in Africa. East Afr Med J 25:10
30. Olsen EGJ, Spry CJF (1979) The pathogenesis of Loffler's endomyocardial disease and its relationship to endomyocardial fibrosis. In: Yu PN, Goodwin JF (eds) Progress in cardiology, vol 8. Lea and Febiger, Philadelphia, p 281

I Hypertrophic Cardiomyopathy

Evolution of Left Ventricular Hypertrophy in Patients with Hypertrophic Cardiomyopathy

B. J. Maron

Introduction

Application of echocardiography to cardiac diagnosis in the 1970s represented a major advance in the non-invasive identification of patients with hypertrophic cardiomyopathy (HCM) [1, 2]. Subsequently, the utilization of two-dimensional echocardiography and other ultrasound modalities in large numbers of patients with HCM over many years have stimulated continued definition of the diverse morphologic expression of the disease, changes in left ventricular morphology which appear to be part of its natural history, and the clinical relevance of left ventricular hypertrophy within the broad spectrum of patients [3–18]. As a result, it has become apparent that the morphology of HCM may not be identical or even similar in different phases of life. With these considerations in mind, the present review is focused on the patterns of left ventricular hypertrophy and the relationship between age and left ventricular anatomy in patients with HCM.

Patterns and Distribution of Left Ventricular Hypertrophy

Left ventricular hypertrophy is the gross anatomic marker and probably the principal determinant of most of the clinical features of HCM [5, 10]. Indeed, it is generally agreed that the characteristic morphologic marker of HCM is an asymmetrically hypertrophied and nondilated left ventricle in the absence of another cardiac or systemic disease capable of producing the degree of left ventricular wall thickening present in that patient. Although a symmetric pattern of left ventricular hypertrophy may occur occasionally [4, 6], the distribution of the hypertrophy is asymmetric in the vast majority of patients [3–5, 7–18] (Fig. 1). Frequently, wall thickening is strikingly heterogeneous, and contiguous segments of the left ventricle may differ greatly in thickness. The transition between regions of the wall that are thickened and regions of normal or mildly increased thickness are often sharp and abrupt, not infrequently creating right-angled contours of the ventricular wall. However, asymmetric patterns of left ventricular wall thickening are not unique to HCM. Asymmetry between septal and posterior free wall thicknesses has been reported in about 5%–10% of adult patients with other congenital or acquired heart diseases

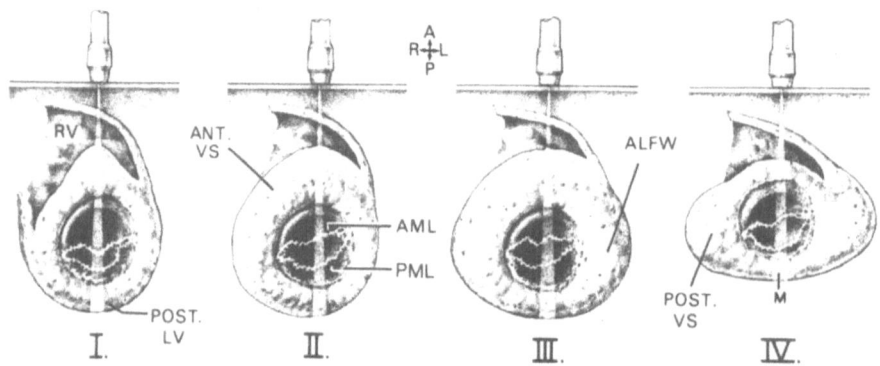

Fig. 1. Artistic representation of morphologic variability in hypertrophic cardiomyopathy, shown here in the short-axis cross-sectional plane at mitral valve level. The expected approximate path of the conventional M-mode echo beam *(M)* through the anterior septum and posterior free wall is shown in each heart. The M-mode echocardiogram would record identical values for wall thicknesses and septal-free wall ratio (i.e., 2.0 in morphologic types I, II and III), although these hearts actually differ considerably with regard to distribution of left ventricular *(LV)* hypertrophy. M-mode echocardiography greatly overestimates the magnitude of hypertrophy in type I (which is quite localized) and underestimates the marked diffuse increase in LV mass in type III; only in type II does the M-mode accurately reflect the distribution of LV hypertrophy. In type IV, the M-mode echo beam does not traverse the thickened portion of LV wall in posterior septum and anterolateral free wall *(ALFW). AML,* anterior mitral leaflet; *A* or *ANT.,* anterior; *L,* left; *LVFW,* LV free wall; *P* or *POST.,* posterior; *PML,* posterior mitral leaflet; *R,* right; *RV,* right ventricle; *VS,* ventricular septum. (From [45])

studied with M-mode echocardiography, particularly those associated with right ventricular hypertension [19]. Specifically, a substantial proportion (about one-third) of patients with long-standing systemic hypertension and marked left ventricular hypertrophy may show asymmetric patterns of left ventricular hypertrophy which are similar to or indistinguishable from many patients with HCM [20].

A great diversity of morphologic forms occur in HCM, and virtually all conceivable patterns of wall thickening have been observed in at least some patients with this disease [4, 7, 8, 10–13, 15–18]. However, in the majority of patients with HCM (about 55%), left ventricular hypertrophy is diffuse and involves both the ventricular septum and large portions of the anterolateral free wall [4] (Fig. 1). The posterior segment of the free wall is least often affected by the hypertrophic process, although occasional patients may show substantial thickening which is confined to, or is most prominent, in this region.

Furthermore, individual patients with HCM may differ considerably with regard to the extent of their left ventricular hypertrophy. Thickness of the left ventricular wall is strikingly increased in many patients, including some who have the most severe hypertrophy observed in any cardiac disease [8]. For example, not uncommonly we have evaluated patients with maximal wall thickness of 35–45 mm (usually in the ventricular septum) with the most extreme dimension observed to date being 52 mm [8]. Such patients with HCM and a

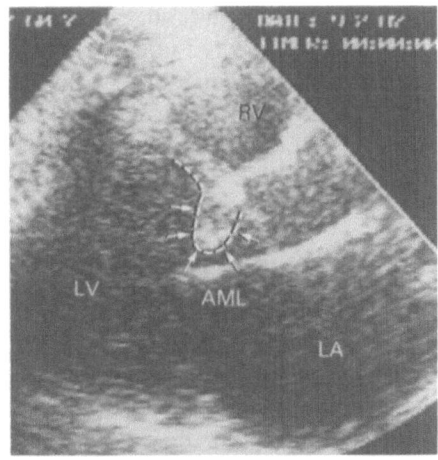

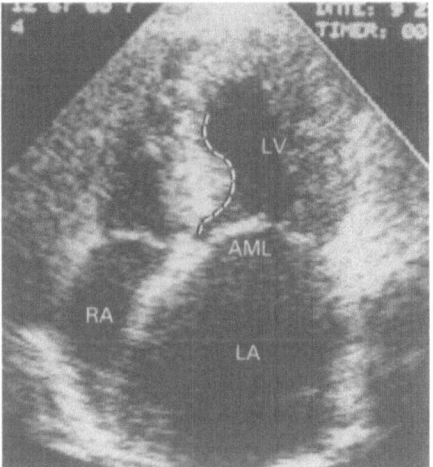

Fig. 2. Segmental hypertrophy in HCM. Two-dimensional echocardiographic stop-frame images in the parasternal long-axis *(upper panel)* and apical four-chamber *(lower panel)* views. Left ventricular wall thickening is confined to the basal portion of anterior ventricular septum *(broken lines* and *arrows)* just below the aortic valve and adjacent to the anterior mitral leaflet *(AML)*. All other regions of the left ventricular wall are of normal thickness. *LA*, left atrium; *LV*, left ventricle; *RV*, right ventricle

"giant heart" exhibit a broad spectrum of clinical manifestations; of note, the majority are without evidence of obstruction to left ventricular outflow under basal conditions.

In contrast, some patients may show wall thickening that is relatively mild and localized to a single segment of myocardium [12, 16] (Figs. 1 and 2). Such mild morphologic expressions of HCM usually selectively involve the anterior basal portion of ventricular septum. It is important to note that these patients can develop important symptoms and show subaortic obstruction [12].

Many affected relatives of patients with HCM who are identified in echocardiographic surveys of pedigrees prove to be asymptomatic, over 50 years of age, without evidence of subaortic obstruction, and usually with a relatively mild degree of localized left ventricular hypertrophy [16]; hence, such individuals appear to have a subclinical form of HCM in which the sole evidence of the disease is the morphologic expression detectable only with echocardiography. In most instances, this expression of HCM probably constitutes a dominant morphologic trait, although in some patients the initial onset of cardiac symptoms may be deferred until the advanced ages of 60–80 years. In young asymptomatic athletic individuals, mild ventricular septal hypertrophy suggestive of HCM (with wall thicknesses of 13–14 mm) may often be difficult to distinguish from the "physiologic" form of left ventricular hypertrophy induced by chronic athletic training [21].

Furthermore, probands and affected relatives within pedigrees having HCM appear to differ distinctly with regard to the clinical and morphologic expression of the disease [11, 16]. This undoubtedly reflects the fact that probands were referred to us for cardiologic evaluation (usually because of marked symptoms), while most relatives were identified as affected by HCM for the first time only by virtue of participating in echocardiographic screening studies at our initiative. For example, probands usually showed evidence of clinically significant disease with symptoms of functional limitation and basal obstruction to left ventricular outflow. In addition, the morphologic expression of the disease was generally substantial with marked ventricular septal thickening and diffuse distribution of left ventricular hypertrophy. In contrast, affected relatives usually demonstrated no or minimal symptoms, absence of outflow obstruction, and less severe hypertrophy with modest septal thickening and more localized and less diffuse patterns of left ventricular hypertrophy.

While segmental hypertrophy in HCM is usually identified in the anterior septum, other forms of localized left ventricular hypertrophy may involve the posterior septum, anterolateral or posterior free wall or the most apical portion of the left ventricle. The latter form has been described most commonly in Japan [22, 23]. Since 1976, Japanese investigators have reported a subgroup of patients with a form of hypertrophic cardiomyopathy that appeared to differ in several important respects from the more typical clinical and morphologic expressions of the disease. Based primarily on angiographic studies, as many as 25% of Japanese patients with hypertrophic cardiomyopathy have been reported to have hypertrophy confined to the true left ventricular apex (below the level of the papillary muscles). This distribution of hypertrophy characteristically creates a "spade" deformity of the left ventricular cavity on contrast angiocardiogram in diastole, and is also associated with a distinctive electrocardiographic pattern of deep ("giant") T wave inversion in the precordial leads. Apical hypertrophy in Japanese patients has been described as clinically benign and nonfamilial, occurring predominantly in older men and frequently associated with systemic hypertension.

Apical hypertrophy appears to assume a somewhat different morphologic appearance in patients form Western countries (e.g., North America and Europe) [9, 15, 24]. In those patients who have been reported from outside of Japan, wall thickening was rarely confined to the true left ventricular apex and was usually more diffuse – i.e., involving greater portions of the septum and free wall in the apical region. In addition, patients with the Western variety of apical hypertrophy uncommonly show marked T wave inversion or the "spade" deformity of the left ventricle, and often incur marked symptoms and occasionally sudden death. Consequently, these latter patients appear to constitute a part of the "usual" morphologic and clinical spectrum of nonobstructive HCM.

For example, of the 965 patients with HCM evaluated by echocardiography at the National Institutes of Health during a 7-year period, only 23 (2%) had wall thickening predominantly in the apical (distal) portion of the left ventricle [15]. Patients ranged in age from 15 to 69 years (mean 37) and were largely male and white (only one was of Asian descent). Of the 23 patients, 15 had significant functional limitation, usually exertional dyspnea and fatigue. Several electrocardiographic patterns were identified, but only four patients showed "giant" negative T waves. Just three patients had the distribution of apical hypertrophy that most closely resembled that described in Japanese patients – i.e., hypertrophy confined to the true left venticular apex (and two of these patients had giant negative T waves).

Relationship of Pattern of Hypertrophy to Clinical Presentation

Extent and distribution of left ventricular hypertrophy also appear to be determinants of the clinical features and course of patients with HCM. For example, in a population of patients with HCM, more marked and diffuse patterns of left ventricular hypertrophy confer not only a predisposition for congestive cardiac symptoms producing functional limitation and basal obstruction to left ventricular outflow, but also for sudden death (or cardiac arrest) [25] and potentially life-threatening arrhythmias such as ventricular tachycardia on ambulatory electrocardiogram [26], or ventricular arrhythmias induced by programmed electrical stimulation in the electrophysiology laboratory. Indeed, it is exceedingly unusual for an adult patient with HCM and mild left ventricular hypertrophy to die suddenly [25]; furthermore, we have only encountered one young patient who we believe had genetically transmitted HCM and sudden death in the absence of left ventricular hypertrophy. However, we should be careful to emphasize that these relationship between left ventricular mass and clinical findings in HCM, while statistically significant, are nevertheless not strong enough to permit the prospective prediction of clinical course in individual patients based on the echocardiographic assessment of magnitude of hypertrophy.

The hypertrophied and stiffened left ventricle, characteristic of HCM is associated with impaired diastolic relaxation, compliance and filling [5, 27] in about 75% of patients [10, 28]. These abnormalities undoubtedly contribute importantly to the congestive symptoms experienced by many patients with nonobstructive as well as obstructive HCM. The early filling phase is prolonged and the rate and volume of rapid filling is decreased. Consequently, there is a compensatory increase in the contribution of atrial systole to overall left ventricular filling. Diastolic dysfunction sufficient to produce symptoms is often associated with considerable left ventricular hypertrophy. However, diastolic abnormalities may also occur in patients with more mild and localized wall thickening [29, 30] (or in regions of the wall which are of normal or only mildly increased wall thickness) [29]. Based on noninvasive studies of diastolic function in a population of patients with HCM, there appears to be little relation between the degree and extent of left ventricular hypertrophy and parameters of diastolic relaxation and filling [30].

Finally, the distribution of hypertrophy appears to be an important determinant of whether left ventricular outflow tract obstruction will occur in patients with HCM [31]. In patients with subaortic obstruction, the basal ventricular septum is usually markedly thickened at the level of the mitral valve, the mitral valve is positioned anteriorly within the left ventricular cavity, and the cross-sectional area of the outflow tract (at end-diastole) is considerably reduced. Conversely, in patients with nonobstructive HCM, the outflow tract at mitral valve level is usually larger and maximal septal thickening is often evident in more distal portions of the ventricle below the mitral valve.

Progression, Development, and Changing Patterns of Hypertrophy

Infancy: HCM has been identified in a small number of infants less than 2 years of age [32, 33]. When clinically overt in infancy, the disease is usuall associated with marked septal hypertrophy relative to body size [32, 33] (Fig. 3), severe progressive congestive heart failure and often obstruction to both left and right ventricular outflow (Fig. 4). Congestive heart failure may prove difficult to treat successfully, but sudden death virtually never occurs in this phase of life. Thus, HCM can represent a congenital heart malformation in which left ventricular wall thickening begins during fetal development and is evident shortly after birth. Autopsy studies have shown that the thickened left ventricular myocardium present in infants who have died of HCM usually show the same histologic abnormalities as children or adults with the disease – i.e., cardiac muscle cell disorganization and abnormal intramural coronary arteries [34].

Childhood: Recent echocardiographic investigations have demonstrated the "dynamic" nature of left ventricular hypertrophy in children with HCM. For example, serial two-dimensional echocardiographic studies in young relatives of patients with HCM have shown that frequently the magnitude, extent or distribution of left ventricular hypertrophy is neither fully expressed at birth

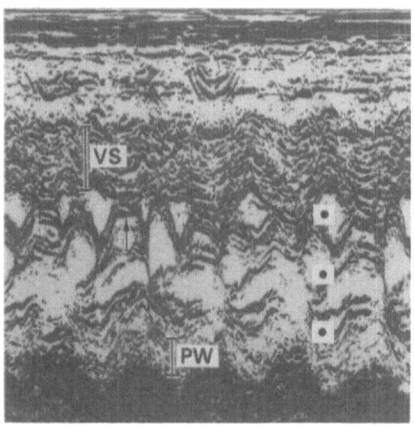

Fig. 3. M-mode echocardiogram from a 2-year-old patient with HCM and marked left ventricular outflow tract obstruction (90 mmHg peak systolic gradient at rest). Ventricular septum *(VS)* is thickened (12 mm) disproportionately with respect to the posterior left ventricular free wall *(PW)*, and there is substantial systolic anterior motion of the mitral valve and prolonged mitral-septal contact *(arrow)*. (From [33])

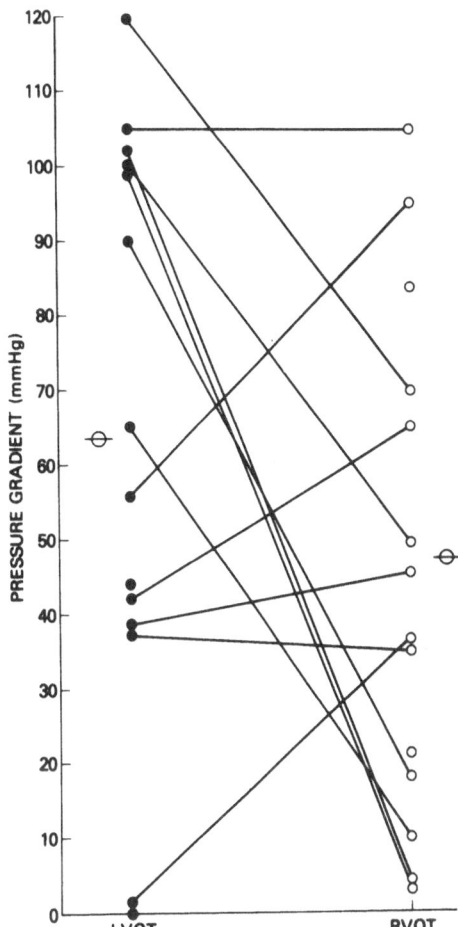

Fig. 4. Left ventricular outflow tract *(LVOT)* and right ventricular outflow tract *(RVOT)* peak systolic pressure gradients in 16 infants with HCM. Data for each of the patients in whom both left and right ventricular outflow gradients were measured are connected by a *line.* Mean values are indicated by ∅. (From [33])

nor fixed early in life [10, 17]. Wall thicknesses may show substantial changes throughout childhood, but particularly during adolescence when growth, development, and maturation are most marked (Figs. 5 and 6). Striking increases in left ventricular wall thickness have been observed in children with pre-existing hypertrophy and hypertrophy may also develop de novo in adolescence. In an investigation at our institution, 39 children with a family history or morphologic evidence of HCM were studied over a 4-year period. Patients were initially investigated at ages 4–15 years (mean 11) and then later at 9–20 years (mean 16) [17]. Seventeen of the study patients showed a marked acceleration in the magnitude and extent of established left ventricular hypertrophy, and five others demonstrated evolution from a morphologically normal-appearing heart to one with substantial asymmetric wall thickening. In these 22 patients, the observed increases in left ventricular wall thickness were striking (6–23 mm; 33%–250% change, mean 100%), and greatly exceeded that which would have been expected to occur as a consequence of normal growth alone. The average absolute increase in wall thickness was 12 mm (maximum increase, 23 mm) and

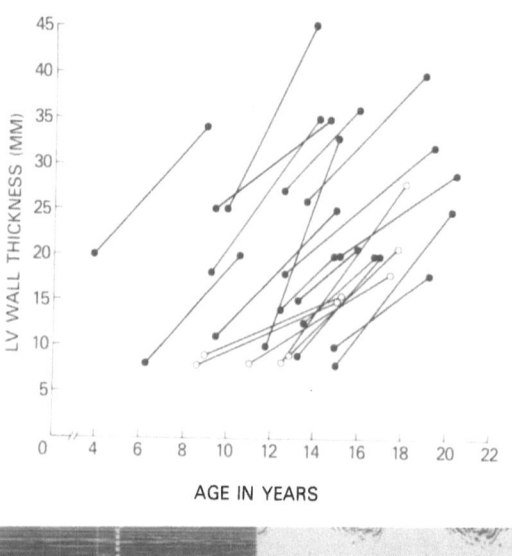

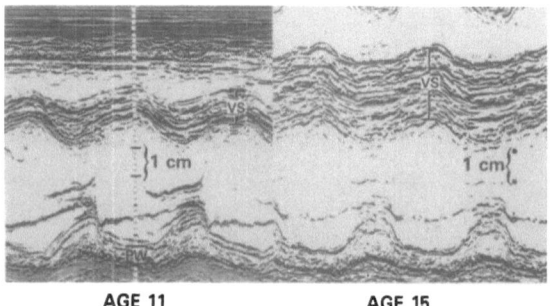

AGE 11   AGE 15

Fig. 5. Development and progression of left ventricular *(LV)* hypertrophy in children with HCM. *Upper panel,* dynamic, striking changes in LV wall thickness with age in 22 children with a family history of HCM who were studied with serial two-dimensional echocardiography; each patient is represented by the left ventricular segment that showed the greatest change in wall thickness. *Open symbols* denote five patients who had a family member with HCM, but themselves had no evidence of hypertrophy in any left ventricular segment at the initial evaluation, but subsequently developed wall thickening typical of HCM *de novo.* *Lower panels,* development of marked hypertrophy of anterior basal ventricular septum *(VS)*. M-mode echocardiograms were obtained at the same cross-sectional level in a young girl with a family history of HCM. At age 11, anterior ventricular septal thickness was at upper limit of normal (10 mm); at age 15, septal thickness markedly increased (to 33 mm), and the appearance became typical of HCM. *PW*, posterior free wall. (From [17])

was ≥ 10 mm in 14 patients (including five ≥ 15 mm). In the 22 patients, 45 (or 41%) of 110 left ventricular segments showed a measurable increase in wall thickness during follow-up; these included 26 segments in which pre-existing hypertrophy increased and 19 previously normal segments in which "new" areas of hypertrophy formed. Therefore, the patterns of hypertrophy became less localized and more diffusely distributed with growth. Ultimately, the region of left ventricular wall most commonly hypertrophied was the anterior ventricular septum, although wall thickening was also frequently identified in the posterior septum and anterior free wall. These changes in left ventricular

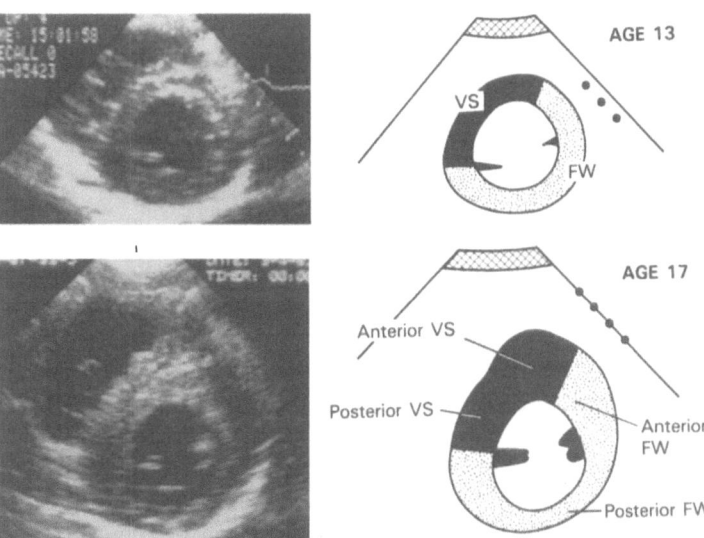

Fig. 6. Development of left ventricular hypertrophy in HCM shown by stop-frame two-dimensional echocardiograms obtained in the short-axis view (at end-diastole) in a boy with a family history of HCM. At age 13, all segments of the left ventricular wall are of normal thickness; at age 17, at the same cross-sectional level, the anterior ventricular septum and contiguous regions of anterior free wall and posterior septum show a marked increase in thickness. *FW*, free wall; *VS*, ventricular septum. (From [17])

mass in children with HCM were generally not associated with symptomatic deterioration, although we have observed development of subaortic obstruction. Indeed, other than those occasional infants with HCM who develop congestive heart failure, the first 10–12 years of life are almost always virtually free of important cardiac symptoms and the risk of sudden death; in the adolescent years, progressive congestive symptoms are uncommon, although the occurrence of sudden death is increased [10, 35, 36].

On the other hand, the striking changes in left ventricular wall thickness that commonly occur during childhood probably represent a morphologic fulfillment of the left ventricular structure genetically predetermined for each patient with this disease. Furthermore, in children with HCM and evolving left ventricular hypertrophy, abnormalities on the 12-lead electrocardiogram may represent the initial clinical manifestation of the disease [37], preceding both onset of symptoms and development and appearance of left ventricular hypertrophy on echocardiogram (Fig. 7). Hence, children with HCM may have some detectable clinical evidence of their cardiomyopathy even before the appearance of left ventricular hypertrophy, and therefore it may be possible to predict in advance which genetically predisposed children will go on to demonstrate the typical morphologic expression of HCM.

Adulthood: Although the onset and progression of symptoms is very common in the third, fourth and fifth decades of life, it has been our experience that adult patients with HCM do not show progression of left ventricular hypertro-

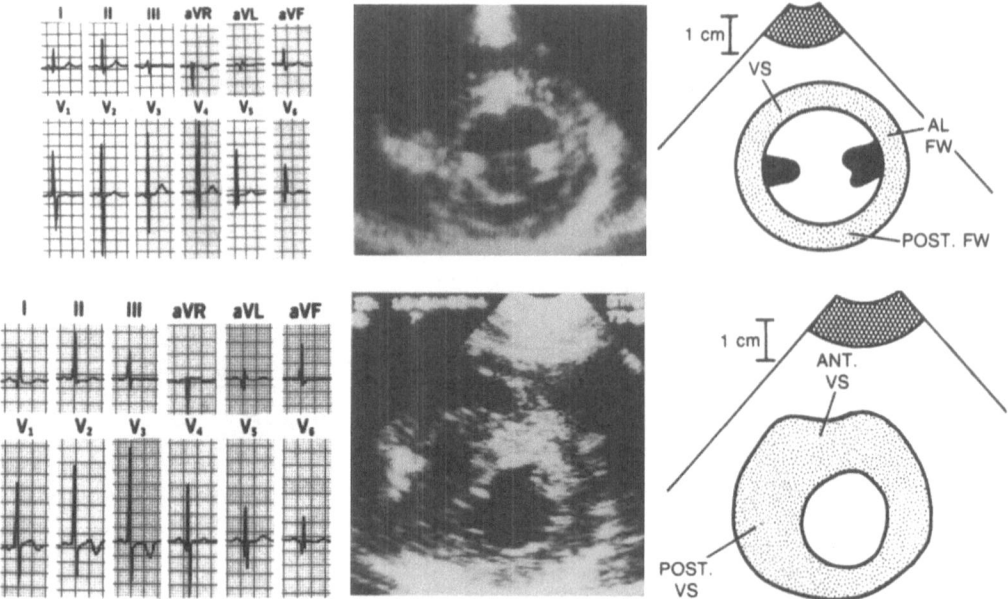

Fig. 7. Twelve-lead ECGs and two-dimensional echocardiograms obtained in the short-axis in diastole in a study patient who developed LVH. ECG alterations precede the appearance of left ventricular wall thickening. *Top panels* show ECG and two-dimensional echocardiogram (accompanied by schematic representation) obtained at age 12. The ECG is abnormal and shows tall voltages in right precordial leads with abnormal R:S ratio in V_1 and narrow abnormal Q waves in V_5 and V_6 even though the echocardiogram demonstrates absence of hypertrophy in each left ventricular segment. *Bottom panels* show the studies performed at age 20. While the echocardiogram demonstrates development of marked LVH involving the anterior and posterior ventricular septum and anterolateral free wall, overall voltage magnitudes on the ECG are virtually the same as at age 12 (overall voltage score 212 mm at age 20 compared to 216 mm at age 12); the pattern of ECG has changed only by virtue of T wave alterations in V_1, V_2, and V_3. *ALFW,* anterolateral free wall; *ANT. VS,* anterior ventricular septum; *POST. FW,* posterior free wall; *POST. VS,* posterior ventricular septum; *VS,* ventricular septum. ECG has been retraced for clarity. (From [37])

phy. In one study, none of the 65 symptomatic adult patients (20–50 years of age) with HCM studied by serial two-dimensional echocardiography showed an unequivocal increase in left ventricular wall thickness over a 3–6-year follow-up period [38]. Therefore, from these observations, we have concluded at this time that the morphologic expression of HCM becomes complete by about age 18 after full physical maturation has been achieved.

Further evidence of the nonstatic nature of the left ventricular hypertrophy in HCM is evident in that minority of patients (about 10%) who show development of severe symptoms and progressive congestive heart failure refractory to medical treatment [10, 12, 13]. These patients show an evolution of the disease through a phase characterized by thinning of previously thickened portions of the left ventricular wall, enlarging cavity size (usually without dilatation in absolute terms), impairment in ventricular contractile function, and occasionally reduction (or disappearance) of a subaortic gradient (Fig. 8). Many of these

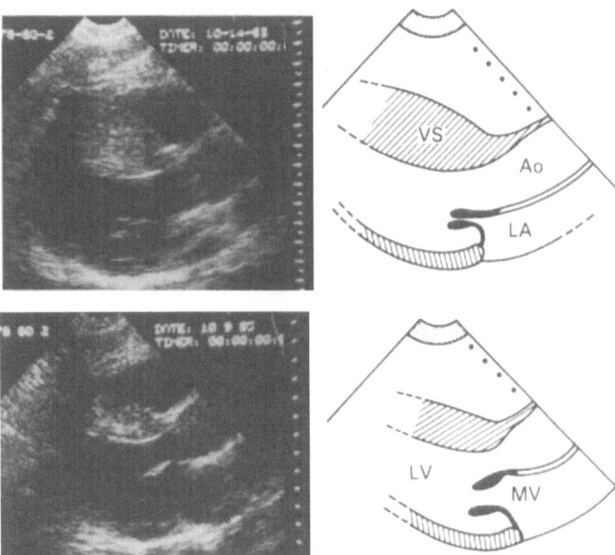

Fig. 8. Stop-frames of two-dimensional echocardiograms, obtained in the parasternal long-axis view during diastole, showing thinning of the anterior ventricular septum *(VS)* in a patient with nonobstructive hypertrophic cardiomyopathy. *Above:* Septal thickness in 32 mm at age 32. *Below:* Two years later, septal thickness has clearly decreased (to 17 mm). The echocardiograms are accompanied by drawings shown to the *right (calibration dots* or *marks* are 10 mm apart). *Ao,* aorta; *LA,* left atrium; *LV,* left ventricle; *MV,* mitral valve. (From [38])

patients with impaired left ventricular systolic function show irreversible abnormalities of myocardial perfusion on thallium-201 studies, probably reflecting extensive myocardial scarring [10]. Patients in this phase of the natural history of HCM have been shown at autopsy to have transmural infarcts [39], and some in this subset have become candidates for cardiac transplantation after all other therapeutic efforts have been exhausted.

Symptomatic patients with end-stage HCM may show cavity enlargement or wall thinning alone, while others show both of these alterations in left ventricular morphology. In whatever form it is expressed, this facet of the natural history of HCM is usually recognized between 20 and 50 years of age (average about 35). Serial echocardiographic studies in this subgroup of patients [13] have shown left ventricular end-diastolic dimension to increase from 44 mm to 49 mm (mean values), usually remaining less than 55 mm. Maximum left ventricular wall thickness decreased from 21 mm to 15 mm, with the largest change in any single patient being 9 mm; radionuclide angiographic ejection fraction was usually less than 50%. These morphologic and functional changes, which are associated with end-stage depression of left ventricular contractile function, could be due to myocardial ischemia or possibly to progression of the intrinsic cardiomyopathic process.

Of note, in a population of symptomatic adult patients with HCM, left ventricular hypertrophy is considerably more severe in younger than in older patients, and an inverse relation between left ventricular wall thickness and age

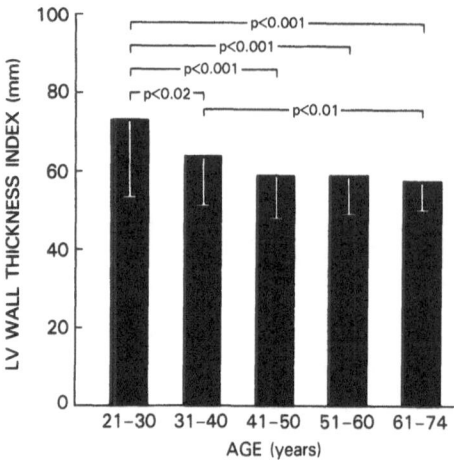

Fig. 9. Comparison of left ventricular (*LV*) wall thickness index in five age groups of 173 patients with HCM. (From [40])

is evident [40] (Fig. 9). For example, particularly marked degrees of hypertrophy (e.g., wall thickness > 30 mm) appear limited largely to patients under age 40, while more elderly patients over age 55–60 generally have more modest degrees of hypertrophy and rarely show marked increases in wall thickness (e.g., > 25 mm). The explanation for this inverse relationship between age and magnitude of left ventricular hypertrophy is not known for certain, but it could be due to a higher rate of premature death in younger patients with severe left ventricular hypertrophy, or alternatively to a process of gradual wall thinning (perhaps due to progressive fibrosis) occurring over a long period of time in a large proportion of patients with HCM.

Hypertrophic Cardiomyopathy in the Elderly

Over the past few years, an increasing number of elderly patients (over the age of 60 years) with many of the morphologic and clinical features of hypertrophic cardiomyopathy have been identified [18]. The echocardiographic features and clinical course demonstrated by many of these patients appear to differ in certain respects from many other patients with more "typical" expressions of hypertrophic cardiomyopathy (Figs. 10 and 11). It is unclear whether such patients truly constitute part of the clinical spectrum of HCM or, alternatively, whether some represent a similar but etiologically distinct clinical entity. In a recent analysis [18], elderly patients with HCM had relatively small hearts and only modest increases in left ventricular wall thickness (most had septal thickness less than 22 mm). Nevertheless, left ventricular morphology was severely distorted as evidenced by the greatly reduced end-diastolic dimension of the outflow tract and exaggerated anterior displacement of the mitral valve within the left ventricular cavity; indeed, in some patients, the mitral valve was situated less than 15 mm from the ventricular septum at end-diastole. Deposits of calcium in the mitral annular region, often sizeable and usually posterior to

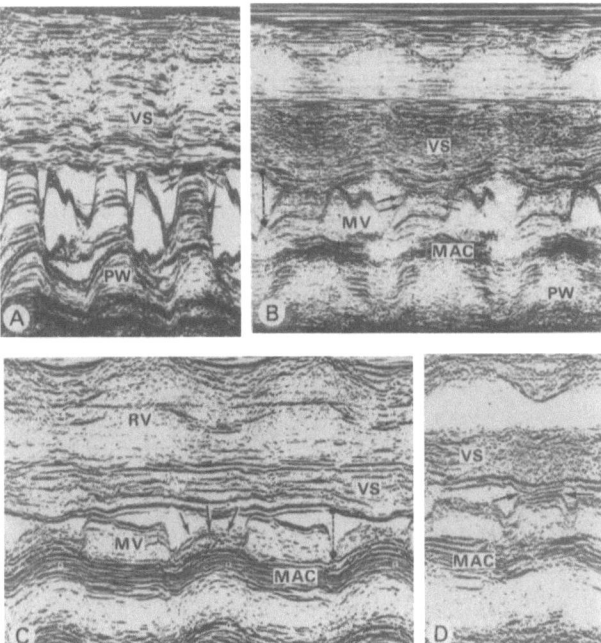

Fig. 10 A–D. M-mode echocardiograms at the mitral valve level in four patients with obstructive HCM; a 21-year-old man **(A)** and three women, aged 74, 65, and 75 years **(B, C, D)**. **A** Marked systolic anterior motion and prolonged contact *(arrows)* between mitral valve and ventricular septum *(VS)* are produced almost entirely by abrupt, marked anterior excursion of mitral valve in early systole; septum shows little posterior excursion toward mitral valve. **B** During systole, anterior excursion of mitral valve *(MV)* toward the septum is much less than shown for young patient in **A,** and posterior septal excursion (toward mitral valve) contributes substantially more to creating contact between mitral valve and septum *(arrows)*. Left ventricular outflow tract dimension at end-diastole is greatly reduced *(vertical broken line)* and considerable mitral annular calcium *(MAC)* is located posterior to the mitral valve between posterior leaflet and posterobasal free wall *(PW)* endocardium. **C** Morphologic features of the left ventricle are similar to those shown in **B,** although mitral systolic anterior motion *(arrows)* does not result in actual mitral-septal contact; outflow tract dimension at end-diastole is greatly reduced *(vertical broken line)*. **D** Systolic contact between mitral valve and septum *(arrows)* begins earlier and is more prolonged than in **B.** *RV,* right ventricle. *Calibration dots* are 1 cm apart. (From [18])

the mitral valve, seemed to contribute to the severe anterior displacement of the mitral valve. It is likely that the mitral valve leaflets are pulled forward toward the ventricular septum during systole (i.e., Venturi phenomenon), as a consequence of the high velocity of blood flow through this narrowed outflow tract.

The mechanism by which systolic contact between mitral valve and septum (and dynamic subaortic obstruction) occurs in many elderly patients with HCM appears to differ from that more typically observed in many other patients with this disease (Figs. 10 and 11). For example, in many younger patients with HCM, systolic outflow tract narrowing occurs predominantly as a consequence of mitral valve motion toward the ventricular septum. The mitral valve exhibits

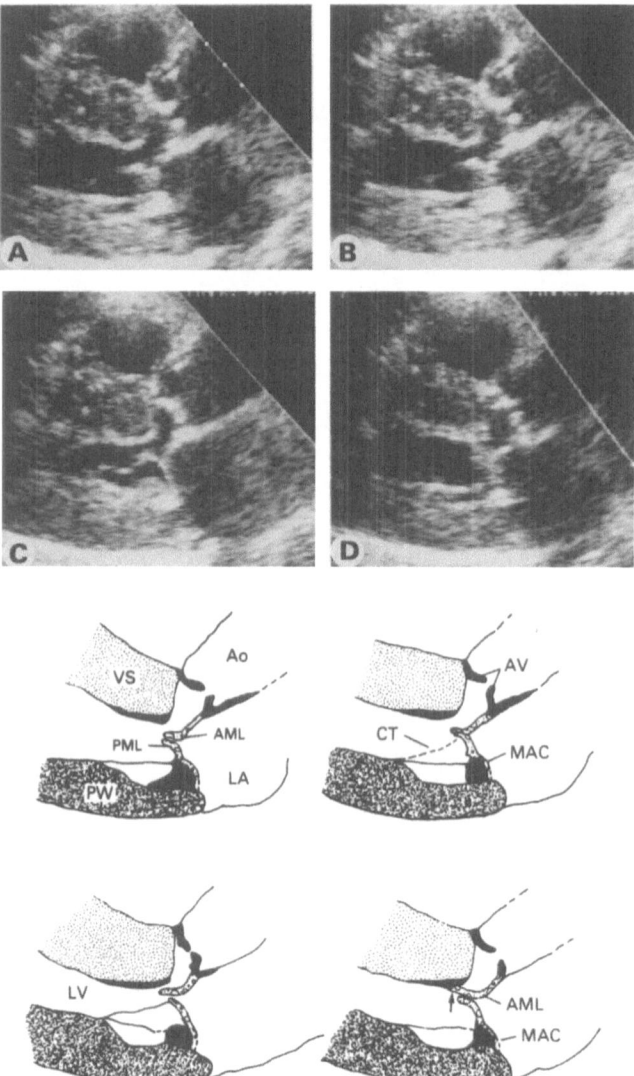

Fig. 11 A–D. Sequential two-dimensional echocardiographic stop-frame images obtained during same cardiac cycle in parasternal long-axis view from an 83-year-old woman with obstructive HCM. Each stop-frame is accompanied by a schematic illustraton *(bottom)*. **A** is image at end-diastole. **B, C** and **D** are images in systole. **A** Anterior and posterior mitral leaflets *(AML* and *PML)* coapt at their distal margins. Mitral annular calcification *(MAC)* located behind posterior leaflet appears to contribute to anterior position of mitral valve within left ventricular *(LV)* cavity. Aortic valve *(AV)* is also calcified, but there was no clinical evidence of hemodynamically significant stenosis. **B, C** Anterior and posterior leaflets remain relatively flat during early systole as they approach ventricular septum *(VS)*. **D** Posterior motion of septum facilitates contact with the distal portion of mitral leaflet during mid-systole. *Ao,* aorta; *CT,* chordae tendineae; *LA,* left atrium; *PW,* posterior wall. *Calibration dots* are 1 cm apart. (From [18])

abrupt and substantial excursion anteriorly from its end-diastolic position as it approaches the septum; contact with the septum is usually made by the distal portion of the mitral valve which bends sharply near its tip during systole. This bend is often so acute that the leaflet assumes an "L" configuration, with as much as a 90° angle forming between the proximal and distal portions of the valve. In these patients, posterior excursion of the ventricular septum usually contributes little to the overall narrowing of the left ventricular outflow tract during systole. In contrast, in many elderly study patients, systolic contact between mitral valve and ventricular septum results from more equal contributions of anterior mitral valve excursion toward the septum and posterior excursion of the ventricular septum toward the mitral valve.

In many elderly patients with HCM, severe symptoms are not present early in life but often develop after 55 years of age. This prolonged period of symptomatic latency is surprising in a disease which is generally expressed morphologically by age 20, and in which symptoms usually occur by 40–50 years of age. While the reason for this particular clinical evolution is not entirely clear, certain dynamic alterations in left ventricular morphology may play an important role in the changing clinical picture. For example, mitral anular calcification which is evident in many elderly patients with HCM undoubtedly develops late in life. With time, this accumulation of calcium posterior to the mitral valve may cause greater anterior displacement of the valve apparatus within the left ventricular cavity, further narrowing of the left ventricular outflow tract, and consequently positioning of the mitral valve leaflets closer to the septum in both diastole and systole. Such an alteration in left ventricular anatomy is likely to create the circumstances in which systolic mitral-septal contact and subaortic obstruction occur. In this way, it is possible that some patients with left ventricular wall thickening but without outflow tract obstruction early in life, might develop obstruction later and consequently incur important symptoms for the first time at advanced ages.

Morphologic Patterns of HCM Within Pedigrees

The morphologic diversity of HCM is underlined by the fact that even closely related first-degree relatives with the genetically transmitted form of the disease [16, 41, 42] usually show great dissimilarities in the pattern of left ventricular wall thickening. In fact, variability in the distribution and pattern of hypertrophy appears to be as great between related members of the same family as between unrelated patients in different families.

In one study, left ventricular morphology was compared in pairs of affected first-degree relatives utilizing a detailed echocardiographic analysis of wall thickness in ten segments of the ventricle [43]. Only 32 (30%) of 105 pairs with HCM showed phenotypically similar hearts with regard to the pattern of left ventricular wall thickening; identical patterns of hypertrophy in these relatives were identified only in identical twins. Morphologic similarities were most common in those relatives who had diffuse hypertrophy involving both the ventricular septum and free wall. The dissimilar morphologic expressions of

HCM present in closely related relatives probably reflect variation in the expressivity of a single gene; however, such phenotypic variability may also imply that inheritance is mediated by more than one gene at a variety of loci.

Applications to Genetic Counseling

Because of the genetic heterogeneity of hypertrophic cardiomyopathy, genetic counseling must be individualized. Families with high gene penetrance have a risk of transmission to future offspring that may approach 50%, but in other families the risk is probably below 25% [16]. In formulating genetic counseling recommendations, it is also important to take into consideration the fact that the morphologic expression of HCM may not be complete until adulthood [17]. Therefore, a single normal echocardiographic examination in a young child with a family history of HCM cannot definitively exclude the disease. If the echocardiogram is initially normal in such children, subsequent echocardiographic studies should be performed at approximately 3-year intervals until the patient attains adult age and mature body size. In addition, after the diagnosis of HCM is made in a patient, it is reasonable to pursue identification of the disease in relatives. This is particularly true for those youthful family members who may contemplate particularly vigorous or competitive athletic activities, since there appears to be some enhanced risk for premature sudden death in patients with HCM under such conditions [44].

The diagnosis of HCM may also be suspected in certain youthful relatives (who are genetically predisposed to HCM) who show abnormalities on the 12-lead electrocardiogram, but have no evidence of left ventricular wall thickening on echocardiogram [37]. However, at present, our convention is to resist making the clinical diagnosis of HCM in such family members in the absence of left ventricular hypertrophy.

References

1. Abbasi AS, MacAlpin RN, Eber LM, Pearce ML (1972) Echocardiographic diagnosis of idiopathic hypertrophic cardiomyopathy without outflow obstruction. Circulation 46:897–904
2. Henry WL, Clark CE, Epstein SE (1973) Asymmetric septal hypertrophy (ASH): Echocardiographic identification of the pathognomonic anatomic abnormality of IHSS. Circulation 47:225–233
3. Maron BJ, Epstein SE (1979) Hypertrophic cardiomyopathy: A discussion of nomenclature. Am J Cardiol 43:1242–1244
4. Maron BJ, Gottdiener JS, Epstein SE (1981) Patterns and significance of distribution of left ventricular hypertrophy in hypertrophic cardiomyopathy. A wide-angle, two-dimensional echocardiographic study of 125 patients. Am J Cardiol 48:418–428
5. Wigle ED, Sasson Z, Henderson MA, et al (1985) Hypertrophic cardiomyopathy. The importance of the site and the extent of hypertrophy. A review. Prog Cardiovasc Dis 28:1–83
6. Shapiro LM, McKenna WJ (1983) Distribution of left ventricular hypertrophy in hypertrophic cardiomyopathy: a two-dimensional echocardiographic study. J Am Coll Cardiol 2:437–444

7. Maron BJ, Gottdiener JS, Bonow RO, Epstein SE (1981) Hypertrophic cardiomyopathy with unusual locations of left ventricular hypertrophy undetectable by M-mode echocardiography: identification by wide-anlge, two-dimensional echocardiography. Circulation 63:409–418

8. Louie EK, Maron BJ (1986) Hypertrophic cardiomyopathy with extreme increase in left ventricular wall thickness: clinical significance functional and morphologic features. J Am Coll Cardiol 8:57–65

9. Keren G, Belhassen B, Sherez J, et al (1985) Apical hypertrophic cardiomyopathy: evaluation by noninvasive and invasive techniques in 23 patients. Circulation 71:45–56

10. Maron BJ, Bonow RO, Cannon RO, Leon MB, Epstein SE (1987) Hypertrophic cardiomyopathy: interrelation of clinical manifestations, pathophysiology, and therapy. N Engl J Med 361:780–789, 844–852

11. Ciró E, Nichols PF, Maron BJ (1983) Heterogeneous morphologic expression of genetically transmitted hypertrophic cardiomyopathy: two-dimensional echocardiographic analysis. Circulation 67:1227–1233

12. Spirito P, Maron BJ, Bonow RO, Epstein SE (1986) Severe functional limitation in patients with hypertrophic cardiomyopathy and only mild localized left ventricular hypertrophy. Am J Coll Cardiol 8:537–544

13. Spirito P, Maron BJ, Bonow RO, Epstein SE (1987) Occurrence and significance of progressive left ventricular wall thinning and relative cavity dilatation in patients with hypertrophic cardiomyopathy. Am J Cardiol 60:123–129

14. Koga Y, Itaya K, Toshima H (1984) Prognosis in hypertrophic cardiomyopathy. Am Heart J 108:351–359

15. Louie EK, Maron BJ (1987) Apical hypertrophic cardiomyopathy: clinical and two-dimensional echocardiographic assessment. Ann Intern Med 106:663–670

16. Maron BJ, Nichols PF, Pickle LW, Wesley YE, Mulvihill JJ (1984) Patterns of inheritance in hypertrophic cardiomyopathy: assessment by M-mode and two-dimensional echocardiography. Am J Cardiol 53:1087–1094

17. Maron BJ, Spirito P, Wesley Y, Arce J (1986) Development and progression of left ventricular hypertrophy in children with hypertrophic cardiomyopathy. N Engl J Med 315:610–614

18. Lewis JF, Maron BJ (1989) Elderly patients with hypertrophic cardiomyopathy: a subset with distinctive left ventricular morphology and progressive clinical course late in life. J Am Coll Cardiol 13:36–45

19. Maron BJ, Epstein SE (1980) Hypertrophic cardiomyopathy. Recent observations regarding the specificity of three hallmarks of the disease: asymmetric septal hypertrophy, septal disorganization and systolic anterior motion of the anterior mitral leaflet. Am J Cardiol 45:141–154

20. Lewis JF, Maron BJ (1989) Diversity of patterns of left ventricular wall thickening in patients with systemic hypertension and marked hypertrophy. Am J Cardiol (in press)

21. Maron BJ (1986) Structural features of the athlete's heart as defined by echocardiography. J Am Coll Cardiol 7:190–203

22. Sakamoto T, Tei C, Murayama M, Ichiyasu H, Hada Y (1976) Giant T wave inversion as a manifestation of asymmetrical apical hypertrophy (AAH) of the left ventricle: echocardiographic and ultrasono-cardiotomographic study. Jpn Heart J 17:611–629

23. Yamaguchi H, Ishimura T, Nishiyma S, et al (1979) Hypertrophic nonobstructive cardiomyopathy with giant negative T waves (apical hypertrophy): ventriculographic and echocardiographic features in 30 patients. Am J Cardiol 44:401–412

24. Maron BJ, Bonow RO, Seshagiri TNR, Roberts WC, Epstein SE (1981) Hypertrophic cardiomyopathy with ventricular septal hypertrophy localized to the apical region of the left ventricle (apical hypertrophic cardiomyopathy). Am J Cardiol 49:1838–1848

25. Spirito P, Maron BJ (1989) Relation between extent of left ventricular hypertrophy and occurrence of sudden cardiac death in hypertrophic cardiomyopathy. J Am Coll Cardiol (in press)

26. Spirito P, Watson RM, Maron BJ (1987) Relation betwen extent of left ventricular hypertrophy and occurrence of ventricular tachycardia in hypertrophic cardiomyopathy. Am J Cardiol 60:1137–1142

27. Sanderson JE, Gibson DG, Brown DJ, et al (1978) Left ventricular filling in hypertrophic cardiomyopathy: an angiographic study. Br Heart J 39:661–670
28. Maron BJ, Spirito P, Green KJ, Wesley YE, Bonow RO, Arce J (1987) Noninvasive assessment of left ventricular diastolic function by pulsed Doppler echocardiography in patients with hypertrophic cardiomyopathy. J Am Coll Cardiol 10:743–747
29. Spirito P, Maron BJ, Chiarella F, et al (1985) Diastolic abnormalities in patients with hypertrophic cardiomyopathy: relation to magnitude of left ventricular hypertrophy. Circulation 72:310–316
30. Spirito P, Maron BJ (1989) Relation between extent of left ventricular hypertrophy and diastolic abnormalities in patients with hypertrophic cardiomyopathy (submitted)
31. Spirito P, Maron BJ (1983) Significance of left ventricular outflow tract cross-sectional area in hypertrophic cardiomyopathy: a two-dimensional echocardiographic assessment. Circulation 67:1100–1108
32. Maron BJ, Edwards JE, Henry WL, Clark CE, Bingle GJ, Epstein SE (1974) Asymmetric septal hypertrophy (ASH) in infancy. Circulation 50:809–820
33. Maron BJ, Tajik AJ, Ruttenberg HD, Graham TP, Atwood GF, Victorica BE, Lie JT, Roberts WC (1982) Hypertrophic cardiomyopathy in infants: clinical features and natural history. Circulation 65:7–17
34. Maron BJ, Wolfson JK, Epstein SE, Roberts WC (1986) Intramural ("small vessel") coronary artery disease in hypertrophic cardiomyopathy. J Am Coll Cardiol 8:545–557
35. Fiddler GI, Tajik AJ, Weidman WH, McGoon DC, Ritter DG, Giuliani ER (1978) Idiopathic hypertrophic subaortic stenosis in the young. Am J Cardiol 42:793–799
36. McKena WJ, Franklin RCG, Nihoyannopoulos P, Robinson KC, Deanfield JE (1988) Arrhythmia and prognosis in infants, children and adolescents with hypertrophic cardiomyopathy. J Am Coll Cardiol 11:147–153
37. Panza JA, Maron BJ (1989) Relation of electrocardiographic abnormalities to evolving left ventricular hypertrophy in hypertrophic cardiomyopathy. Am J Cardiol 63:1258–1265
38. Spirito P, Maron BJ (1987) Absence of progression of left ventricular hypertrophy in adult patients with hypertrophic cardiomyopathy. J Am Coll Cardiol 9:1013–1017
39. Maron BJ, Epstein SE, Roberts WC (1979) Hypertrophic cardiomyopathy and transmural myocardial infarction without significant atherosclerosis of the extramural coronary arteries. Am J Cardiol 43:1086–1102
40. Spirito P, Maron BJ (1989) Relation between extent of left ventricular hypertrophy and age in patients with hypertrophic cardiomyopathy. J Am Coll Cardiol 13:820–823
41. Ten Cate FJ, Hugenholtz PG, van Dorp WJ, Roelandt J (1979) Prevalence of diagnostic abnormalities in patients with genetically transmitted asymmetric septal hypertrophy. Am J Cardiol 43:731–737
42. Greaves SC, Roche AHG, Neutze JM, Whitlock RML (1987) Inheritance of hypertrophic cardiomyopathy: a cross-sectional and M-mode echocardiographic study of 50 families. Br Heart J 58:259–266
43. Ciró E, Maron BJ, Roberts WC (1982) Coexistence of asymmetric and symmetric left ventricular hypertrophy in a family with hypertrophic cardiomyopathy. Am Heart J 104:643–646
44. Maron BJ, Roberts WC, McAllister HA, Rosing DR, Epstein SE (1980) Sudden death in young athletes. Circulation 62:218–229
45. Maron BJ (1985) Asymmetry in hypertrophic cardiomyopathy: The septal to free wall thickness ratio revisited. Am J Cardiol 55:835–838

The Natural History and Clinical Course of Hypertrophic Cardiomyopathy

F. Cecchi, A. Montereggi, G. Squillantini, A. Zuppiroli, and A. Dolara

Definition

Today hypertrophic cardiomyopathy (HCM) can be easily diagnosed from birth to the 8th decade by two-dimensional echocardiography (2D-echo). Abnormal wall thickness of the left and right ventricle can be detected and measured in vivo. A reliable diagnosis of both typical (Fig. 1) and atypical (Fig. 2) patterns of HCM can be made [1], although some pitfalls may be encountered. In the majority of the patients with HCM, hypertrophy is present in the interventricular septum and the anterolateral wall of the left ventricle (LV). Less frequently it can be localized in one or more segments, namely the posterior interventricular septum, the posterior or lateral wall, at the apex, or at midventricular level [2]. Apical HCM may involve only the apical portion of the LV, or be diffuse when additional walls are hypertrophied. A minimal

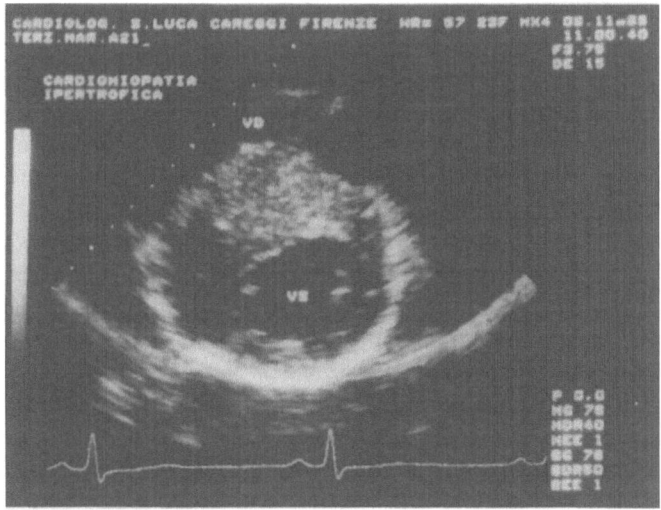

Fig. 1. Patient, age 21, with typical morphologic pattern of HCM. Extreme hypertrophy is present in the interventricular septum (maximal thickness 39 mm), both anteriorly and posteriorly. The anterior LV wall is less hypertrophied, while lateral and posterior LV free walls are normal

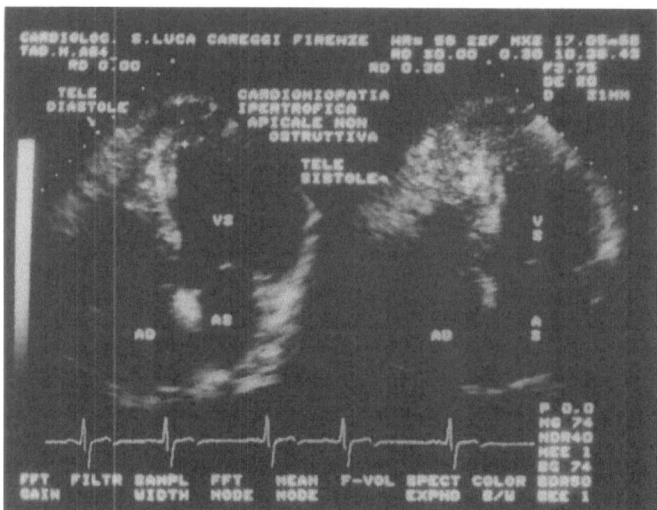

Fig. 2. Patient, age 64, with atypical morphologic pattern of HCM. Hypertrophy is localized at the apex (maximal thickness 21 mm), while basal portion of the LV is normal

thickness of at least 15 mm (and 17 mm in the lateral wall and posterior septum) and a septal to posterior free wall ratio of 1.5 is required for the diagnosis of HCM in adult patients in the absence of other factors which can cause hypertrophy. Symmetric LV hypertrophy is rare [3].

Natural History, Clinical Course and Prevalence

Review of the Literature

The natural history and clinical course of HCM can be defined as "variable." Patients may have few symptoms during their entire life. They may also show progressive deterioration and congestive heart failure or suddenly experience a variety of arrhythmias such as sinus node dysfunction, atrioventricular block, atrial fibrillation or flutter with rapid ventricular rate, ventricular tachycardia (VT), or ventricular fibrillation [4]. Syncopal episodes may be the clinical event, but sudden death may ensue if sinus rhythm is not promptly restored.

Premature death, usually sudden and unexpected, is reported to be common, mostly between 10 and 30 years of age. An annual mortality of 2%–4% has generally been reported in the past, and such a figure is "accepted" by several authors [4–7].

Only a few papers on the natural history of HCM describe a better prognosis in small groups of outpatients, who were diagnosed in district or general hospitals [8, 9]. No deaths were observed after relatively short mean follow-up periods of about 3–4 years.

Nevertheless more than 60% of the cases reported up to now have been observed in referral centers such as the Heart, Lung, and Blood Institute

(National Institutes of Health, Bethesda, USA) and the Hammersmith Postgraduate Medical School (London, UK). It has been suggested that patients that are referred to them have more symptoms and more severe disease [9]. However, even their mean period of observation, usually between 3 and 8 years, does not seem too long for a disease which is genetically determined and is likely to be present at least from adolescence in the majority of the patients [10].

Time of diagnosis is considered for study entry, but now identification of HCM is made earlier by 2D-echo, often in patients without symptoms, with an abnormal electrocardiogram (ECG), and no murmur. It is likely that unselected groups of patients with HCM and few symptoms who are diagnosed in district hospitals are not comparable with those from referral centers.

In addition, epidemiology is of great help in this consideration. True prevalence of HCM is not known in each country, and yet no systematic and specific screening is available. However, Hada et al. [11] showed a prevalence of HCM in the range of 1.7‰ in a large population of Japanese workers screened for health insurance. 2D-echo was performed in those with an abnormal ECG, and a minimum wall thickness of 15 mm was used for the diagnosis. If this prevalence rate was to be applied in our population, it might ensue that patients currently diagnosed as having HCM are probably the tip of the iceberg.

Clinical Experience of HCM in Florence

Our interest started in 1967 with sporadic observations of severely symptomatic patients with HCM who were diagnosed by phonocardiography and/or in the catheterization laboratory. When 2D-echo was extensively used both for in- and outpatients, the number of diagnoses rose dramatically. Patients often had no or few symptoms, but their ECG was often abnormal and the diagnosis had been uncertain for a long time.

In the overall period of 22 years, a total of 157 patients were observed; their mean follow-up was 7.5 years (1 month–22 years). The majority (72%) were male; mean age at diagnosis was 42.5 years ($\pm$ 16.2) with a range of 0.5–78 years. Mean maximal thickness of one LV wall was 23 mm ($\pm$ 5.7) with a range of 16–39 mm.

Distribution of LV hypertrophy was typical in 86% of the cases, while in the remaining patients it was localized to the posterior septum or LV free wall (6%), the apex (6%), midventricular level (2%). Ninety percent of the patients had no or mild symptoms at study entry, while 10% had severe symptoms (NYHA functional class III–IV), and 8% of them had experienced at least one syncopal episode.

Although no systematic screening of the family members was performed, 27% of the patients had a family history of HCM, 13% of sudden death and 9% had both. Cardiac catheterization was performed in 23% of the cases, and in about one third of them a basal left ventricular outflow tract gradient greater than 30 mmHg was present.

Fourty percent of the patients had at least one run of VT at repeated ambulatory Holter monitoring, which was performed in 141 patients for a mean period of 72 h (range 24–382 h). Of the 157 patients, only 71% were treated with drugs such as betablockers (29%), mostly nadolol, verapamil (10%), amiodarone (25%; in about half of the cases in addition to low-dose betablockers), or other antiarrhythmic agents such as propafenone or quinidine (8%). None had cardiac surgery. Diuretics were added for the control of symptoms in 15% of the study patients.

At the last evaluation 143 patients were alive, 12% had improved their symptoms, 17% had worsened, but 71% were stable. Peripheral embolism occurred in 5% of the patients. Fourteen patients had died, five of noncardiac-related causes, six of congestive heart failure (CHF), and three of sudden death. To our surprise, none of the patients who died suddenly had runs of VT at 24 h Holter monitoring. The annual mortality for cardiac causes was 0.7%.

Among the 157, there was a subgroup of 46 patients who received no medical treatment either because of absence of symptoms or drug intolerance. They were younger, their mean age at entry being 37.4 years ($\pm$ 16.3). Mean maximal LV wall thickness was 20 mm ($\pm$ 5.7) with a range of 15 to 32 mm.

Runs of VT at Holter monitoring were detected in 21% of such patients.

No deaths or complications were observed in this subgroup of 46 patients who did not receive medical treatment during a mean follow-up of 6.2 years (with a range of 2.3 to 15 years).

Prognosis

A number of negative prognostic signs have been shown to be associated with higher mortality in patients with HCM [1–4, 12, 13] (Table 1). When present, they seem to identify patients with excess risk of death, although their predictive value is low. The prognostic value of more than one sign has yet to be defined.

In our experience, which is based on the overall group of 157 patients with an annual mortality rate of 0.7% only functional class (FC) at study entry was statistically significant for prognosis. The annual mortality rate was 0,2% for patients with mild or no symptoms and 5.5% for patients with severe symptoms (FC III–IV) ($p < 0.01$).

Moreover, the HCM spectrum is very wide and it would be better to assess the natural history, the clinical course, and the prognosis of specific subsets of HCM. A few such subsets of patients with HCM have already been described in the literature. Some of these are reported here according to age [14–16] (Table 2), to 2D-echo morphology [5, 17–19] (Table 3), to the presence of arrhythmias [20, 21] (Table 4). One of the limitations of these studies is the relatively small number of patients. The great majority were observed in the same referral centers, and the considerations made for the mortality rates can be applied to these specific subsets.

Table 1. HCM: "accepted" negative prognostic signs

Family history of HCM and sudden death
Diagnosis in childhood
Recurrent syncope
Runs of VT at Holter monitoring
Atrial Fibrillation
Severe LV outflow tract gradient and mitral valve regurgitation
Septal thinning and LV cavity dilatation
NYHA functional class at entry and worsening during follow-up

Table 2. HCM: clinical course and mortality of subsets by age

Subset	Mean follow-up (years)	Clinical course	Mortality (%)	Reference
Children	7.4	Variable Sudden death common	3.5	Maron et al. 1976 [14]
Children and adolescents	3	7/53 Cardiac arrest 2/7 Survived	3.1	McKenna et al. 1988 [15]
Elderly	3.4	Good before 60 years Severe symptoms after 60 years	3.4	Lewis and Maron 1989 [16]

Table 3. HCM: clinical course and mortality of subsets by 2D-Echo

Subset	Mean follow-up (years)	Clinical course	Mortality (%)	Reference
Extreme increase of LVH	6	70% Stable or improved 30% Worsened	0	Louie and Maron 1986 [17]
Thinning of LV walls and cavity dilatation	5	Very poor	10	Spirito et al. 1987 [18]
Apical	4.5	Good (no sudden death); CHF rare	?	Koga et al. 1984 [5]
Midventricular obstruction	8	50% LV dilatation and ipokinesia		Fighali et al. 1987 [19]

Among others, new subsets of interest which should be evaluated in the near future are patients with late potentials at ECG signal averaging, or inducible polimorphic ventricular tachycardia at the electrophysiologic study [22], or inducible ischemia without significant coronary artery disease [23].

Table 4. HCM: clinical course and mortality of subsets by arrhythmias

Subset	Mean follow-up (years)	Clinical course	Mortality (%)	Reference
Survivors of cardiac arrest	7	Variable 50% Good 33% Sudden death or recurrent cardiac arrest	3.4	Cecchi et al. 1989 [20]
Runs of VT	3	—	8.6	Maron et al. 1981 [21]

Conclusions

After 30 years of observation, it is clear that the patient population now diagnosed with HCM is different from that seen in the 1960s and 1970s.

Different selection of patients may explain the high annual mortality rates in referral centers and the low ones in general hospitals. A substantial number of patients with LV hypertrophy of unexplained origin and no or few symptoms might still be undiagnosed within the general population. Thus the natural history and the clinical course can be considered benign in the overall patient population with HCM, although some subgroups have a higher risk of experiencing clinical deterioration or sudden and unexpected death. Negative prognostic signs with a low predictive value are well known. The evaluation of the natural history and clinical course of subsets of patients with HCM should better define prognosis. It might also be extremely helpful to the practicing cardiologist in order to assess prognosis in the single patient and take more appropriate clinical decisions such as examinations and therapy for the relief of symptoms and, hopefully, the prevention of sudden death.

References

1. Maron BJ, Bonow RO, Cannon RO, Leon MB, Epstein SE (1987) Hypertrophic cardiomyopathy. Interrelations of clinical manifestations, pathophysiology, and therapy (first of two parts). N Engl J Med 316 (13):780–789
2. Wigle ED, Sasson Z, Henderson MA, Ruddy TD, Fulop J, Rakowski H, Williams WG (1985) Hypertrophic cardiomyopathy: the importance of the site and the extent of hypertrophy. A review. Prog Cardiovasc Dis 28:1
3. Maron BJ (1985) Asymmetry in hypertrophic cardiomyopathy: the septal to free wall thickness ratio revisited. Circulation 71 (1):45
4. Maron BJ, Bonow RO, Cannon RO, Leon MB, Epstein SE (1987) Hypertrophic cardiomyopathy. Interrelations of clinical manifestations, pathophysiology, and therapy (second of two parts). N Engl J Med 316 (14):844–852
5. Koga Y, Itaya K, Toshima H (1984) Prognosis in hypertrophic cardiomyopathy. Am Heart J 108 (32):351–358
6. Frank S, Braunwald E (1968) Idiopathic hypertrophic subaortic stenosis. Clinical analysis of 126 patients with emphasis on the natural history. Circulation 37:759–787

7. Shah PM, Adelman AG, Wigle ED, Gobel FL, Burchell HB, Hardarson T, Curiel R, De la Calzada C, Oakley CM, Goodwin JF (1974) The natural (and unnatural) history of hypertrophic obstructive cardiomyopathy. Circ Res 34–35 [Suppl II]:179–185
8. Shapiro LM, Zezulka A (1983) Hypertrophic cardiomyopathy: a common disease with a good prognosis. Five year experience of a district general hospital. Br Heart J 50:530–533
9. Spirito P, Chiarella F, Carratino L, Zoni Berisso M, Bellotti P, Vecchio C (1989) Clinical course and prognosis of hypertrophic cardiomyopathy in an outpatient population. N Engl J Med 320 (12):749–761
10. Maron BJ, Spirito P, Wesley Y, Arce J (1986) Development and progression of left ventricular hypertrophy in children with hypertrophic cardiomyopathy. N Engl J Med 315 (10):610–614
11. Hada Y, Sakamoto T, Amano K, Yamaguchi T, Takenaka K, Takahashi H, Takikawa R, Hasegawa I, Takahashi T, Suzuki J, Sugimoto T, Saito K (1987) Prevalence of hypertrophic cardiomyopathy in a population of adult Japanese workers as detected by echocardiographic screening. Am J Cardiol 59:183–184
12. McKenna WJ, England D, Doi YL, Deanfield JE, Oakley C, Goodwin JF (1981) Arrhythmia in hypertrophic cardiomyopathy. I: influence on prognosis. Br Heart J 46:168–172
13. Maron BJ, Lipson LC, Roberts WC, Savage DD, Epstein SE (1978) "Malignant" hypertrophic cardiomyopathy: identification of a subgroup of families with unusually frequent premature deaths. Am J Cardiol 41:1133–1140
14. Maron BJ, Henry WL, Clark CE, Redwood DR, Roberts WC, Epstein SE (1976) Asymmetric septal hypertrophy in childhood. Circulation 53:9
15. McKenna WJ, Franklin RCG, Annopoulos PN, Robinson KC, Deanfield JE, Dichie S, Krikler SJ (1988) Arrhythmia and prognosis in infants, children and adolescents with hypertrophic cardiomyopathy. J Am Coll Cardiol 11 (1):147–153
16. Lewis JF, Maron BJ (1989) Elderly patients with hypertrophic cardiomyopathy: a subset with distinctive left ventricular morphology and progressive clinical course late in life. J Am Coll Cardiol 13 (1):36–45
17. Louie EK, Maron BJ (1986) Hypertrophic cardiomyopathy with extreme increase in left ventricular wall thickness: functional and morphologic features and clinical significance. J Am Coll Cardiol 8 (1):57–65
18. Spirito P, Maron BJ, Bonow RO, Epstein SE (1987) Occurrence and significance of progressive left ventricular wall thinning and relative cavity dilatation in hypertrophic cardiomyopathy. Am J Cardiol 59:123–129
19. Fighali S, Krajcer Z, Edelman S. Leachman R (1987) Progression of hypertrophic cardiomyopathy into a hypokinetic left ventricle: higher incidence in patients with mid-ventricular obstruction. J Am Coll Cardiol 9 (2):288–294
20. Cecchi F, Maron BJ, Epstein SE (1989) Long-term outcome of patients with hypertrophic cardiomyopathy successfully resuscitated after cardiac arrest. J Am Coll Cardiol 13 (6):1283–1288
21. Maron BJ, Savage DD, Wolfson JK, Epstein SE (1981) Prognostic significance of 24 hour ambulatory electrocardiographic monitoring in patients with hypertrophic cardiomyopathy: a prospective study. Am J Cardiol 48:252–257
22. Watson RM, Liberati Schwartz J, Maron BJ, Tucker E, Rosing DR, Josephson ME (1987) Inducible polymorphic ventricular tachycardia and ventricular fibrillation in a subgroup of patients with hypertrophic cardiomyopathy at high risk for sudden death. J Am Coll Cardiol 10 (4):761–764
23. Cannon RO, Schenke WH, Maron BJ, Tracy CM, Leon MB, Brush JE, Rosing DR, Epstein SE (1987) Differences in coronary flow and myocardial metabolism at rest and during pacing between patients with obstructive and patients with nonobstructive hypertrophic cardiomyopathy. J Am Coll Cardiol 10 (1):53–62

Left Ventricular Systolic and Diastolic Function in Hypertrophic Cardiomyopathy

P. Spirito

Introduction

Hypertrophic cardiomyopathy is a primary cardiac disease characterized by increased left ventricular wall thickness and normal or decreased cavity dimension [1, 2]. Abnormalities of left ventricular function are common in patients with hypertrophic cardiomyopathy and involve either diastole, systole, or both. The discussion will be focused on the pathophysiologic mechanisms and clinical implications of the diastolic and systolic abnormalities in this disease.

Left Ventricular Diastolic Function

In the early 1960s, shortly after the initial description of hypertrophic cardiomyopathy, the demonstration of elevated left ventricular end-diastolic pressure despite a normal or reduced end-diastolic volume suggested the presence of ventricular filling abnormalities in this disease [1–3]. Subsequent investigations showed that two mechanisms contribute to impaired diastolic filling in hypertrophic cardiomyopathy: abnormal left ventricular relaxation and decreased compliance [4–6].

Relaxation

Following the isovolumic relaxation phase and during the initial filling phase of diastole, active relaxation continues and allows ventricular pressure to decrease despite the rapid increase in ventricular volume. Thus, alterations in the rate and duration of relaxation may result in important abnormalities of ventricular filling dynamics.

Myocardial relaxation is a complex phenomenon due to the interaction of several mechanisms. Inactivation of the actin-myosin cross-bridges (the force generating sites) is a major determinant of relaxation. Inactivation is due to the active reuptake of calcium ions by the sarcoplasmic reticulum which lowers the intracellular calcium concentration and permits the disengagement of the actin-myosin cross-bridges [7]. This process is highly sensitive to ischemia [7–10]. Since myocardial ischemia occurs in hypertrophic cardiomyopathy [11–13], ischemia is probably an important determinant of abnormal ventricular relaxation in this disease. Relaxation is also influenced in a complex manner by ventricular preload and afterload [10]. In hypertrophic cardiomyopathy, both these variables may be altered and may thus contribute to impaired relaxation. Asynchrony of ventricular load and inactivation (actin-myosin dissociation) has also been shown to affect relaxation [10]. In hypertrophic cardiomyopathy, asymmetric distribution of hypertrophy and sparse areas of fibrosis are responsible for marked anatomic nonuniformity, and may create the conditions for regional asynchrony of ventricular load and inactivation.

Chamber Compliance

Left ventricular chamber compliance is a general term that refers to the passive diastolic properties of the ventricle, and is expressed by the relation between changes in volume and pressure during ventricular filling (dV/dP) [4]. Chamber stiffness, which is the reciprocal of chamber compliance (dP/dV), is also frequently used as a descriptor of the passive diastolic behavior of the ventricle. Ventricular chamber stiffness is increased when diastolic pressure during ventricular filling shows an exaggerated increase for a given increase in diastolic volume. Ventricular chamber stiffness is directly related to myocardial stiffness and mass, and inversely related to ventricular volume [4, 14].

In hypertrophic cardiomyopathy, myocardial stiffness is increased (due to myocardial fibrosis and, possibly, cell disorganization), left ventricular mass is also increased and volume is reduced; this leads to an increase in left ventricular chamber stiffness. In addition, since prolonged and incomplete relaxation results in impaired diastolic filling and reduced rate of decline of ventricular pressure, abnormal relaxation also affects the pressure-volume relation and chamber stiffness [9, 14]. However, because of the diverse morphologic expressions of hypertrophic cardiomyopathy, the relative role played by each of these variables in determining the alterations in left ventricular compliance may vary greatly in individual patients.

Clinical Implications of Diastolic Dysfunction

In patients with hypertrophic cardiomyopathy, the increased left ventricular filling pressures secondary to diastolic impairment result in pulmonary congestion and symptoms of cardiac failure. The chronically elevated filling pressures also cause progressive atrial dilatation, and may ultimately lead to atrial fibrillation. Since atrial contraction is of critical importance in ensuring adequate filling of the stiff ventricle, development of atrial fibrillation is usually associated with severe clinical deterioration [15, 16].

Impaired left ventricular diastolic function may also be responsible for the presyncopal and syncopal episodes that occur in some patients with hypertrophic cardiomyopathy. In a stiff, noncompliant ventricle, brief episodes of atrial fibrillation, transitory changes in ventricular preload, or the fall in systemic vascular resistance that accompanies muscular exercise, may each result in a sudden decrease in diastolic filling. In turn, the reduced ventricular filling in the presence of a small end-diastolic volume may lead to an important drop in cardiac output and cause syncope.

Left Ventricular Systolic Function

In the great majority of patients with hypertrophic cardiomyopathy, the left ventricle is characterized by rapid systolic emptying and increased ejection fraction [1, 2, 17]. Although these functional features are often considered to represent an hypercontractile state, they occur in the presence of increased wall thickness (thus, decreased systolic wall stress), small end-diastolic volume, and mild-to-moderate mitral regurgitation. The enhanced systolic function is therefore the expression of reduced systolic stress rather than myocardial hypercontractility. Consequently, in hypertrophic cardiomyopathy, the left ventricle should be more appropriately described as hyperdynamic [18].

In about 20% of the patients with hypertrophic cardiomyopathy, a systolic gradient can be recorded in the left ventricular outflow tract [19, 20]. This gradient is referred to as dynamic, since it is not due to a fixed obstruction to left ventricular ejection and may show large spontaneous variability. The gradient is increased by maneuvers that reduce systemic arterial pressure or left ventricular volume (such as Valsalva or administration of amyl nitrite), and it is reduced or abolished by interventions that decrease left ventricular contractility (such as beta-blockers), or by maneuvers that increase arterial pressure (such as squatting or handgrip) [17].

In almost all patients with hypertrophic cardiomyopathy, the development of the subaortic gradient is associated with the apposition of the mitral valve leaflets to the ventricular septum during systole; the earlier and more prolonged the mitral-septal contact, the more severe the gradient [21, 22]. The mechanisms responsible for this systolic anterior motion of the mitral valve remain to be definitively clarified. In the early 1970s, Wigle first suggested that the high velocity of blood through a narrowed outflow tract could pull the mitral valve leaflets toward the septum by a Venturi effect [23]. This hypothesis still remains the one favored by most investigators, and is supported by a number of observations. For example, any maneuver that changes the velocity of ejection also affects the degree of systolic anterior motion of the mitral valve [17]; the presence of the gradient is generally associated with marked hypertrophy of the subaortic ventricular septum and a severely narrowed left ventricular outflow tract [21, 24, 25]. In addition, some other common morphologic features of hypertrophic cardiomyopathy, such as the elongated mitral valve leaflets and the anterior displacement of the mitral valve toward the ventricular septum (probably due to the greatly hypertrophied and abnormally positioned papillary muscles), may contribute to the anterior movement of the valve during systole [24, 26, 27].

The hemodynamic significance of the subaortic gradient in hypertrophic cardiomyopathy has been a source of debate and controversy. In many patients with a subaortic gradient, the left ventricle empties rapidly and the majority of the stroke volume is ejected during the first half of systole. These functional features have led some authors to question whether the dynamic gradient reflects a true obstruction to left ventricular ejection [28, 29]. However, the great majority of investigators active in this field agree that the gradient represents obstruction to flow.

The following points strongly support this view:

1) while left ventricular ejection time is normal in patients without a gradient, it is prolonged in those with a gradient [17, 30];
2) aortic blood flow decelerates rapidly at the time of mitral-septal contact [31, 32];
3) aortic flow persists throughout systole and the left ventricle continues to shorten after mitral-septal contact [17, 22, 30];
4) in many patients, about 50% of the stroke volume is ejected in the presence of the subaortic gradient [17, 31]:

Clinical Implications of the Outflow Gradient

The clinical significance and prognostic implications of the left ventricular outflow gradient in patients with hypertrophic cardiomyopathy have not been definitively clarified. A prospective investigation comparing the long term clinical course in symptomatic patients with and without outflow gradient has never been performed. Moreover, clarification of the clinical implications of the outflow gradient is complicated by the fact that the presence of the gradient is usually associated with other features, such as a small left ventricular cavity size and marked left ventricular hypertrophy, that could independently affect the clinical course and prognosis of the disease. Nevertheless, indirect evidence of the possible detrimental effects of the outflow gradient may be derived from the general observation that elevated left ventricular systolic pressures are always associated with increased myocardial wall stress and augmented oxygen consumption [33]. The clinical improvement and the increase in exercise capacity experienced by many patients following surgical abolition of the gradient also support the view that the dynamic obstruction to flow may have deleterious pathophysiologic consequences for the left ventricle [34].

References

1. Wigle ED, Heimbecker RO, Gunton RW (1962) Idiopathic ventricular septal hypertrophy causing muscular subaortic stenosis. Circulation 26:325–340
2. Braunwald E, Lambrew CT, Rockoff SD, Ross J Jr, Morrow AG (1964) Idiopathic hypertrophic subaortic stenosis: I. A description of the disease based upon an analysis of 64 patients. Circulation 30 (Suppl 4):IV-3–IV-119
3. Stewart S, Mason DT, Braunwald E (1968) Impaired rate of left ventricular filling in idiopathic hypertrophic subaortic stenosis and valvular aortic stenosis. Circulation 37:8–14

4. Gaasch WH, Levine HJ, Quinones MA, Alexander JK (1976) Left ventricular compliance: mechanisms and clinical implications. Am J Cardiol 38:645–653
5. Sanderson JE, Gibson DG, Brown DJ, Goodwin JF (1977) Left ventricular filling in hypertrophic cardiomyopathy: an angiographic study. Br Heart J 39:661–670
6. Bonow RO, Rosing DR, Bacharach SL et al (1981) Effects of verapamil on left ventricular systolic function and diastolic filling in patients with hypertrophic cardiomyopathy. Circulation 64:787–796
7. Nayler WC, Williams A (1978) Relaxation in heart muscle: some morphological and biochemical considerations. Eur J Cardiol 7 (Suppl):35–50
8. McLaurin LP, Rolett EL, Grossman W (1973) Impaired left ventricular relaxation during pacing induced ischemia. Am J Cardiol 32:751–757
9. Mann T, Goldberg S, Mudge GH, Grossman W (1979) Factors contributing to the altered left ventricular diastolic properties during angina pectoris. Circulation 59:14–20
10. Brutsaert DL, Rademakers FE, Sys SU (1984) Triple control of relaxation: implications in cardiac disease. Circulation 69:190–196
11. Thompson DS, Naqvi N, Juul SM et al (1980) Effects of propranolol on myocardial oxygen consumption, substrate extraction, and haemodynamics in hypertrophic obstructive cardiomyopathy. Br Heart J 44:488–498
12. Pasternac A, Noble J, Streulens Y, Elie R, Henschke C, Bourassa MG (1982) Pathophysiology of chest pain in patients with cardiomyopathies and normal coronary arteries. Circulation 65:778–789
13. Cannon RO III, Rosing DR, Maron BJ et al (1985) Myocardial ischemia in patients with hypertrophic cardiomyopathy: contribution of inadequate vasodilator reserve and elevated left ventricular filling pressures. Circulation 71:234–243
14. Grossman W, McLaurin LP (1976) Diastolic properties of the left ventricle. Ann Intern Med 84:316–326
15. Goodwin JF (1970) Congestive and hypertrophic cardiomyopathies: a decade of study. Lancet 1:731–739
16. Glancy DL, O'Brien KP, Gold HK, Epstein SE (1970) Atrial fibrillation in patients with idiopathic hypertrophic subaortic stenosis. Br Heart J 32:652–659
17. Wigle ED, Sasson Z, Henderson MA et al (1985) Hypertrophic cardiomyopathy: the importance of the site and the extent of hypertrophy: a review. Prog Cardiovasc Dis 28:1–83
18. Pouleur H, Rousseau MF, van Eyll C, Brasseur LA, Charlier AA (1983) Force-velocity-length relations in hypertrophic cardiomyopathy: evidence of normal or depressed myocardial contractility. Am J Cardiol 52:813–817
19. Maron BJ, Nichols PF III, Pickle LW, Wesley YE, Mulvihill JJ (1984) Patterns of inheritance in hypertrophic cardiomyopathy: assessment by M-mode and two-dimensional echocardiography. Am J Cardiol 53:1087–1094
20. Spirito P, Maron BJ (1987) Absence of progression of left ventricular hypertrophy in adult patients with hypertrophic cardiomyopathy. Am J Coll Cardiol 9:1013–1017
21. Henry WL, Clark CE, Glancy DL, Epstein SE (1973) Echocardiographic measurement of the left ventricular outflow gradient in idiopathic hypertrophic subaortic stenosis. N Engl J Med 288:989–993
22. Pollick C, Morgan CD, Gilbert BW, Rakowski H, Wigle ED (1982) Muscular subaortic stenosis: the temporal relationship between systolic anterior motion of the anterior mitral leaflet and the pressure gradient. Circulation 66:1087–1094
23. Wigle ED, Adelman AG, Silver MD (1971) Pathophysiological considerations in muscular subaortic stenosis. In: Wolstenholme GEW, O'Connor M (eds) Hypertrophic obstructive cardiomyopathy. Ciba Foundation Study Group, no 47, Churchill, London, p 63
24. Spirito P, Maron BJ (1983) Significance of left ventricular outflow tract cross-sectional area in hypertrophic cardiomyopathy: a two-dimensional echocardiographic assessment. Circulation 67:100–108
25. Spirito P, Maron BJ, Rosing DR (1984) Morphologic determinants of hemodynamic state after septal myotomy-myectomy in patients with obstructive hypertrophic cardiomyopathy: M-mode and two-dimensional echocardiographic assessment. Circulation 70:984–995

26. Maron BJ, Harding AM, Spirito P, Roberts WC, Waller BF (1983) Systolic anterior motion of the posterior mitral leaflet: a previously unrecognized cause of dynamic subaortic obstruction in patients with hypertrophic cardiomyopathy. Circulation 2:282–293

27. Spirito P, Maron BJ (1984) Patterns of systolic anterior motion of the mitral valve in hypertrophic cardiomyopathy: assessment by two-dimensional echocardiography. Am J Cardiol 54:1039–1046

28. Criley JM, Lewis KB, White RI Jr, Ross RS (1965) Pressure gradients without obstruction: a new concept of "hypertrophic subaortic stenosis". Circulation 32:881–887

29. Murgo JP, Alter BR, Dorethy JF, Altobelli SA, McGranahan GM Jr (1980) Dynamics of left ventricular ejection in obstructive and nonobstructive hypertrophic cardiomyopathy. J Clin Invest 66:1369–1382

30. Wigle ED, Auger P, Marquis Y (1967) Muscular subaortic stenosis: the direct relation between the intraventricular pressure difference and the left ventricular ejection time. Circulation 36:36–44

31. Pierce GE, Morrow AG, Braunwald E (1964) Idiopathic hypertrophic subaortic stenosis: III. Intraoperative studies of the mechanism of obstruction and its hemodynamic consequences. Circulation 30 (Suppl 4):IV-152–IV-213

32. Maron BJ, Gottdiener JS, Arce J, Rosing DR, Wesley YE, Epstein SE (1985) Dynamic subaortic obstruction in hypertrophic cardiomyopathy: analysis by pulsed Doppler echocardiography. Am J Coll Cardiol 6:1–8

33. Maron BJ, Epstein SE (1986) Clinical significance and therapeutic implications of the left ventricular outflow tract pressure gradient in hypertrophic cardiomyopathy. Am J Cardiol 58:1093–1096

34. McIntosh CL, Maron BJ (1988) Current operative treatment of obstructive hypertrophic cardiomyopathy. Circulation 78:487–495

Radionuclide Assessment of Diastolic Function in Hypertrophic Cardiomyopathy: Relation to Symptoms and Prognosis

T. Chikamori, S. Dickie, P. J. Counihan, J. D. Poloniecki, and W. J. McKenna

Introduction

In hypertrophic cardiomyopathy (HCM), abnormal left ventricular diastolic function is considered to be important as a pathophysiologic mechanism [1–3]. There are, however, very few reports which evaluate the relation between diastolic function and prognosis. The purpose of the present study was to evaluate the prognostic implications of diastolic dysfunction derived from equilibrium radionuclide angiography and to compare the significance of these diastolic indices with well-recognized risk factors for an adverse prognosis in HCM.

Method

Patient Selection

One hundred and sixty-one consecutive patients underwent equilibrium radionuclide cineangiography at Hammersmith Hospital between 1983 and 1987. They were aged 8–78 years, mean 42 years; 90 were male and 71 female. The diagnosis of HCM was based upon the echocardiographic demonstration of unexplained left ventricular hypertrophy [4, 5], with systolic and diastolic blood pressures less than 140 and 90 mmHg, respectively. One hundred and seventeen (73%) patients showed asymmetric hypertrophy, 31 (19%) concentric hypertrophy and 13 (8%) distal hypertrophy. Thirty-five patients (22%) had complete systolic anterior motion of the mitral valve. All patients were in sinus rhythm at the time of radionuclide study, and patients with severe mitral regurgitation were excluded.

Equilibrium Radionuclide Angiography

Fifty-eight patients (36%) underwent radionuclide angiography at the time of diagnosis. The mean time from diagnosis and radionuclide examination was 5.4 ± 6.4 years for the remainder.

Left ventricular systolic and diastolic function were assessed by R-wave gated equilibrium radionuclide angiography, acquired in list mode, according to previously published methods [6–9].

A standard count-based method was used for calculation of left ventricular ejection fraction [7]. Peak rates of ejection and filling were computed automatically, by fitting a third-degree polynomial function to the systolic ejection and rapid filling portions of the time-activity curve, using a least-squares technique [6, 8], and were normalized to end-diastolic counts and expressed as change from end-diastolic per second (edv/s) [7, 8]. Time to peak filling rate was defined as the interval from the minimum of the curve to the point of peak filling [7, 9]. Relative filling volume by peak filling rate, relative filling volume during the rapid filling period and atrial contribution were defined as proportional filling volume at each point and were normalized to end-diastolic counts. If diastasis was difficult to define, then the point (that is the inflection point after the peak filling rate) at which rate of filling increased again after the time of peak filling rate [10], was defined as the turning point between rapid filling period and atrial contraction. This inflection point was identified automatically by modifying the method reported previously [11]. The second derivative of the smoothed time-activity curve was evaluated at each point. The first maximum on the second derivative curve occurring after peak filling rate was considered to be the inflection point marking the onset of atrial contribution. With these methods, 140 patients (87%) were recognized to have atrial contribution, but maximum on the second derivative curve after peak filling rate did not occur in the remaining 21 patients (13%).

Statistical Analysis

Results are expressed as mean ± 1 standard deviation. To compare the means of continuous variables, we used Student's t test. Contingency tables were analyzed by chi-square test. Sixteen variables (Tables 1, 2), including five radionuclide indices, were considered as potential predictors for the occurrence of disease-related mortality during follow-up. Relative filling volume during the rapid filling period (RFV2) and atrial contribution (AC) were excluded from multi-variate analysis because these measurements could not be made in 21 patients.

Linear discriminant analysis with stepwise variable selection and Wilks' Lambda as the selection and optimisation criteria was used to assess the potential to predict disease-related mortality. A Bayes rule with equal prior probability was used for the predictions, and the results are presented as sensitivity, specificity, accuracy and positive predictive value. The computations were performed using the SPSS-PC+ computer program.

Table 1. Clinical/prognostic features in 161 patients with HCM: dead versus alive

	Dead (n = 13)	Alive (n = 148)	p value
Age at diagnosis (years)	21 ± 16	37 ± 17	<0.005
Age at radionuclide examination (years)	29 ± 20	42 ± 16	<0.05
Family history			
None	8	90	NS
HCM	2	29	
HCM + sudden death	3	29	
Clinical symptoms at diagnosis			
Angina			
None	8	84	NS
Atypical	1	11	
Exertional	3	35	
Exertional + atypical	1	14	
Dyspnea			
I	7	91	NS
II	5	48	
III + IV	1	7	
Syncope			
None	6	106	< 0.025[a]
Presyncope	0	10	
Syncope	7	28	
Clinical symptoms at the examination			
Angina			
None	8	88	NS
Atypical	1	9	
Exertional	2	35	
Exertional + atypical	1	11	
Dyspnea			
I	6	86	< 0.05[b]
II	1	48	
III + IV	5	11	
Syncope			
None	7	116	< 0.025[a]
Presyncope	0	10	
Syncope	5	17	
VT assessed by ambulatory ECG	4	32	NS
Amiodarone therapy	6	47	NS

Some missing numbers were included in each variable.
[a] p value for no syncope versus presyncope and syncope.
[b] p value for dyspnea I versus dyspnea II, III and IV by NYHA functional class.
Alive, patients without disease-related mortality; *Dead*, patients with disease-related mortality; *ECG*, electrocardiography; *HCM*, hypertrophic cardiomyopathy; *NS*, not significant; *VT*, ventricular tachycardia.

Results

Clinical Status of the Patients After Follow-up

The follow-up period after the radionuclide examination was 3.0 ± 1.9 years. Amiodarone was prescribed for non-sustained ventricular tachycardia in 26,

Table 2. Radionuclide cineangiography in 161 patients with HCM: dead versus alive

	Dead (n = 13)	Alive (n = 148)	p value
PFR (edv/s)	2.87 ± 0.90	3.35 ± 0.98	= 0.089
Time to PFR (ms)	201 ± 55	185 ± 47	NS
RFV1 (%)	41.8 ± 15.2	39.5 ± 11.5	NS
RFV2 (%) (n = 140)	80.0 ± 6.8	75.1 ± 11.7	= 0.061
AC (%) (n = 140)	16.1 ± 8.3	21.3 ± 11.7	= 0.088
EF (%)	71.4 ± 15.0	77.2 ± 10.0	NS
PER (edv/s)	3.61 ± 0.91	4.11 ± 0.88	= 0.083

AC, atrial contribution; *Alive*, patients without disease-related mortality; *Dead*, patients with disease-related mortality; *EF*, ejection fraction; *HCM*, hypertrophic cardiomyopathy; *NS*, not significant; *PER*, peak ejection rate; *PFR*, peak filling rate; *RFV1*, relative filling volume by peak filling rate; *RFV2*, relative filling volume during the rapid filling period.

refractory symptom in 14, paroxysmal atrial fibrillation in 12 and WPW syndrome in one patient. During this period, five patients died suddenly, three were resuscitated from out-of-hospital ventricular fibrillation, four died from heart failure. These 12 patients and another patient who needed cardiac transplantation because of severe cardiac failure were considered to have disease-related mortality.

Univariate Analysis for Disease-Related Mortality

Clinical/prognostic features, ventricular tachycardia on 48-h ambulatory electrocardiography and cardiac indices both in systolic and in diastolic phase are shown in Tables 1 and 2. Patients who had disease-related mortality were younger at the time of diagnosis and at the time of radionuclide examination, more of them had experienced syncope and more had a poorer functional class while radionuclide measurements revealed reduced peak ejection and peak filling rates and greater percentage of filling during the rapid filling period.

Multivariate Analysis for Disease-Related Mortality

A stepwise discriminant analysis in 148 patients without any missing data revealed that young age at diagnosis, reduced peak filling rate, syncope, dyspnea at the radionuclide study, increased relative filling volume by peak filling rate and positive family history best predicted ($p < 0.0001$) disease-related mortality (sensitivity 83%, specificity 80%, accuracy 80%, positive predictive value 26%). Discriminant analysis without diastolic indices or without radionuclide measurements revealed sensitivity, specificity, accuracy and a positive predictive value for disease-related mortality of 75%, 80%, 80%, and 24%, or those of 67%, 80%, 79% and 22%, respectively.

Discussion

Hypertrophic cardiomyopathy has long been recognized as a condition with prominent abnormalities in diastolic function [1–3]. Using radionuclide angiography, Bonow et al. reported prolonged isovolumic period, prolonged time to peak filling rate, reduced relative filling volume during the rapid filling period and increased atrial contribution in HCM [9, 11–13]. Despite many reports about abnormal diastolic function in HCM, few studies focused on the clinical implications between diastolic function and prognosis. In their angiographic study Newman et al. showed both reduced peak ejection and peak filling rate in patients who died suddenly, but no difference between those who died of other cardiac cause when compared with survivors [14]. Bonow et al. reported improvement in left ventricular diastolic filling and increased exercise tolerance in patients treated with verapamil and that this was due to increased peak filling rate, an index of diastolic function [13]. To our knowledge, however, there is no report showing a beneficial effect of verapamil on survival.

In the present study, there was no definite statistical difference in peak filling rate and in relative filling volume by peak filling rate between those with and without disease-related mortality. Although stepwise discriminant analysis revealed these two indices as the important predictors for disease-related mortality, the positive predictive value was low (26%), and the radionuclide measurements failed to improve the over-all predictability, as compared with the predictability without these variables. Newman et al. also reported prognostic significance of peak filling rate in those who died suddenly, but its predictability was also not high [14].

The follow-up period of this study was three years and during this period 13 patients had disease-related mortality. A longer follow-up period, and a correspondingly increased mortality, may increase the importance of diastolic indices as predictors of high risk. Whilst diastolic indices derived from radionuclide angiography may have potential to predict the prognosis in HCM, currently, their importance as predictors of mid-term prognosis are low. The cause of death in HCM is difficult to define clearly; some patients die of heart failure, some die suddenly. Furthermore, the mechanisms of sudden death are complex and have not been fully elucidated [15]. In such a heterogeneous group it is difficult to correctly predict mortality by currently available technique.

In the present study only one radionuclide examination was usually performed in each patient. Although 36% of patients were examined at the time of diagnosis and in the majority of patients there was a time lag between diagnosis and the radionuclide examination, this time lag might have generated variability in the study group. To ascertain prognostic significance of diastolic function, it would be ideal to evaluate the study group with radionuclide examination at diagnosis and follow-up them thereafter. Repeat radionuclide examination, especially in relation to change in clinical status, will clarify the importance of diastolic function, functional limitation and symptoms. To determine its influence on long-term prognosis, further follow-up with repeat radionuclide study is necessary.

References

1. Goodwin JF (1982) The frontiers of cardiomyopathy. Br Heart J 48:1–18
2. Wigle ED (1987) Hypertrophic cardiomyopathy: a 1987 viewpoint. Circulation 75:311–322
3. Maron BJ, Bonow RO, Cannon RO, Leon MB, Epstein SE (1987) Hypertrophic cardiomyopathy: interrelations of clinical manifestations, pathophysiology, and therapy. N Engl J Med 316:780–789, 844–852
4. Braunwald E, Lambrew CT, Rockoff SD, Ross J Jr, Morrow AC (1964) Idiopathic hypertrophic subaortic stenosis. I. A description of the disease based upon an analysis of 64 patients. Circulation 30 [Suppl IV]:3–119
5. Shapiro LM, McKenna WJ (1983) Distribution of left ventricular hypertrophy in hypertrophic cardiomyopathy: a two-dimensional echocardiographic study. J Am Coll Cardiol 2:437–444
6. Thrall JH, Freitas JE, Swanson D, Rogers WL, Clare JM, Brown ML, Pitt B (1978) Clinical comparison of cardiac blood pool visualization with technetium-99m red cells labeled in-vivo and with technetium-99m human serum albumin. J Nucl Med 19:796–803
7. Sugrue DD, McKenna WJ, Dickie S, Oakley CM, Myers MJ, Lavender JP (1983) Equilibrium radionuclide assessment of left ventricular ejection and filling. Comparison of list-mode and multigated frame-mode measurements. Nucl Med Commun 4:323–334
8. Bacharach SL, Green MV, Borer JS, Hyde JE, Farkas SP, Johnston GS (1979) Left ventricular peak ejection rate, filling rate, and ejection fraction: frame rate requirements at rest and exercise. J Nucl Med 20:189–193
9. Bonow RO, Rosing DR, Bacharach SL, Green MV, Kent KM, Lipson LC, Maron BJ, Leon MB, Epstein SE (1981) Effects of verapamil on left ventricular systolic function and diastolic filling in patients with hypertrophic cardiomyopathy. Circulation 64:787–796
10. Spirito P, Maron BJ, Bonow RO (1986) Noninvasive assessment of left ventricular diastolic function: comparative analysis of Doppler echocardiographic and radionuclide angiographic techniques. J Am Coll Cardiol 7:518–526
11. Betocchi S, Bonow RO, Bacharach SL, Rosing DR, Maron BJ, Green MV (1986) Isovolumic relaxation period in hypertrophic cardiomyopathy: assessment by radionuclide angiography. J Am Coll Cardiol 7:74–81
12. Bonow RO, Frederick TM, Bacharach SL, Green MV, Goose PW, Maron BJ, Rosing DR (1983) Atrial systole and left ventricular filling in hypertrophic cardiomyopathy: effect of verapamil. Am J Cardiol 51:1386–1391
13. Bonow RO, Dilsizian V, Rosing DR, Maron BJ, Bacharach SL, Green MV (1985) Verapamil-induced improvement in left ventricular diastolic filling and increased exercise tolerance in patients with hypertrophic cardiomyopathy: short- and long-term effects. Circulation 72:853–864
14. Newman H, Sugrue DD, Oakley CM, Goodwin JF, McKenna WJ (1985) Relation of left ventricular function and prognosis in hypertrophic cardiomyopathy: an angiographic study. J Am Coll Cardiol 5:1064–1074
15. Maron BJ, Roberts WC, Epstein SE (1982) Sudden death in hypertrophic cardiomyopathy: a profile of 78 patients. Circulation 65:1388–1394

Ischemia, Coronary Blood Flow, and Coronary Reserve in Hypertrophic Cardiomyopathy

R. O. Cannon, III

Introduction

Most patients with hypertrophic cardiomyopathy come to medical attention because of symptoms of effort dyspnea, chest pain, fatigue, and alterations in consciousness. Although features of this disease such as abnormal diastolic filling properties and outflow obstruction may account for many of these symptoms, the presence of chest pain may indicate myocardial ischemia. However, unlike patients with coronary artery disease, most symptomatic patients with hypertrophic cardiomyopathy have normal (and often enlarged) epicardial coronary arteries, indicating a different mechanism for ischemia in hypertrophic cardiomyopathy, if present.

Evidence for Ischemia in Hypertrophic Cardiomyopathy

The most convincing evidence for ischemia in heart disease is metabolic evidence of anaerobic metabolism, especially during stress. This might result from an imbalance between myocardial oxygen demands and appropriate oxygen delivery via coronary blood flow, although a primary cellular abnormality involving energy substrate utilization or oxidative metabolism unrelated to supply-demand considerations is possible. Classically, the biochemical marker for ischemia most commonly sought in experimental and clinical studies is myocardial production of lactate. Actual demonstration of lactate production during suspected ischemia is hampered by the necessity in humans of collecting venous drainage from all layers of the myocardium, not just the subendocardium where ischemia is likely to be most severe during stress. In early or mild ischemia, this may result not in lactate production but in a net decrease in myocardial lactate extraction, (or, if multiplied by coronary flow, a decrease in lactate consumption) compared to basal measurements. If myocardial ischemia is more severe and more transmural, then net lactate production may be demonstrable. Thus, although lactate production as demonstrated in coronary venous blood is specific for myocardial ischemia, the sensitivity for demonstration of ischemia is relatively low, but to an unknown degree: [1–3]

Several studies of symptomatic patients with hypertrophic cardiomyopathy have demonstrated unequivocal metabolic evidence of myocardial ischemia,

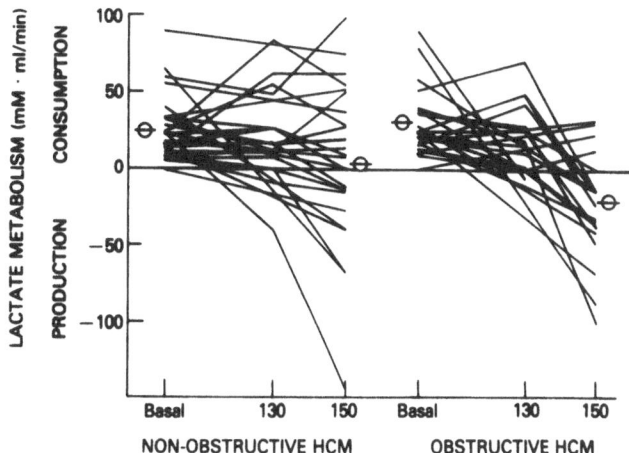

Fig. 1. Lactate consumption in the basal state and during pacing at rates of 130 and 150 beats per minute in patients with hypertrophic cardiomyopathy *(HCM)* with and without obstruction to left ventricular outflow. Lactate consumption < 0 indicates production of lactate by the myocardium. (From [6])

often to a severe degree, during pacing and beta-agonist catecholamine stress [4–9]. Patients with hypertrophic cardiomyopathy, but without a history of chest pain, may not have the same ischemic metabolic response to these stresses [9].

We reported lactate metabolism in 50 symptomatic patients with hypertrophic cardiomyopathy, 23 with basal left ventricular outflow gradients equal to or greater than 30 mmHg, and 27 patients without basal gradients [6]. During atrial pacing to a heart rate of 130, 41 of 50 patients experienced chest pain, and at a heart rate of 150, 46 of 48 patients paced to this heart rate experienced chest pain. At the highest paced heart rate for each patient, great cardiac vein and arterial blood sampling demonstrated myocardial lactate production in 15 of 23 patients with basal obstruction and 11 of 27 patients without basal obstruction (Fig. 1). In five additional patients with basal obstruction and seven patients without obstruction, a decrease in lactate consumption was noted at a heart rate of 150. Thus, overall, 38 of 50 patients demonstrated either lactate production or a decrease in lactate consumption at paced heart rates 130–150 compared to basal measurements. Although patients with basal left ventricular outflow obstruction had more severe metabolic evidence of ischemia in terms of absolute measurements of lactate production during pacing stress, the difference from patients without obstruction was not statistically significant. Isoproterenol infusion resulted in chest pain in 11 of 12 symptomatic patients with obstructive hypertrophic cardiomyopathy associated with metabolic evidence of more severe myocardial ischemia at a heart rate of 130, compared to pacing stress at the same heart rate [7].

Potential Mechanisms of Myocardial Ischemia

Hypertrophic cardiomyopathy is a disease with multiple pathophysiologic and hemodynamic features, including hypertrophy, obstruction to the left ventricular outflow in some patients, morphologically abnormal myocellular architecture and intramural coronary arteries, and abnormal diastolic filling, all of which could influence myocardial oxygen supply/demand relationships, even in the presence of normal epicardial coronary arteries (Table 1). Myocardial oxygen demand considerations include increased muscle mass, a hallmark of this disease. Hypertrophied tissue generally requires greater absolute basal and stress coronary flow because of greater muscle mass and contractile protein content, which require greater rates of oxidative metabolism for providing high energy phosphates. Even though the coronary flow per unit mass may be normal, the higher absolute flow at rest and during stress necessitates greater vasodilatation of autoregulatory arterioles, thus partially exhausting further dilatory capacity and coronary flow reserve. The necessity for greater absolute flow to satisfy the energy requirements of greater myocardial mass is partially offset by decreased regional wall stress, which is inversely related to wall thickness by Laplace's law. Thus, for any diastolic or systolic left ventricular chamber pressure, the wall stress, especially in the mid and outer walls of the hypertrophied myocardium, may be lower than normal. However, wall tension in the subendocardium would still be higher than normal in the presence of increased left ventricular systolic and diastolic pressures.

Several considerations might adversely modify appropriate blood flow and oxygen delivery to the myocardium. Even if the coronary microcirculation remained normal in terms of absolute numbers and maximum cross-sectional area of capillaries, the diffusion distance from capillaries to the center of hypertrophied myocytes might impair appropriate oxygen delivery, especially during stress when oxygen requirements are high. Although new capillary formation that has been demonstrated in some chronic hypertensive animal models might alleviate this concern somewhat by bringing more capillaries in contact with hypertrophied myocytes, diffusion distances might still be greater

Table 1. Potential mechanisms of myocardial ischemia affecting coronary flow reserve in hypertrophic cardiomyopathy

Demand considerations
Increased muscle mass
Increased systolic and diastolic wall stress

Supply considerations
Decreased capillary/myocyte density
Abnormal capillary/myocyte relationships
Fibrous replacement of microcirculation
Systolic compression of epicardial and intramural coronary arteries
Small vessel disease
Effects of abnormal diastolic relaxation on myocardial perfusion
Compression of subendocardial microcirculation

than normal for the most hypertrophied cells. Whether neovascularization occurs in hypertrophic cardiomyopathy in response to the hypertrophic process in unknown. Indeed, fibrous tissue formation and the bizarre myocellular architecture, which are morphologic features of hypertrophic cardiomyopathy, might actually reduce the absolute numbers of small vessels and result in both increased diffusion distance from capillaries to myocytes and impaired peak flow capacity of the microcirculation during stress, thus compromising peak vasodilator reserve. Intimal proliferation and muscular hyperplasia in small, intramural arteries appear capable of compromising the lumen of these vessels ("small vessel disease"), and since resistance is inversely proportional to the radius to the fourth power, small reductions in the radius of a small vessel can have marked effects on flow resistance in the microcirculation. Abnormal small vessels have been seen at necropsy in patients with and patients without obstruction to left ventricular outflow [10, 11].

Two hemodynamic features might also compromise coronary flow delivery. First, systolic compression of epicardial and septal perforator vessels is often noted in patients with hypertrophic cardiomyopathy during angiography [12, 13]. Although the majority of transmural coronary blood flow occurs in diastole, there is a small systolic flow component which might be of considerable importance given the demand/supply concerns discussed in this section, thus limiting peak flow capacity during stress. Further, if there is protracted compression lasting into early diastole when intramyocardial blood flow normally increases, the impact of systolic compression might even be more important with regard to compromising myocardial oxygen delivery during stress. Systolic compression of septal vessels is probably responsible for the "stop and go," or stuttering appearance of contrast dye transit in the coronary arteries frequently noted during angigrapphy of patients with hypertrophic cardiomyopathy, especially those with obstruction, due to cessation of flow during systole followed by rapid dye transit during diastole.

Even in the absence of systolic compression of septal perforating vessels, abnormal diastolic properties of the myocardium, common to most hypertrophic cardiomyopathic ventricles, might impair early diastolic filling of the microcirculation, when coronary flow is normally maximal because of the normal rapid fall in left ventricular tissue pressure [14]. Further, elevated diastolic left ventricular filling pressures might exert compressive effects on the ventricle, limiting appropriate coronary flow delivery within the myocardium, especially the endocardium.

All of the above considerations regarding coronary flow delivery would be expected to be of greatest impact in the subendocardium because of the greater oxygen requirements of the inner regions of the myocardium proximate to high ventricular chamber pressures, compared to the mid and outer walls of the myocardium. Thus the subendocardium is more vulnerable to ischemia if appropriate blood flow cannot meet myocardial oxygen demands.

Invasive Studies of Coronary Blood Flow in Hypertrophic Cardiomyopathy

Classically, myocardial ischemia results from inappropriate matching of myo-cardial demands for oxygen and myocardial oxygen delivery via coronary blood flow. Early studies by Gorlin et al. [15], Brink et al. [16], and Rudolph and Schinz [17] utilizing inert gas washout or xenon-133 methods for measurement of coronary blood flow were performed in patients with hypertrophic cardio-myopathy diagnosed by hemodynamic and contrast ventriculographic studies. Basal left ventricular flow and myocardial oxygen consumption, normalized for mass, were similar to patients with nonhypertrophied ventricles. Weiss et al. [18], utilizing scintillation detection of xenon-133 washout for estimating left coronary artery blood flow, reported that in five patients with ventriculographic determination of hypertrophic cardiomyopathy (three with basal left ventricular outflow gradients), coronary flow per unit mass was lower than normal. How-ever, the absolute basal flows were higher than normal when calculated perfu-sion was multiplied by angiographically determined left ventricular mass. Thompson et al. [4] measured coronary sinus blood flow by thermodilution in 13 symptomatic patients with hypertrophic cardiomyopathy, 11 of whom had significant basal left ventricular outflow gradients. Coronary sinus flow increased from 216 ± 38 ml/min to 374 ± 74 ml/min during pacing to a heart rate of 150. During pacing, the eight patients with normal lactate extraction had increases in coronary sinus flow with each increment in heart rate. In contrast, four out of five patients with lactate production had little or no increase in coronary sinus flow with each pacing increment. Four of five in this group with pacing-induced ischemia also had the highest oxygen consumption at rest and during low paced heart rates. These authors concluded that ischemia in obstruc-tive hypertrophic cardiomyopathy is due to high myocardial oxygen demand or inability of coronary flow to increase with increases in heart rate.

Pasternac et al. [5] measured coronary sinus flow by thermodilution in four symptomatic patients with obstructive hypertrophic cardiomyopathy at rest and during pacing, comparing these findings to five control subjects. Coronary sinus flow was significantly higher than controls at rest, as well as during pacing to a heart rate of 150. However, when flows were divided by mass estimates deter-mined from the RAO ventriculogram, the basal and pacing-induced flows per unit at mass were lower than controls. Likewise, the absolute, but not mass-corrected, myocardial oxygen consumption was higher at rest and during pac-ing in patients with hypertrophic cardiomyopathy compared to controls. All four patients experienced chest pain during pacing, associated with an increase in coronary sinus venous lactate concentration. During pacing, the DPTI/SPTI ratio was significantly lower than controls, which the authors interpreted as causing subendocardial ischemia by virtue of decreased diastolic coronary per-fusion in the setting of increased myocardial oxygen demands.

Cuccurolo et al. [9] performed measurements of coronary sinus flow in the basal state and during isoproterenol infusion (2–4 mcg/min) in 14 patients with obstructive hypertrophic cardiomyopathy and angiographically normal coro-nary arteries, eight of whom had angina by history and six without angina.

Patients with angina developed greater systolic outflow tract gradient (102 ± 8 vs. 52 ± 8 mmHg, $p < 0.001$), higher left ventricular end-diastolic pressures (33 ± 4 vs. 20 ± 6 mmHg, $p < 0.001$), and smaller increases in coronary sinus flow (176 ± 9 vs. 262 ± 34 ml/min, $p < 0.001$), all with lactate production, compared to the six patients without a history of angina. Shimamtasu and Toshima administered dipyridamole 0.56 mg/kg to 19 patients with nonobstructive hypertrophic cardiomyopathy and to seven control subjects [19]. They found that the maximum coronary sinus flow was significantly lower in patients with hypertrophic cardiomyopathy compared to control subjects. These investigators found a significant correlation between the minimum coronary vascular resistance after dipyridamole and left ventricular muscle mass, but no correlation with the left ventricular end-diastolic pressure and the severity of septal perforator compression.

In our initial series of 20 symptomatic patients with echocardiographically determined hypertrophic cardiomyopathy, nine of whom had resting left ventricular outflow tract gradients equal to or greater than 30 mmHg, basal great cardiac vein flow was significantly higher (91 ± 27 vs. 66 ± 17 ml/min, $p < 0.001$) and coronary resistance lower (1.13 ± 38 vs. 1.55 ± 0.45 mmHg $\cdot$ min/ml, $p < 0.001$) compared to 28 control subjects without hypertrophic cardiomyopathy [20]. During pacing, coronary flow rose in both groups, although patients with hypertrophic cardiomyopathy as a group demonstrated an initial rise in flow to 130 beats/min, at which point 12 of 20 patients developed their typical chest pain. With continued pacing to a heart rate of 150 beats per minute, the mean coronary flow actually fell to 114 ± 29 ml/min ($p < 0.002$), with 18 of 20 patients experiencing their typical chest pain, and metabolic evidence of myocardial ischemia. This fall in coronary flow was associated with a substantial rise in left ventricular end-diastolic pressure (30 ± 9 mmHg immediately after peak pacing). In the 14 patients whose great cardiac vein flow actually fell from intermediate to peak pacing, the increase in left ventricular end-diastolic pressure from intermediate to peak pacing was greater than the six patients whose flow remained unchanged or increased (11 ± 8 vs. 2 ± 10 mmHg, $p < 0.01$). In our recently reported series of 50 patients with hypertrophic cardiomyopathy, 23 of whom had basal obstruction to left ventricular outflow, patients with obstruction had significantly greater basal great cardiac vein flow and myocardial oxygen consumption of the anterior left ventricle compared to the 27 patients without basal obstruction (Fig. 2) [6]. Myocardial oxygen consumption and great cardiac vein flow was also significantly higher at a paced heart rate of 100 and 130 beats per minute (the anginal threshold for 41 of the 50 patients). In patients with obstruction, transmural coronary flow reserve was exhausted at a peak rate of 130 beats per minute; higher heart rates resulted in more severe metabolic evidence of ischemia with all patients experiencing chest pain and with an actual increase in coronary resistance. Patients without obstruction also demonstrated evidence of ischemia at heart rates of 130 and 150 beats per minute with 25 of 27 patients experiencing chest pain. In this group, myocardial ischemia occurred at significantly lower coronary flow, higher coronary resistance, and lower myocardial oxygen consumption, suggesting more severely impaired flow delivery in this group compared with those

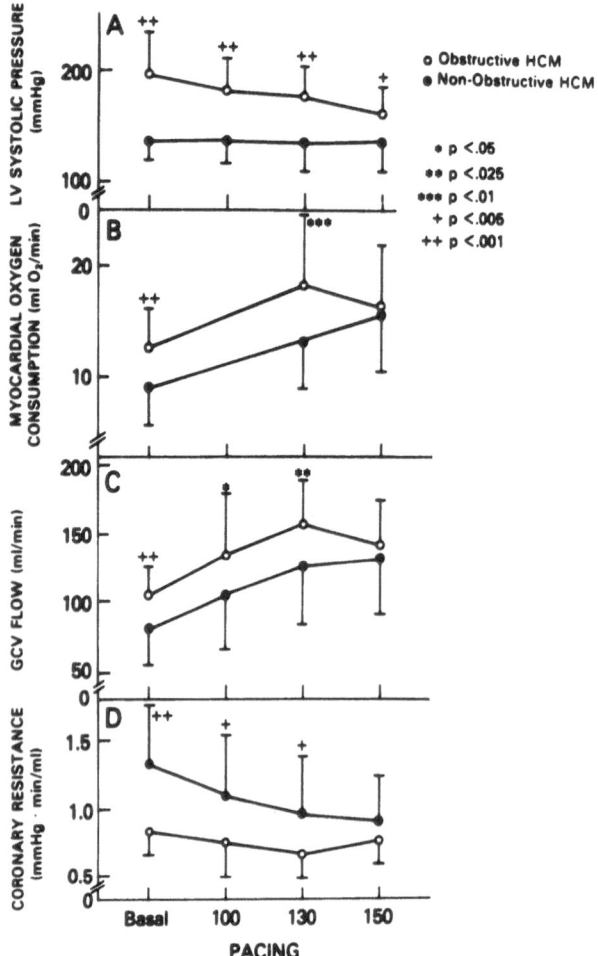

Fig. 2. A Left ventricular *(LV)* systolic pressure; **B** myocardial oxygen consumption in the anterior coronary circulation; **C** great cardiac vein *(GCV)* flow; **D** coronary resistance in the anterior circulation for patients with hypertrophic cardiomyopathy, with *(open circles)* and without *(closed circles)* obstruction to left ventricular outflow. Mean values with 1 SD are plotted in the basal state and during pacing. *$p < 0.05$; **$p < 0.025$; ***$p < 0.01$; + $p < 0.005$; ++ $p < 0.001$ vs. patients without obstruction to left ventricular outflow. (From [6])

with obstruction. Of interest, despite metabolic evidence of severe ischemia (Fig. 1), there was no net increase in myocardial oxygen extraction in patients with hypertrophic cardiomyopathy regardless of whether or not they had basal left ventricular outflow obstruction.

Figure 3 outlines the pathophysiology of ischemia in patients with and patients without obstruction supported by our studies. Although the basal flow and myocardial oxygen consumption per unit mass may be normal, as suggested by previous studies, patients with obstruction to left ventricular outflow have high absolute basal coronary flow and oxygen consumption and rapidly exhaust their coronary flow reserve during stress. These high flows appear to be

Obstructive hyperthrophic cardiomyopathy

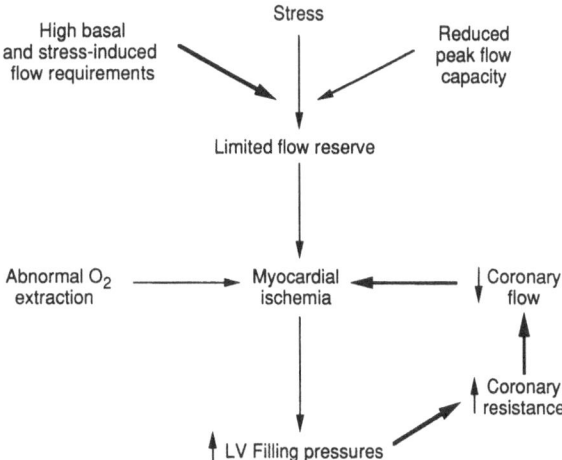

Non-obstructive hyperthrophic cardiomyopathy

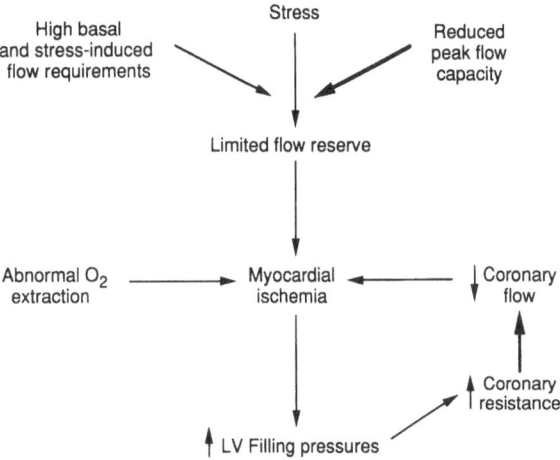

Fig. 3. Proposed mechanisms of myocardial ischemia in hypertrophic cardiomyopathy *(large arrows* indicate mechanisms of greater importance than those indicated by *small arrows).* See text for explanation. (From [6])

particularly vulnerable to increases in left ventricular filling pressures due to compressive effects, with an actual drop in flow and increase in coronary resistance with higher paced heart rates. In contrast, patients without obstruction appear to have more severe impairment in coronary flow delivery, with metabolic evidence of severe ischemia precipitating chest pain at lower peak coronary flows. Abnormal oxygen extraction may contribute to or aggravate ischemia. Undoubtedly, other considerations outlined previously with regard to potential mechanisms of altering myocardial oxygen supply/demand relationships are operative to varying degrees in patients with hypertrophic cardiomyopathy, and may contribute to the atypical features of chest pain experienced by many patients, including prolonged duration of pain, chest pain at rest, and variation in anginal threshold. Unfortunately, because of multiplicity of factors and complex interrelationships amongst them, their relative contribution cannot be ascertained from any one study.

Norepinephrine Kinetics in Hypertrophic Cardiomyopathy

Altered myocardial sympathetic nerve function in hypertrophic cardiomyopathy might also be of importance in the pathophysiology of ischemia in this disease. We have recently reported increased spillover of norepinephrine at the myocardial neuroeffector junction in the basal state in patients with hypertrophic cardiomyopathy, compared to patients with nonhypertrophied ventricles [21]. This augmented spillover of norepinephrine appears to be a consequence of reduced neuronal re-uptake of norepinephrine rather than excessive release. Excess myocardial norepinephrine could explain many of the morphologic features of this disease, including myocardial hypertrophy, coronary vascular smooth muscle hypertrophy and hyperplasia, and myocardial scarring. Additionally, norepinephrine stimulates contractility and may be important in the genesis and propagation of atrial and ventricular arrhythmias. However, the relevance of increased norepinephrine spillover to all of these considerations in hypertrophic cardiomyopathy is unknown at present.

Effect of Operative Reduction in Outflow Gradient

As our studies suggested that patients with obstructive hypertrophic cardiomyopathy had myocardial ischemia because of high metabolic oxygen demands and rapid exhaustion of peak flow capacity, operative reduction of outflow obstruction with reduction in myocardial oxygen demands might be expected to be of benefit and thus of importance in explaining improvement in symptom status and effort tolerance following surgery. In order to assess the impact of operative reduction of left ventricular outflow obstruction in hypertrophic cardiomyopathy, measurements of coronary flow, oxygen and lactate content, left ventricular pressures and cardiac index were measured at rest and during pacing stress in 20 consecutive patients, (13 myotomy/myectomy, six mitral valve replacement, one both myotomy/myectomy and mitral valve replacement) who underwent both preoperative and postoperative studies [22]. All had angiographically normal coronary arteries. Operation resulted in reduction in outflow gradient (64 ± 38 to 4 ± 7 mmHg, $p < 0.001$) and in left ventricular systolic pressure (186 ± 32 to 128 ± 22 mmHg, $p < 0.001$) and was associated with reduction in great cardiac vein flow (101 ± 26 to 78 ± 16 ml/min, $p < 0.001$) and oxygen consumption in the anterior left ventricle and septum (11.9 ± 4.1 to 8.4 ± 1.9 ml O_2/min, $p < 0.001$) in the basal state. Further, the magnitude of the reduction in basal coronary flow and myocardial oxygen consumption correlated with the magnitude of reduction in outflow gradient (Fig. 4).

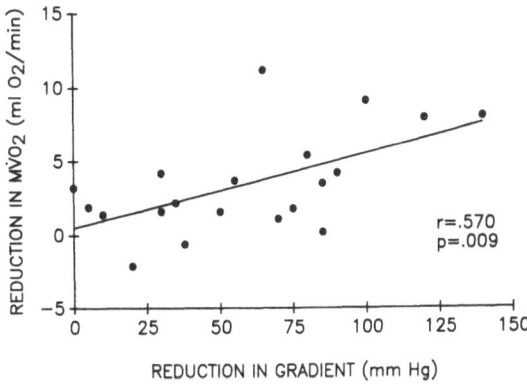

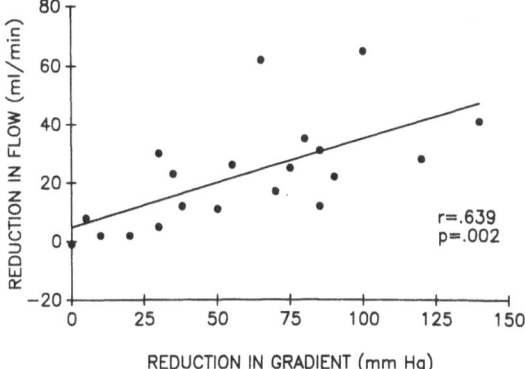

Fig. 4. Correlation of reduction of left ventricular outflow gradient by septal myotomy or mitral valve replacement with reduction in basal myocardial oxygen consumption *(MVO₂)* in the anterior left ventricle and septum *(upper panel)*, and reduction in basal great cardiac vein *(GFV)* flow *(lower panel)*. (From [22])

During rapid atrial pacing, 13 of 20 patients experienced chest pain postoperatively, whereas all 20 developed chest pain during preoperative pacing, with an improvement in pacing anginal threshold (or heart rate 150 if no chest pain was experienced) of 16 ± 18 beats per minute, $p < 0.001$). The peak great cardiac vein flow (161 ± 41 to 131 ± 45 ml/min, $p < 0.025$) and myocardial consumption (19.4 ± 6.1 to 14.3 ± 5.5 ml O_2, $p < 0.005$) during pacing, which correlated directly with the severity of basal left ventricular gradient, were also reduced by operation. Lactate metabolism during pacing changed from net production prior to operation to net consumption after operation (-17 ± 47.6 to 4.4 ± 29.8 micromoles/ml, $p < 0.001$) with six of 20 patients producing lactate following surgery compared to 13 of 20 prior to surgery. Of interest, the six patients with peak great cardiac vein flow greater than 175 ml/min during preoperative pacing had greater symptom and metabolic benefit during pacing following surgery compared to the 14 patients with lower peak coronary flow. Post pacing left ventricular and diastolic pressure (30 ± 7 to 23 ± 7, $p < 0.001$) and pulmonary artery wedge pressure (24 ± 6 to 20 ± 5, $p < 0.001$) were reduced following surgery.

Thus, operative relief of left ventricular outflow obstruction and reduction in left ventricular systolic pressure favorably affects myocardial oxygen consumption and metabolism, due to more advantageous matching of myocardial oxygen delivery to oxygen demands during stress. The particularly marked benefit in those patients with the highest peak flow capacity prior to operation may be due to less intrinsic abnormality in coronary flow delivery, perhaps due to less small vessel coronary disease, thereby favoring restoration of a more normal coronary flow reserve following operation.

Although our studies and others indicate compromised coronary flow responses to stress as being an important component of myocardial ischemia in hypertrophic cardiomyopathy, a primary metabolic abnormality has been proposed. Grover-McKay et al. [23] reported positron emission tomographic (PET) studies in ten mildly symptomatic patients with hypertrophic cardiomyopathy, using flow (N-13 ammonia) and metabolic (C-11 palmitate, F-18 2-deoxyglucose) tracers. After correcting the observed tracer activities for wall thickness (partial volume effect), septal perfusion and glucose utilization was less than the free wall. The relative decrease in septal glucose uptake argued against myocardial ischemia at rest, according to the authors, and instead suggested a primary defect in glucose utilization. A more recent report [24] from this same group performing PET during exercise found increased septal glucose utilization, compatible with ischemia.

Coronary Artery Disease in Patients with Hypertrophic Cardiomyopathy

Of course, patients with hypertrophic cardiomyopathy may have coexisting heart disease unrelated to the hypertrophic process. Several studies have reported coronary artery disease in patients with hypertrophic cardiomyopathy presenting with anginal symptoms [25–28], and improvement in symptom status after surgical revascularization [28]. As is evident in the discussion of studies demonstrating myocardial ischemia and attempting to elucidate mechansims of ischemia presented in this chapter, noninvasive testing is not helpful in separating those patients with coexisting coronary artery disease and thus coronary angiography is the only means of detecting coexisting coronary disease in symptomatic patients.

Left Ventricular Function During Stress

Despite metabolic evidence of ischemia during pacing tachycardia, and elevation of left ventricular diastolic pressures in the majority of patients with hypertrophic cardiomyopathy, the impact of ischemia on exercise may be lessened by beta-adrenergically mediated improvement in diastolic function. We found that isoproterenol infusion to a heart rate of approximately 130 resulted in improved ventricular filling and distensibility in ten of 12 patients, compared to pacing at the same heart rate, despite metabolic evidence of more severe ischemia with isoproterenol [7]. This effect of beta-adrenergic stimulation may be mediated by enhanced inactivation (removal of calcium from the myocyte cytoplasm back into storage sites, with detachment of contractile protein cross-bridges), or restored sensitivity of relaxation to left ventricular systolic pressure. In many respects, isoproterenol simulates catecholamine effects on the heart during exercise, and the beneficial effect of beta adrenergic stimulation on diastolic function may explain preserved effort tolerance despite cardiomyopathy associated with myocardial ischemia during stress in many patients. Whether drugs that improve diastolic filing in hypertrophic cardiomyopathy, such as verapamil, potentiate this effect is unknown. However, a reduction in cytosolic calcium by calcium channel blocker could potentially facilitate beta adrenergically mediated removal of calcium from the cytosol and account for improved effort capacity on this drug. In contrast, beta adrenergic blocking agents, although benefitting diastolic filling by slowing the heart rate response to exercise, could blunt the beneficial effect of beta adrenergic stimulation on relaxation. This may explain the absence of uniform benefit of symptoms of patients with hypertrophic cardiomyopathy to beta adrenergic blocking drugs.

Summary

Patients with hypertrophic cardiomyopathy, especially those symptomatic with angina pectoris, clearly have inducible myocardial ischemia, most likely related to imbalances between myocardial oxygen demands and appropriate coronary flow delivery. Patients with obstruction to left ventricular outflow may have greater metabolic demands during stress with more rapid exhaustion of coronary flow reserve. Patients without obstruction may have greater impairment in coronary flow delivery with rapid exhaustion of a more limited peak flow capacity compared to patients with obstruction. However, in both groups, multiple considerations including factors relating to myocardial oxygen requirements (muscle mass and distribution, systolic and diastolic wall stress) and appropriate coronary flow delivery (abnormal myocellular architecture, capillary/myocyte relationships, fibrosis, effects of abnormal diastolic filling on coronary flow, septal perforator compression, small vessel coronary disease, or coexisting epicardial coronary artery disease) may contribute in varying degrees to the pathogenesis of myocardial ischemia. Unfortunately, at present it is imposible to separate out accurately the most important influences on the induction of myocardial ischemia in a given patient. Also unknown is whether myocardial ischemia may result in extensive regional and global scarring seen in some patients with hypertrophic cardiomyopathy, resulting in either wall motion abnormalities or progression to a dilated, hypocontractile ventricle, or whether these processes are independent of myocardial ischemia. If myocardial ischemia does contribute to myocardial scarring, it is further unknown as to whether medication or operative relief of outflow obstruction alters this process. Also unknown at present is whether metabolic abnormalities in substrate utilization and oxidative metabolism may contribute to myocardial ischemia in some patients with hypertrophic cardiomyopathy.

References

1. Neill WA (1968) Myocardial hypoxia and anaerobic metabolism in coronary heart disease. Am J Cardiol 22:507–515
2. Case RB, Nasser MG, Crampton RS (1969) Biochemical aspects of early myocardial ischemia. Am J Cardiol 24:766–775
3. Gorlin R (1969) Evaluation of myocardial metabolism in ischemic heart disease. Circulation 39–40 (Suppl IV) 155–163
4. Thompson DS, Naqvi N, Juul SM, Swanton RH, Coltart DJ, Jenkins BS, Webb-Peploe MM (1980) Effects of propranolol on myocardial oxygen consumption. Substrate extraction and hemodynamics in hypertrophic cardiomyopathy. Br Heart J 44:488–498
5. Pasternac A, Noble J, Streulens Y, Elie R, Henschke C, Bourassa MG (1982) Pathophysiology of chest pain in patients with cardiomyopathies and normal coronary arteries. Circulation 65:778–789
6. Cannon RO, Schenke WH, Maron BJ, Tracy CM, Leon MB, Brush JE, Rosing DR, Epstein SE (1987) Differences in coronary flow and myocardial metabolism at rest and during pacing between patients with obstructive and patients with nonobstructive hypertrophic cardiomyopathy. J Am Coll Cardiol 10:53–62
7. Udelson JE, Cannon RO, Bacharach SL, Rumble TF, Bonow RO (1989) Betaadrenergic stimulation with isoproterenol enhances left ventricular diastolic performance in hypertrophic cardiomyopathy despite potentiation of myocardial ischemia: comparison to rapid atrial pacing. Circulation 79:371–382
8. Ogata Y, Hiyamuta K, Terasawa M, Ohkita Y, Bekki H, Koga Y, Toshima H (1986) Relationship of exercise of pacing induced ST segment depression and myocardial lactate metabolism in patients with hypertrophic cardiomyopathy. Jpn Heart J 27:145–158
9. Cuccurullo F, Mezzetti A, Lapenna D, Tomassetti V, Parreca E, Paggiopollini G, Guglielmi MD, Mancini M, Marzia L, Lenzi S (1987) Mechanism of isoproterenol-induced angina pectoris in patients with obstructive hypertrophic cardiomyopathy and normal coronary arteries. Am J Cardiol 60:667–673
10. Maron BJ, Wolfson JK, Epstein SE, Roberts WC (1986) Intramural ("small vessel") coronary artery disease in hypertrophic cardiomyopathy. J Am Coll Cardiol 8:545–557
11. Tanaka M, Fujiwara H, Onodera T, Wu D-J, Matsuda M, Hamashima Y, Kawai C (1987) Quantitative analysis of narrowings of intramyocardial small arteries in normal hearts, hypertensive hearts and hearts with hypertrophic cardiomyopathy. Circulation 75:1130–1139
12. Pichard AD, Meller J, Teichholz LE, Lipnick S, Gorlin R, Hermon MV (1977) Septal perforator compression (narrowing) in idiopathic hypertrophic subaortic stenosis. J Am Coll Cardiol 40:310–314
13. Ruddy TD, Henderson MA, Rakowski H, Wigle ED (1981) Systolic constriction of the coronary arteries in hypertrophic cardiomyopathy. Circulation 54:IV-239 (abstr)
14. Brutsaert DL, Housmans PR, Goethals MA (1980) Dual control of relaxation: its role in the ventricular function in the mammalian heart. Circ Res 47:637–652
15. Gorlin R, Cohen LS, Elliott WC, Klein MD, Lane FJ (1964) Hemodynamics of muscular subaortic stenosis (obstructive cardiomyopathy). In: Wolstennhome GEW, O'Connor M (eds) Ciba Foundation Symposium: Cardiomyopathies. Ciba Foundation, London, p 76
16. Brink AJ, Lewis CM, Van Heerden PDR (1967) Coronary blood flow and myocardial metabolism in obstructive cardiomyopathy: observations before and after treatment with a beta adrenergic blocking agent. Am J Cardiol 19:548–555
17. Rudolph W, Schinz A (1973) Studies on myocardial blood flow, oxygen consumption and myocardial metabolism in patients with cardiomyopathy. In: Bajusz E, Rana G (eds) Recent advances in studies on cardiac structure and metabolism: cardiomyopathies, vol 2. University Park Press, Baltimore, p 739
18. Weiss MB, Ellis K, Sciacca RR, Johnson LL, Schmidt DH, Cannon PJ (1976) Myocardial blood flow in congestive and hypertrophic cardiomyopathy. Circulation 54:484–493
19. Shimamatsu M, Toshima H (1987) Impaired coronary vasodilatory capacity after dipyridamole administration in hypertrophic cardiomyopathy. Jpn Heart J 28:387–401

20. Cannon RO, Rosing DR, Maron BJ, Leon MB, Bonow RO, Watson RM, Epstein SE (1985) Myocardial ischemia in patients with hypertrophic cardiomyopathy: contribution of inadequate vasodilator reserve and elevated left ventricular filling pressures. Circulation 71:234–243

21. Brush JE, Eisenhofer G, Garty M, Stull R, Maron BJ, Cannon RO, Panza JA, Epstein SE, Goldstein DS (1989) Cardiac norepinephrine kinetics in hypertrophic cardiomyopathy. Circulation 79:836–844

22. Cannon RO, McIntosh CL, Schenke WH, Maron BJ, Bonow RO, Epstein SE (1989) Effect of surgical reduction of left ventricular outflow obstruction on hemodynamics, coronary flow and myocardial metabolism in hypertrophic cardiomyopathy. Circulation 79:766–775

23. Grover-McKay M, Schwaiger M, Krivokapich J, Perloff JK, Phelps ME, Schelberg HR (1989) Regional myocardial blood flow and metabolism at rest in mildly symptomatic patients with hypertrophic cardiomyopathy. J Am Coll Cardiol 13:317–324

24. Nienaber CA, Gambhir SS, Mady FV, Ratib O, Huang S, Schelbert HR (1988) Quantification of myocardial glucose utilization and flow in hypertrophic cardiomyopathy by positron tomography. Circulation 78:II-599 (abstr)

25. Gulotta SJ, Hamby RI, Aronson AL, Ewing K (1972) Coexistent idiopathic hypertrophic subaortic stenosis and coronary artery disease. Circulation 46:890–896

26. Oran E, Gupta S, Yeo B, et al (1973) Idiopathic hypertrophic subaortic stenosis in patients with coronary artery disease. Importance of recognition and principles of management. Angiology 24:538–547

27. Marcus GB, Popp RL, Stinson EB (1974) Coronary artery disease with idiopathic hypertrophic subaortic stenosis. Lancet 1:901–903

28. Cokkinos DV, Krajcer Z, Leachman RD (1985) Coronary artery disease in hypertrophic cardiomyopathy. Am J Cardiol 55:1437–1438

Left Ventricular Diastolic Function and Myocardial Ischemia in Hypertrophic Cardiomyopathy: Assessment by Radionuclide Methods

R. O. Bonow

Introduction

Impaired diastolic function of the hypertrophied and stiffened left ventricle is a characteristic feature of hypertrophic cardiomyopathy [1–9]. The pathophysiologic basis and clinical significance of altered diastolic performance in this condition has been the subject of intense interest and investigation for the past two decades. Altered left ventricular filling dynamics and reduced left ventricular distensibility are associated with reduced left ventricular stroke volume, increased left ventricular filling pressures, and compressive effects on the coronary microcirculation. These factors contribute importantly to the clinical presentation of many patients, including symptoms of fatigue, dyspnea, and angina pectoris. Abnormal diastolic function has been demonstrated in the vast majority of patients with hypertrophic cardiomyopathy undergoing hemodynamic or noninvasive studies (Fig. 1.) [1–9]. This review will focus on the assessment of left ventricular diastolic function in hypertrophic cardiomyopathy, and the interplay between altered diastolic function and myocardial ischemia, using data derived from radionuclide techniques applied both in the noninvasive laboratory and in the catheterization laboratory.

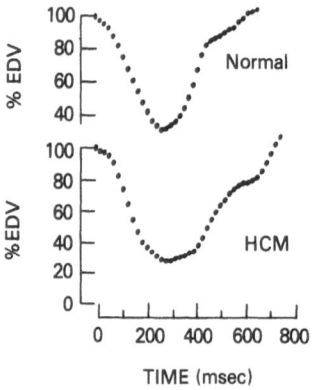

Fig. 1. Left ventricular time-activity curves at rest, representing relative changes in ventricular volume during the cardiac cycle, in a patient with hypertrophic cardiomyopathy and a normal subject matched for age, heart rate, and ejection fraction. Despite well-preserved systolic function, the patient with hypertrophic cardiomyopathy has evidence of impaired diastolic filling, with a prolonged isovolumic relaxation phase, reduced rate and extent of rapid filling, and an increased contribution of atrial systole to ventricular stroke volume. *EDV*, end-diastolic volume

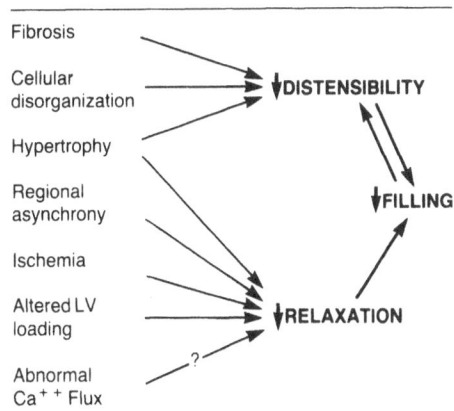

Fibrosis

Cellular disorganization ───────────▶ ↓DISTENSIBILITY

Hypertrophy

Regional asynchrony   ↓FILLING

Ischemia

Altered LV loading ───────────▶ ↓RELAXATION

Abnormal Ca⁺⁺ Flux

Fig. 2. Determinants of impaired left ventricular *(LV)* diastolic function in hypertrophic cardiomyopathy. (From [13])

Evaluation of Left Ventricular Diastolic Function

Left Ventricular Distensibility: Reduced left ventricular diastolic distensibility (or increased left ventricular diastolic chamber stiffness) in hypertrophic cardiomyopathy is responsible for the exaggerated increases in left ventricular pressure that develop in response to small increments in volume during the diastolic filling period [10, 11]. Reduced distensibility results both from factors determining the passive elastic properties of the ventricular chamber (including severity of hypertrophy, fibrosis, and cellular disarray) and from factors influencing the rate and extent of active left ventricular relaxation (Fig. 2). Delayed or incomplete relaxation, with continuing interaction of contractile elements and persistent myocardial tension development during the diastolic filling phase, results in an increase in intracavitary pressure at any level of diastolic volume. Thus, left ventricular distensibility is determined not only by fixed, passive properties of the myocardium but also by potentially reversible alterations in left ventricular filling dynamics resulting from impaired relaxation [11–13].

Left Ventricular Relaxation: As in coronary artery disease, the factors contributing to impaired relaxation in hypertrophic cardiomyopathy are mediated via either inactivation-dependent or load-dependent mechanisms. Myocardial inactivation, the energy-requiring process by which calcium ion is sequestered in the sarcoplasmic reticulum, is reduced in experimental animals with pressure-overload hypertrophy [14–17], resulting in persistent elevation of intracellular calcium concentrations and prolonged interaction of contractile elements. This mechanism may also be operative in hypertrophic cardiomyopathy [18], giving rise to intracellular calcium overload. In addition, there is evidence of an increased number of active calcium antagonist receptors in the sarcolemma in patients with this disease [19], which may lead directly to augmented calcium ion influx and intracellular calcium overload. Finally, there is a growing body of data indicating that myocardial ischemia develops commonly in patients with hypertrophic cardiomyopathy [20–22], which would further hinder myocardial inactivation (and thereby increase filling pressures) in a dynamic and reversible manner analogous to that proposed in patients with coronary artery disease [11, 23–28]. Myocardial ischemia has important implications in hypertrophic cardiomyopathy, as it has also been demonstrated that the effects of hypoxia on ventricular stiffness are compounded in the hypertrophied left ventricle [17, 29, 30].

Reduced rate and extent of left ventricular relaxation in hypertrophic cardiomyopathy may also reflect load-dependent mechanisms, including decreased wall tension at the onset of mitral valve opening [31, 32], altered afterload [31, 33], altered contractile state [34], and altered coronary flow dynamics [31]. In an individual patient, any or all of these possible mechanisms may be operative.

Left Ventricular Nonuniformity: One further factor that may contribute to impaired relaxation is nonuniform or asynchronous regional ventricular function [32, 35–37]. In hypertrophic cardiomyopathy, there may be marked

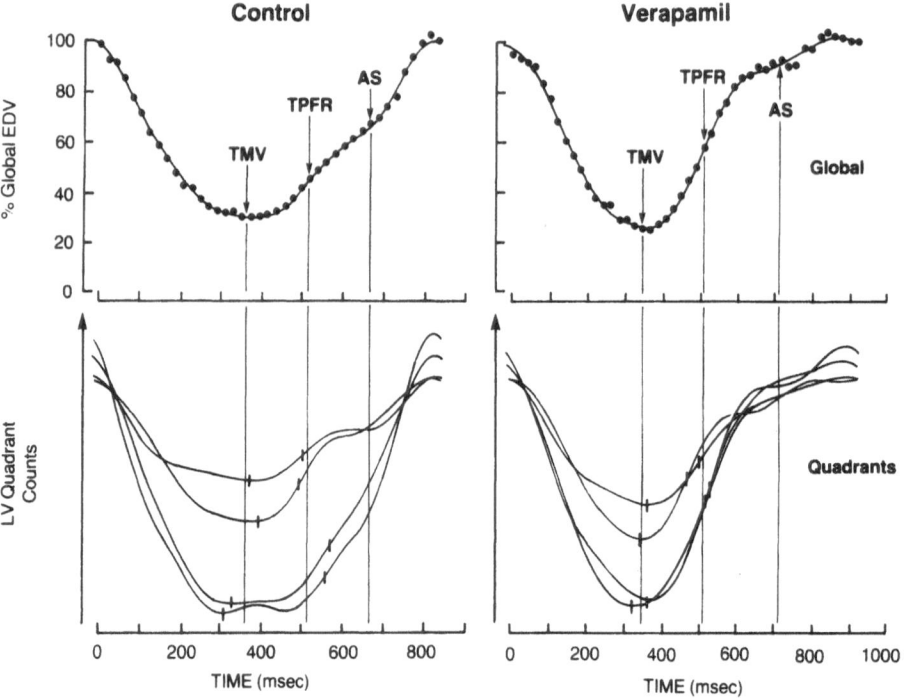

Fig. 3. Regional left ventricular asynchrony in a patient with hypertrophic cardiomyopathy studied at rest by radionuclide angiography before and after oral verapamil therapy. Global left ventricular volume curves are presented in the top panels, indicating time to minimum volume *(TMV)*, time to peak filling rate *(TPFR)*, and onset of mechanical atrial systole *(AS)*. Regional quadrant curves are shown in the bottom panels. Variation among quadrants in TMV and TPFR before verapamil indicates considerable systolic and diastolic asynchrony. Reduction in diastolic asynchrony after verapamil, with greater homogeneity in the relative contributions of rapid filling and atrial systole to regional filling, is associated with improved global rapid diastolic filling. (From [39])

regional heterogeneity in the severity of left ventricular wall thickening, and myocardial ischemia may also affect the left ventricle on a nonuniform, regional basis. These factors result in slowed regional relaxation, increased regional stiffness, and nonuniform loading [38]. The net effect of these many complex and interrelated factors is an asynchronous left ventricular chamber with extreme heterogeneity in the timing, rate, and extent of relaxation and diastolic filling (Fig. 3), which has been demonstrated clinically in patients with hypertrophic cardiomyopathy [1, 3, 39]. the magnitude of regional nonuniformity, in turn, correlates with the severity of impaired global diastolic performance [39].

Effects of Pharmacologic Therapy: In many patients with hypertrophic cardiomyopathy, these abnormalities in regional and global diastolic function are not fixed, but may be modified in a favorable fashion by pharmacologic therapy. In particular, the calcium channel blockers verapamil, nifedipine, and diltiazem have been shown to improve indexes of left ventricular relaxation and filling (Figs. 3, 4) [5, 6, 8, 40–49]. Such effects have not been demonstrated during treatment with beta blocking agents [5, 50]. Among the calcium channel blocking drugs, verapamil and diltiazem appear to be preferable to nifedipine in patients with obstructive hypertrophic cardiomyopathy, as the more potent effects of nifedipine on the peripheral vasculature are more likely to aggravate the outflow gradient [51]. In contrast, the negative inotropic effects of verapamil have the advantage of reducing the degree of outflow obstruction [43, 52]. Although the clinical relevance of altered diastolic properties in the case of nifedipine or diltiazem treatment has not been explored, the changes in indexes of left ventricular filling during treatment with verapamil are related to enhanced exercise tolerance and reduced symptoms [44, 46]. During both

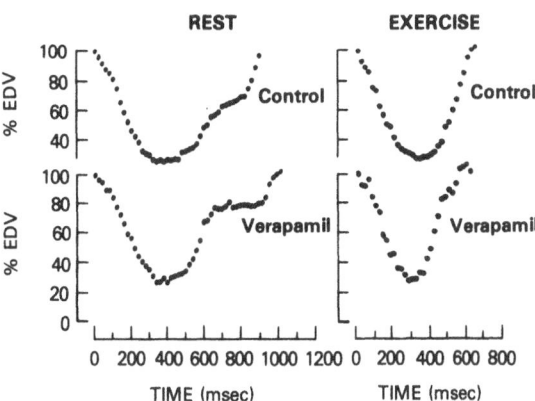

Fig. 4. Left ventricular time-activity curves at rest and during exercise in a patient with hypertrophic cardiomyopathy before (control) and after oral verapamil therapy. At rest, verapamil results in shortening of the isovolumic relaxation period, increased rate and extent of rapid filling, reduced time to peak filling rate, and reduced contribution of atrial systole. Peak filling rate and time to peak filling rate are also improved during exercise with verapamil. (From [47])

short-term and long-term administration of verapamil, over 80% of patients manifesting an improvement in left ventricular filling also manifest an increase in objective exercise tolerance, while such enhanced exercise tolerance is observed in only a minority (approximately 12%) of patients in whom indexes of diastolic filling are not improved by verapamil [46].

The reason for this beneficial correlation between enhanced diastolic filling and improved exercise tolerance is apparent from catheterization studies demonstrating that verapamil augments left ventricular stroke volume without an increase in diastolic pressures at rest (Fig. 5) [43, 44] and with a decrease in left ventricular filling pressures during exercise [44]. Improved indexes of global left ventricular diastolic function with verapamil are also associated with reduction in regional asynchrony and more homogeneous regional diastolic filling (Fig. 3) [39]. Mechanisms for the beneficial effects of verapamil on regional and global diastolic function cannot be determined with certainty, given the complex interrelationships governing altered diastolic properties in hypertrophic cardiomyopathy (Fig. 2). These mechanisms could include alterations in left ventricular loading, increased regional myocardial blood flow, or enhanced inactivation in the hypertrophied myocardium via either direct effects to reduce calcium ion influx or indirect effects mediated by reflex sympathetic stimulation [53] or reduced myocardial ischemia [54].

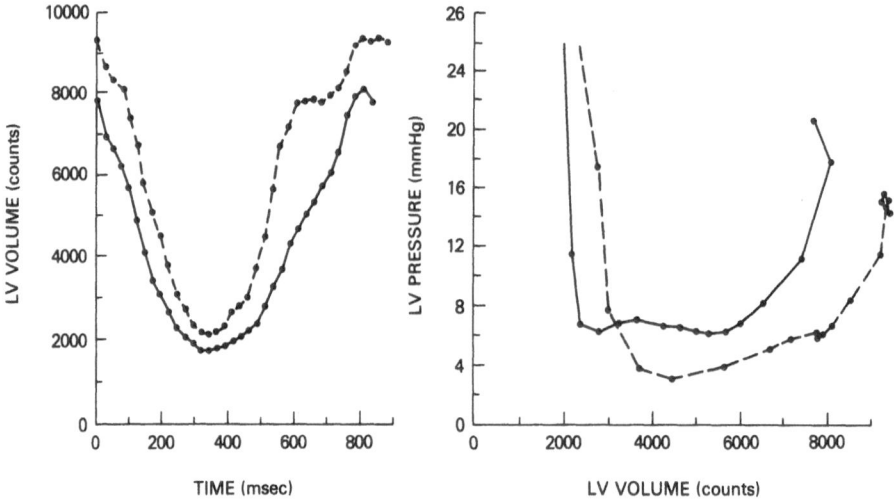

Fig. 5. Left ventricular *(LV)* volume curves *(left panel)* and pressure-volume relations *(right panel)* obtained using radionuclide angiographic techniques in a patient with hypertrophic cardiomyopathy before (control; *solid line*) and during intravenous verapamil infusion *(broken line)*. Verapamil results in increased rate and extent of rapid filling, reduced contribution of atrial systole, and an increase in both end-diastolic volume and stroke volume. These changes are associated with a downward and rightward shift in the pressure-volume relation. (From [43])

Evaluation of Myocardial Ischemia

There is growing awareness that myocardial ischemia occurs commonly in patients with hypertrophic cardiomyopathy in the absence of epicardial coronary artery disease. This concept is supported by several observations, most notable of which is the frequent development of angina pectoris, either at rest or during the increased demands associated with exercise. Angina, when produced in the catheterization laboratory during rapid atrial pacing, is also associated with reduced coronary vasodilator reserve, reduced lactate consumption (or even lactate production), and elevation of left ventricular filling pressures [20, 21]. Necropsy studies demonstrate foci of fibrous tissue deposition, ranging from patchy fibrosis to large regions of transmural scar, which may represent the sequelae of the ischemic process [55, 56].

Thallium-201 Scintigraphy: Exercise thallium-201 scintigraphy has been shown to be a useful method for the noninvasive detection and evaluation of myocardial ischemia in hypertrophic cardiomyopathy [57–61]. Using thallium-201 single photon emission computed tomography (SPECT), we have demonstrated that myocardial perfusion defects, either at rest or during exercise, occur in over 50% of patients (Fig. 6) [61].

In patients with left ventricular systolic dysfunction, the myocardial perfusion defects are almost invariably fixed or only partially reversible, compatible with myocardial fibrosis [61]. This evidence confirms previous studies that impaired systolic function in this subset of patients with hypertrophic cardiomyopathy represents a natural history characterized by progressive myocardial scarring, leading to myocardial wall thinning, left ventricular cavity dilatation, and systolic dysfunction [55, 62–65].

In patients with preserved systolic function, the regional thallium-201 perfusion defects occurring during exercise are usually reversible at rest (Fig. 6) and represent evidence of inducible ischemia. The perfusion abnormalities themselves develop not only in regions of severe hypertrophy, but may also be

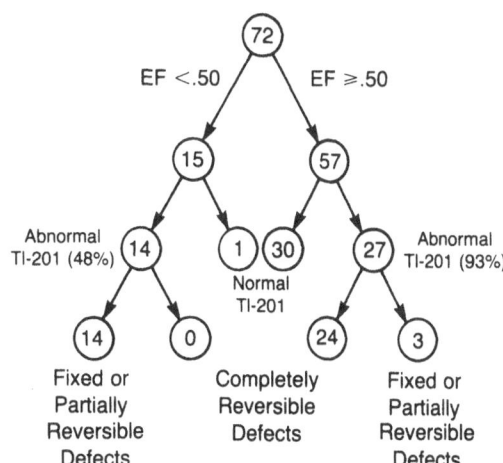

Fig. 6. Flow diagram showing the relation between myocardial perfusion defects during exercise thallium-201 scintigraphy and left ventricular systolic function. *EF,* ejection fraction. (From [61])

observed (less commonly) in regions that are relatively unaffected by the hypertrophic process. The magnitude of myocardial hypertrophy is an important factor related to the thallium-201 defects, however, as patients with perfusion abnormalities induced during exercise have evidence of a greater extent and severity of left ventricular hypertrophy, as well as more severe impairment in left ventricular diastolic filling, than those with normal perfusion patterns during exercise [54, 66]. Thus, ventricular hypertrophy, impaired ventricular diastolic function, and myocardial ischemia appear to be interrelated pathophysiologic features of hypertrophic cardiomyopathy.

Mechanisms for Myocardial Ischemia: There are several possible mechanisms for the development of myocardial ischemia in patients with hypertrophic cardiomyopathy (Fig. 7), related both to inadequate myocardial blood flow and increased myocardial oxygen demand [67]. Impaired left ventricular diastolic relaxation and elevated intracavitary pressures during ventricular filling may result in compressive effects on the coronary microcirculation and restrict diastolic coronary blood flow [21], especially in the subendocardial regions. Patients with hypertrophic cardiomyopathy also manifest limited coronary vasodilator reserve for additional reasons, related to the nonspecific effect of myocardial hypertrophy on vasodilator capacity [68, 69] and to the more specific abnormalities of the small intramural coronary arteries [70, 71] that are characteristic of hypertrophic cardiomyopathy and only rarely present in other forms of myocardial hypertrophy. Myocardial ischemia would be further aggravated by the increases in oxygen demand associated with the hypertrophied left ventricle and, in many patients, the added demands of the greatly elevated systolic pressures resulting from outflow tract obstruction. Once ischemia develops, it may be self-perpetuating, in that ischemia will contribute further to impaired ventricular relaxation [11, 23–28] and elevated diastolic pressures, resulting in a greater compromise of the coronary circulation.

Effects of Verapamil: We have recently demonstrated that exercise-induced myocardial perfusion defects on thallium-201 tomographic studies may be

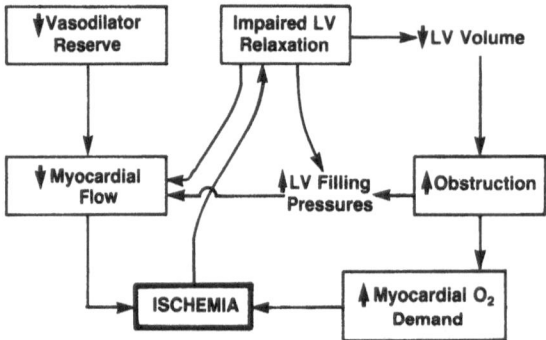

Fig. 7. Influence of reduced coronary vasodilator reserve, impaired left ventricular relaxation, and subaortic obstruction on myocardial ischemia in hypertrophic cardiomyopathy. *LV*, left ventricular. (From [67])

reduced, or in many cases prevented entirely, during oral verapamil treatment (Fig. 8) [54]. This drug effect is observed primarily in patients with more extensive and more severe left ventricular hypertrophy. The improvement in myocardial perfusion does not appear to be related merely to a reduction in myocardial oxygen demands during drug treatment, as patients with either obstructive or nonobstructive hypertrophic cardiomyopathy achieved similar heart-rate blood pressure products during exercise during both baseline and verapamil exercise tests. Although it is impossible to use the rate-pressure product as a clinical index of myocardial demand in patients with obstructive hypertrophic cardiomyopathy, this index is a clinically useful index of demand in nonobstructive patients (as it is in patients with coronary artery disease). Thus, the mechanisms for the verapamil effect on inducible ischemia appear to reflect a preferential increase in myocardial blood flow, related either to coronary dilatation or improved left ventricular relaxation. In keeping with this latter possibility, the patients in whom verapamil improved myocardial perfusion during exercise had evidence of improved ventricular diastolic filling, which was not observed in patients in whom abnormal perfusion patterns persisted during verapamil treatment [54]. Given the intimate relation between ischemia and left ventricular relaxation (Fig. 7), it has not been possible to determine from the currently available data whether a verapamil effect to enhance myocardial relaxation is the primary event, leading to amelioration of ischemia, or whether a primary reduction in ischemia stemming from coronary dilation results in an improvement in left ventricular relaxation and distensibility. It is also uncertain whether the observed effect of verapamil is a relatively specific action of calcium channel blocking agents, or whether other drugs (such as beta blockers) might have similar beneficial effects on inducible myocardial ischemia.

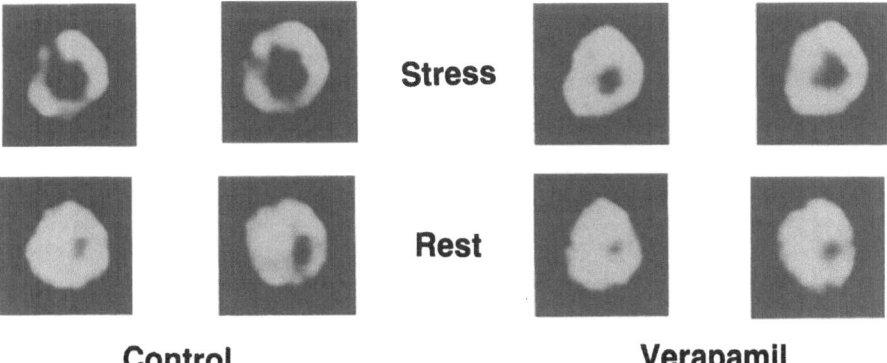

Fig. 8. Short-axis thallium-201 tomograms obtained immediately after maximal treadmill exercise *(top)* and after 3 h rest *(bottom)* in an 18-year-old asymptomatic man with hypertrophic cardiomyopathy. Under control conditions *(left)*, reversible septal and inferoposterior perfusion defects develop during exercise and are improved at rest. There is also apparent reversible cavity dilatation induced by exercise. During oral verapamil *(right)*, myocardial perfusion and apparent cavity dilatation are improved during exercise. (From [54])

Effects of Beta-Adrenergic Stimulation

Beta-adrenergic stimulation enhances relaxation in isolated cardiac muscle studies, even in the absence of a positive effect on contractility [72], related to acceleration of the inactivation process. We therefore hypothesized that beta-adrenergic stimulation might improve left ventricular diastolic performance in patients with hypertrophic cardiomyopathy, despite the detrimental effects of catecholamines associated with increased contractility, which would augment oxygen demands and aggravate ischemia.

Recent data indicate that beta-adrenergic stimulation with isoproterenol may indeed result in favorable effects on left ventricular relaxation and diastolic pressure-volume relations in patients with obstructive hypertrophic cardiomyopathy [73], in comparison to the effects of atrial pacing at similar heart rates (Fig. 9). This improvement in global diastolic ventricular function with isoproterenol occurred despite the expected augmentation of the left ventricular outflow tract gradient and development of worsening myocardial ischemia (as

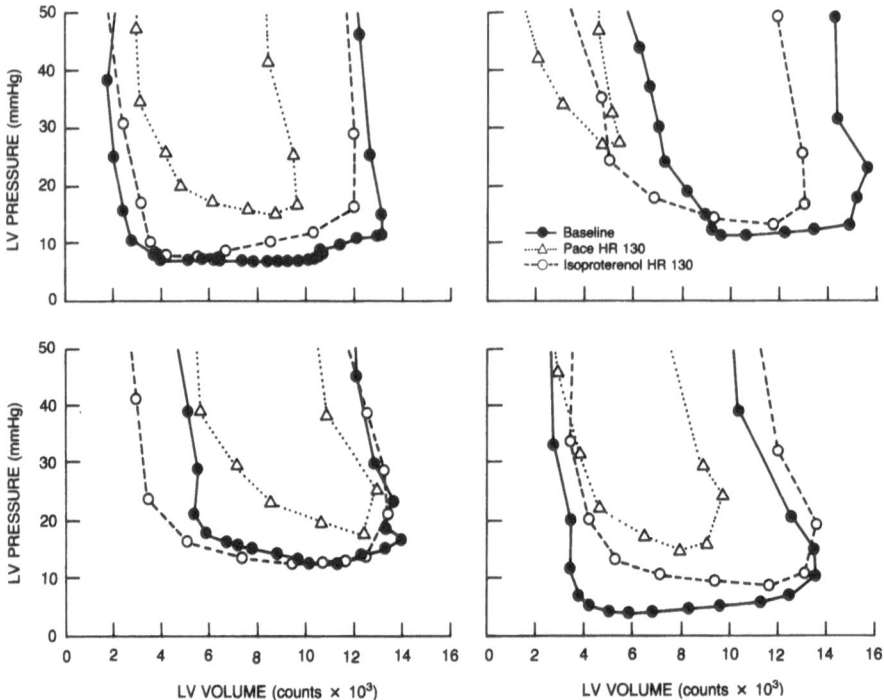

Fig. 9. Effects of isoproterenol infusion on left ventricular *(LV)* diastolic pressure-volume relations in four patients with obstructive hypertrophic cardiomyopathy studied with combined hemodynamic and radionuclide angiographic techniques. During rapid atrial pacing, the curves shift upward and leftward, and pressure continues to decline throughout the filling phase, evidence for impaired relaxation. During isoproterenol to the same heart rate, the curves shift downward and rightward toward the baseline, despite more severe myocardial ischemia in each patient, and there is less evidence of impaired relaxation. (From [73])

reflected by myocardial lactate metabolism). Importantly, isoproterenol also resulted in an increase in systolic shortening with reduced end-systolic volume, suggesting that one mechanism for improved diastolic function, despite ischemia, was related to the beneficial loading effects related to the development of greater restoring forces during contraction and thus greater elastic recoil during diastole. However, since myocardial ischemia would be expected to impair inactivation and thus result in relative load-insensitivity [31, 32], additional effects of isoproterenol must also have played a role. We hypothesize that beta-adrenergic stimulation enhanced the myocardial inactivation process [73], thereby restoring load sensitivity. In addition, another effect of isoproterenol was evident; isoproterenol significantly reduced the marked regional systolic dissynchrony that developed during pacing tachycardia in the absence of beta-adrenergic stimulation. Thus, improvement in regional asynchrony by isoproterenol, despite the effects of ischemia (which would be expected to aggravate regional nonuniformity), is another possible mechanism with which to explain the improvement in diastolic hemodynamics. These findings with beta-adrenergic stimulation, and our previous observations regarding the effects of verapamil, suggest that reduction in regional nonuniformity is one mechanism that may contribute to beneficial effects on left ventricular relaxation and diastolic filling in the treatment of hypertrophic cardiomyopathy.

It is clear that isoproterenol is not a clinically advantageous drug for the treatment of obstructive hypertrophic cardiomyopathy. These data, however, provide further evidence that the disorders of left ventricular diastolic function in this disease are not related merely to the abnormal passive myocardial properties that develop in response to hypertrophy, fibrosis, and cellular disarray, but rather also involve dynamic disturbances in ventricular relaxation, ischemia, asynchrony, and the hypertrophic process itself. These findings suggest that other agents that provide similar mechanisms to enhance myocardial inactivation or to reduce ventricular asynchrony, alone or in combination with calcium channel-blocking drugs, may be beneficial in the management of patients with hypertrophic cardiomyopathy.

References

1. Sanderson JE, Gibson DG, Brown DJ, Goodwin JF (1977) Left ventricular filling in hypertrophic cardiomyopathy: an angiographic study. Br Heart J 39:661–670
2. Sanderson JE, Traill TA, St John Sutton MG, Brown DJ, Gibson DG, Goodwin JF (1978) Left ventricular relaxation and filling in hypertrophic cardiomyopathy: an echocardiographic study. Br Heart J 40:596–601
3. St John Sutton MG, Tajik AJ, Gibson DG, Brown CJ, Seward JB, Giuliani ER (1978) Echocardiographic assessment of left ventricular filling and septal and posterior wall dynamics in idiopathic hypertrophic subaortic stenosis. Circulation 57:512–520
4. Hanrath P, Mathey DG, Siegert R, Bleifeld W (1980) Left ventricular relaxation and filling in different forms of left ventricular hypertrophy: an echocardiographic study. Am J Cardiol 45:15–23
5. Bonow RO, Rosing DR, Bacharach SL, Green MV, Kent KM, Lipson LC, Maron BJ, Leon MB, Epstein SE (1981) Effect of verapamil on left ventricular systolic function and diastolic filling in patients with hypertrophic cardiomyopathy. Circulation 64:787–796

6. Bonow RO, Frederick TM, Bacharach SL, Green MV, Goose PW, Maron BJ, Rosing DR (1983) Atrial systole and left ventricular filling in patients with hypertrophic cardiomyopathy: effect of verapamil. Am J Cardiol 51:1386–1391

7. Alvares RF, Shaver JA, Gamble WH, Goodwin JF (1984) Isovolumic relaxation period in hypertrophic cardiomyopathy. J Am Coll Cardiol 3:71–81

8. Betocchi S, Bonow RO, Bacharach SL, Rosing DR, Maron BJ, Green MV (1986) Isovolumic relaxation period in hypertrophic cardiomyopathy: assessment by radionuclide angiography. J Am Coll Cardiol 7:74–81

9. Maron BJ, Spirito P, Green KJ, Wesley YE, Bonow RO, Arce J (1987) Noninvasive assessment of left ventricular diastolic function by pulsed Doppler echocardiography in patients with hypertrophic cardiomyopathy. J Am Coll Cardiol 10:733–742

10. Gaasch WH, Levine HJ, Quinones MA, Alexander JK (1976) Left ventricular compliance: mechanisms and clinical implications. Am J Cardiol 38:645–653

11. Grossman W, Barry WH (1980) Diastolic pressure-volume relations in the diseased heart. Fed Proc 39:148–155

12. Gaasch WH, Cole JS, Quinones MA, Alexander JK (1975) Dynamic determinants left ventricular pressure-volume relations in man. Circulation 51:317–323

13. Bonow RO (1987) Left ventricular filling in ischemic and hypertrophic heart disease. In: Grossman W, Lorell BH (eds) Diastolic relaxation of the heart. Nijhoff, Boston, pp 231–243

14. Sordahl LA, McCollum WB, Wood WG, Schwartz A (1973) Mitochondria and sarcoplasmic reticulum function in cardiac hypertrophy and failure. Am J Physiol 224:497–502

15. Ito Y, Suko J, Chidsey CA (1974) Intracellular calcium and myocardial contractility. V. Calcium uptake of sarcoplasmic reticulum fractions in hypertrophied and failing rabbit hearts. J Mol Cell Cardiol 6:237–247

16. Lecarptenier Y, Martin L, Gastineau P, Hatt PY (1982) Load dependence of mammalian heart relaxation during cardiac hypertrophy and failure. Am J Physiol 242:H855–861

17. Gwathmey JK, Morgan JP (1985) Altered calcium handling in experimental pressure-overload hypertrophy in the ferrec. Circ Res 57:836–843

18. Gwathmey JK, Copelas L, MacKinnon R, Schoen FJ, Feldman MD, Grossman W, Morgan JP (1987) Abnormal intracellular calcium handling in myocardium from patients with end-stage heart failure. Circ Res 61:70–76

19. Wagner JA, Sax FL, Weisman HF, Portersfield J, McIntosh CL, Weisfeldt ML, Snyder SH, Epstein SE (1989) Calcium antagonist receptors are selectively increased in atrial tissue of patients with hypertrophic cardiomyopathy. N Engl J Med 320:755–761

20. Pasternac A, Noble J, Streulens Y, Elie R, Henschke C, Bourassa MG (1982) Pathophysiology of chest pain in patients with cardiomyopathies and normal coronary arteries. Circulation 65:778–798

21. Cannon RO, Rosing DR, Maron BJ, Leon MB, Bonow RO, Watson RM, Epstein SE (1985) Myocardial ischemia in patients with hypertrophic cardiomyopathy: contribution of inadequate vasodilator reserve and elevated left ventricular filling pressures. Circulation 71:234–243

22. O'Gara PT, Bonow RO, Maron BJ, Damske BA, Van Lingen A, Bacharach SL, Larson SM, Epstein SE (1987) Myocardial perfusion abnormalities in patients with hypertrophic cardiomyopathy: assessment with thallium-201 emission computed tomography. Circulation 76:1214–1223

23. Henry PD, Schuchleib R, David J, Weiss ES, Sobel BE (1977) Myocardial contracture and accumulation of mitochondrial calcium in ischemic rabbit heart. Am J Physiol 233:H677–684

24. Nayler WG, Williams A (1978) Relaxation in heart muscle: Some morphologic and biochemical considerations. Eur J Cardiol 7 (suppl):35–50

25. Nayler WG, Poole-Wilson PA, Williams A (1979) Hypoxia and calcium. J Mol Cell Cardiol 11:683–706

26. Mann T, Goldberg S, Mudge GH, Grossman W (1979) Factors contributing to altered left ventricular diastolic properties during angina pectoris. Circulation 59:14–20

27. Paulus WJ, Serizawa T, Grossman W (1982) Altered left ventricular diastolic properties during pacing-induced ischemia in dogs with coronary stenoses: potentiation by caffeine. Circ Res 50:218–227

28. Carroll JD, Hess OM, Hirzel HO, Krayenbuehl HP (1983) Exercise-induced ischemia: the influence of altered relaxation on early diastolic pressures. Circulation 67:521–528
29. Lorell BH, Wexler LF, Momomura S, Weinberg E, Apstein CS (1986) The influence of pressure hypertrophy on diastolic properties during hypoxia in isovolumically contracting rat hearts. Circ Res 58:653–663
30. Wexler LF, Lorell BH, Monomura S, Weinberg EO, Ingwall JS, Apstein CS (1988) Enhanced sensitivity to hypoxia-induced diastolic dysfunction in pressure-overload left ventricular hypertrophy in the rat: role of high energy phosphate depletion. Circ Res 62:766–775
31. Brutsaert DL, Housmans PR, Goethals MA (1980) Dual control of relaxation: its role in the ventricular function in the mammalian heart. Circ Res 47:637–652
32. Brutsaert DL, Rademakers FE, Sys US (1983) Triple control of relaxation: implications in cardiac disease. Circulation 69:190–196
33. Gaasch WH, Blaustein AS, Andrias CW, Donahue RP, Avitall B (1980) Myocardial relaxation. II. Hemodynamic determinants of rate of left ventricular pressure decline. Am J Physiol 239:H1–6
34. Pouleur H, Rousseau MF, van Eyll C, Brasseur LA, Charlier AA (1983) Force-velocity-length relations in hypertrophic cardiomyopathy: evidence for normal or depressed myocardial contractility. Am J Cardiol 52:813–817
35. Blaustein AS, Gaasch WH (1983) Myocardial relaxation. VI. Effects of beta-adrenergic tone and asynchrony on LV relaxation rate. Am J Physiol 244:H417–422
36. Brutsaert DL (1987) Nonuniformity: a physiologic modulator of contraction and relaxation of the normal heart. J Am Coll Cardiol 9:341–348
37. Zile MR, Blaustein AS, Shimizu G, Gaasch WH (1987) Right ventricular pacing reduces the rate of left ventricular relaxation and filling. J Am Coll Cardiol 10:702–709
38. Bonow RO (1990) Regional left ventricular nonuniformity: effects on left ventricular diastolic function in ischemic heart disease, in hypertrophic cardiomyopathy, and in the normal heart. Circulation (in press)
39. Bonow RO, Vitale DF, Maron BJ, Bacharach SL, Frederick TM, Green MV (1987) Regional left ventricular asynchrony and impaired global ventricular filling in hypertrophic cardiomyopathy: effect of verapamil. J Am Coll Cardiol 9:1108–1116
40. Hanrath P, Mathey DG, Kremer P, Sonntag F, Bleifeld W (1980) Effect of verapamil on left ventricular isovolumic relaxation time and regional left ventricular filling in hypertrophic cardiomyopathy. Am J Cardiol 45:1258–1264
41. Lorell BH, Paulus WJ, Grossman W, Wynne J, Cohn PF (1982) Modification of abnormal left ventricular diastolic properties by nifedipine in patients with hypertrophic cardiomyopathy. Circulation 65:499–507
42. Paulus WJ, Lorell BH, Craig WE, Wynne J, Murgo JP, Grossman W (1983) Comparison of the effects of nitroprusside and nifedipine on diastolic properties in patients with hypertrophic cardiomyopathy: altered left ventricular loading or impaired muscle inactivation? J Am Coll Cardiol 2:879–886
43. Bonow RO, Ostrow HG, Rosing DR, Cannon RO, Lipson LW, Maron BJ, Kent KM, Bacharach SL, Green MV (1983) Effects of verapamil on left ventricular systolic and diastolic function in patients with hypertrophic cardiomyopathy: pressure-volume analysis with a nonimaging scintillation probe. Circulation 68:1062–1073
44. Hanrath P, Schluter M, Sonntag F, Diemert J, Bleifeld W (1983) Influence of verapamil therapy on left ventricular performance at rest and during exercise in hypertrophic cardiomyopathy. Am J Cardiol 52:544–548
45. Suwa M, Hirota Y, Kawamura K (1984) Improvement in left ventricular diastolic function during intravenous and oral diltiazem therapy in patients with hypertrophic cardiomyopathy: an echocardiographic study. Am J Cardiol 54:1047–1053
46. Bonow RO, Dilsizian V, Rosing DR, Maron BJ, Bacharach SL, Green MV (1985) Verapamil-induced improvement in left ventricular diastolic filling and increased exercise tolerance in patients with hypertrophic cardiomyopathy: short- and long-term effects. Circulation 72:853–864
47. Bonow RO (1985) Effect of calcium channel blocking agents on left ventricular diastolic function in hypertrophic cardiomyopathy and in coronary artery disease. Am J Cardiol 55:172B–178B

48. Hess OM, Murakami T, Krayenbuehl HP (1986) Does verapamil improve left ventricular relaxation in patients with myocardial hypertrophy? Circulation 74:530–543
49. Iwase M, Sotobata I, Takagi S, Miyaguchi K, Jing HX, Yokota M (1987) Effects of diltiazem on left ventricular diastolic behavior in patients with hypertrophic cardiomyopathy: evaluation with exercise pulsed Doppler echocardiography. J Am Coll Cardiol 9:1099–1105
50. Speiser KW, Krayenbuehl HP (1981) Reappraisal of the effect of acute beta blockade on left ventricular filling dynamics in hypertrophic obstructive cardiomyopathy. Eur Heart J 2:21–29
51. Betocchi S, Cannon RO, Watson RM, Bonow RO, Ostrow HG, Epstein SE, Rosing DR (1985) Effects of sublingual nifedipine on hemodynamics and systolic and diastolic function in patients with hypertrophic cardiomyopathy. Circulation 72:1001–1007
52. Rosing DR, Kent KM, Borer JS, Seides SF, Maron BJ, Epstein SE (1979) Verapamil therapy: a new approach to the pharmacologic treatment of hypertrophic cardiomyopathy. I. Hemodynamic effects. Circulation 60:1201–1207
53. Walsh RA, O'Rourke RA (1985) Direct and indirect effects of calcium entry blocking agents on isovolumic relaxation in conscious dogs. J Clin Invest 75:1426–1434
54. Udelson JE, Bonow RO, O'Gara PT, Maron BJ, Van Lingen A, Bacharach SL, Epstein SE (1989) Verapamil prevents silent myocardial perfusion abnormalities during exercise in asymptomatic patients with hypertrophic cardiomyopathy. Circulation 79:371–382
55. Maron BJ, Epstein SE, Roberts WC (1979) Hypertrophic cardiomyopathy and transmural myocardial infarction without significant atherosclerosis of the extramural coronary arteries. Am J Cardiol 43:1086–1102
56. St John Sutton MG, Lie JT, Anderson KR, O'Brien PC, Frye RL (1980) Histologic specificity of hypertrophic obstructive cardiomyopathy: myocardial fiber disarray and myocardial fibrosis. Br Heart J 44:433–443
57. Rubin KA, Morrison J, Padrick MB, Binder AJ, Chiaramide S, Margouleff D, Padmanabhan VT, Gulotta SJ (1979) Idiopathic hypertrophic subaortic stenosis: evaluation of anginal symptoms with thallium-201 myocardial imaging. Am J Cardiol 44:1040–1045
58. Pitcher D, Wainwright R, Maisey M, Curry P, Lowton E (1980) Assessment of chest pain in hypertrophic cardiomyopathy using exercise thallium-201 myocardial scintigraphy. Br Heart J 44:650–656
59. Hanrath P, Matthey D, Montz R, Thiel V, Vorbringer H, Kupper W, Schneider C, Bleifeld W (1981) Myocardial thallium-201 imaging in hypertrophic obstructive cardiomyopathy. Eur Heart J 2:177–185
60. Nagata S, Park V-D, Nininikawa T, Yutani C, Kamiya T, Nishimura T, Kozuka T, Sakakibara H, Nimura Y (1985) Thallium perfusion and cardiac enzyme abnormalities in patients with familial hypertrophic cardiomyopathy. Am Heart J 109:1317–1322
61. O'Gara PT, Bonow RO, Maron BJ, Damske BA, Van Lingen A, Bacharach SL, Larson SM, Epstein SE (1987) Myocardial perfusion abnormalities in patients with hypertrophic cardiomyopathy: assessment with thallium-201 emission computed tomography. Circulation 76:1214–1223
62. ten Cate FJ, Roelandt J (1979) Progression to left ventricular dilatation in patients with hypertrophic obstructive cardiomyopathy. Am Heart J 97:762–765
63. Ciro E, Maron BJ, Bonow RO, Cannon RO, Epstein SE (1984) Relation between marked changes in outflow tract gradient and disease progression in patients with hypertrophic cardiomyopathy. Am J Cardiol 53:1103–1109
64. Spirito P, Maron BJ, Bonow RO, Epstein SE (1986) Severe functional limitation in patients with hypertrophic cardiomyopathy and only mild localized left ventricular hypertrophy. J Am Coll Cardiol 8:537–544
65. Spirito P, Maron BJ, Bonow RO, Epstein SE (1987) Occurrence and significance of progressive left ventricular wall thinning and relative cavity dilatation in patients with hypertrophic cardiomyopathy. Am J Cardiol 60:123–129
66. Udelson JE, Maron BJ, O'Gara PT, Bonow RO (1989) Relation between left ventricular hypertrophy, filling, and perfusion in asymptomatic hypertrophic cardiomyopathy. J Am Coll Cardiol 13:80A (abst)

67. Bonow RO, Maron BJ, Leon MB, Cannon RO, Epstein SE (1988) Medical and surgical therapy of hypertrophic cardiomyopathy. In: Shaver JA (ed) Cardiomyopathies: clinical presentation, differential diagnosis, and management. Davies, Philadelphia, pp 221–239
68. Marcus ML, Doty DB, Hiratzka LF, Wright CB, Eastham CL (1982) Decreased coronary reserve: a mechanism for angina pectoris in patients with aortic stenosis and normal coronary arteries. N Engl J Med 307:1362–1366
69. Opherk D, Mall G, Zebe H, Schwarz F, Weihe E, Manthey J, Kubler W (1984) Reduction of coronary reserve: a mechanism for angina pectoris in patients with arterial hypertension and normal coronary arteries. Circulation 69:1–7
70. James TH, Marshall TK (1975) De subitaneis mortibus. XII. Asymmetrical hypertrophy of the heart. Circulation 51:1149–1166
71. Maron BJ, Wolfson JK, Epstein SE, Roberts WC (1986) Intramural ("small vessel") coronary artery disease in hypertrophic cardiomyopathy. J Am Coll Cardiol 8:545–557
72. Morad M, Rolett EL (1972) Relaxing effects of catecholamines on mammalian heart. J Physiol (Lond) 224:537–558
73. Udelson JE, Cannon RO, Bacharach SL, Rumble TF, Bonow RO (1989) Beta-adrenergic stimulation with isoproterenol enhances left ventricular diastolic performance in hypertrophic cardiomyopathy despite potentiation of myocardial ischemia: comparison to rapid atrial pacing. Circulation 79:371–382

Sudden Death in Hypertrophic Cardiomyopathy: Identification and Management of High Risk Patients*

W. J. McKenna, P. J. Counihan, and T. Chikamori

Introduction

The incidence of sudden death in hypertrophic cardiomyopathy is approximately 2%–4% per year in adults and 4%–6% per year in children and adolescents [1]. These data have been generated from referral cardiac centres and may reflect a bias to the more severe patients [2]. The changes in diagnostic criteria and widespread use of more sensitive diagnostic techniques (two-dimensional echocardiography) have not resulted in a significantly different incidence of sudden death. The annual mortality in children followed at the Hammersmith Hospital who were essentially asymptomatic and did not have a family history of sudden death was 3.5%–4% in the 1960s and 1970s and has not changed in the 1980s [3, 4]. The identification and management of patients with hypertrophic cardiomyopathy who are at increased risk of sudden death remains a major problem particularly in younger patients.

Identification of High Risk Adults

During the 1960s and 1970s routine characterization of patients with hypertrophic cardiomyopathy included assessment of symptoms, ECG abnormalities including criteria for left and right ventricular hypertrophy, presence of conduction abnormalities and evidence of atrial overload as well as angiographic and haemodynamic assessment with measurement of left ventricular gradients and filling pressures. Retrospective analysis of this information reveals that this extensive characterisation failed to provide a clinical profile which would identify the majority of patients who subsequently died suddenly (Table 1) [3]. The potential value of M-mode and two-dimensional echocardiographic measurements to this clinical profile has not been rigorously assessed but they would not be expected to be of great predictive value (Fig. 1) [5]. In Maron's study of 78 patients with hypertrophic cardiomyopathy who died suddenly the severity of left ventricular hypertrophy was similar in those who died suddenly and in an age/sex-matched group who survived [5].

---

* Adapted from: McKenna WJ, Camm AJ (1989) Sudden death in hypertrophic cardiomyopathy. Assessment of patients at high risk. *Circulation* 80:1489–92.

Table 1. Prediction of sudden death in adults (> 21 years of age) with hypertrophic cardio-myopathy

	Sensitivity %	Specificity %	Positive predictive accuracy %	Negative predictive accuracy %
Clinical/haemodynamic	70	68	24	94
Angiogram at diagnosis	82	72	32	96
Radionuclide only	83	75	14	99
Radionuclide + clinical/prognostic	83	90	29	99
Nonsustained ventricular tachycardia	69	80	22	97

Clinical assessment from a retrospective series of 254 patients of whom 23 died suddenly during 6 years [3].
Angiographic assessment at diagnosis from a retrospective series of 88 patients of whom 11 died suddenly during 7 years [13].
Radionuclide assessment during follow-up from a prospective series of 161 patients of whom 8 died suddenly during 2 years [7].
Nonsustained ventricular tachycardia was assessed from two independent series (see text for data) [8, 9].

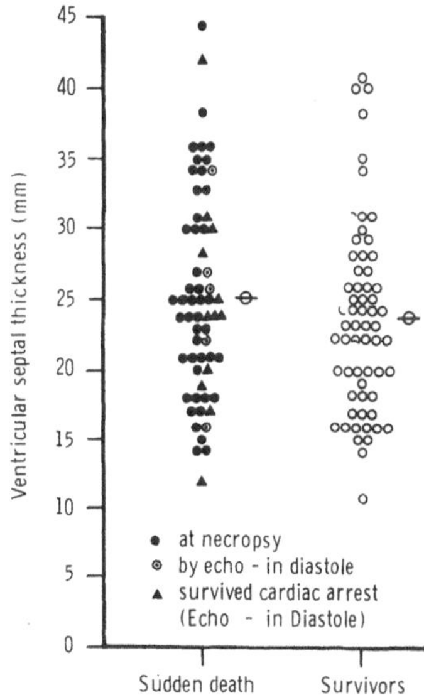

Fig. 1. Ventricular septal thickness in 62 patients with hypertrophic cardiomyopathy who died suddenly or had cardiac arrest, compared with a control group of 62 age- and sex-matched surviving patients with hypertrophic cardiomyopathy. Mean values are indicated. (From [5])

In several centres technetium 99m radionuclide cineangiography has been used to generate indices of systolic and diastolic function [6]. A prospective prognostic study of 161 consecutive patients revealed these radionuclide values to be of no additional value in identifying high risk patients [7]. The single most useful marker of the high risk patient is episodes of nonsustained ventricular tachycardia during 48-h ECG monitoring [8, 9]. These episodes appear benign: they are usually slow, follow periods of relative bradycardia and are not associated with ST segment or QT interval change. Their significance, however, lies in the simultaneous observation from two independent centres that adults with nonsustained ventricular tachycardia have increased mortality from sudden death. Of 170 consecutive unoperated patients from the National Institutes of Health and Hammersmith Hospital, 13 died suddenly during 3 years; 9 of these 13 had nonsustained ventricular tachycardia. In both studies this arrhythmia was significantly more common in those who died suddenly [8, 9]. This does not indicate a causal relationship but does establish that ventricular tachycardia is a marker of the adult who is at particular risk of sudden death.

How useful is the finding of nonsustained ventricular tachycardia during ECG monitoring as a marker of sudden death? It has a sensitivity of 69% and a specifity of 80% for the prediction of sudden death [11]. The reduced sensitivity in part reflects the inclusion of an adolescent who did not have ventricular tachycardia but died suddenly. A recent study reveals that spontaneous arrhythmias are rare in children and adolescents with hypertrophic cardiomyopathy and that other clinical features are of greater predictive value in the young [4, 10]. In addition all four of the patients who did not have nonsustained ventricular tachycardia but died suddenly (two from National Institutes of Health and two from Hammersmith) had only 24 h of ECG monitoring and thus a sampling error is possible, particularly as ventricular arrhythmias in hypertrophic cardiomyopathy are known to exhibit marked biological variability [12]. We perform 48-h ECG monitoring at the time of diagnosis and usually annually thereafter. During the past 6 years sudden death has occurred in adults who did not have ventricular tachycardia during ECG monitoring but it is rare. The finding of nonsustained ventricular tachycardia during ECG monitoring identifies adults at high risk with a sensitivity that is probably greater than 69%.

Of the 41 patients with nonsustained ventricular tachycardia in the two studies 32 survived 3 years; this is reflected in the low positive predictive accuracy (22%) of ventricular tachycardia for sudden death and it raises the possibility that not all patients with ventricular tachycardia are at increased risk. Though the number of patients in the subset with ventricular tachycardia in each study was small there did not appear to be features that distinguished patients who survived from those who died suddenly. In the National Institutes of Health study patients with ventricular tachycardia and sudden cardiac catastrophe did not differ from survivors with regard to age or sex distribution, ventricular septal thickness or recurrence of an abnormal electrocardiogram [8]. In the Hammersmith study, the symptomatic status, the proportion with left ventricular gradients and the incidence of supraventricular and ventricular arrhythmias were similar in the survivors and the patients who died suddenly [9]. In another study of the relation of left ventricular function and prognosis in a subset of 14 patients with ventricular tachycardia digitized angiographic analysis revealed that peak left ventricular ejection rate was significantly reduced in patients with ventricular tachycardia who died suddenly compared with those who survived [13]. Impaired left ventricular function may be an important predictor of which patients with ventricular tachycardia are at increased risk and prospective evaluation is warranted.

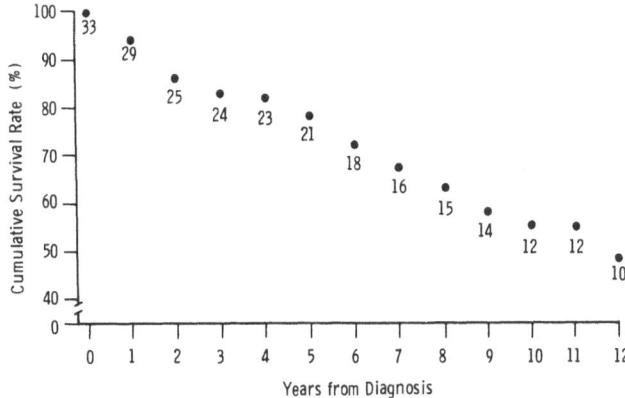

Fig. 2. Cumulative survival curve from the year of diagnosis for 33 medically treated patients. The probability of death = the total number of deaths for the year divided by the adjusted number at risk minus the number of deaths due to other causes. (From [4])

Identification of High Risk Children and Adolescents

Patients with a family history of multiple sudden deaths are recognised to be at particular risk [3, 14]. Children and adolescents without such a malignant family history still have an annual mortality from sudden death of over 4% (Fig. 2) [4]. Apart from syncopal episodes which are associated with sudden death other clinical features and electrocardiographic and haemodynamic measurements are similar in those who die suddenly and survive and do not help identify the high risk young patient. The majority of children and adolescents who die suddenly do not have any limitation of exercise tolerance nor have they experienced syncope; when syncope does occur this is ominous and in a retrospective analysis of 37 patients it was 86% specific for subsequent sudden death [4]. In addition arrhythmias during electrocardiographic monitoring are uncommon in children and adolescents and do not appear to be of predictive prognostic value [20]. Thus, in the patients with hypertrophic cardiomyopathy who are at greatest risk, many of whom are not only young but also asymptomatic, current clinical and haemodynamic evaluation is of limited value in the identification of most of those who died suddenly. This underscores the need to better characterize patients with hypertrophic cardiomyopathy in relation to likely mechanisms of sudden death.

Mechanisms of Sudden Death

There are numerous potential mechanisms of sudden death to consider in the identification of high risk patients (Fig. 3). Both impaired and accelerated atrioventricular conduction have been documented [15, 16]. It is well recognised that a tachycardia, whether physiological or secondary to an arrhythmia, may be associated with hypotension, ischaemia and symptoms of angina or impaired consciousness. A recent case report by Stafford et al. is of interest in

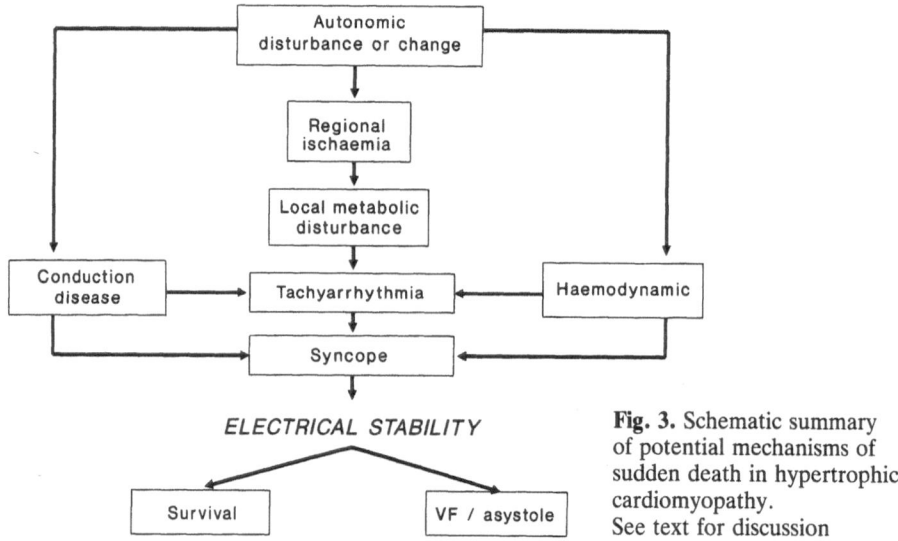

Fig. 3. Schematic summary of potential mechanisms of sudden death in hypertrophic cardiomyopathy. See text for discussion

this regard [17]. A 15-year-old youth, who presented with cardiac arrest and documented ventricular fibrillation, was found to have nonobstructive hypertrophic cardiomyopathy with diffuse left ventricular hypertrophy. Electrophysiological study demonstrated inducible sustained atrial fibrillation with a ventricular response of 180 to 190 beats/min. This rhythm which was associated with hypotension and evidence of myocardial ischaemia degenerated into ventricular fibrillation. There was no evidence of an accessory pathway and no ventricular arrhythmias were inducible during programmed ventricular stimulation. It has long been claimed that patients with hypertrophic cardiomyopathy are unable to maintain stroke volume and increase cardiac output during exercise or tachycardia presumably because of the shortened time for filling of a poorly relaxing and noncompliant left ventricle [18]. Recently we have demonstrated hypotension during exercise in a third of over 100 consecutive patients with falls in blood pressure of 20–110 mmHg (median 40 mmHg) from peak pressure recorded [19]. In general two hypotensive responses were observed. In the majority blood pressure rose initially and then fell, while in the minority the blood pressure failed to rise at all during exercise. A possible cause of these findings is that during exercise these patients are unable to increase or maintain stroke volume. To test this hypothesis we performed invasive haemodynamic studies in 10 hypotensive responders and 10 normal blood pressure responders [19]. Cardiac output increased appropriately and similarly in both groups but there was an exaggerated fall in systemic vascular resistance which was observed to take place in association with the fall in blood pressure (Fig. 4). This indicates abnormal peripheral vascular responses which may be an important determinant of not only exercise blood pressure but also the haemodynamic response to arrhythmias in the condition. Preliminary observations in over 50 patients reveal abnormal forearm blood flow responses during supine exercise in the patients with exercise hypotension but not in those with normal blood pressure response during exercise. The prognostic

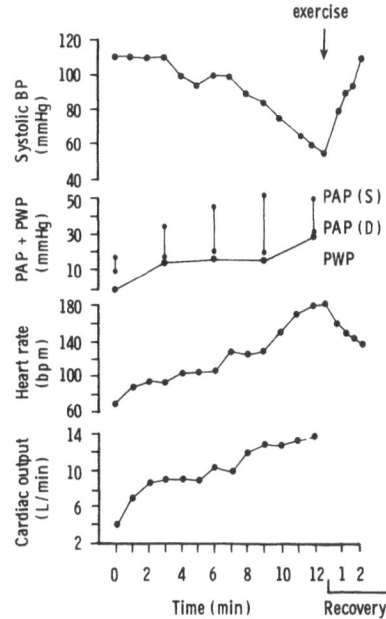

Fig. 4. Haemodynamic monitoring with intra-arterial blood pressure recording during maximal treadmill exercise in a 24-year-old asymptomatic man with mild asymmetric septal hypertrophy and a family history of hypertrophic cardiomyopathy and sudden death. Blood pressure falls progressively despite appropriate increases in heart rate, filling pressures and cardiac output. (*BP*, blood pressure; *D*, diastolic; *PAP*, pulmonary artery pressure; *PWP*, pulmonary wedge pressure; *S*, systolic)

significance of exercise hypotension and abnormal control of peripheral blood flow remains to be determined. To date follow-up is short and there have only been three events: one patient died suddenly and two experienced out of hospital ventricular fibrillation. All three of these patients had marked exercise hypotension in the absence of premonitory symptoms.

In addition to haemodynamic factors the electrical stability of the myocardium must also be an important determinant of sudden death. In the adult nonsustained ventricular tachycardia during electrocardiographic monitoring may be a marker of this while in children and adolescents to date no such marker has been identified. The extent and severity of myocardial disarray must be an important determinant of the electrical stability of the myocardium. Myocardial disarray is greater in young patients who die suddenly than in adults who die suddenly or from other causes, but the severity and distribution of disarray is not closely related to the severity and distribution of hypertrophy and at present can only be reliably assessed at post-mortem examination [20].

What is the role of electrophysiological testing in the identification of high risk patients with hypertrophic cardiomyopathy? Several groups have done electrophysiological studies in adults, many of whom were at "high risk" with previous syncopal episodes or cardiac arrest. Anderson et al. performed right ventricular programmed electrical stimulation in the operating room in 17 symptomatic patients with left ventricular outflow tract gradients who were undergoing myotomy/myectomy and in five control patients who were undergoing coronary artery bypass grafting [21]. In their protocol, which included three premature ventricular stimuli, 14 of the 17 patients had inducible sustained ventricular tachycardia ($n = 9$) or ventricular fibrillation ($n = 5$) which was not seen in the five control patients. Their findings indicate that with an aggressive stimulation protocol, inducible life-threatening arrhythmias are more common in patients with hypertrophic cardiomyopathy than in patients without a primary heart muscle disorder.

Watson et al. from the National Institutes of Health performed right ventricular programmed electrical stimulation in 17 "high risk" patients with hypertrophic cardiomyopathy who had experienced cardiac arrest ($n = 2$) or syncope ($n = 4$), had a malignant family history ($n = 2$), or had nonsustained ventricular tachycardia during ECG monitoring ($n = 9$). Ventricular fibrillation was induced in eight patients (47%) with up to three premature stimuli during programmed ventricular stimulation and in an additional patient during atrial stimulation [22]. Fananapazir from the same institution performed right and left ventricular programmed stimulation in 155 patients, many of whom had demonstrated either electrical and/or haemodynamic vulnerability: 22 had experienced cardiac arrest and 55 had syncopal episodes [23]. Sustained ventricular arrhythmias were initiated in 66 (43%) using two premature stimuli in 19 and three premature stimuli in 47. Fifty of these 66 patients had sustained polymorphic ventricular tachycardia or primary ventricular fibrillation. Other centres have also shown that programmed electrical stimulation can initiate sustained polymorphic ventricular tachycardia or fibrillation in a significant proportion of patients (20 of 95,21%, using two premature ventricular stimuli; 16 of 41,39%, using three premature ventricular stimuli or incremental atrial pacing) [11]. The high rate of inducible ventricular tachycardia and fibrillation observed by these workers supports the contention that patients with hypertrophic cardiomyopathy may be unusually vulnerable to spontaneous ventricular tachyarrhythmias, particularly in the presence of ischaemia or haemodynamic collapse. The prognostic significance of these findings, however, will be uncertain until the clinical outcome has been determined in more patients.

What is the potential for programmed electrical stimulation to improve upon the sensitivity (> 69%) of electrocardiographic monitoring for the identification of the high risk adult with hypertrophic cardiomyopathy? As electrocardiographic monitoring identifies most of the adults who are at high risk, electrophysiological studies may he more profitably performed in selected "high risk" patient populations. As discussed above, the predictive accuracy of ventricular tachycardia is low (22%). Programmed stimulation as well as assessment of left and right ventricular function may provide measurements that will improve the predictive accuracy and identify those patients with episodes of nonsustained ventricular tachycardia during electrocardiographic monitoring who are at greatest risk and warrant more vigorous treatment. A broader application of programmed ventricular stimulation in adults with hypertrophic cardiomyopathy, however, does not seem warranted.

The cause of sudden death in hypertrophic cardiomyopathy is uncertain. The low incidence of spontaneous arrhythmias in the young suggests that in this subgroup of patients, a primary arrhythmia is unlikely. We speculate that in some adults, but particularly in the young, the precipitating event is most often haemodynamic with hypotension in relation to emotion or exercise related tachycardia; a primary supraventricular tachyarrhythmia as the cause of the tachycardia is possible but less likely. The outcome, survival versus sudden death, is then determined by the vulnerability of the myocardium to ventricular fibrillation.

In the assessment of adults and particularly children and adolescents with hypertrophic cardiomyopathy future studies should evaluate patients in relation to likely mechanisms of sudden death. This should include an assessment of both propensity for haemodynamic collapse as well as the vulnerability of the myocardium to life-threatening arrhythmias. The optimal method of acquiring this information has not been determined and may differ in patient subgroups, particularly in relation to age and perhaps in relation to the severity of both left ventricular hypertrophy and functional impairment. Noninvasive tests which simulate or record events during normal daily life, such as stress testing, response to physiological manoeuvres and electrocardiographic monitoring, can be broadly applied while invasive investigations, particularly electrophysiological studies, are more appropriate in selected subgroups. It is important that patients with hypertrophic cardiomyopathy are better characterized in relation to likely mechanisms of sudden death as the pharmacological and surgical treatments may significantly improve prognosis if they are applied appropriately.

The role of surgery in the prevention of sudden death remains to be defined. At present it is reserved for symptomatic patients with features of left ventricular outflow tract "obstruction". Whether myotomy/myectomy will prevent haemodynamic collapse and improve prognosis requires evaluation. Though there is no convincing evidence to suggest that symptomatic therapy with beta-blockers or calcium antagonists improves prognosis [1], the use of low dose amiodarone in patients with nonsustained ventricular tachycardia during electrocardiographic monitoring is associated with improved survival [24]. There have been no deaths in 38 patients who received amiodarone between 1978 and 1982 and who have now been followed for at least 5 years, compared with a 7% annual mortality at 3 years in well-matched control patients [25]. The use of amiodarone in other potentially high risk patients, such as children who may require therapy for many years, is limited by dose/duration-related side effects. The role of amiodarone in these high risk patients in currently under evaluation.

References

1. McKenna WJ, Goodwin JF (1981) The natural history of hypertrophic cardiomyopathy. In: Harvey P (ed) Current problems in cardiology, vol VI. Year Book Medical Publishers, Chicago, pp 5–26
2. Spirito P, Chiarella F, Carratino L, Zoni Berisso M, Bellotti P, Vecchio C (1989) Clinical course and prognosis of hypertrophic cardiomyopathy in an outpatient population. N Engl J Med 320:749–755
3. McKenna WJ, Deanfield J, Faruqui A, England D, Oakley CM, Goodwin JF (1981) Prognosis in hypertrophic cardiomyopathy. Role of age, and clinical, electrocardiographic and hemodynamic features. Am J Cardiol 47:532–538
4. McKenna WJ, Deanfield JE (1984) Hypertrophic cardiomyopathy: an important cause of sudden death. Arch Dis Childhood 59:971–975
5. Maron BJ, Roberts WC, Epstein SE (1982) Sudden death in hypertrophic cardiomyopathy: a profile of 78 patients. Circulation 65:1388–1394

6. Bonow RO, Rosing DR, Bacharach SL, Green MV, Kent KM, Lipson LC, Maron BJ, Leon MB, Epstein SE (1981) Effects of verapamil on left ventricular systolic function and diastolic filling in patients with hypertrophic cardiomyopathy. Circulation 64:787–796

7. Chikamori T, Dickie S, Poloniecki JD, Myers MJ, Lavender JP, McKenna WJ (1990) Prognostic significance of diastolic function in hypertrophic cardiomyopathy: a radionuclide study. Am J Cardiol (in press)

8. Maron BJ, Savage DD, Wolfson JK, Epstein SE (1981) Prognostic significance of 24 hour ambulatory electrocardiographic monitoring in patients with hypertrophic cardiomyopathy. A prospective study. Am J Cardiol 48:252–257

9. McKenna WJ, England D, Doi YL, Deanfield JE, Oakley CM, Goodwin JF (1981) Arrhythmia in hypertrophic cardiomyopathy. 1. Influence on prognosis. Br Heart J 46:168–172

10. McKenna WJ, Franklin RCG, Nihoyannopoulos P, Robinson KR, Deanfield FE (1988) Arrhythmia and prognosis in infants, children and adolescents with hypertrophic cardiomyopathy. J Am Coll Cardiol 11:147–153

11. McKenna WJ (1987) Sudden death in hypertrophic cardiomyopathy: identification of the "high risk" patient. In: Brugada P, Wellens HJJ (eds) Cardiac arrhythmias: Where to go from here? Futura, Mount Kisco, New York, pp 353–365

12. Mulrow JP, Healy MJR, McKenna WJ (1986) Variability of ventricular arrhythmia in hypertrophic cardiomyopathy and implications of treatment. Am J Cardiol 58:615–618

13. Newman H, Sugrue DD, Oakley CM, Goodwin JF, McKenna WJ (1985) Relation of left ventricular function and prognosis in hypertrophic cardiomyopathy: an angiographic study. J Am Coll Cardiol 5:1064–1074

14. Maron BJ, Lipson LC, Roberts WC, Savage DD, Epstein SE (1978) "Malignant" hypertrophic cardiomyopathy: identification of a subgroup of families with unusually frequent premature death. Am J Cardiol 41:133–1140

15. Chmielewzki CA, Riley RS, Mahendran A, Most AS (1977) Complete heart block as a cause of syncope in asymmetric septal hypertrophy. Am Heart J 93:91–93

16. Krikler DM, Davies MJ, Rowland E, Goodwin JF, Evans RC, Shaw DB (1980) Sudden death in hypertrophic cardiomyopathy: associated accessory atrioventricular pathways. Br Heart J 43:245–251

17. Stafford WJ, Trohman RG, Bilsker M, Zaman L, Castellanos A, Myerburg RJ (1986) Cardiac arrest in an adolescent with atrial fibrillation and hypertrophic cardiomyopathy. J Am Coll Cardiol 7:701–704

18. Goodwin JF, Oakley CM (1972) The cardiomyopathies. Br Heart J 34:545–552

19. Frenneaux MP, Counihan PJ, Webb D, McKenna WJ (1989) Evidence for an abnormal vasodilator response in hypertrophic cardiomyopathy. J Am Coll Cardiol 13:117A

20. Maron BJ, Roberts WC (1979) Quantitative analysis of cardiac muscle cell disorganisation in the ventricular septum of patients with hypertrophic cardiomyopathy. Circulation 59:689–706

21. Anderson KP, Stinson EB, Derby GC, Oyer PE, Mason JW (1983) Vulnerability of patients with hypertrophic obstructive cardiomyopathy to ventricular arrhythmia induction in the operating room. Am J Cardiol 51:811–816

22. Watson RM, Liberati Schwartz J, Maron BJ, Tucker E, Rosing DR, Josephson ME (1987) Inducible polymorphic ventricular tachycardia and ventricular fibrillation in a subgroup of patients with hypertrophic cardiomyopathy at high risk for sudden death. J Am Coll Cardiol 10:761–774

23. Fananapazir L, Tracy CM, Leon MB, Winkler JB, Cannon III RO, Bonow RO, Maron BJ, Epstein SE (1989) Electrophysiologic abnormalities in patients with hypertrophic cardiomyopathy: a consecutive analysis in 155 patients. Circulation 80:1259–1268

24. McKenna WJ, Oakley CM, Krikler DM, Goodwin JF (1985) Improved survival with amiodarone in patients with hypertrophic cardiomyopathy and ventricular tachycardia. Br Heart J 53:412–416

25. McKenna WJ, Adams KM, Poloniecki JD, Dickie S, Oakley CM, Krikler DM, Goodwin JF (1989) Long term survival with amiodarone in patients with hypertrophic cardiomyopathy and ventricular tachycardia. Br Heart J 61:472

Electrophysiologic Studies in Patients with Hypertrophic Cardiomyopathy: Safety and Relation of Results to Clinical Findings

L. Fananapazir

Introduction

Patients with hypertrophic cardiomyopathy have a varied clinical presentation. This includes symptoms that suggest an arrhythmic etiology: sudden cardiac arrest, syncope, presyncope, and palpitations. Since early studies linked ventricular tachycardia recorded during Holter monitoring with subsequent sudden cardiac death [1–3], many asymptomatic hypertrophic cardiomyopathy patients are also referred for evaluation due to the presence of ventricular tachycardia (most nonsustained) during 24–48 h Holter monitoring. Electrophysiologic studies have an established role in elucidating possible arrhythmic cause of sudden cardiac arrest, syncope and palpitation and guiding therapy in many other cardiac disease states. Programmed electrical stimulation in hypertrophic cardiomyopathy patients has unfortunately resulted in death in isolated patients [4, 5] and programmed ventricular stimulation has been reported to result in the induction of non-specific ventricular arrhythmias.

The purpose fo this presentation is therefore

1) to describe the precautions that may add to the safety of electrophysiologic studies in hypertrophic cardiomyopathy patients; and
2) report on the prevalence of abnormal electrophysiologic findings in these patients, and relation of induced ventricular arrhythmias to clinical presentation.

Methods

Study Population

Electrophysiologic studies were performed prospectively on 106 patients with hypertrophic cardiomyopathy referred for evaluation of out-of-hospital cardiac arrest (13 patients), syncope (41 patients), presyncope (29 patients), and asymptomatic ventricular tachycardia (23 patients). All patients had full hemodynamic assessment prior to electrophysiologic study. None of the patients had coronary artery disease.

Hypertrophic cardiomyopathy was defined as the presence of a hypertrophied, nondilated left ventricle demonstrated by echocardiography, in the absence of another cardiac or systemic disease that might produce left ventricular hypertrophy [6]. Patients were categorized according to clinical presentation and presence or absence of ventricular tachycardia on 24–48 h Holter monitoring.

Electrophysiologic Study

All cardioactive drugs were discontinued five half-lives or more before study. Electrophysiologic study was performed with the patient fasting and sedated with 10 mg oral diazepam. Informed consent was obtained in accordance with a study protocol approved by the Institute Review Board of the National Heart, Lung, and Blood Institute. Three multiple electrode catheters (5F or 6F, USCI or Mansefield) were introduced percutaneously into a femoral vein and positioned under fluoroscopic guidance in the high right atrium, across the tricuspid valve in the region of the His bundle and at the right ventricular apex. In patients with supraventricular tachycardia, a quadripolar catheter was also placed in the coronary sinus via a subclavian vein. A femoral artery was cannulated (8F Cordis sheath) for continuous recording of the systemic arterial pressure and in some patients for left ventricular stimulation. Following programmed atrial stimulation, the high right atrial catheter was repositioned in the right ventricular outflow tract for programmed ventricular stimulation. Intracardiac electrograms were filtered at 30–500 Hz and standard electrocardiographic leads I, II and V_1 or V_6 were filtered at 0.1–20 Hz, and displayed on a multichannel oscilloscope (Electronic for Medicine, VR16) and recorded on light sensitive paper at 100 mm/s. Twelve-lead electrocardiograms were recorded during induced arrhythmia. Programmed stimulation was performed using a digital programmable stimulator (Bloom Associates Ltd.) using a 2.0-ms rectangular pulse at twice late diastolic thresholds.

Stimulation Protocol

The following pacing protocol was used:

1) introduction of single atrial premature stimuli during sinus rhythm that scanned diastole 10–20 ms decremental intervals;
2) atrial overdrive continuous pacing at cycle length of 700, 650, 600, 550, 500, 450, 400 and 350 ms (unless limited by symptoms or hypotension at the shorter pacing cycle lenghts) for 30 s and with > 30 s rest in between each pacing drive;
3) introduction of atrial premature stimuli (S_2) after eight driven (S_1) atrial beats at pacing cycle length (PCL) of 600 ms (700 ms if atrioventricular block occurred at PCL of 600 ms) – the premature interval (S_1-S_2) was decreased in 10–20-ms intervals;

4) atrial pacing at progressively shorter cycle lenghts using 5–10-ms decremental steps until atrioventricular block occurred or until limited by symptoms or hypotension; and

5) programmed ventricular stimulation. In patients with pre-excitation syndrome, the site and characteristics of the accessory pathway were determined by standard methods [7, 8].

Programmed ventricular stimulation protocol involved a stepwise increase in "aggressiveness" as follows:

1) insertion of one, two, and three premature stimuli during sinus rhythm at the right ventricular apex;

2) introduction of one and two premature stimuli after three ventricular drive PCL of 600 ms, 500 ms, and 400 ms, first at the right ventricular apex and second, at the right ventricular outflow tract;

3) introduction of three premature stimuli after the three ventricular drive PCLs at the right ventricular apex and right ventricular outflow tract; and

4) introduction of one, two, and three premature stimuli after the three ventricular drive PCLs at a left ventricular site. The end-point of the stimulation protocol was refractoriness or induction of a sustained ventricular arrhythmia.

The following were determined: basic intervals (AH, HV, QRS, QT, QTc), sinus node recovery time [43], sinoatrial conduction time [44, 45], atrial effective and functional refractory periods, atrioventricular nodal effective and functional refractory period, Wenckebach cycle length, maximum atrial rate with 1:1 atrioventricular conduction, ventricular refractory periods at the three ventricular PCLs, determined at the three ventricular sites, and the prematurity index; shortest premature coupling intervals ($S_2+S_3+S_4$ and $V_2+V_3+V_4$) that failed to induce or resulted in the induction of sustained ventricular arrhythmia.

Definitions

Abnormal sinus node function: prolonged sinoatrial conduction time (SACT): > 120 ms () *prolonged sinus node recovery time* (SNRT) and *corrected sinus node recovery time* (CSNRT): > 1500 ms and > 525 ms, respectively [9, 10].

Prolonged AH interval: > 125 ms [11].

Abnormal atrioventricular nodal effective refractory period: > 425 ms [11].

Abnormal Wenckebach cycle lenght: > 500 ms.

Enhanced atrioventricular nodal conduction: 1:1 atrioventricular conduction at atrial pacing cycle lengths of < 300 ms, associated with a < 50-ms increase in the AH interval.

Delayed HV intervals: > 55 ms [11]. Prolongation of HV interval or infra-His block in response to atrial premature stimulation during right atrial refractory period measurement or during incremental atrial pacing at cycle lengths of > 400 ms were also considered abnormal.

Nonsustained ventricular tachycardia: 5–29 consecutive ventricular beats, at ≥ 120 beats per minute and terminating spontaneously.

Sustained ventricular tachycardia: ventricular tachycardia of ≥ 30 beats duration or requiring termination because of hemodynamic compromise. Ventricular tachycardia with continuous changing QRS morphology was termed polymorphic and one with QRS complexes was termed monomorphic.

Ventricular fibrillation: ventricular arrhythmia with no discernable discrete ventricular beats identifiable on the surface 12-lead electrocardiogram and with continuous intracardiac ventricular electrical activity.

Sudden cardiac arrest: history of a resuscitation attempt with required direct current cardioversion within 2 h of collapse.

Statistics

Data are expressed as mean ± 1 SD. Continuous variables were analyzed using Student's t test for unpaired data. Contingency tables were evaluated by Fisher's exact test. A probability value of $p < 0.05$ was considered significant.

Results

Safety of Electrophysiologic Studies

There have been no deaths. The only serious complication has consisted of a femoral arteriovenous fistula that required surgical repair.

The following measures are believed to have contributed to the safety of the electrophysiologic studies:

1) The hemodynamic state of patients is ascertained – the severity of left ventricular outflow obstruction and filling pressures just prior to the electrophysiologic study. Dehydration following the overnight fast is corrected by infusion of fluids, as in these patients it frequently results in sinus tachycardia and aggravates the left ventricular outflow tract obstruction.
2) Patients are well sedated to reduce anxiety-related increase in catecholamine levels.
3) Patients are fitted with two self-adhesive R2 ECG/Defibrillation Pads (R2 Corporation) that are attached to two independent defibrillators (Physiocontrol, Lifepak 6s, Cardiac monitor). If an arrhythmia is induced that results in loss of consciousness both defibrillators are charged simultaneously to 200 J for rapid sequential direct current shocks if the first shock failed

to terminate the arrhythmia, thereby reducing the period of time that the hypertrophied myocardium suffers ischemia in between shocks from > 10 s to < 3 s. This may not only result in increased cardioversion success but also prevents intractable ventricular fibrillation developing secondary to myocardial ischemic damage.

4) An adequate interval is allowed to lapse between stimulation steps to allow the arterial pressure to recover.

5) Induced ventricular arrhythmias are usually rapid and polymorphic. Time is therefore not wasted in trying to terminate the arrhythmia by overdrive pacing.

6) If sinus asystole or bradycardia complicates the immediate postcardioversion period atrioventricular sequential pacing should be instituted promptly to ensure early return of satisfactory systemic arterial pressure.

Electrophysiologic Abnormalities and Relation of Morphology of Induced Sustained Ventricular Arrhythmia to Symptoms, Ventricular Tachycardia, and Aggressiveness of Programmed Ventricular Stimulation

Electrophysiologic abnormalities were demonstrated in 84/106 (79%) of patients. A high prevalence of prolonged SACT and/or SNRT and HV interval was noted (48% and 37%, respectively). Abnormally delayed and rapid AV node conduction was noted in 20% of patients and was unrelated to presenting symptoms.

Sustained ventricular arrhythmia was induced in 44 (42%) patients. The ventricular arrhythmia was polymorphic ventricular tachycardia in 32 (73%) patients, monomorphic ventricular tachycardia in ten (23%) patients and ventricular fibrillation in two (5%) patients.

Sustained ventricular tachycardia was induced with $\leq$ two premature stimuli in 13/44 (30%) patients and with three premature stimuli in 31/44 (70%) patients. In only 1/13 (8%) of sudden cardiac arrest patients was sustained ventricular tachycardia induced with two premature stimuli.

The relation between presenting symptoms and inducibility of sustained ventricular arrhythmia, including polymorphic ventricular tachycardia, was significant ($p < 0.02$); cardiac arrest patients 85%, syncope (68%), presyncope (41%), and asymptomatic ventricular tachycardia (26%).

Polymorphic ventricular tachycardia was not induced as a result of a more aggressive programmed stimulation compared with monomorphic ventricular tachycardia – the number of ventricular sites tested, drive cycle lengths, number of premature stimuli used and premature intervals achieved were not significantly different for the two arrhythmias.

For the group as a whole, the incidence of nonsustained ventricular tachycardia recorded during ambulatory monitoring was unrelated to symptoms or inducibility of sustained ventricular tachycardia.

Discussion

Sudden cardiac death and syncope are well-known complications of hypertrophic cardiomyopathy [13–19]. Although several mechanisms may contribute to these events, it is suspected that the primary etiology in most cases is an arrhythmia [20–29]. In this respect, nonsustained episodes of ventricular tachycardia during Holter monitoring have been associated with increased risk for sudden cardiac death [1–3]. Although this finding is not very specific or sensitive, it does indicate that left ventricular electrical instability may be an important cause of at least some of the episodes of sudden cardiac arrest/death. It is unfortunately rare to have direct electrocardiographic evidence of responsible arrhythmia during episodes of sudden cardiac arrest or syncope. Electrophysiologic studies have been shown to be of value in establishing the nature of arrhythmias in patients with other cardiac diseases who present with sudden cardiac arrest or syncope [30, 31]. A number of workers have reported on electrophysiologic findings in patients with hypertrophic cardiomyopathy [32–39]. However, due to the relatively small numbers of patients studied and heterogeneity of clinical presentation, the role of electrophysiologic studies, and in particular, relevance of induced ventricular arrhythmias in these patients remains controversial. It has been reported that in hypertrophic cardiomyopathy patients programmed ventricular stimulation with a maximum of two ventricular stimuli does not distinguish between patients with cardiac arrest or syncope and asymptomatic patients and that use of three premature stimuli may result in the induction of nonspecific arrhythmias [39]. In common with previous reports [38, 39] we found that the commonest sustained ventricular arrhythmia induced in hypertrophic cardiomyopathy patients was polymorphic ventricular tachycardia. This arrhythmia is rarely induced in patients with normal or mildly diseased left ventricles despite aggressive programmed ventricular stimulation using three to four premature stimuli [40–47]. Few of our severely symptomatic patients – sudden cardiac arrest survivors or patients with recurrent syncope with ventricular tachycardia during Holter monitoring had sustained ventricular arrhythmia induced with two or less premature stimuli. The frequency with which sustained ventricular arrhythmia was induced (polymorphic ventricular tachycardia in most patients), using up to three premature stimuli did correlate closely with the clinical presentation indicating that the induction of these arrhythmia may indicate left ventricular electrical instability in symptomatic patients and guide therapy. Electrophysiologic studies also reveal a variety of other mechanisms for sudden cardiac arrest/death and syncope in patients with hypertrophic cardiomyopathy that also may require to be addressed. These studies are challenging but safe in experienced hands.

References

1. McKenna WJ, England D, Doi YL, Deanfield JE, Oakley C, Goodwin JF (1981) Arrhythmia in hypertrophic cardiomyopathy I: influence on prognosis. Br Heart J 46:168–172
2. Savage DD, Sedes SF, Maron BJ, Myers DJ, Epstein SE (1979) Prevalence of arrhythmias during 24-hour electrocardiographic monitoring and exercise testing in patients with obstructive and non-obstructive hypertrophic cardiomyopathy. Circulation 59:866–875
3. Maron BJ, Savage DD, Wolfson JK, Epstein SE (1981) Prognostic significance of 24 hour ambulatory monitoring in patients with hypertrophic cardiomyopathy: a prospective study. Am J Cardiol 48:252–257
4. Krikler DM, Davis MJ, Rowland E, Goodwin JF, Evans RC, Shaw DB (1980) Sudden death in hypertrophic cardiomyopathy: associated atrioventricular pathways. Br Heart J 43:245–251
5. Wellens HJJ, Bar FW, Vanagt EJ (1980) Death after ajmaline administration. Am J Cardiol 45:905
6. Maron BJ; Epstein SE (1979) Hypertrophic cardiomyopathy: a discussion of nomenclature. Am J Cardiol 434:1242–1244
7. Gallagher JJ, Pritchett ELC, Sealy WC, Kasell H, Wallace AG (1978) The preexcitation syndromes. Prog Cardiovasc Dis 20:285–325
8. Gallagher JJ, Pritchett ELC, Benditt DG, Tonkin AM, Cambell RWF, Dugan FA, Bashore TM, Wallace AG (1977) New catheter techniques for analysis of the sequence of retrograde atrial activation in man. Eur J Cardiol 6:1–14
9. Strauss HC, Bigger JT Jr, Saroff AL, Giardina EG (1976) Electrophysiological evaluation of sinus node function in patients with sinus node dysfunction. Circulation 53:763–776
10. Reiffel JA, Bigger JT Jr, Cramer M, Reid DS (1977) Ability of Holter electrocardiographic recording and atrial stimulation to detect sinus node dysfunction in symptomatic and asymptomatic patients with sinus bradycardia. Am J Cardiol 40:189–194
11. Josephson ME (1979) Atrioventricular conduction. In: Josephson ME, Seides SF (eds) Clinical cardiac electrophysiology. Techniques and interpretations. Lea and Febiger, Philadelphia, pp 79–101
12. Fananapazir L, Tracy C, Winkler JB, Leon MB, Cannon RO, Epstein SE (1989) Relation of inducibility of ventricular arrhythmias to symptoms in patients with hypertrophic cardiomyopathy – relevance of induced polymorphic ventricular tachycardia. J Am Coll Cardiol 13:19A
13. Frank S, Braunwald E (1968) Idiopathic hypertrophic subaortic stenosis, clinical analysis of 126 patients with emphasis on natural history. Circulation 37:759–788
14. Swan DA, Bell B, Oakley CM, Goodwin JF (1971) Analysis of symptomatic course and prognosis and treatment of hypertrophic obstructive cardiomyopathy. Br Heart J 33:671–685
15. Hardarson T, de la Calzada CD, Curiel R, Goodwin JF (1973) Prognosis and mortality of hypertrophic cardiomyopathy. Lancet 2:1462–1467
16. Shah PM, Adelman AG, Wigler ED, Globel FL, Burchett HB, Hardarson T, Curiel R, Calzada C, Oakley CM, Goodwin J (1974) The natural (and unnatural) history of hypertrophic cardiomyopathy. Circ Res 35 (Suppl II):179–195
17. Maron BJ, Lipson LC, Roberts WC, Savage DD, Epstein SE (1978) "Malignant" hypertrophic cardiomyopathy: identification of a subgroup of families with unusually frequent premature deaths. Am J Cardiol 14:1130–1140
18. McKenna WJ, Harris L, Deanfield J (1982) Syncope in hypertrophic cardiomyopathy. Br Heart J 47:177–179
19. Maron BJ, Roberts WC, Epstein SE (1982) Sudden death in hypertrophic cardiomyopathy; a profile of 78 patients. Circulation 65:1388–1394
20. Goodwin JF, Krikler DM (1976) Hypothesis: arrhythmia as a cause of sudden death in hypertrophic cardiomyopathy. Lancet 2:937–940
21. Joseph S, Balcon R, McDonald L (1972) Syncope in hypertrophic obstructive cardiomyopathy due to asystole. Br Heart J 34:974–976

22. Chmielewski CA, Riley RS, Mahendtan A, Most AS (1977) Complete heart block as a cause of syncope in asymmetric septal hypertrophy. Am Heart J 93:91–93
23. Canedo MI, Frank MJ, Abdulla AM (1989) Rhythm disturbances in hypertrophic cardiomyopathy: prevalence, relation to symptoms an management. Am J Cardiol 45:848–855
24. Stafford WJ, Trohman RG, Bilsker M, Zamal L, Castellanous A, Myerburg RJ (1986) Cardiac arrest in an adolescent with atrial fibrillation and hypertrophic cardiomyopathy. J Am Coll Cardiol 7:701–704
25. Nicod P, Pollikar R, Peterson KL (1988) Hypertrophic cardiomyopathy and sudden death. N Engl J Med 318:1255–1257
26. Louie EK, Maron BJ (1986) Familial spontaneous complete heart block in hypertrophic cardiomyopathy. Br Heart J 55:469–474
27. Glancy DL, O'Brien KP, Gold HK, Epstein SE (1970) Atrial fibrillation in patients with idiopathic hypertrophic subaortic stenosis. Br Heart J 32:652–659
28. Bjarnason I, Hardarson T, Jonsson S (1982) Cardiac arrhythmias in hypertrophic cardiomyopathy. Br Heart J 48:198–203
29. Frank MJ, Watkin LD, Prisant ML, Stefadouros MA, Abdulla A (1984) Potentially lethal arrhythmias and their management in hypertrophic cardiomyopathy. Am J Cardiol 53:1608–1613
30. Morady F, Schienman MM, Hess DS, Sung RJ, Shen E, Shapiro W (1983) Electrophysiologic testing in the management of survivors of out-of-hospital cardiac arrest. Am J Cardiol 51:85–89
31. Morady F, Shen E, Schwartz A, Hess D, Bhandari A, Sung RJ, Schienman MM (1983) Long-term follow-up of patients with recurrent unexplained syncope evaluated by electrophysiologic testing. J Am Coll Cardiol 2:1053–1056
32. Ingham RE, Mason JW, Rossen RM, Harrison DC (1978) Electrophysiologic findings in patients with idiopathic hypertrophic subaortic stenosis. Am J Cardiol 41:811–816
33. Anderson KP, Stinson EB, Derby GC, Oyer PE, Mason JW (1983) Vulnerability of patients with hypertrophic cardiomyopathy to ventricular arrhythmia induction in the operating room. Am J Cardiol 51:811–815
34. Kowey PR, Eisenberg R, Engel TR (1984) Sustained arrhythmias in hypertrophic obstructive cardiomyopathy. N Engl J Med 310:1566–1569
35. Schiavone WA, Maoloney JD, Lever HM, Castle LW, Sterba R, Morant V (1986) Electrophysiologic studies of patients with hypertrophic cardiomyopathy with syncope of undetermined etiology. PACE 9:476–481
36. Borggrefe M, Podczeck A, Breithardt G (1986) Electrophysiologic studies in hypertrophic cardiomyopathy. Circulation 74 (Suppl II):II-1922
37. Geibel A, Brugada P, Zehender M, Kersschot I, Wellens HJJ (1986) Results of a standardized ventricular stimulation protocol in patients with hypertrophic cardiomyopathy. J Am Coll Cardiol 7:2, 195 A
38. Kuck K-H, Kunze K-P, Geiger M, Costard A, Schuter M (1987) Programmed electrical stimulation in patients with hypertrophic cardiomyopathy: results in patients with and without cardiac arrest or syncope. In: Brugada P, Wellens HJJ (eds) Cardiac arrhythmias: where to go from here? Futura, New York, pp 367–376
39. Watson R, Schwartz JL, Baron BJ, Tucker E, Rosing DR, Josephson ME (1988) Inducible polymorphic ventricular tachycardia and ventricular fibrillation in a subgroup of patients with hypertrophic cardiomyopathy at high risk for sudden death. J Am Coll Cardiol 10:761–774
40. Brugada P, Abdollah H, Heddle B, Wellens HJJ (1983) Results of a ventricular stimulation protocol using a maximum of 4 premature stimuli in patients without documented or suspected ventricular arrhythmias. J Am Coll Cardiol 52:1214–1218
41. Livelli FD, Bigger JT, Reiffel JA, Gang ES, Patton JN, Noethling PM, Rolnitzky LM, Gliklich JI (1982) Response to programmed ventricular stimulation: sensitivity, specificity and relation to heart disease. Am J Cardiol 50:452–458
42. Mann DE, Luck JC, Griffin JC, Herre JM, Limacher MC, Magro SA, Robertson NW, Wyndham CRC (1983) Induction of clinical ventricular tachycardia using programmed stimulation: value of third and fourth extra stimuli. Am J Cardiol 52:50–61

43. Buxton AE, Waxman HL, Marchlinski FE, Untereker WJ, Waspe LE, Josephson ME (1984) Role of triple extra stimuli during electrophysiologic study of patients with documented sustained ventricular tachyarrhythmias. Circulation 69:532–540
44. Brugada P, Green M, Abdollah H, Wellens HJJ (1984) Significance of ventricular arrhythmias initiated by programmed ventricular stimulation: the importance of the type of ventricular arrhythmia induced and the number of premature stimuli required. Circulation 69:87–92
45. Morady F, DiCarlo L, Winston S, Davis JC, Sheinman MM (1984) A prospective comparison of triple extra stimuli and left ventricular tachycardia induction. Circulation 70:52–57
46. Wellens HJJ, Brugada P, Stevenson WG (1985) Programmed electrical stimulation of the heart in patients with life-threatening ventricular arrhythmias: what is the significance of induced arrhythmias and what is the correct stimulation protocol. Circulation 72:1–7
47. Anderson JL, Mason JW (1986) Criteria for selection of patients for programmed electrical stimulation. Circulation 73 (Suppl II):50–58

Cerebral Embolic Risk
in Hypertrophic Cardiomyopathy

G. Di Pasquale, A. Andreoli, A. M. Lusa, S. Urbinati, P. Grazi, G. Carini,
M. Ruffini, and G. Pinelli

Hypertrophic cardiomyopathy (HCM) is characterized by a broad spectrum of clinical manifestations [1–4]. Systemic embolism is a recognized complication in the natural history of the disease [4–8]. In most cases reported in the larger series, embolism involves the cerebral circulation. However, cerebral embolism is almost never the presenting manifestation of HCM. It has always been tacitly assumed that embolism can occur in patients with HCM, but the stratification of the embolic risk has not received much attention up to the present time.

We observed six patients in whom cerebral embolism was the onset manifestation of previously unrecognized HCM. Through an analysis of these cases and a review of the literature, we tried to assess the risk of embolism in patients with HCM. On the same basis, in order to obtain a risk stratification, an analysis was made of the determinant factors of the embolic risk in HCM.

Patients and Methods

In the period between September 1981 and December 1988, 380 consecutive patients with cerebral ischemia, aged 3–75 years (mean 53.6) were referred to the neurosurgery department and underwent a complete cardiologic evaluation.

The diagnosis of cerebral ischemia was made by the neurologist on the basis of neurological examination, CT scan of the brain, and cerebral angiography or carotid echotomography. The neurological deficit was classified as transient ischemic attack (TIA), reversible ischemic neurological deficit (RIND), or stroke. In order to detect embolic cardiac disorders, all patients underwent clinical evaluation, standard ECG, and two-dimensional echocardiography (ATL MK 300 IC, phased-array sector scanner).

Cardiac abnormalities were detected by two-dimensional echocardiography in 75 patients (20%); in 27 of these (7%) the cardiac lesions were considered responsible for the cerebral ischemia through an embolic mechanism. Among these cases, six patients with HCM, aged 21–68 years, were identified. In two of them cardiac catheterization was also performed. In no case had the HCM been recognized before. All patients but one, who had suffered from peripheral embolism, were asymptomatic until the cerebral event.

The diagnosis of cardiogenic cerebral embolism was based on the criteria proposed by the Cerebral Embolism Task Force [9], mainly the absence of atherosclerotic vascular disease on cerebral angiography.

Results

The data pertinent to the six patients with HCM and cerebral embolism are summarized in Table 1. They were two males and four females, aged 21–68 years; all were normotensive. Two patients had a family history of sudden death (Nos. 1, 3); all patients were in NYHA class I. On admission four patients presented a stroke and two patients a carotid TIA.

Paroxysmal atrial fibrillation (AF) was revealed by repeated Holter monitoring performed in the acute phase of cerebral ischemia in two patients (Nos. 1, 2), while it was suspected, but never documented, in patient No. 3 who complained of episodes of palpitation. Mild to moderate left atrial enlargement (4.1, 4.2, 4.5 cm) was observed at two-dimensional echocardiography in all these three patients. Patient No. 4 had suffered before from a brachial artery embolism during an episode of suspected endocarditis 1 year earlier. She was admitted to our hospital for sudden right hemiparesis occurring after a few

Table 1. Characteristics of six patients with HCM and cerebral embolism

Pa-tient No.	Age Sex	Type of CVA	Cerebral CT scan	Cerebral angiography or carotid echotomo-graphy	Contributing factors for embolism	Treatment	Follow-up
1	60 F	Stroke	Ischemia	Normal	Paroxysmal AF	Amiodarone, anticoagulant	Alive, permanent AF pacemaker
2	65 M	Stroke	Ischemia	Normal	Paroxysmal AF	Amiodarone, anticoagulant	Alive, permanent AF
3	68 F	TIAs	Normal	Normal	Episodes of palpitation (AF?)	Amiodarone	Alive
4	56 F	Stroke	Ischemia	Normal	Infective endocarditis	Penicillin + gentamicin diuretics	Alive
5	21 M	Stroke	Normal	Normal	LV dilata-tion, gene-ralized hypokinesia, thrombus	Digoxin, anti-coagulant	CHF, sudden death
6	36 F	TIA	Normal	Normal	–	Beta-blockers	Alive

CHF, congestive heart failure; *CT*, computed tomography; *CVA*, cerebrovascular accident; *LV*, left ventricle

days of fever, asthenia, and polyarthralgias; blood cultures were found to be positive for Enterococcus, and two-dimensional echocardiography showed endocarditis vegetation on the anterior mitral leaflet.

Patient No. 5 was a 21-year-old man with HCM who had developed asymptomatically a dilated form; two-dimensional echocardiography revealed a moderate left ventricular enlargement, with diffuse wall thickening and global hypokinesia; an apical pedunculated thrombus was present.

Patient No. 6 was admitted because of a TIA; neurological and cardiac evaluation failed to reveal any cause of cerebral ischemia other than HCM.

Three patients (two with documented paroxysmal AF and one with HCM who had developed a dilated form) were placed on anticoagulant treatment with warfarin. In no case was there a recurrence of embolism in a follow-up period ranging from 1 to 5 years. Permanent AF developed in two patients (Nos. 1, 2) despite treatment with amiodarone. Patient No. 5 became severely symptomatic from congestive heart failure after 1 year and eventually died suddenly while awaiting heart transplantation.

Discussion

HCM has never been considered a high risk disease for embolism. However, our observations and the data from the literature demonstrate that the risk of cerebral and peripheral embolism in HCM is not negligible. HCM per se is not an embolic cardiac condition; the rapid flows and lack of opportunity for stasis do not predispose to the formation of left ventricular thrombi. The risk of embolism is almost always related to the occurrence of any of three major events, i.e., AF, infective endocarditis, or evolution toward dilatation with

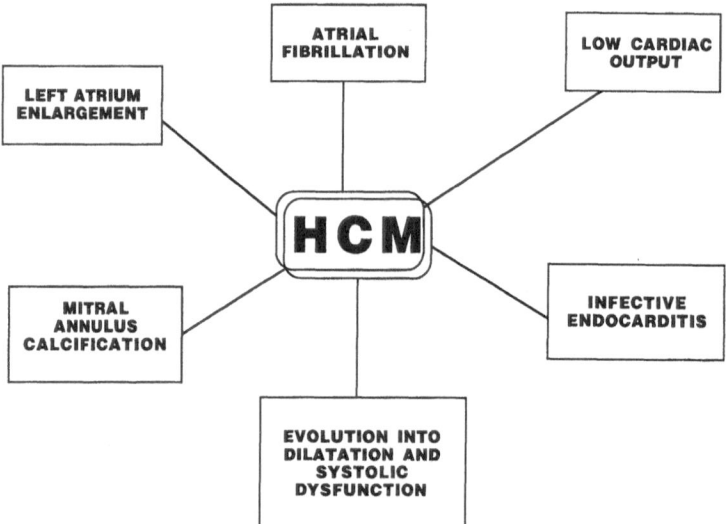

Fig. 1. Determinant factors of the risk of systemic embolism in HCM

Table 2. Complications associated with HCM

Reference	n	Follow-up (years)	Infective Endo-carditis (n) (%)	Atrial Fibril-lation (n) (%)	Embolism (n) (%)	Embolic Risk %/years	Type of embolism and associated factors
Frank and Braunwald 1968 [1]	126	12	6 4.8	10 7.9	–	–	
Swan et al. 1971 [2]	85	4	4 4.7	4 4.7	–	–	
Hardarson et al. 1973 [3]	119	4.6	4 3.4	10 8.4	11 9.2	2	Systemic or pulmonary embolism (3 cerebral); 3 with stable AF, 1 with probable paroxysmal AF, 3 with probable WPW
Shah et al. 1974 [4]	190	5.2	2 1	13 6.8	–	–	
Furlan et al. 1984 [5]	150	5.5	–	7 4.6	11 7	0.6	All cerebral embolism; 4 with AF, 1 with AF + MAC, 2 with LA enlargement without AF
Koga et al. 1984 [6]	136	5.1	–	15 11	3 2.2	0.4	All cerebral embolism; 2 with persistent AF, 1 with paroxysmal AF
Kogure et al. 1986 [7]	66	3.7	–	15 22.7	6 9	2.4	4 cerebral, 1 femoral; all with AF (1 paroxysmal), 1 with CHF
Cohen et al. 1986 [8]	60	6.3	1 1.6	11 18	9 15	2.4	6 cerebral, 2 peripheral, 1 splenic; 6 with AF and severe LA enlargement

AF, atrial fibrillation; *CHF*, congestive heart failure; *LA*, left atrium; *MAC*, mitral annulus calcification; *WPW*, Wolff Parkinson White.

systolic dysfunction and congestive heart failure (Fig. 1). In Table 2 the incidence of AF, infective endocarditis, and embolism in larger series of HCM is reported; the risk factors for embolism are specified in the last column.

In our series of patients with cerebral ischemia referred to a neurosurgical department, cardiac lesions which could be the source of embolism, were documented by two-dimensional echocardiography in 27 patients (7%). Patients with HCM (6/27) represent a significant fraction (22%) of all these cardioembolic strokes.

An analysis of the larger series of HCM, published in the literature in the last 2 decades, indicates that in the natural history of HCM systemic embolism occurs in 2%–15% of patients (Table 2). In most cases embolism involved the brain; in the remaining cases embolism was peripheral, splenic, or pulmonary. The estimated incidence of embolism is between 0.4%–2.4% yearly, which is not trivial, and in some series the risk of embolism is similar to corresponding figures in patients with valvular heart disease [3–8].

The vast majority of embolic events occurred in the presence of AF. Also in our experience, two out of six patients had a documented paroxysmal AF and one had a suspected AF. AF occurs in 5%–10% of patients with HCM, usually late in the course of the disease, and it is associated with clinical deterioration [3, 6, 10]. A higher incidence of AF has been reported in recent series [7, 8]. At the time of diagnosis approximately 7% of the patients have AF. On continuous 72-h ECG monitoring about 40% will be found to have AF or supraventricular arrhythmias [11].

Glancy et al. [10] reported a 25% rate of cerebral emboli in a subgroup of 16 patients with HCM and AF. In the series of Koga et al. [6] cerebrovascular accidents occured in two of eight cases with HCM and persistent AF and in two of seven cases with paroxysmal AF. In the series of Kogure et al. [7] six of 15 patients with persistent or paroxysmal AF experienced a systemic embolism during a 3.7-year observation period. Finally, Samukawa et al. [12] observed six cases of arterial embolism among 18 patients with HCM and AF. These data emphasize that HCM associated with AF involves a very high risk of systemic embolism.

In the presence of AF, the embolic risk is particularly high when significant left atrial enlargement and a decrease in cardiac output are concomitant [6, 7]. In the study of Kogure et al. [7] the echocardiographically determined left atrial dimension tended to be greater and the cardiac index tended to be lower in patients with HCM and embolism than in those without systemic embolism with or without AF. Left atrial enlargement was severe in the series of Cohen et al. [8]. In our cases, left atrial enlargement was only mild to moderate.

Another factor which, in association with AF, may predispose to cerebral embolism is mitral annulus calcification, as was found in one patient by Furlan et al. [5]. A relation between mitral annulus calcification and HCM is well established, and a relation between isolated mitral annular calcium and stroke has been suggested [13, 14].

Infective endocarditis is another major complication of HCM predisposing to systemic embolism. The incidence of infective endocarditis in HCM is not low, being around 5% [15]. The risk of embolism in such cases is definitely high, probably the same as it is when infective endocarditis occurs on rheumatic or myxomatous cardiac valves. Embolic stroke occurs in about 20% of patients with infective endocarditis, and peripheral embolism occurs in about 15%–35%

of patients [9, 16]. Patients at higher risk for infective endocarditis are those with mitral valve regurgitation and with a higher pressure gradient. Most of the reported cases were symptomatic before the infectious complication developed. Vegetations may implant at any level of the malformation, i.e., mitral, aortic valves, or left ventricular outflow tract. In our case of Enterococcus endocarditis the vegetations implanted at the level of anterior mitral leaflet; obvious signs of mitral valve regurgitation were present, but neither physical nor echocardiographic signs of outflow obstruction were evident.

The third major complication favoring systemic embolism could be the progression of HCM toward left ventricular dilatation and systolic dysfunction. This event is not as unusual as previously thought, occuring in about 10% of patients with HCM, with a rate of progression close to 1% patient per year [17–19]. In this setting the risk of embolism might be extremely high, as in patients with dilated cardiomyopathy. These functional and morphologic changes are usually associated with congestive heart failure. However, a possible subtle evolution of HCM into a hypokinetic left ventricle, without corresponding symptoms of clinical deterioration, can also be assumed. A striking example of this event is the case of our 21-year-old patient with HCM, who had developed a dilated form with left ventricular thrombus, and had been asymptomatic until the cerebral embolism.

Management implications regarding the prevention of the embolic risk in HCM are long-term anticoagulation treatment in patients with AF and the antibiotic prophylaxis of infective endocarditis.

In the presence of long-standing AF, long-term anticoagulation treatment with warfarin is certainly necessary. Even in the presence of paroxysmal AF, the embolic risk is not negligible. Repeated Holter monitoring is therefore advisable in order to detect even asymptomatic episodes of AF. In the presence of paroxysmal AF, electrical or pharmacological cardioversion, followed by antiarrhythmic prophylaxis of recurrences, is advisable. The concomitance of left atrial enlargement or a decrease in cardiac output seems to be a determining element for anticoagulation.

As far as the risk of infective endocarditis is concerned, it is conceivable that patients with HCM should benefit from infective endocarditis prophylaxis as do patients with valvular heart disease. Antibiotic prophylaxis is recommended in the case of dental manipulation and other procedures involving risk of bacteriemia. Finally, patients with HCM should be monitored echocardiographically for a possible progression into left ventricular hypokinesia.

No data are available regarding the risk of embolism at this stage of the disease, but it is likely to be the same as in patients with primary dilated cardiomyopathy. Anticoagulation is probably mandatory. In conclusion, systemic embolism, particularly involving the cerebral circulation, is another possible burden in the natural history of HCM. Among the risk factors for embolism, AF and infective endocarditis play a significant role.

Acknowledgement: This study was supported in part by CRS research grant 336/85 from Regione Emilia-Romagna, Italy.

References

1. Frank S, Braunwald E (1968) Idiopathic hypertrophic subaortic stenosis: clinical analysis of 126 patients with emphasis on the natural history. Circulation 37:759–788
2. Swan AD, Bell B, Oakley CM, Goodwin JF (1971) Analysis of symptomatic course and prognosis and treatment of hypertrophic obstructive cardiomyopathy. Br Heart J 31:671–685
3. Hardarson T, de la Calzada CS, Curiel R, Goodwin JF (1973) Prognosis and mortality of hypertrophic obstructive cardiomyopathy. Lancet 2:1462–1467
4. Shah PM, Adelman AG, Wigle ED, Gobel FL, Burchell HB, Hardarson T, Curiel R, de la Calzada CS, Oakley C, Goodwin JF (1974) The natural (and unnatural) history of hypertrophic obstructive cardiomyopathy. Circ Res 34–35 (Suppl II):179–195
5. Furlan AJ, Craciun AR, Raju NR, Hart N (1984) Cerebrovascular complications associated with idiopathic hypertrophic subaortic stenosis. Stroke 15:282–284
6. Koga Y, Itaya K, Toshima H (1984) Prognosis in hypertrophic cardiomyopathy. Am Heart J 108:351–359
7. Kogure S, Yamamoto Y, Tomono S, Hasegawa A, Suzuki T, Murata K (1986) High risk of systemic embolism in hypertrophic cardiomyopathy. Jpn Heart J 27:475–480
8. Cohen S, Benichou M, Larbi MB, Bory M, Serradimigni A (1986) Myocardiopathie hypertrophique: évolution et pronostic. Soixante observations. Presse Med 15:423–427
9. Cerebral Embolism Task Force (1986) Cardiogenic brain embolism. Arch Neurol 43:71–84
10. Glancy DL, O'Brein KP, Gold HK, Epstein SE (1970) Atrial fibrillation in patients with idiopathic hypertrophic subaortic stenosis. Br Heart J 32:652–659
11. McKenna WJ, Kleinebenne A (1985) Arrhythmien bei hypertropischer Kardiomyopathie. Bedeutung und therapeutische Konsequenzen. Herz 10 (2):91–101
12. Samukawa M, Hasegawa K, Harada Y, Nakao M, Tadaoka S, Yoneda M, Fujiwara T, Nakamura T, Nezuo S, Sawayama T (1987) Clinical features and significance of hypertrophic cardiomyopathy with atrial fibrillation. J Cardiol 17 (3):465–474
13. Motamed HE, Roberts WC (1987) Frequency and significance of mitral annular calcium in hypertrophic cardiomyopathy: analysis of 200 necropsy patients. Am J Cardiol 60:877–884
14. De Bono P, Warlow CP (1979) Mitral-annulus calcification and cerebral or retinal ischemia. Lancet 2:383–385
15. Chagnac A, Rudniki C, Loebel H, Zahavi I (1982) Infectious endocarditis in idiopathic hypertrophic subaortic stenosis. Chest 81:346–349
16. Le Jemtel TH, Factor SM, Koengsberg M, O'Reilly M, Frater EH (1979) Mural vegetations at the site of endocardial trauma in infective endocarditis complicating idiopathic hypertrophic subaortic stenosis. Am J Cardiol 44:569–574
17. Ten Cate FS, Roelandt J (1979) Progression to left ventricular dilatation in patients with hypertrophic obstructive cardiomyopathy. Am Heart J 97:762–765
18. Spirito S, Maron BJ, Bonow RO, Epstein SE (1987) Occurrence and significance of progressive left ventricular wall thinning and relative cavity dilatation in hypertrophic cardiomyopathy. Am J Cardiol 59:123–129
19. Fighali S, Krajcer Z, Edelman S, Leachman R (1987) Progression of hypertrophic cardiomyopathy into a hypokinetic left ventricle: higher incidence in patients with mid-ventricular obstruction. J Am Coll Cardiol 9:288–294

Cytogenetic Studies in Familial Hypertrophic Cardiomyopathy: Identification of a Fragile Site on Human Chromosome 16

M. Ambrosini, M. Ferraro, M. C. Maccaglia, R. Santoro, C. Gaudio, R. Ricci, G. Scartòn, and A. Reale

Introduction

A familial origin of hypertrophic cardiomyopathy was postulated from the first observations of the disease. In 1949 Evans described a syndrome having a distinct clinical, electrocardiographic, and pathological pattern and emphasized the diagnostic importance of family history, frequent arrhythmias, and tendency to sudden death. He concluded that the etiology of this condition might be familial and hereditary and proposed to name it familial cardiomegaly [1].

In 1957 Bridgen first used the term cardiomyopathy to indicate isolated noncoronary myocardial disease. He explored the congenital form and reviewed the pedigrees of the families (eight from the literature, two from his series) showing that in all cases more than one member was affected, and that usually the maternal parent was diseased when members from two generations are involved. He concluded that this evidence suggested a genetic origin and that familial cardiomyopathy was probably inherited as a mendelian dominant [2].

Before the echocardiographic era, when the diagnosis was obtained from physical findings, chest radiography, and ECG, Emanuel et al. suggested in 1971 that in idiopathic cardiomyopathy both dominant and recessive mode of inheritance can be demonstrated [3].

In the last decade, the genetic origin of hypertrophic cardiomyopathy has been widely accepted, and in 1980 Goodwin affirmed that the lack of difference in proven familial and nonfamilial cases suggests that there is a genetic basis even though it may not be detectable in many cases [4]. The pattern of inheritance was consistent as an autosomal dominant trait [5] with a high degree of penetrance [6, 7] or of reduced penetrance [8].

Using M-mode and cross-sectional echocardiography Maron described that in genetically transmitted hypertrophic cardiomyopathy a variety of morphologic expression may be observed, including symmetric as well as asymmetric left ventricular hypertrophy, and that these forms may coexist in the same family [9–11].

Also, Emanuel noted that, in familial hypertrophic cardiomyopathy, isolated asymmetrical septal hypertrophy is a part of the clinical spectrum of hypertrophic cardiomyopathy and has the same genetic implications [12].

All the investigations on the patterns of inheritance obviously aim at a speculative knowledge but also at the genetic counseling recommendation to the families with hypertrophic cardiomyopathy regarding the risk of hypertrophic cardiomyopathy transmission to future offspring [13]. Nevertheless, in the literature extended cytogenetic studies have not been described. Therefore, we performed cytogenetic studies in a large family with marked occurrence of hypertrophic cardiomyopathy and a high incidence of premature sudden death through three generations.

Patients

The family taken into consideration was a three-generation family comprising a total of 23 members (Fig. 1). Physical examination, 12-lead electrocardiogram, chest X-ray, and M-mode and cross-sectional echocardiography were performed in all living members. Moreover, heart catheterization was performed in three (II-2, II-4, II-6), magnetic resonance in three (II-4, II-6, III-9), and necropsy in two (II-3, III-5). M-mode and cross-sectional echocardiography were performed using a Hewlett Packard 77020 A, phased array, ultrasonic scanner with a 2.5-MHz hand-held transducer. Images were recorded on reel-to-reel videotape (Panasonic AG 6200) for subsequent review both in real-time on slow motion and stop-action mode, and on hard copy paper speeding at 100 mm/s.

Five sudden deaths had occurred in the family: I-1 (not examined) died suddenly at 41 years, II-2 and II-3, respectively, died suddenly at 29 and 31 years, III-5 died suddenly at 10 years, the last one, III-4, was successfully resuscitated from ventricular fibrillation at 21 years.

Echocardiographic data allowed the diagnosis in ten living members of the family: seven of them had clinical signs of hypertrophic cardiomyopathy with mild to severe symptoms while three had a "subclinical" form (abnormal echo with morphologic features of hypertrophic cardiomyopathy, abnormal or normal ECG but without overt clinical expressions of the disease). It is important to note that, as previously reported in literature [5, 14], also in this family two young members, III-12 and III-15, had been found normal in previous clinical, ECG, and echographic examinations. Echocardiography ruled out hypertrophic cardiomyopathy in nine individuals.

Cytogenetic Studies

Cytogenetic studies were carried out in ten individuals of the family, namely, I-2, II-4, II-5, II-6, III-7, III-9, III-10, III-11, III-14, III-15, including members who were healthy (II-5, III-11, III-14) and who had clinical or subclinical expressions of hypertrophic cardiomyopathy. Chromosome preparations were obtained by standard methods from short-term lymphocyte cultures. R-banding with chromomycin A3 and C-banding were performed. In all ten individuals examined, R-banding allowed the exclusion of the presence of any numerical or structural chromosome aberration. On the contrary, it was found that seven out of the ten examined individuals displayed spontaneous expression of a

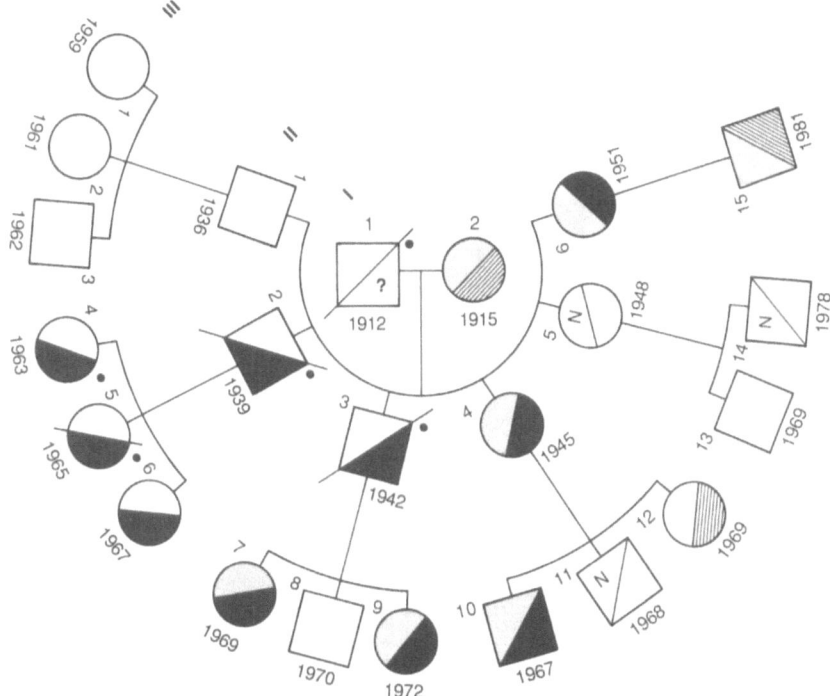

Fig. 1. Genetic tree of the family. Each family member has an index number shown above the symbol, and the year of birth is shown below. Symbols:

Men	Women	
◩	◑	With clinical hypertrophic cardiomyopathy
▨	◓	With subclinical hypertrophic cardiomyopathy
◿	⊘	Dead
•	•	Sudden death
▨	⊘	Fragile site
▨	⊘	Fragile site not found

fragile site that, according to R-and C-banding, was located on the long arm of chromosome 16. In Fig. 2 one partial C-banded metaphase presenting the fragile site is shown. C-banding was carried out since it allows an easier identification of chromosome 16. In fact, besides the centromeric regions of all chromosomes, in the human karyotype this technique preferentially stains the heterochromatic areas of chromosomes 1, 9, and 16.

Fragile sites in human chromosomes are cytologically recognized as a region on the chromosome where nonstaining gaps, breaks, or rearrangements do not occur randomly, both spontaneously or when cells are cultured under appro-

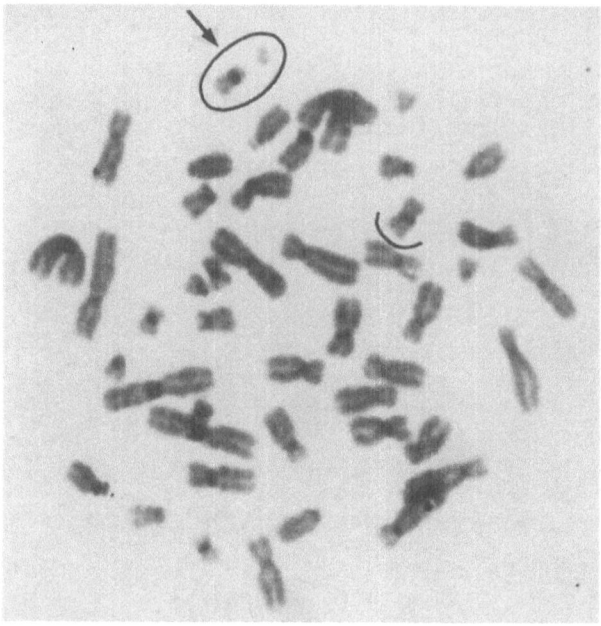

Fig. 2. Partial C-banded metaphase showing the fragile site *(arrow)*.
The normal homologue is indicated with a *curved line*

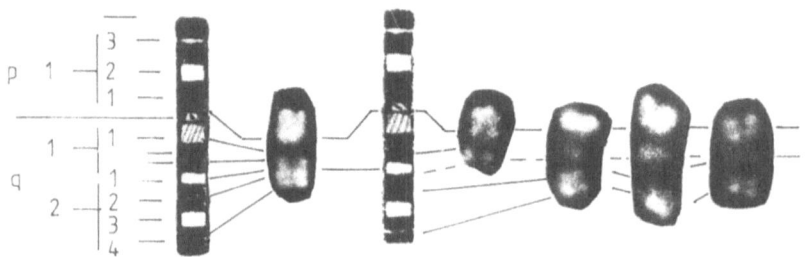

Fig. 3. Identification of the break-points of the fragile site by R-banding with
chromomycin A3

priate conditions. Two major groups of fragile sites are described, namely those
which are "rare" and those which are "common." Yet spontaneous expression
does not allow the assignment of a fragile site to any of these two groups [15].
By combined R- and C-banding the break-points of the fragile site observed in
this family were located on the long arm of chromosome 16, at band q2 1 at the
interface of 16q2 1 and q2 2 (Fig. 3). All the individuals presenting the fragile
site were affected by hypertrophic cardiomyopathy, though with variable morphologic and clinical expression. The frequencies of expressions of the fragile
site varied from 3% to 16%, without any relation to the clinical seriousness of

the disease. On the contrary, the unaffected individuals that were examined did not show spontaneous expression of the fragile site in any of the 100 meta-phases scored for each individual.

Discussion and Conclusion

Previous studies have shown that in families with high gene penetrance and consistent autosomal dominant pattern of inheritance, the probability of trans-mission of the disease to future offspring approaches to 50% [10–13]. In the family we studied, hypertrophic cardiomyopathy was transmitted in 66% of the members in the second generation. A possible explanation is that both mother and father were affected, the first by a subclinical form, the second by hyper-trophic cardiomyopathy as suggested from juvenile premature sudden death. The occurrence of both parents being diseased may also be, in part, responsible for the high degree of malignancy. The frequency and the modality of occur-rence of the disease in the third generation are consistent with the proposed autosomal dominant mode of transmission.

The finding of a fragile site on chromosome 16 in all the individuals affected by hypertrophic cardiomyopathy and its absence in the unaffected ones may suggest that in this family a correlation exists between the presence of this fragile site and hypertrophic cardiomyopathy, also in the subclinical form. The percentage of expression of the fragile site does not seem to be correlated with the seriousness of clinical expression, since the highest value (16%) is found in individuals III-7, with minimal symptoms, and in III-9 presenting moderate symptoms.

We conclude that it is worthwhile studying the remaining components of this family, and other families with both familial or sporadic hypertrophic cardio-myopathy with the aim of verifying the possible correlation between the pres-ence of the fragile site on chromosome 16 and hypertrophic cardiomyopathy.

References

1. Evans W (1949) Familial cardiomegaly. Br Heart J 11:68–81
2. Bridgen W (1957) Uncommon myocardial disease – the non coronary cardiomyopathies. Lancet ii:1179–1184, 1243–1249
3. Emanuel R, Whithers R, O'Brien K (1971) Dominant and recessive modes of inheritance in idiopathic cardiomyopathy. Lancet ii:1065–1067
4. Goodwin JF (1980) Hypertrophic cardiomyopathy: a disease in search of its own identity. Am J Cardiol 45:177–180
5. Bridgen W (1987) Hypertrophic cardiomyopathy. Br Heart J 58:299–302
6. Clark EC, Henry LW, Epstein ES (1973) Familial prevalence and genetic transmission of idiopathic hypertrophic subaortic stenosis. N Engl J Med 289:709–714
7. van Dorp GW, ten Cate FJ, Vletter BW, Dohmen H, Roelandt J (1976) Familial preva-lence of asymmetric septal hypertrophy. Eur J Cardiol 4:349–357
8. Csanàdy M, Högye M, Forster T (1987) Hypertrophic cardiomyopathy associated with congenital deaf-mutism. Eur Heart J 8:528–534

9. Cirò E, Maron BJ, Roberts WC (1982) Coexistence of asymmetric and symmetric left ventricular hypertrophy in a family with hypertrophic cardiomyopathy. Am Heart J 104:643–646

10. Cirò E, Nichols PF III, Maron BJ (1983) Heterogeneous morphologic expression of genetically transmitted hypertrophic cardiomyopathy – two dimensional echocardiographic analysis. Circulation 67:1227–1233

11. Maron BJ, Nichols PF III, Pickle LW, Wesley YE, Mulvihill JJ (1984) Patterns of inheritance in hypertrophic cardiomyopathy: assessment by M-mode and two-dimensional echocardiography. Am J Cardiol 53:1087–1094

12. Emanuel R, Marcomichelakis J, Whithers R, O'Brien K (1983) Asymmetrical septal hypertrophy and hypertrophic cardiomyopathy. Br Heart J 49:309–316

13. Maron BJ, Mulvihill JJ (1986) The genetics of hypertrophic cardiomyopathy. Ann Intern Med 105:610–613

14. Maron BJ, Spirito P, Wesley Y, Arce J (1986) Development and progression of left ventricular hypertrophy in children with hypertrophic cardiomyopathy. N Engl J Med 315:610–614

15. Sutherland G, Hecht F (1985) Fragile sites on human chromosomes. Oxford University Press, Oxford

Medical Treatment of Hypertrophic Cardiomyopathy

R. Hopf and M. Kaltenbach

Introduction

In 1907 Schmincke [93] was the first to describe diffuse "hyperplasia" of the heart muscle, involving predominantly the wall of the left ventricular outflow tract, in two female patients. In 1958 Teare [104] presented pathologic findings of asymmetrical hypertrophy of the heart in young adults, eight of whom died from sudden death, seven of them during physical activity. In 1964 Braunwald et al. [9] described the findings in 64 patients with hypertrophic cardiomyopathy (HCM), emphasizing angiographically determined normal or even supernormal left ventricular function and hemodynamically documented large variations of outflow tract gradient. Today, there seems to be no doubt that impaired diastolic function of the left ventricle is the predominant hemodynamic characteristic in HCM [106, 107].

By 1962, it had been demonstrated that drugs with positive inotropic action augment outflow tract gradient in hypertrophic obstructive cardiomyopathy (HOCM) [8], so that various degrees of obstruction were thought to be under beta-adrenergic modulation, as, for example, during physical activity [27]. After it had been shown that the positive inotropic effects of isoprenaline administration could be acutely counteracted by pronethalol [26], beta-blockade seemed be a rational modality of medical treatment of hypertrophic cardiomyopathy.

The importance of the calcium ion in the pathogenesis of hypercontraction and impaired relaxation had been repeatedly emphasized; we therefore initiated calcium antagonist therapy in patients with hypertrophic cardiomyopathy in 1973 and first presented our results in 1976 and in 1979 [40, 49, 50]. The effect of the combined therapy with nifedipine and propranolol we described in 1987 [45]. With regard to the role of ventricular arrhythmia associated with sudden death [70], antiarrhythmic drugs, especially amiodarone have been given to patients with hypertrophic cardiomyopathy since 1981 [73].

Therapy with Beta-Adrenergic Blocking Agents

It has been discussed that increased activity of sympathetic nerves in the heart or a disorder of inotropic catecholamine stimulation might be closely associated with the systolic features in hypertrophic cardiomyopathy [26, 58]. Hemodynamic measurements seemed to confirm this hypothesis, because exercise, tachycardia, emotion, and circulatory active drugs augmented contractility as well as outflow tract obstruction [8, 9]. It therefore appeared to be a rational concept to treat patients with hypertrophic cardiomyopathy with beta-adrenergic blocking agents.

A reduction in heart rate at rest and a modulation of rate increase during exertion is expected because of the negative chronotropy which in turn may improve exercise tolerance [26]. The effects of pronethalol had not been marked at rest, but, owing to negative inotropic action, hemodynamic studies uncovered a slight decrease in ventricular systolic pressure and outflow obstruction [103]. A reduction in the basal gradient in the left ventricle was observed only in a few patients [16, 25], whereas an increase in gradient with sympathetic stimulation could usually be prevented, the spontaneous variation of the obstruction decreased, and the effective outflow orifice presumably widened [20, 32, 80, 98]. Left ventricular end-diastolic and end-systolic volume showed a significant increase, and ejection fraction was reduced [103], but cardiac index usually did not change [20, 26]. Depending on early hemodynamic or noninvasive studies, it was suggested that propranolol might decrease left ventricular filling pressure and improve left ventricular diastolic function by shortening the isovolumic relaxation time and increasing myocardial distensibility [15, 98, 103]. In contrast, other investigators could demonstrate that beta-blocking agents did not greatly influence ventricular diastolic function, but could increase filling pressure at rest and during exercise [33, 63, 80].

In HOCM, as well as in the nonobstructive form (HNCM), beta-blocking agents can relieve typical symptoms such as dyspnea and angina, but they seldom improve lightheadedness or syncope [11, 12]. Exercise tolerance was improved only in some patients [12, 62]. In contrast, some patients were described as feeling better under placebo [98]. Long-term observations showed symptomatic benefit [20] in some cases, but more often complaints remained unaffected or reappeared during therapy [2, 24, 25]. In addition, the favorable hemodynamic effects following acute intravenous administration of beta-blockers could not be reproduced during long-term oral therapy, where the obstruction was seen to partly reappear [100]. End diastolic pressure and mean pulmonary artery pressure were not influenced by long-term therapy [4, 63, 100]. Perhaps owing to relatively low doses of beta-blockers, the overall clinical course was not influenced and the mortality remained high [53, 60]. More satisfying results were reported by Frank et al. [21, 22], who administered a mean oral dose of 500 mg propranolol per day, and whose results were interpretated as "complete beta-blockade". Unfortunately, it appears, however, that beta-blockers influence neither the disease progression nor the incidence of sudden death [1, 19].

Our own experience is related to the observation of 17 (two female and 15 male) patients (age: 24–59 years, mean: 44 years). They had been treated for 3–106 (mean: 31) months with beta-blockers, given doses as high as subjectively tolerated, i.e., up to 480 mg propranolol per day. In only three cases could initial and temporal improvement be seen, but in all cases slow progressive or recurrent deterioration was reported, and exercise tolerance did not improve in any case. The Sokolow index remained unchanged (4.9 and 4.8 mV, respectively). Heart size, calculated by X-ray techniques [34, 77, 78], showed an enlargement from 850 to 915 ml/1.73 m^2 (for reasons of better comparability, the heart volume was calculated for a body surface area of 1.73 m^2; normal: men < 800, and women < 700 ml/1,73 m^2), paralleled by an echocardiographic increase of left atrial diameter from 42 to 44 mm, whereas left ventricular wall thickness remained unchanged (interventricular septum 24 vs. 25 mm and posterior left ventricular wall 15 mm at the beginning and at the end of the follow-up period).

Therapy with Calcium Antagonists

In 1976 we presented the first data describing therapeutic results achieved with verapamil in 20 patients with HCM. During the 14 months treatment, most patients reported impressive relief of symptoms, accompanied by reduction in QRS amplitude and heart volume [40, 49]. In 1979, we could confirm these results through longer studies with 22 patients [50]. Also in 1979, Rosing et al. [87] were able to show that intravenously administered verapamil significantly decreased outflow obstruction in hypertrophic obstructive cardiomyopathy and, given orally, improved exercise capacity and symptomatic status compared with placebo and propranolol [88]. In 1980, Hanrath et al. [30] verified that verapamil improved left ventricular relaxation and filling. These results could be confirmed by radionuclide angiograms [6, 7, 43] and by hemodynamic investigations following acute and chronic verapamil administration [3] or after nifedipine [61]. Furthermore, we have presented our results of long-term verapamil treatment (up to more than 10 years) [35, 36, 38, 39, 41, 42, 44, 46–48, 50], and experience following nifedipine and diltiazem therapy were also published.

Studies on Verapamil

For more than 10 years now, verapamil has been shown to be an effective therapeutic agent in the medical treatment of HCM, relieving dyspnea and angina, and achieving sustained improvement in exercise capacity [38, 44, 65, 89]. Following intravenous administration of verapamil, left ventricular outflow tract gradient, filling pressure, and contractility were significantly reduced [37, 87]. An oral dose of 160 mg verapamil reduced the filling pressure [37]. Hemodynamic effects have also been evident during exercise [31, 36, 37, 52, 63]. The good clinical results from verapamil in patients with HCM can probably be explained by the improvement in systolic and particularly in diastolic left ventricular function, irrespective of whether there is an outflow tract obstruction or not [6, 10, 31, 33, 38, 52, 54, 90]. We investigated the hemodynamic effects of verapamil following intracoronary, intravenous, and oral administration.

Effects of Intracoronary Administration (Fig. 1): To evaluate its exclusive myocardial effects, verapamil was administered into the left coronary artery in seven patients with HOCM (five males and two females; age: 41–65 years, mean: 49 years). The mean dose was 1.6 mg (1.5–2.0 mg). Following slow administration, no verapamil could be detected in the plasma. Hemodynamic measurements were performed after 5 min. Heart rate fell from 75.4 to 71 beats per minute (not significant), and systolic left ventricular pressure went down from 128.3 to 107.9 mmHg (not significant). Left ventricular filling pressure was 25.7 mmHg before and 21.6 mmHg after verapamil ($2 p < 0.02$). The basal left ventricular outflow tract gradient was reduced from 45.4 to 25.9 ($2 p < 0.02$) and the maximal gradient (following provocation: nitroglycerine, Valsalva maneuver, and postextrasystolic augmentation) from 107 to 63.9 mmHg ($2 p < 0.01$). dp/dt_{max} was reduced from 2107 to 1650 mmHg/s (not significant).

Effects of Intravenous Administration: In 15 patients (14 male and one female; age: 29–62 years, mean: 45 years) we investigated the effects of slow intravenous verapamil administration (10 mg over 10 min). Heart rate increased from 67.7 to 75.6 beats per min ($2 p < 0.03$) while dp/dt_{max} remained unaffected (2243 vs. 2231 mmHg/s (not significant). Systolic left ventricular pressure fell from 118.7 to 110.6 mmHg ($2 p < 0.02$). Left ventricular filling pressure was 19.5 mmHg before and 16.6 mmHg after verapamil ($2 p < 0.05$). In nine patients with obstructive cardiomyopathy, the basal left ventricular outflow tract gradient was reduced from 45.3 to 32.9 (not significant), and the maximal gradient dropped markedly from 117.1 to 80.4 mmHg ($2 p < 0.01$). In ten of the 15 patients, ergometry was performed before and after verapamil. The increase of systolic blood pressure and of left ventricular filling pressure was found to be reduced after verapamil (left ventricular systolic pressure from 158.5 to 153.6 (not significant)), while end-diastolic pressure was reduced from 36.3 to 27.5 mmHg ($2 p < 0.05$).

Effects of Oral Administration (Fig. 2): The effects of oral verapamil are of greatest interest. We investigated a total of 18 patients, 12 of whom (three females and nine males) had HOCM. The age ranged from 16–59 years (mean 39 years). Measurements were performed before and 50 min after 160 mg oral verapamil was given and diagnostic angiography and myocardial biopsy were carried out. To take into account the hemodynamic effects of radiopaque medium, hemodynamic changes were measured before and after angiography in six patients without medication. This group consisted of two female and four male patients, whose ages ranged from 26 to 57 years (mean 48 years); all had HOCM. In the control group, heart rate (67.3 vs. 70.5 beats per minute), systolic blood pressure (141.2 vs. 135.7 mmHg), dp/dt_{max} (2880 vs. 2740 mmHg/s), and the degree of outflow tract obstruction (basal gradient 58.2 vs. 52.0, maximal gradient 129.2 vs. 124.2 mmHg) were reduced, whereas left ventricular filling pressure increased from 25.7 to 28.2 mmHg. In the 12 patients receiving oral verapamil medication, heart rate (74.6 vs. 72.8 beats per minute) and systolic blood pressure (131.0 vs. 117.5 mmHg) tended to show reductions; these changes were not significant, however, when compared to the

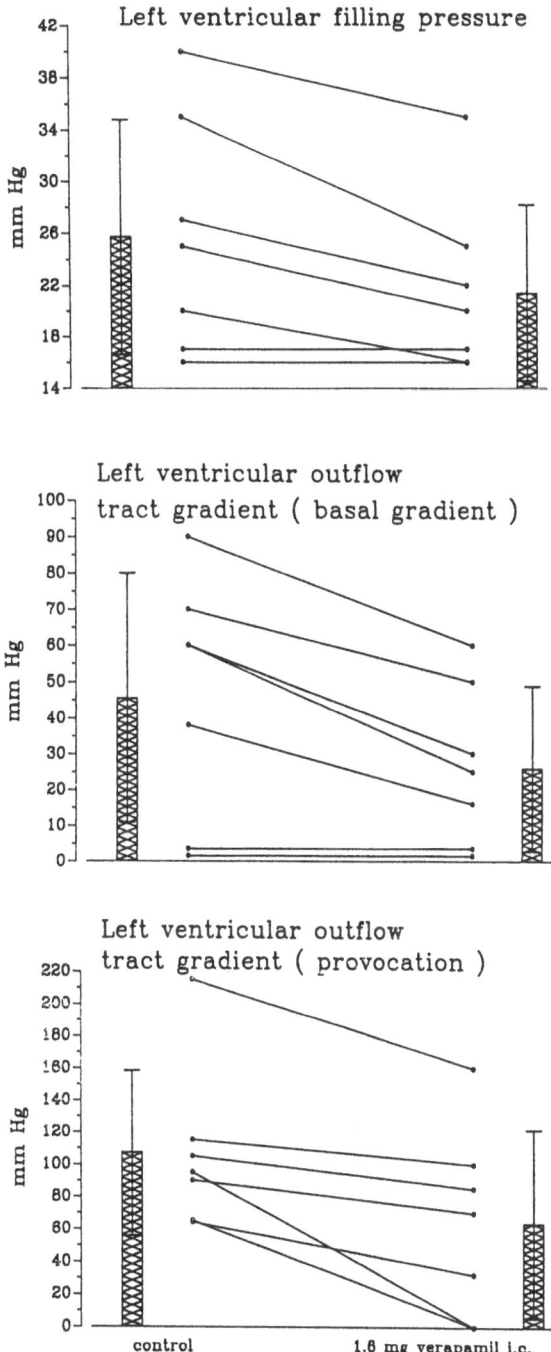

Fig. 1. Hemodynamic effects of intracoronary administration of 1.6 mg verapamil in seven patients with HCM. There was a significant reduction in left ventricular filling pressure ($2\,p < 0.02$) as well as in left ventricular outflow tract gradient (basal gradient: $2\,p < 0.02$; following provocation: $2\,p < 0.01$)

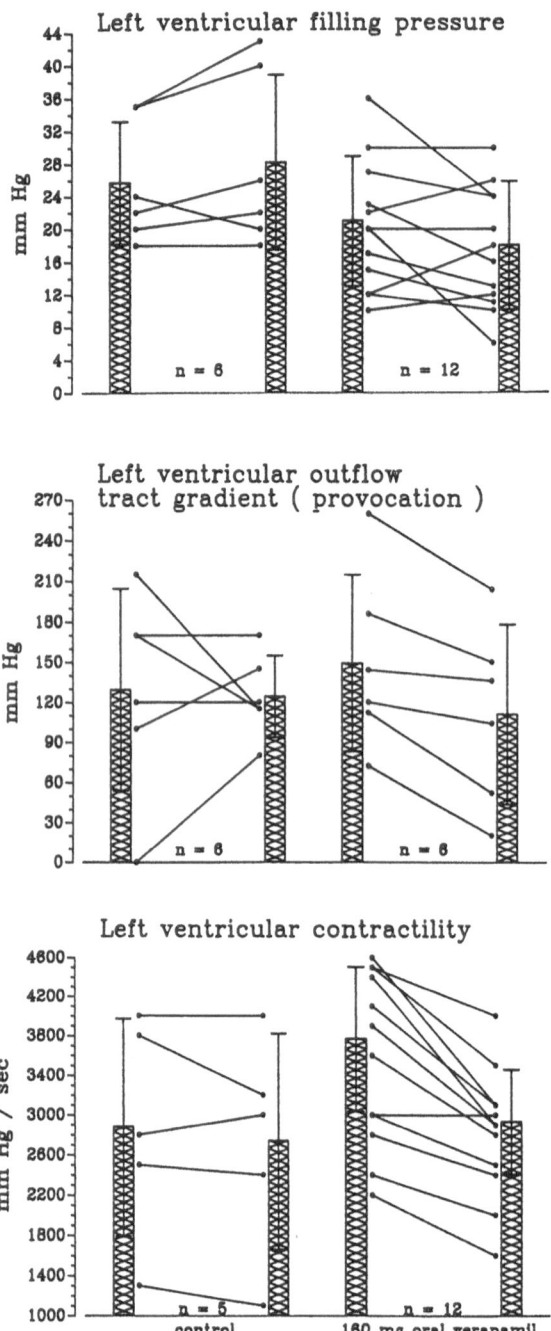

Fig. 2. Left ventricular filling pressure, outflow tract gradient, and contractility before and after routine heart catheterization in 18 patients with HCM: six control patients received no medication; in 12 patients hemodynamic effects of 160 mg oral verapamil were studied. Verapamil significantly reduced filling pressure ($2\,p < 0.05$) and contractility ($2\,p < 0.02$), and in tendency the outflow tract gradient in the six patients with obstruction

control group. But left ventricular filling pressure was significantly reduced from 20.3 to 17.5 mmHg (2 $p < 0.05$) as well as dp/dt$_{max}$ from 3770 to 2935 mmHg/s (2 $p < 0.02$). In the subgroup of six patients with HOCM, there was only a trend towards a reduction of the obstruction (basal gradient 51.0 vs. 42.7 mmHg and maximal gradient 149.0 vs. 111.0 mmHg), when compared to the control group (not significant). These results confirm other experience: verapamil predominantly improves diastolic left ventricular function, but can also reduce high contractility and the degree of the left ventricular obstruction.

Our Clinical Experience: Our clinical experience with verapamil covers 101 consecutive patients (21 women and 80 men; age: 12–61 years, mean: 43 years), with HNCM in 31 and the obstructive form (left ventricular outflow tract pressure gradient exceeding 30 mmHg) in 70 cases. The patients were treated with mean oral daily doses of 506 mg verapamil in 76 cases, with 166 mg gallopamil in 22, and 30 mg nifedipine in three cases, with the follow-up period being between 6 and 175 months (mean 78.3 months); 29 patients had been treated for more than 10 years. Thus, our experience is based on a total of 659 patient treatment years (Table 1). For each patient the mean values for all data acquired during calcium antagonist therapy were calculated and then compared with individual primary values. Complete echocardiographic measurements are available in patients included in the study since 1976.

Results: Prior to therapy with calcium antagonists, 90% of patients were symptomatic, mostly with effort-induced dyspnea and angina pectoris (Table 2).

Table 1. Data of 101 patients with proven HCM and treated with calcium antagonists

Sex female: 21; male: 80
Age (years) 43 ± 11.8 (range: 12–61)

HNCM 31	(definition: max. LV gradient ≤ 30 mmHg)
HOCM 70	max. gradient: 102 ± 56 (32–290) mmHg
RV gradient	(definition: max. LV gradient ≥ 10 mmHg)
	HOCM: 15; HNCM: 5
	14.6 ± 6.3 (10–32) mmHg
LVEDP (mmHg)	19.3 ± 9.2 (5–48)
	HOCM: 20.2 ± 9.9 (5–48)
	HNCM: 17.3 ± 6.9 (8–32)
Treatment period	78.3 (6–175) months
	659 patient treatment years

Medication
Verapamil	76:	506 ± 93 (240–720) mg
Gallopamil	22:	166 ± 24 (150–200) mg
Nifedipine	3:	30 mg
Concomitant medication		
Saluretics	16	
Antiarrhythmic agents	9	
Digitalis	1	
Salicylates/anticoagulants	4	

Only ten patients were symptom free. During therapy, 85% of the previously symptomatic patients reported improvement or even complete relief of symptoms. There was no change in 12 patients. In only three patients had symptoms and stress tolerance slightly deteriorated. According to the New York Heart Association (NYHA) classification, an improvement from functional class 2.73 to 1.95 was achieved in the mean of all 101 patients (Fig. 3).

Follow-up electrocardiograms during calcium antagonist treatment were available in 99 patients. The mean Sokolow index significantly decreased from 4.87 to 4.5 mV within the first 24 months and was 4.37 mV at the end of the treatment period (Fig. 4). The cardiac configuration, evaluated by conventional chest X-rays in the standing position as well as the cardiac size remained unchanged during calcium antagonist treatment. Heart volume measurements were available in 100 patients and showed a reduction from 960.9 to 900.3 ml/1.73 m^2 within 24 months. Heart volume was 910.7 ml/1.73 m^2 at the end of observation (Fig. 4.)

Table 2. Symptoms of 101 patients with HCM before and during therapy with calcium antagonists

Before therapy	During therapy					
	(n)	Disap-peared	Improved	Unchanged	Worsened	Newly Appeared
Dyspnea	72	23	36	11	2	5
Angina pectoris	69	9	49	9	2	3
Arrhythmias/ palpitations	45	14	22	8	1	7
Syncope/ collapse	17	12	3	2	–	2
Vertigo	20	10	7	2	1	7
Weakness	17	12	4	1	–	6

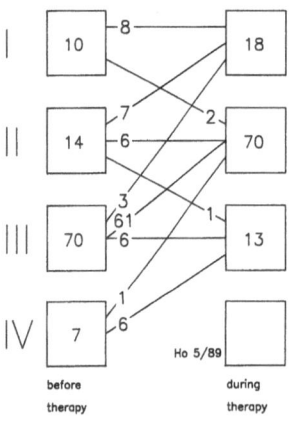

Fig. 3. Symptomatic status of 101 patients with HCM before and during therapy with calcium antagonists according to NYHA classification (I–IV)

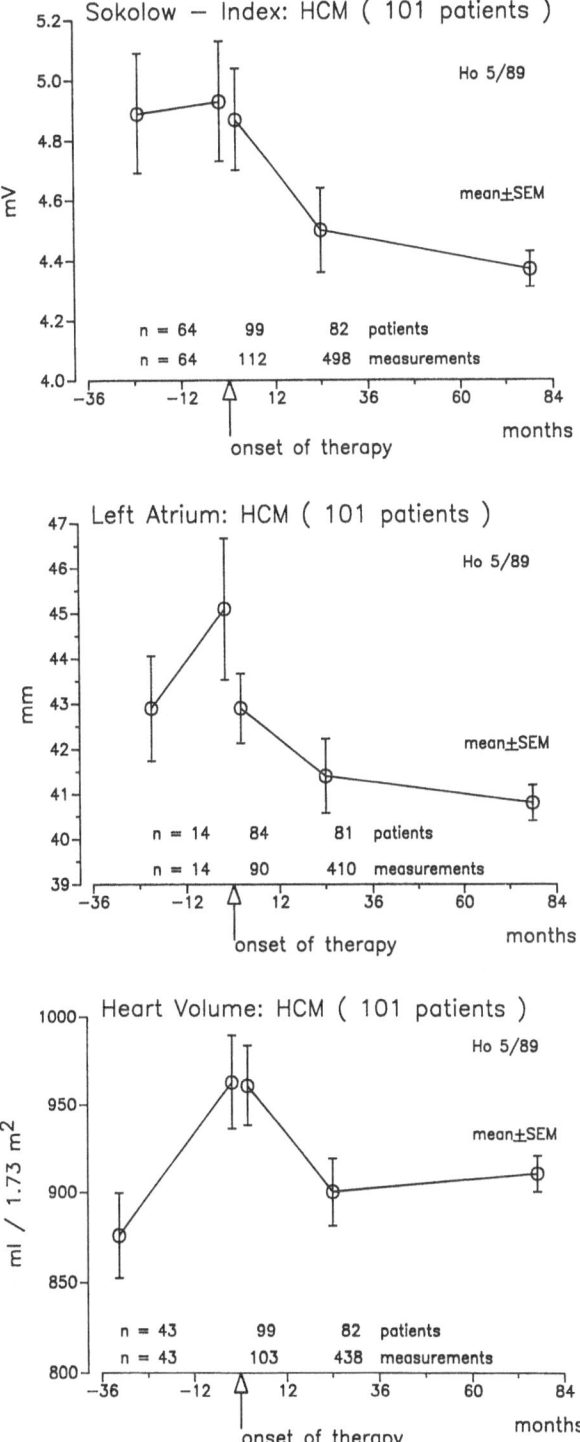

Fig. 4. Behaviour of Sokolow index, echocardiographic left atrial diameter and radiologic heart volume before and during therapy with calcium antagonists in 101 patients with HCM

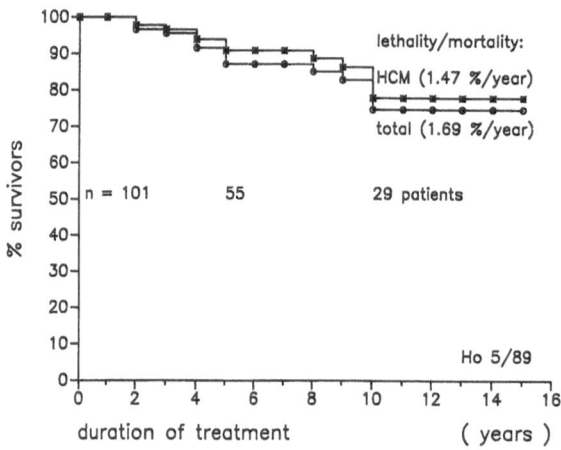

Fig. 5. Survival probability in 101 patients with HCM treated with calcium antagonists; 10-year survival probability (calculated by the method of Kaplan and Meier) is 74.7%

Paralleling the changes in heart volume during therapy with calcium antagonists, left atrial diameter decreased from 42.9 to 41.4 mm within the first 24 months and was 40.8 at the end of observation. There were no significant changes in left ventricular wall thickness (intraventricular septum: 22.5 vs. 21.4 and posterior wall 14.1 vs. 13.6 mm).

The annual mortality in our patients, related to cardiomyopathy, was 1.5%. The cardiac 10-year survival probability (Kaplan-Meier test) was 74.7% (Fig. 5).

Studies on Diltiazem

In 1983, Nagao et al. [79] demonstrated with echocardiography in 11 patients that intravenously administered diltiazem decreased isovolumic left ventricular relaxation time and thus might improve impaired diastolic filling patterns in hypertrophic cardiomyopathy. Suwa et al. [102] compared diltiazem and propranolol, and found left ventricular diastolic function only improved following acute intravenous or chronic oral diltiazem administration. Although no controlled clinical trials have been reported as yet, it could be expected that diltiazem, because of its similar hemodynamic actions, might have effects on hypertrophic cardiomyopathy similar to those of verapamil.

Studies on Nifedipine

Nifedipine has also been reported to improve diastolic ventricular function in patients with hypertrophic cardiomyopathy. Lorell et al. [61] first demonstrated modification of left ventricular filling pattern in a patient with HNCM. This could be confirmed by systematic studies [62, 94]. In contrast, Betocchi et al. were unable to see these effects on systolic and diastolic function in 36 patients with HCM, including 17 with HOCM [5]. Nifedipine diminishes peripheral vascular resistance and can thereby produce hemodynamic instability with provocation or augmentation of outflow tract obstruction [5, 52]. Following acute administration or short-term therapy with sublingual nifedipine, cardiac index usually increases in association with a fall in blood pressure and filling pressure [5, 82, 90, 92], whereas the behavior of left ventricular outflow tract gradient is nonuniform [90, 92].

Combination of Calcium Antagonists and Beta-Blockers

It could be supposed that the hemodynamic effects of propranolol on supernormal left ventricular systolic function and those of nifedipine on impaired diastolic function together might improve cardiac function and consequently the symptoms as well. Although clinical investigations with beta-blockers only showed minor effects on ventricular systolic function at rest, augmentation of obstruction following provocation could be prevented. Calcium antagonists predominantly improve diastolic left ventricular function. Therefore, it has been suggested that the combination of beta-blockers and calcium antagonists might constitute a beneficial therapeutic approach [14, 23, 55]. Combined therapy should be especially effective with the beta-blocker propranolol because there is no intrinsic sympathomimetic activity which could produce an attenuation of the desired effects. It seems to be rational to use nifedipine as a calcium antagonist, thereby improving especially the diastolic function without additional negative chronotropic or dromotropic effects. In addition, data have shown that nifedipine has beneficial short-term effects on ventricular dynamics which are further improved by propranolol and vice versa [28].

Our Clinical Experience: Our study comprised 15 patients with hypertrophic cardiomyopathy (14 male, one female; age 22–67 years, mean 45.5 years). HNCM was present in five and HOCM in ten patients. Left ventricular filling pressures ranged from 5 to 32 (mean: 16) mmHg. Twelve patients had undergone pretreatment with verapamil, one with propranolol; two had no previous therapy. Combined medication was initiated with a daily oral dose of 30 mg nifedipine and 240 mg propranolol. The duration of combined therapy was 6–24 (mean: 18) months. Owing to side effects, premature termination became necessary in three patients after 6 months, and in two patients after 12 months. The other ten patients tolerated the combined treatment well. The study was stopped when eight patients had been treated for 24 months and two for 18 months.

During treatment with nifedipine and propranolol, improvement occurred in two patients, no change in five, and deterioration in eight patients. Two patients exhibited syncope for the first time while under this therapy. The symptomatic status, according to the NYHA classification, was 1.9 before and 2.1 at the end of therapy.

The Sokolow index of all patients showed no significant change during nifedipine-propranolol therapy, but the heart volume increased significantly from 887 to 947 ml/1.73 m^2 body surface area. On echocardiography, a significant increase in left atrial diameter from 40 to 42 mm was evident, whereas left ventricular wall thickness did not change (intraventricular septum: 20.5 vs. 21.5 mm; posterior wall: 13.1 vs. 13.6 mm).

Our results indicate that the combination of nifedipine and propranolol has no favorable clinical effects in patients with hypertrophic cardiomyopathy [45].

Therapy with Antiarrhythmic Agents

Arrhythmias, including supraventricular tachyarrhythmias, bradyarrhythmias, and heart block, are frequent in patients with hypertrophic cardiomyopathy [70, 97]. Nonsustained ventricular tachycardia can be present even in patients with normal exercise tolerance and without symptomatic episodes and may be associated with cardiac arrest [64, 68, 69, 71]. The aim of antiarrhythmic therapy is prevention of sudden cardiac death, but conventional agents, such as quinidine or mexiletine, when used alone or in combination with moderate doses of beta-blockers were unsuccessful and not well tolerated [67].

Studies on Disopyramide

Disopyramide has also been proven to be potentially effective in the treatment of supraventricular and ventricular arrhythmias in patients with hypertrophic cardiomyopathy. The observation that this drug with its negative inotropic action is able to reduce the degree of outflow tract obstruction seemed to be an additional argument for the introduction into the therapeutic regimen [84]. However, part of the reduction in the pressure gradient is related to an increase in peripheral resistance and blood pressure. Following short-term administration, improvement in symptoms and exercise capacity could be seen [85, 86, 96], but long-term experience is not yet available. Effectiveness of disopyramide on rhythm disturbances has been reported to be poor in patients with hypertrophic cardiomyopathy [67].

Studies on Amiodarone

Because amiodarone is effective in preventing and converting supraventricular as well as serious ventricular arrhythmias, it can be assumed to play an important role in the therapy of hypertrophic cardiomyopathy [68, 72]. Supraventricular arrhythmias have been suppressed or even abolished. Ventricular tachycardia was almost completely prevented [74]. In comparison to conventional antiarrhythmic treatment, amiodarone reduced the mortality rate [75]. However, inefficacy and potential increase in the rate of sudden death has also been described [57]. Independently of antiarrhythmic effects, systolic anterior motion of the mitral valve was seen to disappear after treatment [17], and improvement of symptoms and prolongation of exercise tolerance was described in some patients [56]; this was, however, not seen during long-term treatment [83]. In addition, hemodynamic measurements as well as radionuclide angiography did not show beneficial effects [83, 101]. Side effects are well documented, so that an individual dose titration is advised [76]. Amiodarone might thus be useful in patients with refractory arrhythmias [65]; the combination with calcium antagonists seems, in our experience, to be useful and without major complications.

Other Medications

Formerly, diuretics were assumed to be dangerous in HOCM because of a possible reduction in preload and subsequent augmentation of outflow tract obstruction. In our experience, however, these agents have proved to be useful, especially in patients with pulmonary congestion and peripheral edema. Today, diuretics are usually included in the therapeutic regimen, and their beneficial effects are mainly attributed to the reduction in left ventricular filling pressure [65].

However, drugs which cause rapid reduction in preload, such as nitroglycerine, or with positive inotropy are potentially dangerous in HOCM, but in some special events during tachyarrhythmia, digitalis might become necessary to delay atrioventricular conduction.

There are HCM patients with normal systolic ventricular function who suffer from pulmonary congestion due to "diastolic heart failure." In these cases, it can be helpful to administer sublingual verapamil or nifedipine in addition to saluretic basic medication. In later stages of the disease, some patients with HCM may have severely impaired systolic left ventricular function and, therefore, congestive heart failure. Our experience indicates that, even for these patients, the combination of verapamil with diuretics is able to improve symptoms and exercise tolerance.

Comparison of Different Treatment Regimens and Conclusions

There are the following goals of therapeutic intervention which are the basis in the comparison of treatment regimens and their value: a reduction in symptoms and thereby an improvement of exercise tolerance, a retardation or even prevention of disease progression, and an improvement of the patients' prognosis.

High-risk patients with the obstructive form of hypertrophic cardiomyopathy are characterized by a familial history or episodes of syncope and/or rapid subjective and objective progression, and manifestation in childhood. In these cases, surgery with myotomy/myectomy must be discussed, although in many of them impressive improvement can be seen following verapamil treatment. Kober et al. [51] conducted a multicenter study comparing verapamil with propranolol in a 2-year treatment in matched pairs of patients with HCM. On the basis of symptoms and electrocardiograms, verapamil showed better results than high doses of propranolol. Side effects and deterioration were also seen more often in the propranolol group. Severe side effects following verapamil described by Epstein and Rosing [19] cannot be confirmed by us. Usually, verapamil was well tolerated. Only one of our patients developed first-degree atrioventricular block, and we did not observe pulmonary edema due to verapamil in any patient, including those with high outflow tract gradients or very high left ventricular filling pressures [38]. Verapamil improved maximum exercise tolerance and hemodynamics; no comparable effects were brought about by propranolol [63]. This is in agreement with the results of Suwa et al. [102], who found diastolic left ventricular function improved only after long-term diltiazem therapy, but not with long-term propranolol therapy. Similar results were reported when verapamil was compared to pindolol, with the calcium antagonist clearly considered superior to the beta-blocker [66]. In contrast, nifedipine alone was not seen to be more effective than propranolol [14], but the combined short-term administration of both drugs had favorable hemodynamic effects [55].

The clinical results of amiodarone therapy are contradictory; thus, it is considered as a therapeutic option only in those patients in whom conventional treatment has failed [65].

It is not yet clear if any therapeutic intervention is potent enough to stop the process of hypertrophy or hyperplasia in HCM, but results indicate at least a probable retardation of the disease progression with surgery or verapamil therapy [49, 54]. Perhaps this is only the consequence of the hemodynamic effects which can also be shown in children and adolescents [99]. The disease may be – analogous to the model of calcium overload in the myocardium of Syrian hamsters [81] – the results of increased intracellular calcium concentrations or may be due to increased calcium receptors [105].

The natural history of HCM is characterized by slow progression, but sudden death may occur independently of objective findings and symptomatic status. It has been shown that annual mortality is about 3.5% in untreated symptomatic patients [29, 59, 95]. Medical or surgical treatment may improve prognosis [91]. Only Frank et al. [22, 23] have reported a better prognosis in patients treated with propranolol; others have seen no improvement [53, 59, 60] or only minor effects [91]. Prognosis was significantly better in patients who successfully underwent surgery or were treated with verapamil [29, 53, 59, 60, 100]. It has been shown that verapamil beside improving left ventricular function has antiarrhythmic effects [13]. When compared to verapamil, amiodarone was shown to have the more pronounced antiarrhythmic effects [67], but it has not been clearly demonstrated to improve life expectancy in HCM [57, 65]. It therefore seems rational to treat patients with HCM with calcium antagonists, especially with verapamil or gallopamil also. With regard to a probable improvement in life expectation, we consider that it is, in addition, reasonable to treat patients early, even those without symptoms. Rhythm disturbances should be treated with supplementary antiarrhythmics, for example, amiodarone. We saw no problems with this combination, but repeat studies of its effectiveness are necessary. If patients do not respond to medical treatment, surgery can be considered an alternative in the obstructive form of cardiomyopathy.

References

1. Adelmann AG, Shah PM, Gramiak R, Wigle ED (1970) Long-term propranolol therapy in muscular subaortic stenosis. Br Heart J 32:804–811
2. Adelman AG, Wigle ED, Ranganathan R, Webb GD, Kidd BSC, Bigelow WG, Silver MD (1972) The clinical course of muscular subaortic stenosis. Ann Intern Med 77:515–525
3. Anderson DM, Raff GL, Ports TA, Brundage BH, Parmley WW, Chatterjee K (1984) Hypertrophic obstructive cardiomyopathy: effects of acute and chronic verapamil treatment on left ventricular systolic and diastolic function. Br Heart J 51:523–529

4. Assmann H, Assmann I, Fiehring H, Dittrich P, Eger H (1975) Verlaufsbeobachtungen bei der idiopathischen hypertrophischen subaortalen Stenose unter Propranololbehandlung. Dtsch Gesundheitswes 30:918–920

5. Betocchi S, Cannon RO, Watson RM, Bonow RO, Ostrow HG, Epstein SE, Rosing DR (1985) Effects of sublingual nifedipine on hemodynamics and systolic and diastolic function in patients with hypertrophic cardiomyopathy. Circulation 72:1001–1007

6. Bonow RO, Rosing DR, Bacharach SL, Green MV, Kent KM, Lipson LC, Maron BJ, Epstein SE (1981) Effects of verapamil on left ventricular systolic function and diastolic filling in patients with hypertrophic cardiomyopathy. Circulation 64:787–796

7. Bonow RO, Dilsizian V, Rosing DR, Maron BJ, Bacharach SL, Green MV (1985) Verapamil-induced improvement in left ventricular diastolic filling and increased exercise tolerance in patients with hypertrophic cardiomyopathy: short- and long-term effects. Circulation 72:853–864

8. Braunwald E, Ebert PA (1962) Hemodynamic alterations in idiopathic hypertrophic subaortic stenosis induced by sympatho-mimetic drugs. Am J Cardiol 10:489–491

9. Braunwald E, Lambrew CT, Rockoff SD, Ross J Jr, Morrow AG (1964) Idiopathic hypertrophic subaortic stenosis: A description of the disease based upon an analysis of 64 patients. Circulation [Suppl 4] 30:IV 3 – IV 213

10. Bryhn M, Eskilsson J (1987) Effects of verapamil on left ventricular diastolic function at rest and during isometric exercise in patients with hypertrophic cardiomyopathy. Clin Cardiol 10:31–36

11. Cherian G, Brockington IF, Shah PM, Oakley CM, Goodwin JF (1966) Beta-adrenergic blockade in hypertrophic obstructive cardiomyopathy. Br Med J 1:895–898

12. Cohen LS, Braunwald E (1967) Amelioration of angina pectoris in idiopathic hypertrophic subaortic stenosis with beta adrenergic blockade. Circulation 35:847–851

13. Cranefield PF, Aronson RS, Wit AL (1974) Effect of verapamil on the normal action potential and on a calcium dependent slow response of canine Purkinje fibers. Circ Res 34:204–213

14. Cserhalmi L, Aßmann I, Glavanow M, Rev J, Kelecseneyi Z (1984) Langzeittherapie der hypertrophischen obstruktiven und nichtobstruktiven Kardiomyopathie mit Nifedipin im Vergleich zu Propranolol. Z Gesamte Inn Med 39:330–335

15. De la Calzada CS, Ziady GM, Hardarson T, Curiel R, Goodwin JF (1976) Effect of acute administration of propranolol on ventricular function in hypertrophic obstructive cardiomyopathy measured by non-invasive techniques. Br Heart J 38:798–803

16. El Gamal M, Schasfort GBA, Schrijvers LCM (1975) Relief of severe left ventricular outflow obstruction in a case of hypertrophic obstructive cardiomyopathy treated with practolol. Br Heart J 37:225–228

17. Enia F, Comparato C, DiFranca F, Ledda A, Mizio G (1987) Systolic anterior motion of the mitral valve in patients with hypertrophic cardiomyopathy: disappearance after treatment with amiodarone. Chest 91:277–278

18. Epstein SE, Maron BJ (1980) Hypertrophic cardiomyopathy: an overview. Clin Invest Med 3:185–193

19. Epstein SE, Rosing DR (1981) Verapamil: its potential for causing serious complications in patients with hypertrophic cardiomyopathy. Circulation 64:437–441

20. Flamm MD, Harrison DC, Hancock EW (1968) Muscular subaortic stenosis: prevention of outflow obstruction with propranolol. Circulation 38:846–858

21. Frank MJ, Abdulla AM, Canedo MI, Saylors RE (1978) Long-term medical management of hypertrophic obstructive cardiomyopathy. Am J Cardiol 42:993–1001

22. Frank MJ, Abdulla AM, Watkins LO, Prisant L, Stefadouros MA (1983) Long-term medical management of hypertrophic cardiomyopathy: usefulness of propranolol. Eur Heart J [Suppl F] 4:155–164

23. Frank MJ, Watkins LO, Abdulla AM (1985) Management with beta-adrenergic blocking drugs. In: Ten Cate FJ (ed) Hypertrophic cardiomyopathy: clinical recognition and management. Dekker, New York, pp 155–172

24. Goodwin JF (1970) Congestive and hypertrophic cardiomyopathies. A decade of study. Lancet 1:731–739

25. Goodwin JF (1973) Treatment of cardiomyopathies. Am J Cardiol 32:341–351

26. Goodwin JF, Shah M, Oakley CM, Cohen J, Yipintsoi T, Pocock W (1964) The clinical pharmacology of hypertrophic obstructive cardiomyopathy. In: Wolstenholme GEW, O'Connor M (eds) Cardiomyopathies. Churchill, London, pp 189–213
27. Gorlin R, Cohen LS, Elliott WC, Klein MD, Lane FJ (1964) Haemodynamics of muscular subaortic stenosis (obstructive cardiomyopathy). In: Wolstenholme GEW, O'Connor M (eds) Cardiomyopathies. Churchill, London, pp 76–99
28. Gotsman MS, Lewis BS (1974) Left ventricular volumes and compliance in hypertrophic cardiomyopathy. Chest 66:498–505
29. Haberer T, Hess OM, Jenni R, Krayenbühl HP (1983) Hypertrophe obstruktive Kardiomyopathie: Spontanverlauf im Vergleich zur Langzeittherapie mit Propranolol und Verapamil. Z Kardio 72:487–493
30. Hanrath P, Mathey DG, Kremer P, Sonntag F, Bleifeld W (1980) Effect of verapamil on left ventricular isovolumic relaxation time and regional left ventricular isovolumic relaxation time and regional left ventricular filling in hypertrophic cardiomyopathy. Am J Cardiol 45:1258–1264
31. Hanrath P, Schlüter M, Sonntag F, Diemert J, Bleifeld W (1983) Influence of verapamil therapy on left ventricular performance at rest and during exercise in hypertrophic cardiomyopathy. Am J Cardiol 52:544–548
32. Harrison DC, Braunwald E, Glick G, Mason DT, Chidsey CA, Ross J Jr (1964) Effects of beta adrenergic blockade on the circulation, with particular reference to observations in patients with hypertrophic subaortic stenosis. Circulation 29:84–98
33. Hess OM, Grimm J, Krayenbühl HP (1983) Diastolic function in hypertrophic cardiomyopathy: effects of propranolol and verapamil on diastolic stiffness. Eur Heart J [Suppl F] 4:47–56
34. Hopf R, Kaltenbach M (1977) Röntgenologische Herzvolumenbestimmung: Beschreibung einer neuen Methode mit Durchführung im Sitzen. Fortschr Geb Röntgenstr 127:167–169
35. Hopf R, Kaltenbach M (1982) Verapamil treatment of hypertrophic cardiomyopathy. In: Kaltenbach M, Epstein SE (eds) Hypertrophic cardiomyopathy. The therapeutic role of calcium antagonists. Springer, Berlin Heidelberg New York, pp 163–178
36. Hopf R, Kaltenbach M (1982) Die hypertrophische Kardiomyopathie: Möglichkeiten der kalziumantagonistischen Behandlung. Thieme, Stuttgart, pp 129–137
37. Hopf R, Kaltenbach M (1984) Einfluß hoher Dosen von Verapamil auf die linksventrikuläre Hämodynamik. In: Gross F (ed) Die Bedeutung der Kalzium-Antagonisten für die Hochdrucktherapie. MMW Medizin, München, pp 41–57
38. Hopf R, Kaltenbach M (1987) 10-year results and survival of patients with hypertrophic cardiomyopathy treated with calcium antagonists. Z Kardiol [Suppl 3] 76:137–144
39. Hopf R, Kaltenbach M (1988) Medical treatment of hypertrophic cardiomyopathy: Influence on outflow obstruction and filling pressure. In: Toshima H, Maron BJ (eds) Cardiomyopathy update 2: Hypertrophic cardiomyopathy. University of Tokyo Press, Tokyo, pp 189–205
40. Hopf R, Keller M, Kaltenbach M (1976) Die Behandlung der hypertrophen obstruktiven Kardiomyopathie mit Verapamil. Verh Dtsch Ges Inn Med 82 (2):1054–1057
41. Hopf R, Kaltenbach M, Kober G (1981) Verapamil in the treatment of hypertrophic obstructive cardiomyopathy. In: Zanchetti A, Krikler DH (eds) Calcium antagonism in cardiovascular therapy – Experience with verapamil. Excerpta Medica, Amsterdam, pp 353–362
42. Hopf R, Kober G, Kaltenbach M (1983) Die Behandlung der hypertrophen Kardiomyopathie mit Kalziumantagonisten. In: Olsen EG, Schrey A (eds) Expertengespräche Venedig 1981 – Medikamentöse Behandlung ausgewählter kardiovaskulärer Krankheiten. Klett, Stuttgart, pp 226–244
43. Hopf R, Richter H, Kaltenbach M, Maul FD, Standke R, Hör G (1985) Radionuklidventrikulographie nach akuter und chronischer Verapamil-Medikation bei Patienten mit hypertropher Kardiomyopathie. In: Hör G, Kaltenbach M, Maul FD, Pabst HW (eds) Interventionelle Nuklearkardiologie. Kern und Birner, Frankfurt, pp 368–377
44. Hopf R, Rodrian S, Kaltenbach M (1986) Behandlung der hypertrophen Kardiomyopathie mit Kalziumantagonisten: Eine Zehnjahresbilanz. Therapiewoche 36:1433–1454

45. Hopf R, Thomas J, Klepzig H, Kaltenbach M (1987) Behandlung der hypertrophischen Kardiomyopathie mit Nifedipin und Propranolol in Kombination. Z Kardiol 76:469–478
46. Kaltenbach M, Hopf R (1984) Use of calcium-channel blockers in the treatment of hypertrophic cardiomyopathy. Pract Cardiol 10:197–215
47. Kaltenbach M, Hopf R (1984) Long-term treatment of hypertrophic myocardiopathy with calcium antagonists. In: Althaus U, Burckhardt D, Vogt E (eds) Calcium-Antagonismus. International symposium on calcium-antagonism. Uni Versi Med, Frankfurt, pp 259–271
48. Kaltenbach M, Hopf R (1985) Treatment of hypertrophic cardiomyopathy: Relation to pathological mechanism. J Mol Cell Cardiol [Suppl 2] 17:59–68
49. Kaltenbach M, Hopf R, Keller M (1976) Calciumantagonistische Therapie bei hypertroph obstructiver Kardiomyopathie. Dtsch Med Wochenschr 101:1907–1911
50. Kaltenbach M, Hopf R, Kober G, Bussmann WD, Keller M, Petersen Y (1979) Treatment of hypertrophic obstructive cardiomyopathy with verapamil. Br Heart J 42:35–42
51. Kober G, Hopf R, Biamino G, Bubenheimer P, Förster K, Kuck KH, Hanrath P et al (1987) Long-term treatment of hypertrophic cardiomyopathy with verapamil or propranolol in matched pairs of patients. Results of a multicenter study. Z Kardiol [Suppl 3] 76:113–118
52. Krayenbühl HP, Hirzel HO, Hess OM, Senn M (1983) Behandlung der hypertrophen Kardiomyopathie mit Kalzium-Antagonisten. In: Fleckenstein A, Hashimoto K, Herrmann M, Schwartz A, Seipel L (eds) New calcium antagonists: recent developements and prospects. Fischer, Stuttgart, pp 199–210
53. Kuhn H, Loogen F (1978) Die Anwendung von Beta-Rezeptorenblockern bei hypertrophischer obstruktiver Kardiomyopathie (HOCM). Internist (Berlin) 19:527–531
54. Kuhn H, Thelen U, Leuner C, Köhler E, Bluschke V (1980) Langzeitbehandlung der hypertrophischen nicht obstruktiven Kardiomyopathie (HNCM) mit Verapamil. Z Kardiol 69:669–675
55. Landmark K, Sire S, Thanlow E, Amlie JP, Nitter-Hange S (1982) Haemodynamic effects of nifedipine and propranolol in patients with hypertrophic obstructive cardiomyopathy. Br Heart J 48:19–26
56. Leon MB, Rosing DR, Maron BJ, Bonow RO, Lesko LL, Epstein SE (1984) Amiodarone in patients with hypertrophic cardiomyopathy and refractory cardiac symptoms: an alternative to current medical therapy. Circulation [Suppl 2] 70:II-18
57. Leon MB, Tracy CM, Winkler J, Bergamo C, Bonow RO, Epstein SE (1987) Amiodarone does not prevent, and may increase, sudden death in patients with hypertrophic cardiomyopathy (Abstr). Circulation [Suppl 4] 76:248
58. Linden RJ (1964) Related physiology of cardiac contraction. In: Wolstenholme GEW, O'Connor M (eds) Cardiomyopathies. Churchill, London, pp 100–131
59. Loogen F, Kuhn H, Krelhaus W (1978) Natural history of hypertrophic cardiomyopathy and the effect of therapy. In: Kaltenbach M, Loogen F, Olssen EG (ed) Cardiomyopathy and myocardial biopsy. Springer, Berlin Heidelberg New York, pp 286–299
60. Loogen F, Kuhn H, Gietzen F, Lösse B, Schulte HD, Bircks W (1983) Clinical course and prognosis of patients with typical and atypical hypertrophic obstructive and with hypertrophic non-obstructive cardiomyopathy. Eur Heart J [Suppl F] 4:145–153
61. Lorell BH, Paulus WJ, Grossman W, Wynne J, Cohn PF, Braunwald E (1980) Improved diastolic function and systolic performance in hypertrophic cardiomyopathy after nifedipine. N Engl J Med 303:801–803
62. Lorell BH, Paulus WJ, Grossman W, Wynne J, Cohn PF (1982) Modification of abnormal left ventricular diastolic properties by nifedipine in patients with hypertrophic cardiomyopathy. Circulation 65:499–507
63. Lösse B, Kuhn H, Loogen F, Schulte HD (1983) Exercise performance in hypertrophic cardiomyopathies. Eur Heart J [Suppl F] 4:197–208
64. Maron BJ, Savage DD, Wolfson JK, Epstein SE (1981) The prognostic significance of 24 hour ambulatory electrocardiographic monitoring in patients with hypertrophic cardiomyopathy. Am J Cardiol 48:252–257

65. Maron BJ, Bonow RO, Cannon RO, Leon MB, Epstein SE (1987) Hypertrophic cardiomyopathy: interrelations of clinical manifestations, pathophysiology, and therapy. N Engl J Med 316:780–789, 844–852
66. Masini V, Ceci V, Malinconico U, Milazzotto F (1981) Therapeutic evaluation of pindolol and verapamil in hypertrophic obstructive cardiomyopathy. G Ital Cardiol 11:1729–1737
67. McKenna WJ (1983) Arrhythmia and prognosis in hypertrophic cardiomyopathy. Eur Heart J [Suppl F] 4:225–234
68. McKenna WJ, Kleinebenne A (1985) Arrhythmien bei hypertrophischer Kardiomyopathie: Bedeutung und therapeutische Konsequenzen. Herz 10:91–101
69. McKenna WJ, Chetty S, Oakley CM, Goodwin JF (1980) Arrhythmia in hypertrophic cardiomyopathy: exercise and 48 hour ambulatory electrocardiographic assessment with and without beta adrenergic blocking therapy. Am J Cardiol 45:1–5
70. McKenna WJ, England D, Oakley C, Goodwin J (1980) Detection of arrhythmia in hypertrophic cardiomyopathy: prospective study (Abstr). Circulation [Suppl 3] 62:187
71. McKenna WJ, England D, Oakley C, Goodwin JF (1981) Detection of arrhythmia in hypertrophic cardiomyopathy. I. Influence on prognosis. Br Heart J 46:168–172
72. McKenna WJ, Harris L, Perez G, Krikler DM, Oakley C, Goodwin JF (1981) Arrhythmia in hypertrophic cardiomyopathy. II. Comparison of amiodarone and verapamil in treatment. Br Heart J 46:173–178
73. Deleted
74. McKenna WJ, Harris L, Rowland E, Kleinebenne A, Krikler DM, Oakley CM, Goodwing JF (1984) Amiodarone for long-term management of patients with hypertrophic cardiomyopathy. Am J Cardiol 54:802–810
75. McKenna WJ, Oakley CM, Krikler DM, Goodwin JF (1985) Improved survival with amiodarone in patients with hypertrophic cardiomyopathy and ventricular tachycardia. Br Heart J 53:412–416
76. McKenna WJ, Harris L, Mulrow JP, Rowland E, Holt DW (1986) Amiodarone dose titration: a method to minimise side effects during long-term therapy. Br J Clin Proctol [Suppl 44] 40:121–127
77. Mushoff K, Reindell H (1956) Zur Röntgenuntersuchung des Herzens in horizontaler und vertikaler Körperstellung. I Mitteilung: Der Einfluß der Körperstellung auf das Herzvolumen. Dtsch Med Wochenschr 81:1001–1008
78. Mushoff K, Reindell H (1957) Zur Röntgenuntersuchung des Herzens in horizontaler und vertikaler Körperstellung: II Mitteilung: Der Einfluß der Körperstellung auf die Herzform. Dtsch Med Wochenschr 82:1075–1080
79. Nagao M, Omote S, Takizawa A, Yasue H (1983) Effect of diltiazem on left ventricular isovolumic relaxation time in patients with hypertrophic cardiomyopathy. Jpn Circ J 47:58
80. Oakley CM (1973) Beta-adrenergic blocking agents in hypertrophic cardiomyopathy (HOCM). Singapore Med J 14:408–409
81. Olbrich HG, Borgers M, Thone F, Frotscher M, Mutschler E, Schneider M, Kober G, Kaltenbach M (1988) Ultrastructural localization of calcium in the myocardium of cardiomyopathic Syrian Hamsters. J Mol Cell Cardiol 20:753–762
82. Paulus WJ, Lorell BH, Craig WE, Wynne J, Murgo JP, Grossman W (1983) Comparison of the effects of nitroprusside and nifedipine on diastolic properties in patients with hypertrophic cardiomyopathy: altered left ventricular loading or improved muscle inactivation? J Am Coll Cardiol 2:879–886
83. Paulus WJ, Nellens P, Heyndrickx GR, Andries E (1986) Effects of long-term treatment with amiodarone on exercise hemodynamics and left ventricular relaxation in patients with hypertrophic cardiomyopathy. Circulation 74:544–554
84. Pollik C (1982) Muscular aortic stenosis: hemodynamic and clinical improvement after disopyramide. N Engl J Med 307:997–999
85. Pollik C (1988) Disopyramide in hypertrophic cardiomyopathy. II. Noninvasive assessment after oral administration. Am J Cardiol 62:1252–1255
86. Pollik C, Kimball B, Henderson M, Wigle ED (1988) Disopyramide in hypertrophic cardiomyopathy. I. Hemodynamic assessment after intravenous administration. Am J Cardiol 62:1248–1251

87. Rosing DR, Kent KM, Borer DJ, Seides SF, Maron BJ, Epstein SE (1979) Verapamil therapy: a new approach to the pharmacologic treatment of hypertrophic cardiomyopathy. I. Hemodynamic effects. Circulation 60:1201–1207

88. Rosing DR, Kent KM, Maron BJ, Epstein SE (1979) Verapamil therapy: a new approach to the pharmacologic treatment of hypertrophic cardiomyopathy. II. Effects on exercise capacity and symptomatic status. Circulation 60:1208–1213

89. Rosing DR, Condit JR, Maron BJ, Kent KM, Leon MB, Bonow RO, Lipson LC, Epstein SE (1981) Verapamil therapy: a new approach to the pharmacologic treatment of hypertrophic cardiomyopathy. III. Effects of long-term administration. Am J Cardiol 48:545–553

90. Rosing DR, Idänpään-Heikkilä U, Maron BJ, Bonow RO, Epstein SE (1985) Use of calcium-channel blocking drugs in hypertrophic cardiomyopathy. Am J Cardiol [Suppl 1] 55:185 B – 195 B

91. Rothlin ME, Gobet D, Haberer T, Krayenbühl HP, Turina M, Senning A (1983) Surgical treatment versus medical treatment in hypertrophic obstructive cardiomyopathy. Eur Heart J [Suppl F] 4:215–223

92. Schanzenbächer P, Schick KD, Kochsiek K (1982) Nifedipin bei hypertrophisch obstruktiver Kardiomyopathie. Dtsch Med Wochenschr 107:1842–1846

93. Schmincke A (1907) Über linksseitige muskuläre Conusstenosen. Dtsch Med Wochenschr 33:2082–2083

94. Senn M, Hess OM, Krayenbühl HP (1982) Nifedipin in der Behandlung der hypertrophen, nicht obstruktiven Kardiomyopathie. Schweiz Med Wochenschr 112:1312–1317

95. Shah PM, Adelman AG, Wigle Ed, Gobel FL, Burchell HB, Hardarson T, Curiel R et al (1973) The natural (and unnatural) history of hypertrophic obstructive cardiomyopathy. A multicenter study. Circ Res [Suppl 2] 34:179–195

96. Sherrid M, Delia E, Dwyer E (1988) Oral disopyramide therapy for obstructive hypertophic cardiomyopathy. Am J Cardiol 62:1085–1088

97. Sonntag F, Hanrath P, Saal M, Diemert J, Mathey D, Kupper W, Bleifeld W (1980) Untersuchungen zur Frage der Häufigkeit und Vorhersehbarkeit von ventrikulären Herzrhythmusstörungen bei Patienten mit hypertropher Kardiomyopathie. Herz Kreislauf 12:481–489

98. Sowton E (1976) Betarezeptorenblocker bei hypertropher Kardiomyopathie. In: Schweizer W (ed) Die Betablocker-Gegenwart und Zukunft. Huber, Bern, pp 239–258

99. Spicer RL, Rocchini AP, Crowley DC, Vasiliades J, Rosenthal A (1983) Hemodynamic effects of verapamil in children and adolescents with hypertrophic cardiomyopathy. Circulation 67:413–420

100. Stenson RE, Flamm MD Jr, Harrison DC, Hancock EW (1973) Hypertrophic subaortic stenosis: clinical and hemodynamic effects of long-term propranolol therapy. Am J Cardiol 31:763–773

101. Sugrue DD, Dickie S, Myers MJ, Lavender JP, McKenna WJ (1984) Effect of amiodarone on left ventricular ejection and filling in hypertrophic cardiomyopathy as assessed by radionuclide angiography. Am J Cardiol 54:1054–1058

102. Suwa M, Hirota Y, Kawamura K (1984) Improvement in left ventricular diastolic function during intravenous and oral diltiazem therapy in patients with hypertrophic cardiomyopathy: an echocardiographic study. Am J Cardiol 54:1047–1053

103. Swanton RH, Brooksby IAB, Jenkins BS, Webb-Peploe MM (1977) Hemodynamic studies of beta-blockade in hypertrophic obstructive cardiomyopathy. Eur J Cardiol 5(4):327–341

104. Teare D (1958) Asymmetrical hypertrophy of the heart in young adults. Br Heart J 20:1–8

105. Wagner JA, Sax FL, Weisman HF, Porterfield J, McIntosh C, Weisfeld ML, Snyder SH, Epstein SE (1989) Calcium-antagonist receptors in the atrial tissue of patients with hypertrophic cardiomyopathy. N Engl J Med 320:755–761

106. Wigle ED, Wilansky S (1987) Diastolic dysfunction in hypertrophic cardiomyopathy. Heart Failure 2:82–93

107. Wigle ED, Heimbecker RO, Gunton RW (1962) Idiopathic ventricular septal hypertrophy causing muscular subaortic stenosis. Circulation 26:325–340

Surgical Results in Patients with Hypertrophic Obstructive Cardiomyopathy

H. D. Schulte, W. Bircks, and B. Lösse

Introduction

Hypertrophic obstructive cardiomyopathy (HOCM) – a disease of unknown etiology – is characterized by a hypertrophied left ventricle (LV) with a relatively small cavity, an asymmetric subaortic and/or midventricular or apical septal hypertrophy which may cause a considerable systolic obstruction of the left ventricular outflow-tract (LVOT) and diastolic LV dysfunction by delayed relaxation and filling impairment. In many cases a mitral regurgitation of different degrees and clinical importance can be found. Data of the natural history of the disease clearly indicate a slow continuing clinical deterioration. Sudden death – mainly in younger age groups and often after acute physical exertion – is a typical complication. Patients are additionally endangered by arrhythmias, systemic embolism, endocarditis, and congestive heart failure (CHF). The most important diagnostic procedures are listed in (Table 1). In our experience, clinical examination, carotid pulse tracings, echocardiography, Doppler echochardiography, transseptal left heart catheterization, and cineangiocardiography are the most important diagnostic tools. Management of clinically symptomatic HOCM (Table 2) was started medically using β-adrenergic blocking agents (propranolol [16], mainly to prevent provocation of the obstruction by beta-agonists [59]). Later Kaltenbach et al. [22] reported a good clinical response by using the calcium antagonist verapamil. Antiarrhythmic drugs were introduced by Wigle et al. [50] (disopyramide) or by McKenna et al. [32] (amiodarone). Cleland [9] introduced surgical management in London 1958 by performing a transaortic subvalvular myotomy. Morrow and colleagues [33–35] adopted this technique in 1961 adding a second myotomy and resection

Table 1. Diagnostic procedures in HOCM

Physical examination (systolic murmur), ECG, PCG
Art. carotis pulse tracing (spike and dome configuration)
Echocardiography: septal hypertrophy, SAM, midsystolic closure of aortic leaflets
Doppler echocardiography: flow characteristics, gradient
Catheterization: pressure gradient at rest, after provocation
Ventriculography: localization of obstruction, angulation, mitral regurgitation
Computed tomography, magnetic resonance tomography

Table 2. Management of HOCM

Medical	β-Receptor-blocking agents [16]
	Calcium antagonists [22]
	Antiarrhythmic drugs [50]; [32]
Surgical	Myotomy [9]; [33]; [4]
	Myectomy-transaortic [34]
	Myectomy-trans-LV [23]
Pacemaker	VVI mode [18]
	Dual chamber [13, 14]

of the hypertrophied septal muscle between both myotomies – the new classical type of transaortic subvalvular myectomy [33]. Kirklin and Ellis [23], Barratt-Boyes [2], and Senning [44] performed successfully the trans-left ventricular approach with or without additional opening of the ascending aorta. In contrast to Cleland and Morrow, Bigelow et al. [4] placed their myotomy exactly below the commissure between the left and right coronary cusps of the aortic valve, expanding the incision by finger compression to a broader channel. A completely different way of solving the problem of functional and anatomical LVOT obstruction (LVOTO) was to change the mode and direction of stimulation of the cardiac conduction system from the ventricular apex to the basis by implanting a pacemaker system [13, 14, 18] which is not generally accepted. We tried this technique in few patients; however, it failed.

Indication for Surgery

In symptomatic patients we usually begin treatment with the Ca-antagonist verapamil up to 480 mg per day (Table 3). Only in case of inadequate response or when after an initial improvement there is a clinical deterioration reaching NYHA class III we consider surgery indicated. Only in very few cases of HOCM the operative indication was accepted in less symptomatic patients if family history showed evidence of early and sudden deaths, or the patient had a history of severe arrhythmias or reanimation. The systolic gradient at rest or after provocation between the left ventricle and the ascending aorta or, an intraventricular gradient were considered of minor importance, however, intraoperatively the main aim is to enlarge the LVOT or to remove the midventricular obstructive tissue in order to abolish the gradients as complete as possible.

Table 3. Indication for surgery in HOCM

Reliable diagnosis
Clinical deterioration despite long-term medical therapy
Clinical (NYHA) class III or IV
Clinical class I or II: Family history
                            History of reanimation
Considerable systolic gradient at rest (LV aorta)
Postextrasystolic increased gradient (paradoxical pressure behavior)

Aims of Surgical Treatment

An effective enlargement of the subvalvular region by myectomy and excision of the thickened fibrotic endocardial layer is necessary to give access to the midventricular portion, using cardioplegia and a careful introduction of a special set of angled instruments. This technique allows a partial reconstruction of the LV long axis angulation, a better diastolic function, and a decrease of the amount of mitral regurgitation. In many cases with considerable preoperative mitral insufficiency we found an additional marked hypertrophic lateral LV wall, especially opposite the anterior (lateral) papillary muscle which, during systole, seems to be deviated towards the thickened septum and thus may prevent a complete closure of the mitral leaflets. Whether this mechanism also supports systolic anterior movement of the anterior mitral leaflet (SAM) in echocardiography is not yet clarified. Other aims of effective surgical procedure are the prevention of arrhythmias, infective endocarditis, congestive heart failure, and perhaps sudden death.

Surgical Therapy and Techniques

Since 1958 many different surgical approaches and techniques have been reported (Table 4). Most centers have accepted the techniques of Morrow and his colleagues [34, 35] (transaortic subvalvular myectomy) or of Kirklin and Ellis [23] (transventricular myectomy). The earlier recommendations of Johnson [20] and especially of Cooley et al. [11] to solve the problem of LVOTO by resection of the mitral valve and implantation of a prosthetic valve found no general acceptance. We completely agree with the statement of Roberts [27] not to add a second disease to the original one if not necessary for severe mitral insufficiency. The trans-RV approaches may be of value for additional severe muscular RVOTO; however, the significance for relief of the LVOT has not yet been demonstrated except in a few cases.

The Düsseldorf Procedure

Since the beginning in 1963 we have adopted the Cleland and Morrow techniques. With more intraoperative experience and simultaneous pressure recordings before and after the surgical procedure, it became necessary to extend the transaortic subvalvular myectomy leading to a combination of the Morrow [35] and Bigelow et al. [4] incisions and a far more extended myectomy, which often includes parts of the lateral hypertrophied LV wall.

The surgical procedure (Table 5): After setting the cannulas for extracorporeal circulation (ECC) simultaneous pressure tracings from the right atrium (RA): right ventricle (RV), left atrium (LA): left ventricle (LV): ascending aorta at rest and after provocation are registered. ECC is started with hypothermic perfusion (5 min with blood temperature below 27 °C) and insertion of a LV vent. The superior and inferior venae cavae are closed around the venous cannulas

Table 4. Surgical procedures for relief of HOCM

Reference	Procedure
Cleland 1963 [9]	Transaortic ventriculomyotomy
Morrow et al. 1960 [33]	Transaortic ventriculomyotomy
Kirklin and Ellis 1961 [23]	Combined transaortic and trans-left ventricular myectomy
Morrow et al. 1963 [34]	Transaortic ventriculomyectomy
Julian et al. 1963 [21]	Fish-mouth incision LV
Lillehei and Levy 1963 [26]	Left transatrial approach with detachment of aortic mitral leaflet
Trimble et al. 1964 [46]	Aimed transaortic myotomy
Dobell and Scott 1964 [12]	Left transatrial approach to LVOT with medial incision of the aortic mitral leaflet and myectomy with cautery loop
Johnson 1964 [20]	Transaortic approach and MVR
Harken 1964 [17]	Transaortic + right ventricular approach and myectomy
Stinson and Shumway 1968 [45]	Heart transplantation
Cooley et al. 1970 [11]	Mitral valve replacement
Rastan and Koncz 1975 [36]	
Konno et al. 1975 [25]	Aortoventriculo-plasty
Hassenstein et al. 1975 [18]	Right ventricular pacing
Bernhard et al. 1975 [3],	
Cooley et al. 1976 [10]	Apicoaortic valved conduit
Vouhé et al. 1984 [49]	Aortoseptal approach through RV and myectomy
Alvarez-Diaz et al. 1984 [1]	Aortoseptal approach through RV with resection of septum and patch-plasty
Duch et al. 1984 [13]	Atrial synchronized ventricular stimulation
Isner et al 1984 [19]	Laser myoplasty
Erwin et al. 1985 [14]	Dual chamber pacing

Table 5. Performance of myocardial protection in HOCM patients using crystalloid cardioplegic solution [8]

General hypothermia by perfusion (ECC) (5 min blood temperature $< 27°$C)

Cardioplegic solution $6–8°$C for coronary perfusion and pericardial surface cooling of the heart

Coronary perfusion pressure until cardiac arrest 80–100 mmHg, during cardiac arrest 40 mmHg

Coronary perfusion time 8–10 min

Coronary perfusion volume 2000–4000 ml

Retrocardial temperature $9–15°$C

Intramyocardial temperature (calculated) $12–15°$C

Repeated coronary perfusion in case of electrical ventricular activity

High paracoronary blood flow: after 30–45 min, in expected long-term procedures: after 45–60 min

Before declamping of the aorta: reduction of perfusion pressure to 40 mmHg for 1–2 min

Postischemic reperfusion without myocardial burden 12 min, until rewarming at least 15–30 min (rectal temperature $34°$C)

Table 6. Composition and condition of crystalloid Bretschneider cardioplegic solution[a]

Sodium chloride	15.0 mmol/l
Potassium chloride	9,0 mmol/l
Magnesium chloride 6 H_2O	4,0 mmol/l
Histidine	180.0 mmol/l
Histidine-HCl H_2O	18.0 mmol/l
Tryptophan	2.0 mmol/l
Potassium hydrogen-2-oxoglutarate	1.0 mmol/l
Mannitol	30.0 mmol/l
pH (25°C)	7.2 mmol/l
Osmolality	290 mosmol/kg
Oxygen	0.6 vol%

[a] Manufactored and distributed by Dr. F. Köhler Chemie GmbH, D-6146 Alsbach, Berg-straße.

with snares. Cross clamping of the aorta is followed by an oblique aortic incision into the noncoronary cusp sinus. Inspection and finger palpation of the beating or fibrillating heart allows a good impression of the LVOTO. Cardioplegia is started immediately by selective perfusion of the coronary arteries using metallic hand-held cannulas occluding the ostia. Cold crystalloid Bretschneider solution [8] is perfused under pressure and volume control for a minimum of 8 min (Table 6). Some auxiliary techniques may facilitate the subsequent procedure significantly: because of the usually very small and narrow entrance to the LV, the surgeon should wear a head-light; and the operating table is tilted to the left, which improves the view into the aortic ring and LV. Despite the cooling procedure, the myocardium is completely relaxed. A flexible brain spatulum is inserted into the LV cavity to protect the mitral valve, chordae, and papillary muscles. In addition, the septum is pushed backwards into the LVOT using a spongestick. The aortic cusps are protected and withdrawn by special hooks, thus preparing the incisions for myectomy. The first incision is made maximum of 2 mm to the right of the nadir of the right coronary cusp in direction of the LV apex (Morrow); the second incision is made in the same direction starting below the commissure of the left and right coronary cusps [4]. Then the myectomy is performed by excision of the obstructing septal part in one piece.

The LVOT can then be opened using specially angled and modified Langenbeck hooks of different lengths, which allow a good approach to the midventricular and apical regions. By inspection and repeated finger palpation, further resections can be controlled to abolish muscular obstructions nearly down into the apex of the LV. Then the thickened fibrotic endocardial layer is carefully removed from the residual LVOT. Special attention is paid to the papillary muscles which often demonstrate atypical connections to the septum or lateral LV wall which should be cut. In case of severe bulging of the hypertrophied lateral LV wall, a myectomy is added starting below the lateral part of the left coronary cusp. The incisions are rounded and tissue roughnesses are smoothed using angled pliers. Rewarming is started. The LV cavity is rinsed at least twice to remove possible muscle particles and to control the aortic cusps. After closure of the aortotomy, opening of the aortic clamp, and careful debubbling of the aorta and the LV cavity by apical introduction of a needle vent, reperfusion for about 20 min is performed with cardiac defibrillation after 5 min if necessary. The circulatory behavior and the cardiac output as well as the simultaneous control pressure tracings after coming off bypass demonstrate the result of the surgical procedure. All patients receive retractable bipolar atrial and ventricular pacemaker electrodes for at least 10 days.

Postoperatively the patients have bed rest for 10 days. The medical treatment is continued at a considerably reduced dosage in accordance with the preoperative clinical condition and the results of the surgical procedure. In all patients anticoagulation with dicumarol starts in the afternoon of the day of surgery for a 4-week period.

Results of Surgical Treatment

Because of the scientific and clinical interests of our cardiological group for cardiomyopathies for many years, the number of investigated and medically treated patients with diagnosed HOCM is relatively high. Therefore, the number of operated patients is also unusually high for one center. However, the relatively good and long-term results of the patients surviving after surgery led to increasing expectations of cardiologists and patients, giving both surgeons (WB, HDS) the chance of gaining more and more experience and improving our results.

An overview concerning the frequency of HOCM during the last 5 years (1984–1988) (Table 7) demonstrates a continuous increase of HOCM patients: 124 out of 6003 pump cases (2.1%). A survey of our total surgical experience (1963 – May 15, 1989) with 261 typical HOCM cases and 32 atypical cases is summarized in Table 8. The male: female ratio was nearly 3:2. The total hospital mortality was 4.6% ($n = 12$) for typical and 6.3% ($n = 2$) for atypical HOCM. With more experience, the hospital mortality could be significantly reduced resulting in an operative risk of 1% for the last 100 consecutive patients (Table 9).

Table 7. Frequency of HOCM patients. Cardiological patients (1961–1988), $n > 650$; surgical patients (1963–1988), $n = 283$

Surgical frequency	1984	1985	1986	1987	1988	Total
Surgery with ECC (n)	1171	1166	1178	1232	1256	6003
Surgery for HOCM (n)	16	23	28	28	29	124
(%)						2.1
HOCM: early mortality (n)	1	0	1	0	0	2
(%)						1.6

Table 8. Surgical results in HOCM (January 1963 – May 15, 1989)

(n = 293)	Typical HOCM		Atypical HOCM
Patients (n)	261		32
Male : female (n)	158 : 103		21 : 11
Mean age (years)	44.9		44.1
Age range (years)		6–74	
Clinical class II	6		1
Clinical class III	244		30
Clinical class IV	11		1
Hospital mortality (n)	12		2
(%)	4.6		6.3

Table 9. HOCM: Hospital mortality related to different time periods and additional surgical procedures

Years	Patients	Early mortality	
	(n)	(n)	(%)
1963–1969	12	3	25.0
1970–1980	87	6	5.9
1981–1989 (May 15)	194	5	2.6
Last consecutive patients	100	1	1.0
1963–1989 (May 15)	293	14	4.8
TSM	218	6	2.7
TSM + additional procedures	75	8	10.6

TSM transaortic subvalvular myectomy.

There was also a risk difference in our experience between patients who needed transaortic subvalvular myectomy (TSM) only (2.7) in contrast to patients with additional cardiac procedures (mortality 10.6%) (Table 10).

Intra- and Postoperative Complications

Despite a very careful operative technique, a number of intraoperative injuries and complications occurred which were classified as HOCM related when they were correlated to the original disease and to the special surgical approach, or as HOCM nonrelated when more general surgical complications were present (Tables 11 and 12).

Intraoperative injuries caused no immediate problems, but during the post-operative period one patient died because of problems partly related to a technical injury which needed mitral valve replacement, and congestive heart failure. One patient had a LV wall perforation which could be easily treated, however, 10 days after surgery and immediately after a very exciting telephone

Table 10. HOCM: Surgical treatment and additional cardiac procedures

		Deaths	
	(*n*)	(*n*)	(%)
Transaortic myectomy (typical, atypical)	218	6	2.7
TSM + additional cardiac procedures	75	8	10.6
TSM + ligation of LCA-PA fistula	1		
TSM + closure of ASD II	2		
TSM + splitting of LAD muscle bridge	4	1	
TSM + WPW syndrome	1		
TSM + LV ventriculotomy (thrombus, diverticle, aneurysm)	6		
TSM + RV ventriculotomy (without TSM 2)	6 (+2)	1	
TSM + aortic valve reconstructions	10		
TSM + mitral valve reconstructions	5		
TSM + AVR	6		
TSM + MVR	18	5	
TSM + TVR	1		
TSM + ACBG	19		
TSM + ascending aorta aneurysm repair (postoperative rupture)	1	1	

TSM, transaortic subvalvular myectomy; LCA-PA, left coronary artery-pulmonary artery; ASD, atrial septal defect; LAD, left anterior descending coronary artery; WPW, Wolff-Parkinson-White syndrome; AVR, aortic valve replacement; MVR, mitral valve replacement; TVR, tricuspid valve replacement; ACBG, aortocoronary bypass grafting.

Table 11. HOCM-related perioperative complications

Complications	Procedures	(*n*)	Deaths (*n*)
Intraoperative injuries			
Aortic valve	Repair	2	
Mitral valve	Repair	1	
	Replacement	1	1
Tricuspid valve	Replacement	1	
LV wall perforation	Repair	1	1 (VF)
Septal perforations	Repair (*n* = 5)	9	
Total atrioventricular block	Pacemaker implantation	10	
	Before pacemaker implantation	1	1
Septal infarction		1	
Left bundle branch block		166	
Intra- and postoperative complications			
Intraoperative remyectomy		22	
Reoperation for insufficient primary myectomy		4	1
Late postoperative endocarditis : AVR + MVR		2	
Acute tachyarrhythmias (ventricular fibrillation)		2	2
Postoperative defibrillator implantation		2	
Myocardial insufficiency		17	5
Cerebral embolism		5	

Table 12. HOCM nonrelated perioperative complications

Complications	(n)	Deaths (n)
Pulmonary embolism	2	1
Gastrointestinal bleeding	2	1
Septicemia	1	1
Rethoracotomy (bleeding)	11	
Sternal wound dehiscence	4	
Postoperative pneumothorax	4	
Acute renal insufficiency (hemodialysis)	2	
Hepatitis B	3	
Intrapericardial lymph fistula	1	

call with her family, she suddenly died on the ward and could not be resuscitated. A man with a postoperative total atrioventricular block was scheduled for pacemaker implantation the following morning when the external pacemaker system failed.

Septal perforations during myectomy occurred in nine patients of which three could be repaired intraoperatively via the RV, two patients had later reoperations for closure, while in four cases the secondary ventricular septal defect (VSD) was very small and without any hemodynamic relevance.

Intraoperative remyectomy is necessary if the postsurgical gradient at rest exceeds 30 mmHg and after provocation is more than 50 mmHg. In these cases ($n = 22$) remyectomy was successfully added.

In four patients, with one postoperative death, a reoperation had to be performed because sufficient relief of the LVOTO had not been originally achieved. A real relapse of a LVOTO in HOCM patients after surgery was never observed. Two further patients had repeated acute tachyarrhythmias which finally led to ventricular fibrillation and death. Two other patients had postoperative catheter stimulation which could evoke tachycardias and ventricular fibrillation. Therefore in both patients an automatic defibrillator had to be implanted as preventative measure.

During the 1 st decade several patients had postoperative cerebral embolism. Since that time all patients have been postoperatively anticoagulated with dicumarol for at least 4 weeks, and we have never again observed any cerebral attacks postoperatively.

In the group of HOCM-nonrelated complications, there were three deaths after septicemia, severe gastrointestinal bleeding, and after pulmonary embolism, which, after the use of ECC, was quite unusual. The other complications caused no life-threatening problems.

Late Results

Clinical and Hemodynamic Follow-up Data

Surgery of HOCM patients is a symptomatic procedure which has no influence on the underlying cardiomyopathy. Therefore, it seemed necessary to collect data on the late outcome of the patients operated. Our latest follow-up (May 1989) included all patients ($n = 258$) operated until April 1988, with 261 surgical procedures (three reoperations after 6–8 years). The follow-up rate was 100% ($n = 244$ survivors after the first operation). The postoperative observation time was a minimum of 1 year, and a maximum of 23 years; mean 6.2 years.

During the follow-up time 34 patients died. The cause of death was HOCM related in 17 patients (eight sudden deaths, four congestive heart failures, four cases of embolism in atrial fibrillation, one after reoperation because of myocardial insufficiency). In 17 patients death was not related to HOCM [four cardiac deaths for coronary or valvular reasons, 13 were extracardiac (accidents, malignant tumors, abdominal diseases)]. An evaluation of all the late postoperative deaths with regard to age at surgery and years after surgery demonstrated absolutely no correlation.

In a comparison of patients after propranolol ($n = 12$), verapamil ($n = 25$), and myectomy ($n = 21$), the postoperative clinical classification after 1 year and after 4 years demonstrated superior results after myectomy despite the fact that the patients operated were at a more advanced stage of the disease at the time of surgery. The patients reinvestigated invasively after myectomy not only had the best results regarding heart rate, stroke volume index, cardiac index, and mean pulmonary pressure reduction but maintained their improvement [28].

The cumulative survival rate of patients treated surgically ($n = 258$) was 90% $\pm 2\%$ after 5 years, and 82% $\pm 3\%$ after 10 years. The data of a group of patients in NYHA clinical classes III and IV who were treated medically and were not operated on for several reasons ($n = 59$), revealed a survival rate after 5 years of 81%, and after 10 years of 54%.

Arrhythmias

A pre- and postoperative 48-h ECG monitoring has been performed 2–4 days before and 10–12 days after surgery in nearly all patients since 1985 [8a, b]. The long-term follow-up of 57 patients after a mean of 40 ± 18.7 months revealed that 53 patients were alive with no postoperative syncope, resuscitation, or sudden death. There were two perioperative deaths in this group of patients who were investigated early as well as two late deaths caused by congestive heart failure and one for a noncardiac reason.

From these studies of pre- and postoperative arrhythmia evaluation the following conclusions can be drawn:

– Complex ventricular arrhythmias are common in patients with HOCM before and after myectomy (47%).

- The frequency and complexity of ventricular arrhythmias are not influenced by myectomy.
- During long-term follow-up of 40 ± 18.7 months, no patient had syncope, resuscitation, or sudden death.
- Complex ventricular arrhythmias seem to have no prognostic significance after surgical treatment of HOCM.
- Possibly, myectomy may provide protection and complex arrhythmias are better tolerated and easier to treat after surgery.

Results of programmed ventricular stimulation (PVS) pre- and postoperatively after myectomy demonstrated in six out of seven patients an increased ventricular vulnerability preoperatively, whereas postoperatively ventricular fibrillation could be evoked in only one patient.

The origin of monomorphic ventricular tachycardia could be localized in one patient by catheter and intraoperative mapping in the hypertrophied subvalvular portion of the septum, which could be eliminated by routine myectomy.

Data from the Literature

Larger series of surgically treated patients with HOCM during the last 15 years are summarized in Table 13. In general, these data clearly demonstrate the continuing improvement of early surgical results concerning transaortic subval-

Table 13. Surgical treatment of HOCM: early and late mortality

Reference	Pati-ents (n)	Surgical proce-dure	Hospital mortality (%)	Late mortality (%)	HOCM-related morta-lity/year (%)
Bigelow et al. 1974 [4]	39	TSMT/E	7.5	2.4	
Björk and Radegran 1976 [7]	32	TSME	6.3	2.9	
Cooley et al. 1976 [11]	27	MVR	3.7		
Maron et al. 1983 [29]	240	TSME	8.0	2.7	1.6
Binet et al. 1983 [5]	75	TSME	9.2	2.8	
Bircks and Schulte 1983 [6]	137	TSME	6.6		
Rothlin et al. 1983 [38]	64	TLVM	1.6	2.1	1.9
Von der Lohe et al. 1984 [48]	33	TSME	3.0		
Barratt-Boyes 1985 [2]	75	TLVM	5.3		1.6
Kirklin and Barratt-Boyes 1986 [24]	76	TSME	7.0		1.3
Williams et al. 1987 [51]	61	TSME	1.6	6.6	
McIntosh et al. 1989 [31]	58	MVR	8.6	11.3	
Düsseldorf 1989	293	TSME	4.8	2.2	1.1
Last consecutive patients	100	TSME	1	–	–

TSMT, transaortic subvalvular myotomy; TSME, transaortic subvalvular myectomy; TLVM, trans-LV myectomy; MVR, mitral valve replacement.

vular myectomy (48, 51, own experience). Subsequently there is a long-term clinical improvement with an almost constant HOCM-related annual late mortality of about 1.1% to 1.6%, which seems to be acceptable in relation to the natural history and the severity of the underlying disease in all surgically treated patients.

Conclusion

Taking into consideration the preoperative clinical condition, in relation to the early and late postoperative results in comparison to medical treatment, the following conclusions may be drawn. The progression of HOCM is slow. In many patients, long-term medical therapy is sufficient, but in a certain number it is inappropriate. The operative risk could be reduced to 1%. The incidence of perioperative complications is relatively low. Surgical treatment indicates a high probability of subjective, hemodynamic, and physical improvement.

Up to now, there have been no reports on a real relapse or restenosis after surgery. The incidence of preoperative arrhythmias with the risk of sudden death requires a careful analysis and localization, which in certain patients can be of definite value for surgical treatment. There is a trend – but not yet a proof – that after myectomy the rate of sudden death and late mortality is reduced.

Acknowledgement: This work was supported by grants from the Deutsche Forschungsgemeinschaft Sonderforschungsbereich 242 (Düsseldorf).

References

1. Alvarez-Diaz F, Cabo J, Cordovilla G, Greco R, Sanz E, Berches D, Alvarado F, Garcia-Aguado A (1984) Surgical correction of diffuse subaortic stenosis by an infundibular septal resection. 33rd Congress of the European Society of Cardiovascular Surgery. Madrid, Abstracts, p 118
2. Barratt-Boyes BG (1985) Operative management. In: ten Cate FJ (ed) Hypertrophic cardiomyopathy. Clinical recognition and management. Dekker, New York, pp 209–230
3. Bernhard FW, Poirier V, La Farge CG (1975) Relief of congenital obstruction to left ventricular outflow with a ventricular-aortic prosthesis. J Thorac Cardiovasc Surg 69:223
4. Bigelow WG, Trimble AS, Wigle ED, Adelmann AG, Felderhof C (1974) The treatment of muscular subaortic stenosis. J Thorac Cardiovasc Surg 68:384–391
5. Binet JP, David P, Pirot JD (1983) Surgical treatment of hypertrophic obstructive cardiomyopathies. Eur Heart J 4 (Suppl F):191–195
6. Bircks W, Schulte HD (1983) Surgical treatment of hypertrophic obstructive cardiomyopathy with special reference to complications and to atypical hypertrophic obstructive cardiomyopathy. Eur Heart J 4 (Suppl F):187–190
7. Björk VO, Radegran K (1976) Obstructive cardiomyopathie. J Cardiovasc Surg (Torino) 17:376–379
8. Bretschneider HJ (1980) Myocardial protection. J Thorac Cardiovasc Surg 28:295–302
8a. Borggrefe M, Kuhn H, Königer HH, Stöter H, Loogen F, Schulte HD, Bircks W (1983) Arrhythmias in hypertrophic obstructive and nonobstructive cardiomyopathy. Eur Heart J 4 (Suppl V), 245–251
8b. Borggrefe M, Breithardt G, Lösse B, Loogen F (1989) Hypertrophische Kardiomyopathie. In: Breithardt G, Hombach V (eds) Plötzlicher Herztod (Sudden death). Steinkopff, Darmstadt, pp S 39–47

9. Cleland WP (1963) The surgical management of obstructive cardiomyopathy. J Cardiovasc Surg (Torino) 4:489–491

10. Cooley DA, Norman JC, Mullins CE, Grace RR (1975) Left ventricle to abdominal aorta conduits for relief of aortic stenosis. Cardiovasc Dis 2:376–380

11. Cooley DA, Wukasch DC, Leachman RD (1976) Mitral valve replacement for idiopathic subaortic stenosis. Results in 27 patients. J Cardiovasc Surg (Torino) 17:380–387

12. Dobell ARC, Scott AJ (1964) Hypertrophic subaortic stenosis. Evolution of a surgical technique. J Thorac Cardiovasc Surg 47:26

13. Duch HJ, Hutschemeiter W, Paneau H, Trenckmann H (1984) Atrioventricular stimulation with reduced av-delay time as a therapeutic principle in hypertrophic obstructive cardiomyopathy. Z Gesamte Inn Med 391:437–447

14. Erwin J, McWilliams E, Geary G, Maurer B (1985) Haemodynamic and symptomatic improvement using dual chamber pacing in hypertrophic cardiomyopathy. Br Heart J 54:641 (Abstr)

15. Goodwin JF (1985) Recent views on hypertrophic cardiomyopathy. In: Van der Wall E, Lie KI (eds) Recent views on hypertrophic cardiomyopathy. Nijhoff, Boston, pp 1–10

16. Harrison DC, Braunwald E, Glick G, Mason DT, Chidsey CAL, Ross J Jr (1964) Effects of beta adrenergic blockade on circulation with particular reference to observations in patients with hypertrophic subaortic stenosis. Circulation 29:84–98

17. Harken DE (1964) Discussion. J Thorac Cardiovasc Surg 47:33

18. Hassenstein P, Storch HH, Schmitz W (1975) Erfahrungen mit der Schrittmacherdauerbehandlung bei Patienten mit obstruktiver Kardiomyopathie. Thoraxchirurgie 23:496–499

19. Isner JM, Clark RH, Pandian NG (1984) Laser myoplasty for hypertrophic cardiomyopathy. In vitro experience in human postmortem hearts, and in vivo experiments in a canine model (transarterial) and human patients (intraoperative). Am J Cardiol 53:1620–1625

20. Johnson J (1964) Discussion of Dobell and Scott [13] J Thoracic Cardiovasc Surgery 47, 29

21. Julian OC, Dye WS, Javid H, Hunter JA, Muenster JJ, Najafi H (1965) Apical left ventriculotomy in subaortic stenosis due to fibromuscular hypertrophy. Circulation 31 (Suppl I):45

22. Kaltenbach M, Hopf R, Keller M (1976) Calciumantagonistische Therapie bei hypertropher obstruktiver Kardiomyopathie. Dtsch Med Wochenschr 101:1284–1287

23. Kirklin JW, Ellis FW (1961) Surgical relief of diffuse subvalvular aortic stenosis. Circulation 24:739–742

24. Kirklin JW, Barratt-Boyes BG (1986) Cardiac surgery. Wiley, New York

25. Konno S, Imai Y, Jida Y, Makajima M, Tetsuno K (1974) A new method for prosthetic valve replacement in congenital aortic stenosis associated with hypoplasia of the aortic ring. J Thorac Cardiovasc Surg 70:109

26. Lillehei CW, Levy MJ (1963) Transatrial exposure for correction of subaortic stenosis. J Am Med Assoc 186:8

27. Lösse B, Kuhn H, Loogen F, Schulte HD (1983) Exercise performance in hypertrophic cardiomyopathies. Eur Heart J 4 (Suppl F):197–208

28. Lösse B, Loogen F, Schulte HD (1983) Hemodynamic long-term results after medical and surgical therapy of hypertrophic cardiomyopathies. Z Kardiol 76 (Suppl 3):119–130

29. Maron BJ, Epstein SE, Morrow AG (1983) Symptomatic status and prognosis of patients after operation for hypertrophic obstructive cardiomyopathy: efficacy of ventricular septal myotomy and myectomy. Eur Heart J 4 (Suppl F):175–185

30. McIntosh CHL, Maron BJ, Leon MB, Cannon RO (1988) Clinical and hemodynamic results following mitral valve replacement in patients having idiopathic hypertrophic subaortic stenosis. 24th Annual meeting: Society of Thoracic Surgeons. New Orleans, Lousiana, September 26–28, 1988

31. McIntosh CHL, Greenberg GJ, Maron BJ, Leon MB, Cannon III RO, Clark RE (1989) Clinical and hemodynamic results after mitral valve replacement in patients with obstructive hypertrophic cardiomyopathy. Ann Thorac Surg 47:236–246

32. McKenna WJ, Harris L, Perez G, Krikler DM, Oakley CM, Goodwin JF (1981) Arrhythmia in hypertrophic cardiomyopathy: II. Comparison of amiodarone and verapamil in treatment. Br Heart J 46:173–178

33. Morrow AG, Brockenbrough EC (1961) Surgical treatment of idiopathic hypertrophic subaortic stenosis: technique and hemodynamic results of subaortic ventriculotomy. Ann Surg 154:181–189
34. Morrow AG, Lambrew CT, Braunwald E (1964) Idiopathic hypertrophic subaortic stenosis. II. Operative treatment and the results of pre- and postoperative hemodynamic evaluations. Circulation 29 (Suppl 4):120–151
35. Morrow AG (1978) Hypertrophic aortic stenosis. Operative methods utilized to relieve left ventricular outflow obstruction. J Thorac Cardiovasc Surg 76:423–430
36. Rastan H, Koncz J (1975) Plastische Erweiterung des linken Ausflußtraktes – eine neue Operationsmethode. Thoraxchirurgie 3:169–175
37. Roberts WC (1973) Operative treatment of hypertrophic obstructive cardiomyopathy: the case against mitral valve replacement. Am J Cardiol 32:377–381
38. Rothlin M, Gobet D, Haberer T, Krayenbühl HP, Turina M, Senning A (1983) Surgical treatment versus medical treatment in hypertrophic obstructive cardiomyopathy. Eur Heart J 4 (Suppl F):215–223
39. Schulte HD, Bircks W, Körfer R, Kuhn H (1981) Surgical aspects of typical subaortic and atypical midventricular hypertrophic obstructive cardiomyopathy (HOCM). Thorac Cardiovasc Surg 29:375–380
40. Schulte HD, Lösse B (1985) Hypertrophische obstruktive Kardiomyopathie: Chirurgische Behandlung und Ergebnisse. Herz 10:102–111
41. Schulte HD, Bircks W, Lösse B (1985) Ursachen und Bedeutung der Mitralklappeninsuffizienz bei der chirurgischen Behandlung der hypertrophischen obstruktiven Kardiomyopathie. Wien Klin Wochenschr 135:489–493
42. Schulte HD, Bircks W, Lösse B (1987) Techniques and complications of transaortic subvalvular myectomy in patients with hypertrophic obstructive cardiomyopathy (HOCM). Z Kardiol 76 (Suppl 3):145–151
43. Schulte HD, Lösse B, Bircks W (1988) Früh- und Spätergebnisse nach transaortaler Myektomie bei hypertrophischer obstruktiver Kardiomyopathie (HOCM). Z Herz-Thorax-Gefäßchir 2:149–156
44. Senning A (1976) Transventricular relief of idiopathic hypertrophic subaortic stenosis. J Cardiovasc Surg (Torino) 17:371–375
45. Stinson EB, Shumway NE (1978) Transplantation of the heart. In: Longmore DB (ed) Modern cardiac surgery. MTP-Press, Lancaster, pp 3–18
46. Trimble AS, Bigelow WG, Wigle ED, Chrysohon A (1964) Simple and effective surgical approach to muscular subaortic stenosis. Circulation 29 (Suppl):125
47. Van der Wall E (1985) Recent views on left ventricular function in hypertrophic cardiomyopathy: hemodynamic concepts and their clinical implication. In: Van der Wall E, Lie KI (eds) Recent views on hypertrophic cardiomyopathy. Nijhoff, Boston, pp 71–99
48. Von der Lohe E, Müller-Hake C, Minale C, Von Essen R, Effert S, Messmer BJ (1984) Septumresektion bei hypertrophierter obstruktiver Kardiomyopathie. Dtsch Med Wochenschr 109:1749–1753
49. Vouhé PR, Pulain H, Block G, Loisance DY, Gamain J, Lombaer M, Quiret JC, Lesbre JP, Bernasconi P, Pietri J, Cachera JP (1984) Aortoseptal approach for optimal resection of diffuse subvalvular aortic stenosis. J Thorac Cardiovasc Surg 87:887–893
50. Wigle ED, Sasson Z, Handerson MA, Ruddy TD, Fulop J, Rakowski H, Williams WG (1985) Hypertrophic cardiomyopathy. The importance of the site, and the extent of hypertrophy. A review. Prog Cardiovasc Dis 28:1–83
51. Williams WG, Wigle ED, Rakowski H, Smallhorn J, LeBlanc J, Trusler GA (1987) Results of surgery for hypertrophic obstructive cardiomyopathy. Circulation 76 (Suppl V):104–108

Utility of Intraoperative Echocardiography in Planning Surgical Strategy in Obstructive Hypertrophic Cardiomyopathy*

B. J. Maron, G. Greenberg, and C. L. McIntosh

Operative intervention has been an important part of the therapeutic strategy for patients with obstructive hypertrophic cardiomyopathy (HCM) for the past 30 years [1–16]. Cleland [1], in 1958, was the first to successfully perform a transaortic myectomy operation in a patient with this disease by resecting a small amount of muscle from the thickened upper portion of ventricular septum. Shortly thereafter, Morrow [2, 3] modified and refined the ventricular septal myotomy-myectomy operation (also known as left ventricular myotomy-myectomy, ventriculomyectomy, or the Morrow procedure), which he ultimately performed on 350 patients at the National Institutes of Health. Abouth the same time, in Toronto, Bigelow et al. [4] successfully pioneered the myotomy operation (ventriculomyotomy) which was similar to the myotomy-myectomy except that no muscle was ultimately removed from the ventricular septum.

Over the past 3 decades, operation for patients with obstructive HCM has continued to be performed frequently, but primarily in only a few selected referral centers [1–16]. Operative intervention has achieved symptomatic benefit and improved the quality of life for considerable periods of time in many patients with HCM (in whom medical therapy has failed), by virtue of relieving the subaortic pressure gradient and reducing or normalizing left ventricular pressures [17–20]. The experience gained from the clinical appraisal of these patients over a long period of time, as well as from technical advances in echocardiographic techniques, have considerably enhanced our understanding of the role of operation in HCM and have altered our concepts regarding the intraoperative management of such patients.

Obstruction to Left Ventricular Outflow in Hypertrophic Cardiomyopathy

Operative intervention in HCM is predicated on the premise that true mechanical impedance to left ventricular outflow is present in these patients. Indeed, there is substantial evidence available from a series of hemodynamic, contrast

* Adapted from C. L. McIntosh and B. J. Maron, *Circulation* 78:487–495, 1988, with permission of the American Heart Associaton.

and radionuclide angiographic, Doppler and echocardiographic studies that supports the principle that systolic anterior motion of the mitral valve (and prolonged systolic contact between the mitral valve and ventricular septum) creates true obstruction to left ventricular outflow [17–27]. For example, the gradient develops at the same time in mid-systole that the mitral valve makes initial contact with the ventricular septum; the earlier and more prolonged this mitral-septal apposition, the more severe the outflow gradient. Indeed, it has been the clinical experience of our institution and others [18] that in individual patients with HCM a left ventricular outflow gradient under basal conditions is, with only very rare exception, associated with marked mitral systolic anterior motion and mitral-septal contact. Although the left ventricle in HCM is hypderdynamic and ejects a considerable proportion of its stroke volume rapidly and early in systole, a large proportion of left ventricular emptying (about 50%) does occur in the presence of the subaortic gradient and systolic contact between mitral valve and ventricular septum. Hence, the left ventricle is not truly devoid of blood when the outflow gradient is present; the gradient and forward blood flow coexist in midsystole, flow persists throughout the prolonged period of left ventricular ejection in most patients, and the left ventricle continues to shorten even after increased intraventricular pressures appear. Doppler investigations (including color flow mapping) [27] confirm that the site of jet formation is at or near the point of maximum mitral systolic anterior motion, blood flow-velocity is increased in the left ventricular outflow tract, and the magnitude of this velocity shows a linear relationship with the measured subaortic gradient [28].

Indications for Operation in Hypertrophic Cardiomyopathy

About 1800 operations (primarily ventricular septal myotomy-myectomy) have been performed on patients with obstructive HCM of virtually all ages from about 10 to 75 years, largely at ten major institutions throughout the world that have active surgical experience with this disease [1–20]. Operative mortality has been about 5%. The usual indications for operation are:

1) marked symptoms unrelieved by adequate medical trials of beta-blockers, calcium antagonists or other drugs; and
2) obstruction to left ventricular outflow under basal conditions (subaortic gradient $\geq$ 50 mmHg), or with provocative maneuvers alone (at some institutions).

However, there are no conclusive studies demonstrating whether or not operation prolongs life; therefore, surgery is only recommended and performed to improve severe symptoms and the quality of life. Owing to the uncertainty regarding whether operation influences longevity and because of the risks of the procedure, asymptomatic or mildly symptomatic patients with large gradients are not usually considered to be candidates for myotomy-myectomy even through they could theoretically benefit hemodynamically from this procedure.

Operative Techniques

The standard ventricular septal myotomy-myectomy operation [2] is performed through an aortotomy, largely without the benefit of direct anatomic visualization of the operative field (Figs. 1–7). Two vertical and parallel incisions are made in the basal ventricular septum about 1 cm apart and 1.0–1.5 cm deep into muscle (Fig. 1) and are extended toward the apex for about 3–4 cm. A third transverse incision connects the first two incisions at their distal extent, and the bar of septal muscle is excised. Generally, a rectangular channel is created, extending from a point near the aortic anulus to a point beyond the site of mitral-septal systolic contact (Figs. 1 and 2E). This channel is made in the

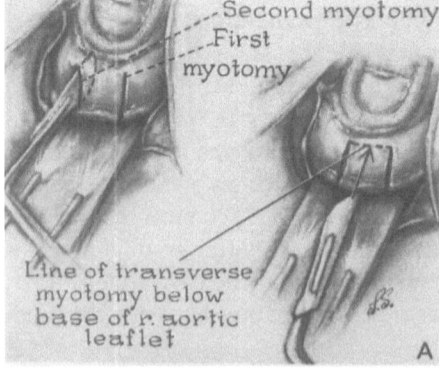

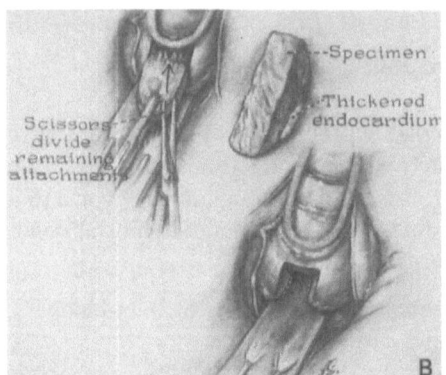

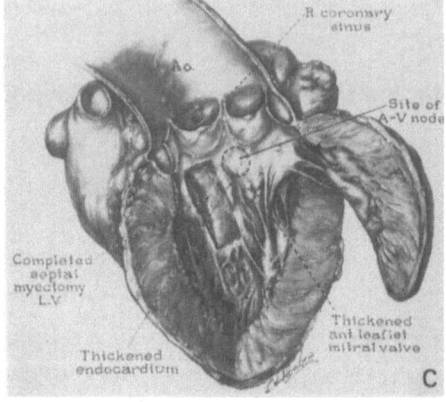

Fig. 1 A–C. The ventricular septal myotomy-myectomy operation (performed through an aortotomy), the standard operative procedure to relieve the subaortic gradient in patients with obstructive HCM. **A** Two vertical and parallel incisions are made in the most basal portion of ventricular septum about 1 cm apart, with an angled knife. A third incision is made transversely, connecting the initial two parallel myotomies. Attachments of the muscle bar to the septum are divided. **B** This segment of muscle is isolated, excised and removed either intact (as shown) or in several pieces. **C** At completion of the myotomy-myectomy operation, a rectangular channel is created, about 1 cm wide, 1 cm deep, and 4 cm long, extending from a point 5–10 mm below the aortic anulus to a point just distal to the region of systolic contact between the distal portion of mitral valve leaflets and ventricular septum. In some patients additional tissue may be resected from the margins of the channel to achieve grater enlargement of the left ventricular outflow tract. (From [40])

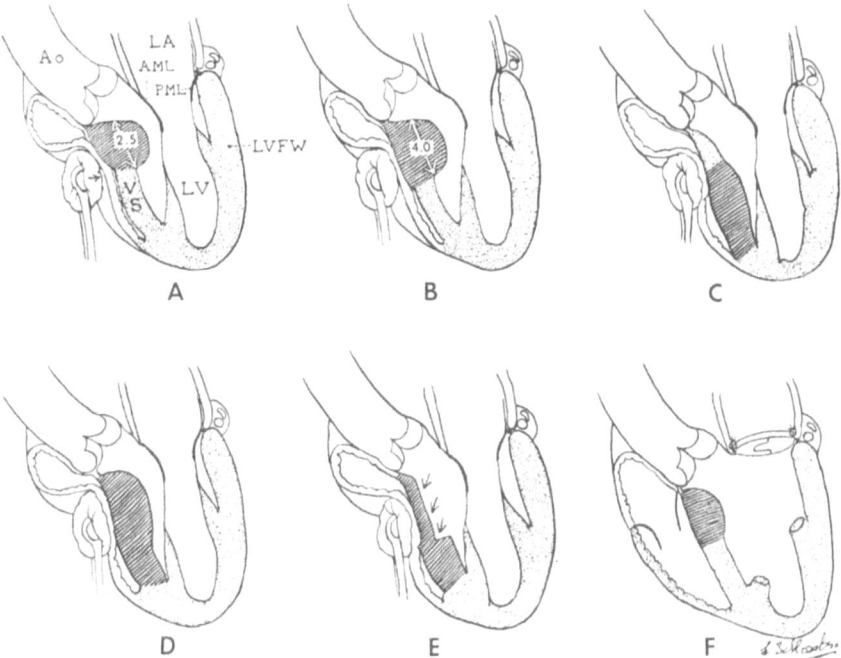

Fig. 2 A–F. Morphologic spectrum of obstructive HCM and importance of the distribution of ventricular septal *(VS)* thickening to the myotomy-myectomy operation. **A–D** show different distributions of ventricular septal hypertrophy in the longitudinal cross-sectional plane; thickened areas of septum are denoted by parallel slanted lines. **A** Septal hypertrophy is quite localized to the most proximal 2 cm of the anterior basal septum. **B** Hypertrophy involves the upper and mid-septal areas, extending over the proximal 4 cm of anterior septum. **C** Basal portion of the anterior ventricular septum is relatively thin, while substantially increased septal thickness is evident at the point of systolic contact between mitral valve and septum, as well as in the more distal portion of septum. **D** Hypertrophy is more diffuse and involves the entirely septum homogeneously. **E** Completed myotomy-myectomy channel *(arrows)* created in the same left ventricle that is depicted in **D**, extending from near the aortic anulus to just beyond the mitral valve tips. **F** Low-profile disc prothesis implanted in the mitral position after the native mitral valve has been removed from a patient with relatively thin ventricular septum (i.e., < 18 mm). *AML*, anterior mitral leaflet; *Ao*, aorta; *LA*, left atrium; *LV*, left ventricle; *LVFW*, left ventricular free wall; *PML*, posterior mitral leaflet; *RV*, right ventricle. (From [40])

12 o'clock position (on the echocardiographic short-axis orientation), avoiding portions of the conducting system and the membranous septum which are located more medially toward the 11 o'clock position. By two-dimensional echocardiography in the short-axis view, the muscular resection appears as a "notch," with each of the three sides usually at sharp right angles (Fig. 3). If the resection is precisely at 12 o'clock in the short-axis plane, its cephalad-caudal extent can be easily visualized in the long-axis view.

In addition to myotomy-myectomy, a number of other operations have been proposed through the years for patients with obstructive HCM, including myotomy alone, or mitral valve replacement [5, 15, 20]. Although these operations

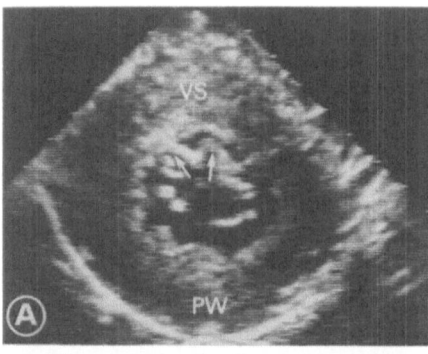

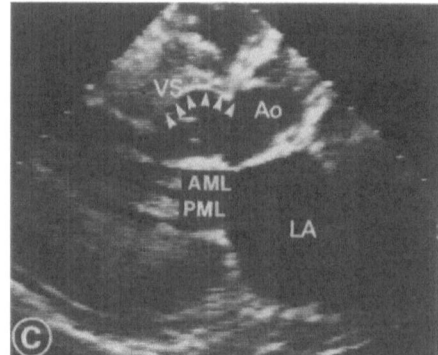

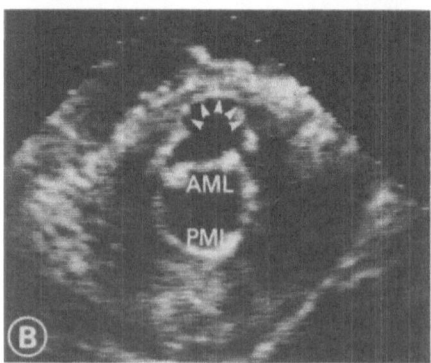

Fig. 3 A–C. Stop-frames of a two-dimensional echocardiogram from a patient with obstructive HCM, obtained in short-axis view at the level of the mitral valve before (**A**) and after (**B and C**) septal myotomy-myectomy. **A** Left ventricular outflow tract *(LVOT)* cross-sectional area is virtually obliterated in systole; points of mitral-septal contact with ventricular septum *(VS)* are identified by *arrows.* **B** Myotomy-myectomy appears as a "notch" *(arrow)* in the anterior ventricular septum *(arrowheads),* and the cross-sectional area of the left ventricular outflow tract and distance between anterior mitral leaflet *(AML)* and septum has been greatly increased by operation. **C** Appearance of myotomy-myectomy in parasternal long-axis view *(arrowheads).* *Ao*, aorta; *LA*, left atrium; *PML*, posterior mitral leaflet; *PW*, posterior wall. *Calibration dots* are 1 cm apart

differ in design, the immediate objective has been the same in each case – i.e., to abolish or substantially reduce the subaortic gradient and systolic anterior motion of the mitral valve and thereby normalize left ventricular systolic pressure. With septal myotomy-myectomy, this goal is achieved under basal conditions in about 95% of patients [17, 20] without importantly compromising global left ventricular function [29]; in the vast majority of these patients the basal gradient is abolished, and in the remainder only small gradients (≤ 20 mmHg) are evident postoperatively.

Although the amount of muscle excised (usually 1.5–3.0 g) constitutes only a small fraction of overall left ventricular mass, it is removed from a particularly critical site in the left ventricular outflow tract where mitral-septal contact and increased outflow tract velocities occur. Consequently, operation has the effect of widening and enlarging the left ventricular outflow tract and increasing the distance between septum and mitral valve (Figs. 3–5, 7), and thereby substan-

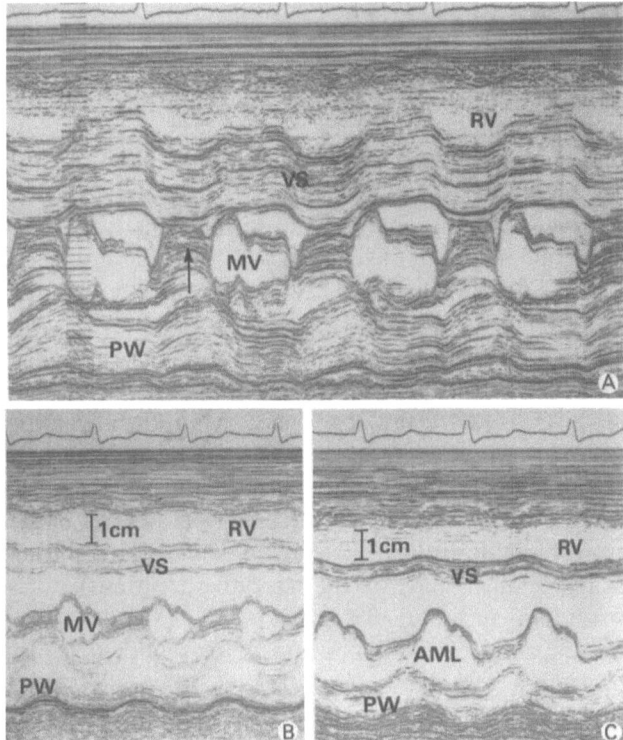

Fig. 4 A–C. Transthoracic M-mode echocardiogram obtained from a 24-year-old woman with HCM at the level of the mitral valve *(MV)* before myotomy-myectomy (**A**) and after myotomy-myectomy at the level of the mitral valve (**B**) and just below the aortic valve (**C**). **A** Preoperatively, ventricular septum is thickened (21 mm), septum to mitral valve distance is reduced (17 mm), and marked systolic anterior motion of the mitral valve is present *(arrow)*. *Calibration lines* are 2 mm apart. **B** Postoperatively, ventricular septum now appears normal in thickness (9 mm), septum to mitral valve distance is greatly increased (24 mm), and systolic anterior motion of the mitral valve is absent. **C** Just below the aortic valve, septal thickness has been greatly reduced (to 5 mm). *AML*, anterior mitral valve leaflet; *PW*, posterior wall; *RV*, right ventricle. (From [30])

tially reducing the high outflow tract velocities and presumably the Venturi forces that create mitral systolic anterior motion and mechanical impedance to outflow [9, 17, 30–33]. Because mitral regurgitation is usually a consequence of systolic anterior motion of the valve, it is also relieved or reduced by operation [18].

Morphologic Spectrum of HCM and Significance to Operative Treatment

The application of two-dimensional echocardiographic imaging to a large number of patients within the broad clinical spectrum of HCM has emphasized the great morphologic diversity present in this disease, particularly with respect to the distribution of left ventricular hypertrophy [17, 18, 34, 35]. Frequently, in patients with HCM, the pattern of wall thickening is strikingly heterogeneous (Figs. 2, 6, and 7). Contiguous segments of the left ventricular wall may differ greatly in thickness and wall thickness may show abrupt change, often within only a few millimeters (Fig. 7); in fact, it is not uncommon for markedly thickened left ventricular segments to be adjacent to portions of the wall that are of normal thickness (Fig. 7). Such heterogeneity may occur within the ventricular septum and even within the relatively confined region of the potential septal myotomy-myectomy – i.e., the basal portion of septum extending for about 3–4 cm from the aortic anulus distally toward the left ventricular apex (Figs. 2 and 7).

Our appreciation of the morphologic and clinical spectrum of those patients with obstructive HCM referred for operative therapy has evolved through the years, and we are now cognizant of a more diverse expression of the disease than perhaps was the case in the 1960s and 1970s. Certainly, since 1980, we have been exposed to more varied patterns of left ventricular hypertrophy by virtue of expanding and diversifying patterns of patient referral as well as our extensive utilization of diagnostic echocardiography. This experience has had an important impact on the operative treatment of patients with HCM at our institution, including the selection of patients for septal myotomy-myectomy and the precise techniques utilized to relieve the left ventricular outflow tract gradient.

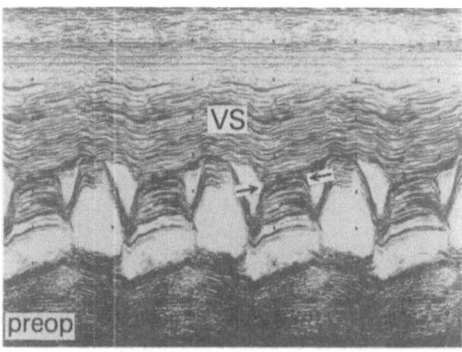
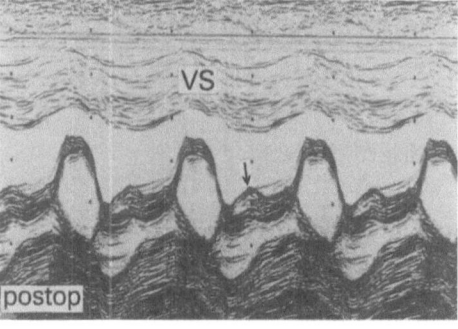

Fig. 5. M-mode echocardiograms obtained in the operating room before and after ventricular septal myotomy-myectomy in a patient with obstructive hypertrophic cardiomyopathy. Preoperatively, marked systolic anterior motion of the mitral valve with prolonged mitral-septal contact *(arrows)* is present. Postoperatively, after relief of the outflow gradient, the left ventricular outflow tract is widened, the ventricular septum *(VS)* is thinner, and only trivial mitral systolic anterior motion remains *(arrow). Calibration dots* are 1 cm apart

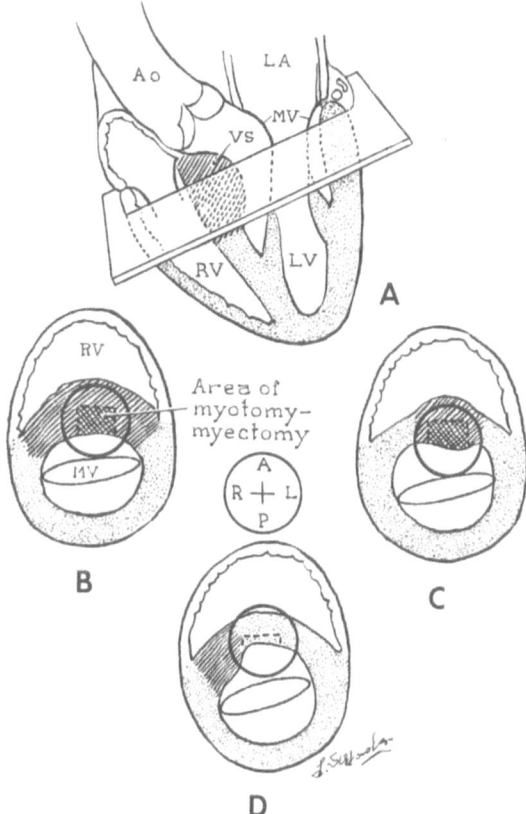

Fig. 6 A–D. Morphologic spectrum of obstructive HCM and importance of the distribution of ventricular septal *(VS)* thickening to the myotomy-myectomy operation. **A** Longitudinal cross-sectional plane through left ventricle *(LV)* showing hypertrophy of the ventricular septum. **B–D** Short-axis views of left ventricle in a plane perpendicular to the ventricular long axis (as in **A**) at mitral valve *(MV)* level and shown in the echocardiographic orientation (as viewed from the position of the left ventricular apex). Three different patterns of ventricular septal hypertrophy are illustrated; thickened areas of septum are denoted by parallel slanted lines. **B** Homogeneous marked thickening of anterior ventricular septum permits myectomy to be performed through conventional aortotomy in the 12 o'clock position; *circle* indicates superimposed location of the aortic ring (anulus) which would be the surgeon's field of view from above (i.e., "operative window"). **C** Septal thickening is at the 12 o'clock position, but portions of septum to each side are much thinner. Myectomy can still be performed, but care must be taken to confine resection to the thickened segment. **D** Thickening of anterior basal septum shows an inhomogeneous pattern; medial portion (toward patient's right) is thick, but the lateral (toward patient's left) and central 12 o'clock regions are of normal thickness. Myectomy cannot be performed in the conventional 12 o'clock position because of the risk for septal perforation; also, muscle usually cannot be resected from the extreme medial portion of septum because technical factors often prohibit the operative exposure that would be necessary. Mitral valve replacement would be an alternative operation in such a patient. *A*, anterior; *Ao*, aorta; *L* (patient's) left; *LA*, left atrium; *P*, posterior; *R*, (patient's) right; *RV*, right ventricle

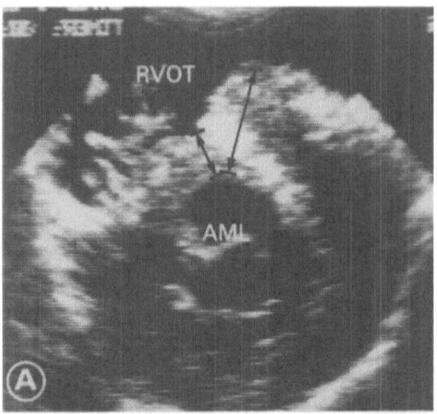

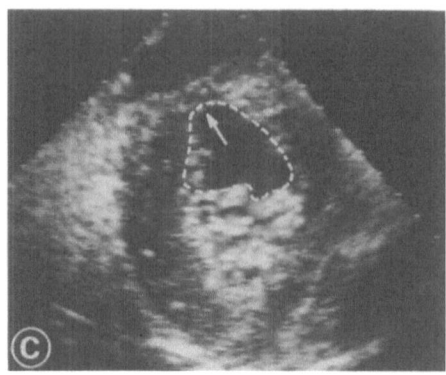

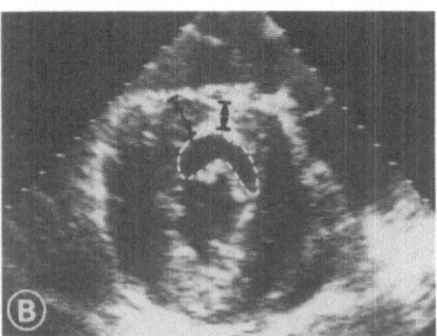

Fig. 7 A–C. Variations in distribution of ventricular septal thickening identified by intraoperative echocardiography, influencing operative strategy in obstructive HCM. **A** Patient who received mitral valve replacement. Abrupt change in wall thickness near 12 o'clock region of anterior ventricular septum; medially (toward 11 o'clock and the patient's right) the wall is too thin for a muscular resection to be performed without unacceptable risk for perforation while laterally (toward 1 o'clock and the patient's left) the wall is about twice as thick. **B** Patient with heterogeneous thickening of anterior ventricular septum who underwent myotomy-myectomy. Note that medially (toward 11 o'clock) the wall is thicker than it is at 12 o'clock (*broken line* outlines the limits of the left ventricular outflow tract). **C** Same patient as in **B**, after completion of muscular resection which was directed toward thicker region of anterior septum at 11 o'clock *(arrow)*. Note enlargement of left ventricular outflow tract cross-sectional area which was accomplished without producing ventricular septal defect

Application of Intraoperative Echocardiography to Ventricular Septal Myotomy-Myectomy

Two major complications of the myotomy-myectomy operation that may contribute importantly to mortality and morbidity are iatrogenic complete heart block and ventricular septal defect [3, 8, 14]. Complete heart block results when the integrity of the conducting system is interrupted by improper placement of the myotomy incisions (or even with appropriate myectomy in those rare patients with pre-existing right bundle branch block). This complication can now usually be treated adequately with implantation of atrioventricular sequential or rate-responsive pacemakers.

Ventricular septal defect, produced by removal of an excessive amount of muscle from the septum (or by excessively deep myotomy incisions), is probably the most profound complication of septal myotomy-myectomy. Septal defects usually occur when myectomy is performed in areas of the septum which are of normal or only mildly increased thickness, either by virtue of direct perforation or by creating an area of necrosis that in turn predisposes to perforation. Therefore, we believe that it is critical for the surgeon to be aware of any heterogeneity in the thickness of the ventricular septum so that relatively thin areas of the septum can be excluded from the myectomy.

Since ventricular septal morphology is not identical in all patients with obstructive HCM who are candidates for myotomy-myectomy (Figs. 2, 6, and 7), the precise mode of muscular resection should not necessarily be identical in all patients. Consequently, we have found detailed echocardiographic mapping of septal hyertrophy by echocardiography to be crucial for the safe and efficacious performance of this operation. However, in an important minority of patients, conventional transthoracic echocardiography cannot provide the precise definition of septal thickness that is required in this clinical circumstance (Fig. 8); this may be due to a number of variables including unfavorable body habitus or chest configuration, or the presence of pulmonary disease. It was such considerations that ultimately led us to routinely utilize intraoperative echocardiography to define septal morphology in patients with obstructive HCM [36]. Consequently, over the past 6 years, each patient undergoing operation for HCM at the National Institutes of Health has had the distribution and magnitude of septal hypertrophy mapped in the operating room with an integrated two-dimensional and M-mode echocardiographic examination (Fig. 9). For this purpose, we have utilized commercially available ultrasound units

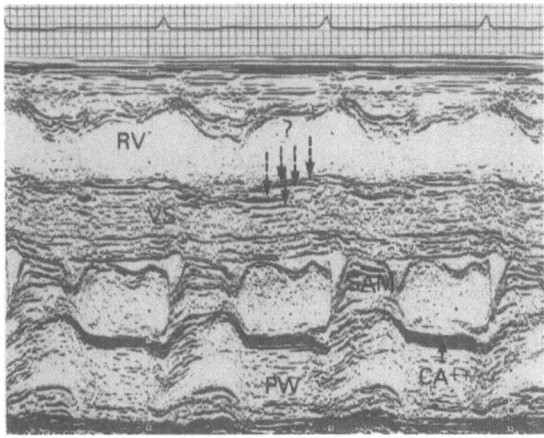

Fig. 8. M-mode echocardiogram showing difficulty often encountered with transthoracic echocardiography in imaging and quantitative measurement of ventricular septal *(VS)* thickness. Note that several echo-dense lines *(arrows)* could conceivably represent the interface of the right septal surface. Ca^{++}, calcium in mitral anulus; *PW*, posterior left ventricular free wall; *SAM*, systolic anterior motion; *VS*, ventricular septum

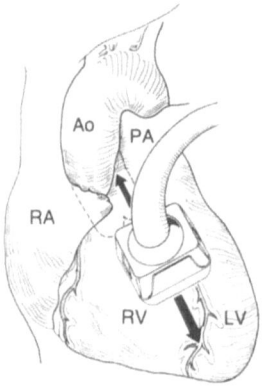

Fig. 9. Position of transducer on exposed heart surface for intraoperative echocardiography. For short-axis imaging of the left ventricle, the transducer is initially placed at or near the junction of aortic root with the base of left ventricle *(LV)* and then moved slowly toward the apex maintaining the transducer head flat on the heart surface. The long-axis is obtained by orienting the transducer at 90° to the short-axis plane. *RV*, right ventricle, *RA*, right atrium; *Ao*, aorta; *PA*, pulmonary artery

(currently Hewlett-Packard) with 3.5–5.0-mHz transducers which are enclosed in a sterile sleeve with a small amount of ultrasound transmission gel placed between the transducer head and sleeve; the transducer is positioned directly on the surface of the right ventricle of the beating heart prior to the institution of cardiopulmonary bypass.

The information obtained from this intraoperative echocardiographic assessment is used to determine if myotomy-myectomy should be performed and, if so, whether the standard muscular resection needs to be tailored to the individual patient's septal anatomy (Figs. 2, 6, and 7). At our institution, it is relatively uncommon to encounter a patient with obstructive HCM at operation in whom septal hypertrophy is both particularly marked and homogeneously distributed, so that the standard myotomy-myectomy can be undertaken with virtually no preoperative deliberation regarding the pattern and magnitude of septal thickness. Instead, a variety of "atypical" patterns of septal hypertrophy are often encountered. Such forms of septal hypertrophy include those in which the thickening of the septum is displaced laterally (Figs. 2, 6, and 7), medially or distally. *Hence, the most crucial information provided by the intraoperative echocardiographic examination is whether the most basal portion of ventricular septum at or near the 12 o'clock position on the short-axis orientation is thick enough to permit septal muscle to be safely resected without incurring undo risk for iatrogenic ventricular septal defect.*

Based on the information derived from intraoperative echocardiographic studies, it is now the routine at our institution to avoid beginning the proximal portion of the myectomy resection directly beneath the aortic anulus (Figs. 1 and 2). Outflow obstruction does not occur at this point, the most proximal 5–10 mm of ventricular septum is frequently quite thin, and support for the aortic valve anulus (and avoidance of iatrogenic aortic regurgitation) may well depend upon leaving this area of the septum intact. If echocardiography reveals that the area of most marked septal hypertrophy is located at or near the point of systolic mitral-septal contact, but the most basal portion of septum is relatively thin, then the resection of muscle is begun farther from the aortic anulus than usual, bypassing the proximal thin area of septum (Fig. 2). Because of these considerations, it is our routine practice to assess the distance from aortic anulus to the point of mitral-septal contact in the parasternal long-axis view. This distance is usually about 20–25 mm, and if this is the case the surgeon has no particular difficulty in extending the myotomy-myectomy resection far enough distally from the aortotomy incision to include the region of mitral-septal contact where obstruction occurs. Occasionally, this systolic contact point on the ventricular septum is displaced more distally; this usually occurs in the presence of particularly long mitral leaflets and often systolic anterior motion of the posterior mitral leaflet [37]. It is necessary for the surgeon to have prior knowledge of this fact so that the resection can be extended more distally. On the other hand, some patients with HCM have relatively mild hypertrophy which is localized to the anterior basal septum, and the contact point is much closer to the aortic valve (about 12–20 mm). In the latter instance, it is relatively easy for the surgeon to resect muscle up to and beyond the point of mitral-septal contact and obstruction; however, in such patients it is also important to avoid the resection of muscle much beyond this point where septal thickness often decreases abruptly.

In another variation of anterior septal morphology, the medial portion is markedly thickened, but the lateral portion and central 12 o'clock areas are relatively thin or even of normal thickness (Fig. 6). The precise localization of the muscular resection can sometimes be shifted slightly laterally in this circumstance; however, should the surgeon judge this revision to be impractical due to the limited exposure permitted through the aortotomy (i.e., between the 11 and 1 o'clock positions in the echocardiographic short-axis orientation), the myotomy-myectomy is abandoned and mitral valve replacement is adopted as a more appropriate alternative. The same considerations apply when the medial and 12 o'clock portions of the septum are thinner than the more lateral segment (Fig. 7). Similarly, if the entire basal septum is relatively thin (< 18 mm) and the risk of incurring a ventricular septal defect with a myotomy-myectomy is judged to be unacceptably high, mitral valve replacement is undertaken (Figs. 2 and 7). At our institution, we have found that intraoperative echocardiography plays an important role in determining the precise operative approach in about one-third of the operations performed on patients with HCM.

In addition, after myotomy-myectomy, intraoperative echocardiography [36] provides the surgeon with the capability of immediately assessing the site and adequacy of the muscular resection and its impact on mitral systolic anterior motion (and, hence, subaortic obstruction), as well as visualizing iatrogenically produced ventricular septal defect or damage to the mitral valve apparatus. Consequently, in the event that operative relief of obstruction is judged to be incomplete, the myotomy-myectomy can be revised in the operating room and additional septal muscle removed, or the mitral valve replaced.

Potential Role of Mitral Valve Replacement

Currently, virtually all investigators agree that ventricular septal myotomy-myectomy is the preferred operation for most patients with obstructive HCM. However, mitral valve replacement [38] with a low-profile disc or bileaflet prosthesis may have an application in certain patients with obstructive HCM, despite the inherent risks for thromboembolic or anticoagulant complications and prosthetic valve dysfunction. Patients most suited to valve replacement are those in whom the risk of resection of septal tissue is judged to be unacceptably high – i.e., with relatively thin basal anterior septum (< 18 mm; usually 15–17 mm) or when the regions of greatest septal thickness are inaccessible to a conventional myotomy-myectomy performed through an aortotomy. Additional indications for mitral valve replacement include inadequate relief of subaortic obstruction following myotomy-myectomy, severe mitral regurgitation secondary to an intrinsic abnormality of the valve, and coexistent coronary artery disease associated with relatively thin ventricular septum [39].

Conclusions

Operation is a important and rational therapeutic alternative when drug therapy is unsuccessful in relieving or controlling the severe symptoms experienced by many patients with obstructive HCM. Following operative relief of outflow obstruction and normalization of left ventricular systolic pressure, the vast majority of patients experience important relief of symptoms and functional limitation and an improved quality of life, which is often long-lasting. Greater awareness and understanding of the morphologic spectrum of HCM afforded by the application of two-dimensional echocardiography has had an important impact on the operative management of patients with this disease. In particular, characterization of the distribution of ventricular septal hypertrophy with intraoperative echocardiography before operation permits myotomy-myectomy to be planned and performed so that muscle is resected only from sufficiently thickened regions of the septum. Consequently, the risk of iatrogenic ventricular septal defect is minimized. Therefore, those patients with HCM and modest degrees of septal hypertrophy (maximum wall thickness of < 18 mm) or particularly heterogeneous patterns of septal thickening may be judged to be more appropriate candidates for mitral valve replacement than for myotomy-myectomy.

References

1. Cleland WP (1963) The surgical management of obstructive cardiomyopathy. J Cardiovasc Surg 4:489–491
2. Morrow AG (1978) Hypertrophic subaortic stenosis: operative methods utilized to relieve left ventricular outflow obstruction. J Thorac Cardiovasc Surg 76:423–430
3. Morrow AG, Reitz BA, Epstein SE, Henry WL, Conkle DM, Itscoitz SB, Redwood DR (1975) Operative treatment in hypertrophic subaortic stenosis: techniques, and the results of pre- and postoperative assessment in 83 patients. Circulation 52:88–102
4. Bigelow WG, Trimble AS, Wigle ED, Adelman AG, Felderhof CH (1967) The treatment of muscular subaortic stenosis. J Thorac Cardiovasc Surg 68:384–392
5. Wigle ED, Trimble AS, Adelman AG, Bigelow WG (1967) Surgery in muscular subaortic stenosis. Prog Cardiovasc Dis 11:83–112

6. Agnew TM, Barratt-Boyes BC, Brandt PWT, Roche AHG, Lowe JB, O'Brien KG (1977) Surgical resection in idiopathic hypertrophic subaortic stenosis with a combined approach through aorta and left ventricle. J Thorac Cardiovasc Surg 74:307–316
7. Reis RL, Hannah H, Carley JE, Pugh DM (1977) Surgical treatment of idiopathic hypertrophic subaortic stenosis (IHSS). Postoperative results in 30 patients following ventricular septal myotomy and myectomy (Morrow procedure). Circulation [Suppl 2] 56:II-128–II-132
8. Maron BJ, Merrill WH, Freier PA, Kent KM, Epstein SE, Morrow AG (1978) Long-term inimical course and symptomatic status of patients after operation for hypertrophic subaortic stenosis. Circulation 57:1205–1213
9. Schapira JN, Stemple DR, Martin RP, Rakowski H, Stinson EB, Popp RL (1978) Single and two-dimensional echocardiographic visualization of the effects of septal myectomy in idiopathic hypertrophic subaortic stenosis. Circulation 58:850–860
10. Bircks W, Schulte HD (1983) Surgical treatment of hypertrophic obstructive cardiomyopathy with special reference to complications and to atypical hypertrophic obstructive cardiomyopathy. Eur Heart J [Suppl F] 4:187–190
11. Binet JP, David PH, Piot JD (1983) Surgical treatment of hypertrophic obstructive cardiomyopathies. Eur Heart J [Suppl F] 4:191–195
12. Rothlin ME, Gobet D, Haberer T, Krayenbuehl HP, Turina M, Senning A (1983) Surgical treatment versus medical treatment in hypertrophic obstructive cardiomyopathy. Eur Heart J [Suppl F] 4:215–223
13. Beahrs MM, Tajik AJ, Seward JB, Giuliani ER, McGoon DC (1983) Hypertrophic obstructive cardiomyopathy: 10–21 year follow-up after partial septal myectomy. Cardiology 51:1160–1166
14. Maron BJ, Epstein SE, Morrow AG (1983) Symptomatic status and prognosis of patients after operation for hypertrophic obstructive cardiomyopathy: Efficacy of ventricular septal myotomy and myectomy. Eur Heart J [Suppl F] 4:175–185
15. Fighali S, Krajcer Z, Leachmen RD (1984) Septal myomectomy and mitral valve replacement for idiopathic hypertrophic subaortic stenosis: short and long-term follow-up. J Am Coll Cardiol 3:1127–1134
16. Williams WG, Wigle Ed, Rakowski H, Smallhorn J, LeBlanc J, Trusler GA (1987) Results of surgery for hypertrophic obstructive cardiomyopathy. Circulation [Suppl 5] 76:V104–V108
17. Maron BJ, Bonow RO, Cannon RO, Leon MB, Epstein SE (1987) Hypertrophic cardiomyopathy. Interrelations of clinical manifestations, pathophysiology, and therapy. N Engl J Med 316:780–789
18. Wigle Ed, Sasson Z, Henderson MA, Ruddy TD, Fulop J, Rakowski H, Williams WG (1985) Hypertrophic cardiomyopathy. The importance of the site and the extent of hypertrophy: a review. Prog Cardiovasc Dis 28:1–83
19. Wigle ED (1987) Hypertrophic cardiomyopathy: A 1987 viewpoint. Circulation 75:311–322
20. Maron BJ, Epstein SE (1986) Clinical significance and therapeutic implications of the left ventricular outflow tract pressure gradient in hypertrophic cardiomyopathy. Am J Cardiol 58:1093–1096
21. Pollick C, Morgan CD, Gilbert BW, Rakowski H, Wigle ED (1982) Muscular subaortic stenosis. The temporal relationship between systolic anterior motion of the anterior mitral leaflet and the pressure gradient. Circulation 66:1087
22. Maron BJ, Gottdiener JS, Arce J, Rosing DR, Wesley YE, Epstein SE (1985) Dynamic subaortic obstruction in hypertrophic cardiomyopathy: Analysis by pulsed Doppler echocardiography. J Am Coll Cardiol 6:115
23. Pierce GE, Morrow AG, Braunwald E (1964) Idiopathic hypertrophic subaortic stenosis. III. Intraoperative studies of the mechanism of obstruction and its hemodynamic consequences. Circulation [Suppl 4] 30:IV-152–IV-207
24. Maron BJ, McIntosh CL, Seipp HWL (1985) Evidence favoring existence of true subaortic obstruction in hypertrophic cardiomyopathy: Intraoperative aortic flow studies before and after operation (Abstr). Circulation 72 [Suppl 3]:III-447

25. Yock PG, Hatle L, Popp RL (1986) Patterns and timing of Doppler-detected intracavitary and aortic flow in hypertrophic cardiomyopathy. J Am Coll Cardiol 8:1047–1058
26. Spirito P, Maron BJ (1984) Patterns of systolic anterior motion of the mitral valve in hypertrophic cardiomyopathy: Assessment by twodimensional echocardiography. Am J Cardiol 54:1039–1046
27. Rakowski H, Sasson Z, Wigle ED (1988) Echocardiographic and Doppler assessment of hypertrophic cardiomyopathy. J Am Soc Echo 1:31–47
28. Sasson Z, Yock PG, Hatle LK, Alderman EL, Popp RL (1988) Doppler echocardiographic determination of the pressure gradient in hypertrophic cardiomyopathy. J Am Coll Cardiol 11:752–756
29. Borer JS, Bacharach SL, Green MV, Kent KM, Rosing DR, Seides SF, Morrow AG, Epstein SE (1979) Effect of septal myotomy and myectomy on left ventricular systolic function at rest and during exercise in patients with IHSS. Circulation [Suppl 1] 60:I82–I87
30. Spirito P, Maron BJ, Rosing DR (1984) Morphologic determinants of hemodynamic state following ventricular septal myotomy-myectomy in patients with hypertrophic cardiomyopathy; M-mode and two-dimensional echocardiographic assessment. Circulation 70:984–995
31. Shah PM, Gramiak R, Adelman AG, Wigle ED (1972) Echocardiographic assessment of the effects of surgery and propranolol on the dynamics of outflow obstruction in hypertrophic obstructive cardiomyopathy. Circulation 45:516–521
32. Turina J, Jenni R, Krayenbuehl HP, Turina M, Rothlin M (1986) Echocardiographic findings late after myectomy in hypertrophic obstructive cardiomyopathy. Eur Heart J 7:685–692
33. Bolton MR, King JF, Polumbo RA, Mason DT, Pugh DM, Reis RL, Dunn MI (1974) The effects of operation on the echocardiographic features of idiopathic hypertrophic subaortic stenosis. Circulation 50:897–900
34. Maron BJ, Gottdiener JS, Epstein SE (1981) Patterns and significance of the distribution of left ventricular hypertrophy in hypertrophic cardiomyopathy: a wide-angle, two-dimensional echocardiographic study of 125 patients. Am J Cardiol 48:418–428
35. Maron BJ (1985) Asymmetry in hypertrophic cardiomyopathy: The septal to free wall thickness ration revisited. Am J Cardiol 55:835–838
36. Maron BJ, McIntosh CL, Wesley YE, Arce J (1984) Application of intraoperative two-dimensional echocardiography to patients with hypertrophic cardiomyopathy undergoing ventricular septal myotomy-myectomy (Abstr). J Am Coll Cardiol 3:565
37. Maron BJ, Harding AM, Spirito P, Roberts WC, Waller BF (1983) Systolic anterior motion of the posterior mitral leaflet: a previously unrecognized cause of dynamic subaortic obstruction in hypertrophic cardiomyopathy. Circulation 68:282–293
38. Cooley DA, Wukasch DC, Leachman RD (1976) Mitral valve replacement for idiopathic hypertrophic subaortic stenosis: results in 27 patients. J Cardiovasc Surg 17:380–387
39. Siegman IL, Maron BJ, Permut LC, McIntosh CL, Clark RE (1989) Results of operation for coexistent obstructive hypertrophic cardiomyopathy and coronary artery disease. J Am Coll Cardiol (in press)
40. McIntosh CL, Maron BJ (1988) Current operative treatment of obstructive hypertrophic cardiomyopathy. Circulation 78:487–495

Rational Choice of Medical and/or Surgical Therapy in Hypertrophic Cardiomyopathy

E. D. Wigle, W. G. Williams, B. Kimball, Z. Sasson, and H. Rakowski

Introduction

A rational choice between medical and surgical therapy in any disease entity can only exist when both forms of therapy are possible. In hypertrophic cardiomyopathy (HCM), there is a choice between medical and surgical therapy in the clinical syndromes listed in Table 1. In this review, we will discuss the various forms of medical and surgical therapy that are available to patients with HCM, but will focus on the Toronto experience, which is based on the hemodynamic classification of this disease [1–6]. We will not discuss those forms of HCM that are only amenable to medical therapy, because in those there is no rational choice between medical and surgical therapy.

Hemodynamic Classification

A hemodynamic classification of HCM is listed in Table 2. It has been traditional to equate obstructive HCM with muscular (hypertrophic) subaortic stenosis, but as indicated in Table 2, both midventricular obstruction and right ventricular outflow tract obstruction are also forms of obstructive HCM. Although we recognize these three different forms of obstructive HCM, in this discussion, for reasons of tradition, we will continue to equate obstructive HCM with muscular subaortic stenosis unless otherwise specified.

In the usual form of obstructive HCM due to mitral leaflet-septal contact, the subaortic pressure gradient may be persistent (gradient at rest), labile (sponta-

Table 1. Clinical syndromes in HCM in which there is a choice between medical and surgical therapy

---

Obstructive HCM
  1) Muscular (hypertrophic) subaortic stenosis
     Special situations: – Atrial fibrillation
                    – Ventricular arrhythmia
  2) Midventricular obstruction
  3) Right ventricular outflow obstruction
Severe mitral regurgitation in nonobstructive HCM
End-stage HCM

Table 2. Hemodynamic classification of HCM

Obstructive HCM
1) Muscular (hypertrophic) subaortic stenosis due to mitral leaflet-septal contact
   – Resting obstruction
   – Labile (variable) obstruction
   – Latent (provocable) obstruction
2) Midventricular obstruction due to midventricular hypertrophy (papillary muscle level)
3) Right ventricular outflow obstruction
Nonobstructive HCM

neously variable) or latent (provocable) (Table 2). In nonobstructive HCM there is no systolic pressure gradient either at rest or on provocation. Because our treatment of HCM is based on the presence or absence of obstruction to left ventricular outflow, in the next few sections, we will review the Toronto viewpoint with regard to the nature and significance of the different types of intraventricular pressure differences that may be encountered in HCM. As well, we will review the pathophysiological significance of the subaortic obstruction caused by mitral leaflet-septal contact in obstructive HCM.

Types of Systolic Pressure Difference in HCM

Prior to discussing the characteristics of obstructive HCM due to mitral leaflet-septal contact (muscular or hypertrophic subaortic stenosis), it is necessary to define the four different types of systolic pressure difference that may be encountered in this condition [3–5] (Fig. 1, Tables 1, 3). An early systolic impulse gradient across the aortic valve results from flow acceleration in early systole.

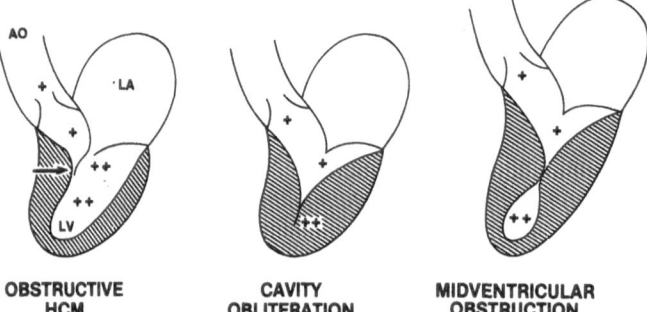

Fig. 1. The left ventricular (LV) inflow tract pressure concept [11, 12]. In obstructive HCM, all LV pressures proximal to the outflow tract obstruction, caused by mitral leaflet-septal contact *(arrow)*, are elevated, including the inflow tract pressure, just inside the mitral valve. In cavity obliteration and midventricular obstruction, the pressure at the apex of the LV is elevated, but the inflow tract pressure is not (see text). *AO*, aorta; *LA*, left atrium. (From [5])

This gradient may be greater than normal in HCM, due to very rapid, early systolic ejection, but it ends by mid-systole, when flow acceleration decreases [7]. A second type of systolic pressure difference within the left ventricle in HCM is that produced by midventricular obstruction at the level of the papillary muscles (Fig. 1, right) [3, 5, 8]. This hemodynamic variant of HCM may occur with or without apical myocardial infarction and aneurysm formation [3]. In midventricular obstruction, the apical systolic pressure is elevated, but both the left ventricular inflow and outflow tract pressures are low, and equal to aortic systolic pressure [3–5] (Fig. 1, right; Table 1). Left ventricular cineangiography reveals midcavity obliteration (occlusion) at the level of the papillary muscles [3]. It is important to distinguish the cineangiographic appearance in midventricular obstruction from end-systolic papillary muscle approximation (without obstruction) that occurs in HCM when there is extensive left ventricular and papillary muscle hypertrophy. An impulse gradient and the gradient that occurs in midventricular obstruction should be readily recognizable [3–5] (Fig. 1, Tables 1, 3).

The third type of pressure difference that may be encountered in HCM is the intraventricular pressure difference that may be associated with cavity obliteration [9] (Fig. 1, centre; Table 1). In this situation, the apical cavity obliteration occurs early in systole [10], and at the catheter recording the elevated apical systolic pressure is usually observed to be outside the end-systolic cineangiographic silhouette of the left ventricle [9]. The apical left ventricular pressure is elevated (Fig. 1, centre), whereas all other pressures in the left ventricle, including the left ventricular inflow tract pressure, are low and equal to the outflow tract and aortic systolic pressures [11, 12]. The intraventricular pressure difference of cavity obliteration is not associated with echocardiographic or cineangiographic evidence of mitral leaflet-septal contact [3–5] (Tables 1, 3).

The elevated apical systolic pressure in cavity obliteration was originally attributed to the apical catheter being enfolded [9], engulfed [9] or entrapped [11, 12] by isometrically contracting myocardium in the obliterated apex of the ventricle. More recently, it has been suggested that the intraventricular pressure difference in cavity obliteration is the result of a high pressure being generated by the rapidly contracting apex, and that this pressure is somehow not transmitted to the hypocontractile base of the left ventricle [13]. However, Doppler velocity signals recorded at the junction between the rapidly contracting apex and the poorly contracting base (D in Fig. 2, right) do not correlate in time or magnitude with the measured intraventricular pressure difference [4]. Thus, it would seem most likely that the elevated left ventricular systolic pressure in cavity obliteration is due to the apical catheter being entrapped [11, 12], by isometrically contracting myocardium as was originally suggested [9]. In these circumstances, the high pressure recorded may be a reflection of intramyocardial tissue pressure [11, 12]. The elevated systolic pressure in cavity obliteration is usually associated with various catheter entrapment phenomenon [12].

The fourth type of intraventricular pressure difference that may be encountered in HCM is the subaortic pressure gradient due to mitral leaflet-septal contact in obstructive HCM (Fig. 1, left; Fig. 2; Table 1). In this situation (Fig.

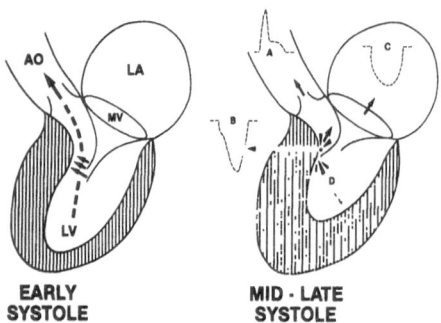

EARLY   MID - LATE
SYSTOLE   SYSTOLE

Fig. 2. *Left,* in obstructive HCM there is rapid, early systolic ejection *(dashed line)* through the outflow tract that is narrowed by septal hypertrophy. This results in Venturi forces *(three short oblique arrows in the outflow tract)* drawing the anterior *(upper two arrows)* and/or posterior *(lower arrow)* mitral leaflet(s) toward the septum (systolic anterior motion) [14]. Subsequent mitral leaflet-septal contact results in obstruction to left ventricular *(LV)* outflow and concomittant mitral regurgitation, as seen on the right. *Right,* by mid-systole, anterior mitral leaflet-septal contact causes obstruction to LV outflow resulting in a decreased forward aortic flow *(smaller arrow)* and mitral regurgitation *(oblique arrow arising from the mitral orifice).* Converging and diverging lines represent color flow imaging abnormalities at site of obstruction (see text). A, B, C and D indicate Doppler velocity recordings throughout systole in the ascending aorta [18, 32, 35] *(A)* (flow toward the transducer), at the level of mitral leaflet-septal contact [3, 20, 24, 26] *(B),* in the left atrium [3, 20, 23] *(C),* and near LV apex [20] *(D).* In B, C, and D, flow is away from the transducer. Peak velocities recorded at B correlate accurately with simultaneously measured obstructive subaortic pressure gradients [3, 20, 24, 26], whereas late peaking velocities at D do not. *AO,* aorta; *LA,* left atrium; *MV,* mitral valve; *LV,* left ventricle (see text). (From [4])

1, left), the left ventricular outflow tract pressure, distal to mitral leaflet-septal contact (and proximal to the aortic valve) is low and equal to aortic systolic pressure, whereas all ventricular pressures proximal to the obstruction, including the left ventricular inflow tract pressure just inside the mitral valve, are elevated [11, 12]. This type of subaortic pressure gradient is associated with echocardiographic and cineangiographic evidence of mitral leaflet-septal contact (Fig. 1, left; Fig. 2, right; Fig. 3, Table 1), and an elevated left ventricular inflow tract pressure (Fig. 1, left), whereas in cavity obliteration, or in midventricular obstruction, the left ventricular inflow tract pressure is not elevated (Fig. 1, centre and right), and there is no evidence of mitral leaflet-septal contact [3–5, 11, 12] (Table 1). It is essential in the management of patients with HCM to distinguish an obstructive subaortic pressure gradient due to mitral leaflet-septal contact, from the other three types of intraventricular pressure difference that may be encountered in this condition (Fig. 1, Tables 1, 3).

Mechanism of Mitral Leaflet Systolic Anterior Motion and Mitral Leaflet-Septal Contact in Obstructive HCM

In 1971, we first suggested that mitral leaflet systolic anterior motion could result from Venturi forces acting on the mitral leaflets, due to the rapid, nonobstructed early systolic ejection jet passing closer to the mitral leaflets than is normal, as a result of the outflow tract being narrowed by ventricular septal hypertrophy [14] (Fig. 2, left). The evidence in support of this concept has recently been summarized [3–5].

Evidence That Mitral Leaflet-Septal Contact is the Cause of the Obstructive Subaortic Pressure Gradient and Mitral Regurgitation in Obstructive HCM

1) HCM patients with severe systolic anterior motion with early and prolonged mitral leaflet-septal contact have obstructive subaortic pressure gradients (Fig. 3), whereas patients with moderate, mild or no systolic anterior motion do not [15].

2) Combined hemodynamic-echocardiographic [16, 17] and hemodynamic-cineangiographic [10] studies reveal that the onset of the obstructive subaortic pressure gradient (defined as the peak of the aortic percussion wave) begins just before or simultaneously with the onset of echocardiographic or cineangiographic mitral leaflet-septal contact (Fig. 3). The mitral leaflet strikes the septum with considerable force, as is evidenced by the septal fibrotic plaque, the fibrous thickening on the ventricular surface of the mitral leaflet that strikes the septum, and the occasional occurrence of an audible sound at the onset of mitral leaflet-septal contact [3].

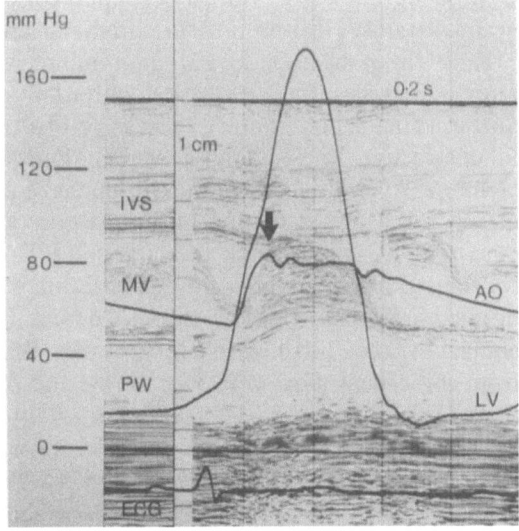

Fig. 3. Simultaneous hemodynamic and one-dimensional echocardiographic recordings in a patient with severe obstructive HCM (gradient = 86 mmHg). The *arrow* indicates the onset of mitral leaflet-septal contact and the onset of the pressure gradient (defined as the peak of the aortic percussion wave), which are virtually simultaneous. Note how early in systole the onset of mitral leaflet-septal contact and the pressure gradient occur in patients with severe outflow tract obstruction. *IVS,* intraventricular septum; *MV,* mitral valve; *PW,* posterior wall; *AO,* central aortic pressure; *LV,* left ventricular pressure. (From [16])

3) A number of characteristic features of obstructive HCM occur in close time proximity to the onset of mitral leaflet-septal contact: the peak of the aortic percussion wave [16, 17], the onset of flow deceleration in the ascending aorta [18], the point of inflection on the rising left ventricular pressure tracing [19] (Fig. 3) and on the continuous wave Doppler recording from the level of mitral leaflet-septal contact [20], the onset of partial aortic valve closure, as well as an abrupt midsystolic slowing of left ventricular emptying [21] and velocity of inward left ventricular wall movement [22]. This combination of near simultaneous events strongly suggest a sudden alteration of systolic hemodynamics, i.e., the onset of outflow tract obstruction.

4) The time of onset in systole of mitral leaflet-septal contact determines the magnitude of the obstructive pressure gradient, the degree of prolongation of left ventricular ejection time, the degree of mitral regurgitation and the percentage of left ventricular stroke volume that is ejected in the presence of the pressure gradient [3, 17]. Thus, early, and prolonged mitral leaflet-septal contact is associated with a high pressure gradient, marked prolongation of left ventricular ejection time, a significant amount of mitral regurgitation, and a large percentage of left ventricular stroke volume is ejected against the obstruction. In contrast, mitral leaflet-septal contact of late onset and short duration is associated with small pressure gradient, mild prolongation of left ventricular ejection time, a lesser degree of mitral regurgitation, and only a small percentage of left ventricular stroke volume is ejected against the obstruction [3, 17]. If mitral leaflet-septal contact occurs after 55% of the systolic ejection period [3] or if the duration of mitral leaflet-septal contact is less than 30% of echocardiographic systole [15], no pressure gradient develops.

Recently, pulsed [3, 20, 23], continuous wave [20, 23, 24] and color [23–26], Doppler studies have provided important new confirmatory evidence that mitral leaflet-septal contact causes the obstructive subaortic pressure gradient in obstructive HCM (Fig. 2, right). Pulsed and continuous wave Doppler techniques permit accurate measurement of peak flow velocity across a stenotic orifice, allowing calculation of the pressure gradient by the modified Bernoulli equation (PG = 4 × peak velocity^2) [20]. Both pulsed Doppler and sequential continuous wave and color Doppler studies in obstructive HCM localize the origin of the high outflow tract velocities to the site of mitral leaflet-septal contact [3, 20, 23–26] (B in Fig. 2, right). When pressure gradients are derived from these peak flow velocities across the outflow tract in obstructive HCM, there is a highly significant correlation with the simultaneously measured hemodynamic pressure gradients, whether recorded in the heart catheterization laboratory [3, 26] or intraoperatively [24]. This close correlation between flow velocity measured by pulsed or continuous wave Doppler and the simultaneously measured pressure gradient, represents strong, confirmatory evidence of the obstructive nature of the left ventricular outflow tract pressure gradient in HCM. The same strong correlations between flow velocity and pressure are present in valvular aortic stenosis.

Color Doppler studies demonstrate two other important features in obstructive HCM:

(a) acceleration of the jet just proximal to the obstruction, i.e., mitral leaflet-septal contact (in valvular aortic stenosis the jet accelerates just proximal to the valve);
(b) significant systolic narrowing of the jet at the level of mitral leaflet-septal contact, presumably caused by mitral leaflet systolic anterior motion [23, 25] (Fig. 2, right).

5) Mitral regurgitation invariably accompanies the obstructive subaortic pressure gradient in obstructive HCM, and in the absence of an independent mitral valve abnormality, the severity of the obstruction and the mitral leak are directly related to the degree of mitral leaflet systolic anterior motion [3, 4, 27] (Fig. 2). Cineangiography [3, 28] and color Doppler [23] studies reveal an eject/obstruct/leak sequence in systole in obstructive HCM, i.e., there is rapid nonobstructed early systolic ejection into the aorta (Fig. 2, left), the onset of mitral leaflet-septal contact and the obstruction (Fig. 2, right; Fig. 3), followed by posteriorly directed, predominantly mid-to-late systolic mitral regurgitation, that is the principal determinant of the end-systolic size of the left ventricle [3, 23, 28]. A decrease or abolition of mitral leaflet systolic anterior motion by pharmacological or surgical means results in a decrease or abolition of both the outflow tract obstruction and the mitral regurgitation [2–4, 27] (Fig. 4).

The presence of an independent mitral valve abnormality in obstructive HCM often results in the mitral regurgitation becoming pansystolic and more severe [2–4, 27].

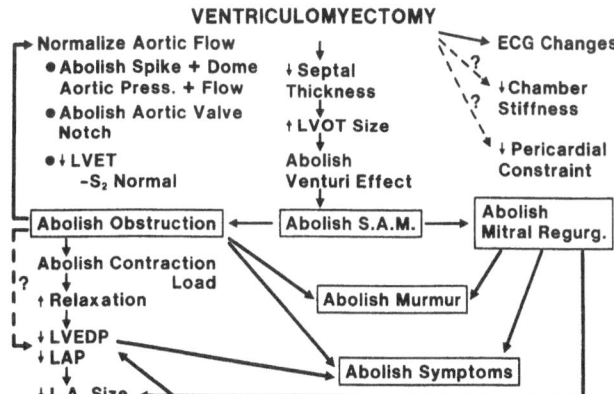

Fig. 4. Diagram indicating the proposed mechanism(s) by which the ventriculomyectomy operation affects the hemodynamics and clinical findings in patients with obstructive HCM (see text). (From [3])

The Obstructive Nature of the Subaortic Pressure Gradient in Obstructive HCM

All Ventricular Systolic Pressures Proximal to Mitral Leaflet-Septal Contact Are Elevated

As in the case with valvular aortic stenosis, in obstructive HCM all ventricular systolic pressures proximal to the subaortic obstruction, caused by mitral leaflet-septal contact, are elevated, including the left ventricular inflow tract pressure [3–5, 11, 12, 29] (Fig. 1, left). Catheters recording these high pressures can be freely moved about within the left ventricular cavity without altering the high systolic pressures, and, indeed, multiple catheters may be placed in the left ventricle, proximal to the obstruction and equally elevated pressures are recorded [11, 12, 29]. When the proximal end of these catheters are open, blood "shoots out" in systole, indicating that the distal tip of the catheter is in a high pressure, blood-filled area of the left ventricle [12].

Prolongation of Left Ventricular Ejection Time

One of the most characteristic features of any form of obstruction to left ventricular outflow, is a prolongation of left ventricular ejection time. We have previously demonstrated that the degree of prolongation of left ventricular ejection time in obstructive HCM is directly related to the magnitude of the pressure gradient [30, 31] and that both are related to the time of onset of mitral leaflet-septal contact in systole [3–5, 17]. This direct relationship between the magnitude of the pressure gradient and the degree of prolongation of left ventricular ejection time is maintained whether the gradient is increased or decreased by pharmacological or surgical means [3–5, 30, 31].

Percentage of Left Ventricular Stroke Volume Ejected in the Presence of the Obstructive Subaortic Pressure Gradient

It is recognized that there is rapid, nonobstructed, early systolic ejection in obstructive HCM (Fig. 2, left). If this were not the case, there would be no Venturi effect to cause mitral leaflet systolic anterior motion [14]. The question we are addressing here is: what percentage of left ventricular stroke volume leaves the left ventricle after the onset of mitral leaflet-septal contact and the pressure gradient?

Five different techniques have been used to study this question, and the results are rather similar. Thus, cineangiographic [3], echocardiographic [18], and combined micromanometric and nuclear angiographic [19], as well as Doppler [32] and electromagnetic [29, 33] flow studies have indicated that between 40% and 70% of left ventricular stroke volume leaves the left ventricle after the onset of mitral leaflet-septal contact and/or the subaortic pressure gradient. With the onset of the obstruction to outflow, the calculated resistance across the outflow tract increases dramatically [34], and this is accompanied by a sudden deceleration in ascending aortic flow [35] (A in Fig. 2, right), a decrease in the rate of left ventricular emptying [19] and a sudden decrease in inward left ventricular wall motion [22]. Ascending aortic and left ventricular outflow tract velocity flow studies indicate continued but reduced ejection into the left ventricular outflow tract and aorta (A and B in Fig. 2, right) during the presence of the subaortic pressure gradient [32–36]. Cineangiographic [3, 28] as well as color [23, 25] and continuous wave [20] Doppler studies (C in Fig. 2, right) indicate that the major portion of mitral regurgitation occurs in the last half of systole, after the onset of mitral leaflet-septal contact and the subaortic obstruction. Thus, there is a large volume of evidence to indicate that a very significant percentage of left ventricular stroke volume leaves the left ventricle as forward or regurgitant flow during the presence of the obstructive subaortic pressure gradient. The actual percentage of left ventricular stroke volume that is ejected in the presence of the subaortic obstruction is determined by the time of onset of mitral leaflet-septal contact in systole, which also determines the magnitude of the pressure gradient, the amount of mitral regurgitation, and the degree of prolongation of left ventricular ejection time [3, 17].

This systolic overload to the left ventricle in obstructive HCM is not only of hemodynamic significance as discussed above, but also has metabolic and clinical implications. Thus, large pressure gradients are associated with increased myocardial oxygen consumption and metabolic evidence of myocardial ischemia, which are reversed with surgical abolition of the pressure gradient [27]. In a similar vein, we have recently demonstrated that patients with obstructive HCM have more severe symptomatology than do those with the nonobstructive form of the disease [3–5].

Treatment

The rational choice of medical and/or surgical therapy in HCM is based on the hemodynamic abnormality that is present in any given patient (Tables 1–3).

Obstructive HCM (Muscular Subaortic Stenosis)

Prior to discussing therapy for obstructive HCM, it is important to review the pharmacodynamics of the subaortic obstruction. Traditionally, it has been thought that left ventricular preload, afterload, and contractility affect the magnitude of the subaortic pressure gradient. Although this is true, we believe that these three factors may act through their effect on the velocity of early systolic ejection and the Venturi forces acting on the mitral leaflets to cause systolic anterior motion [4] (Fig. 2, left). Thus, increased contractility (positive inotropes) or decreased afterload (vasodilators) would increase the early systolic ejection velocity and hence the severity of mitral leaflet systolic anterior motion, the pressure gradient, and the mitral regurgitation. Decreased contractility (negative inotropes) and increased afterload (vasopressors) would have

Table 3. Differentiation of intraventricular pressure differences that may be encountered in hypertrophic cardiomyopathy

	Obstructive HCM	Cavity obliteration	Impulse gradient	Midventricular obstruction
Hemodynamics				
Elevated LV inflow pressure	+	–	+	–
Entrapment criteria[a]	–	+	–	–
Time of peak systolic gradient	Late	Late	Early	Late
Spike-and-dome aortic pressure	+	–	–	–
Spike-and-dome aortic flow	+	–	–	–
LV ejection time	Increased	Normal (or short)	Normal (or short)	Increased
Cineangiography				
Mitral-leaflet-septal contact (ML-SC) (radiolucent line)	+	–	–	–
LV end-systolic volume	Variable	Small	Normal	Base small Apex large
Mitral regurgitation (MR)	++	+	–	–
LV cavity obliteration	+/– Late if +	+ Early	–	–
Echocardiography				
1D Severe SAM	+	–	–	–
Left atrial enlargement	+	–	–	+
Aortic valve notch	+	–	–	–
2D Mitral leaflet-septal contact	+	–	–	–
Doppler				
LV peak velocity at	ML-SC (pressure gradient)	Papillary muscle level (late peak)	–	Midventricular (pressure gradient)
Left atrium	Posteriorly directed MR	MR +	–	MR +
Clinical				
Apical murmur	3–4/6	0–2/6	+	2–4/6
Reversed split S_2	+	–	–	+

[a] See text.
LV, left ventricle; SAM, systolic anterior motion of mitral leaflet; 1D, 2D, one- and two-dimensional echocardiography.

the opposite effect on the severity of the systolic anterior motion, the pressure gradient and the mitral regurgitation, by decreasing early systolic ejection velocity and the Venturi forces acting on the mitral leaflets [4].

Increased preload and the ventriculomyectomy operation (Fig. 4) decrease or abolish mitral leaflet systolic anterior motion and the obstruction, by widening the left ventricular outflow tract, thus reducing the early systolic ejection velocity and/or displacing the ejection path away from the mitral leaflets.

Medical Therapy: For resting or labile obstructive HCM medical therapy consists of administering negative inotropic agents (beta-blockers, calcium antagonists, or disopyramide) to reduce or abolish mitral leaflet systolic anterior motion, the obstruction, and the concomitant mitral regurgitation [6]. Table 4

Table 4. Propranolol therapy in HCM, Toronto Experience 1976

	Resting obstruction	Latent obstruction
Patients (*n*)	40	15
Improved (*n*)	11	15
(%)	27.5	100
Deaths (*n*)	5	0
(%)	12.5	
Ventriculomyectomy (*n*)	15	0
(%)	37.5	
Average follow-up (months)	25	32

depicts our experience in the 1970s in administering propranolol (in a dose to give a resting heart rate of 60 beats per minute) to patients with resting and latent obstruction. Although patients with latent obstruction uniformly did well, most patients with a resting obstruction did not do well, required surgery, or died. The patients in this group who did improve were those with mild outflow obstruction and mild symptoms. Subsequently, other authors have reported beneficial results with high-dose beta-blocker therapy [38]. Our patients with severe outflow tract obstruction have not been able to tolerate large doses of these drugs, in that this therapy has led to increased presyncope and dyspnea.

Kaltenbach in the Federal Republik of Germany [39, 40] and the investigators at the National Institutes of Health (NIH) in the United States [41–43] have championed the use of verapamil in both obstructive and nonobstructive HCM and have reported beneficial results in large numbers of patients. Intravenous verapamil usually reduced the magnitude of the subaortic pressure gradient presumably by its negative inotropic effect, but, on occasion, the pressure gradient increases due to the vasodilating actions of this drug [41]. The NIH investigators have reported that about 50% of patients with obstructive HCM can defer surgery because of the beneficial effects of verapamil [42]. However, some of their patients on oral verapamil have developed intensified outflow tract obstruction, pulmonary edema, cardiogenic shock, and have died, presumably due to the vasodilating effect of the drug. Although we use verapamil to treat patients with nonobstructive HMC, we have chosen not to use calcium antagonists in the therapy of obstructive HCM because of this unpredictable occurrence of intensification of the outflow tract obstruction. We believe that nifedipine is particularly to be avoided in this respect because of its potent vasodilator action.

Having been unimpressed with the results of beta-blocker therapy, and concerned about the potential for calcium antagonists to unpredictably worsen the outflow tract obstruction, we have chosen to use the negative inotropic, antiarrhythmic agent, disopyramide as medical therapy for obstructive HCM [3, 6, 44, 45]. In acute hemodynamic studies, this drug uniformly reduced or abolished the subaortic pressure gradient [45]. When 100 mg disopyramide administered intravenously over 10 min does not markedly reduce or abolish the pressure gradient during the acute hemodynamic study, the patient is unlikely to do well on oral therapy with this agent. Patients in whom the subaortic pressure gradient is abolished in the acute study tend to initially do well on oral therapy and have both clinical and echocardiographic evidence of reduced outflow tract obstruction. This initial beneficial response is maintained in some, but in a significant percentage of these patients, the effect wears off in one to 3 years. Because disopyramide does not block intensification of the obstruction by vasodilators or sympathetic stimulants, recently we have combined beta blocker therapy (to achieve a resting heart rate of 60 beats per minute) with disopyramide. We believe this combination of drugs in our hands represents optimal medical therapy for obstructive HCM.

Surgical Therapy: When patients with obstructive HCM remain symptomatic on optimal medical therapy, are dissatisfied with their disease imposed limitations, or are intolerant to their drug regimen, we recommend the ventriculomyectomy operation which, in our hands, provides far more hemodynamic and symptomatic benefit than any form of medical therapy currently available [4, 6].

The mechanism by which the ventriculomyectomy operation provides these dramatic benefits to patients with obstructive HCM is depicted in Fig. 4. By decreasing septal thickness, this operation increases the size of the left ventricular outflow tract (LVOT) and results in the early systolic ejection path being displaced away from the mitral leaflets, thus reducing or abolishing the Venturi forces on these leaflets. As a result, mitral leaflet systolic anterior motion (SAM), the obstruction to outflow, and the mitral regurgitation are abolished (Fig. 4). The abolition of the obstruction normalizes aortic flow with the result that the spike and dome aortic flow and pressure profiles and aortic valve notch are abolished. Left ventricular ejection time (LVET) is no longer prolonged and splitting of the second heart sound (S_2) becomes normal. The abolition of the obstruction results in a reduction in left ventricular end-diastolic (LVEDP), and left atrial pressures (LAP) directly and possibly indirectly, through improved left ventricular relaxation. Abolition of the mitral regurgitation would also decrease LVEDP and LAP as well as left atrial (LA) size, thus rendering the patient less liable to atrial arrhythmias. The abolition of the apical systolic murmur results from the abolition of the obstruction and the mitral regurgitation, whereas these two factors plus the lowering of LVEDP and LAP result in a lessening or abolition of the patient's symptoms (Fig. 4). It is not known whether a decrease in chamber stiffness or in the degree of pericardial constraint could also favor symptomatic benefit after the ventriculomyectomy operation (Fig. 4). There is evidence that surgically induced ventricular conduction defects do not explain the beneficial effects of this surgery.

The ventriculomyotomy/myectomy surgery in Toronto was carried out by Dr. W. G. Bigelow from 1961 to 1977. The results of this experience have been previously documented [2, 46, 47]. Since 1978 Dr. W. G. Williams has performed 110 ventriculomyectomies. In 81 patients (74%) ventriculomyectomy was the only surgical procedure; there were no operative deaths in these patients. In 29 patients (26%) various associated surgical procedures were performed, including aortic valve replacement (three patients), right ventriculomyectomy (six patients), cutting of a myocardial bridge (five patients), miscellaneous procedures including mitral valve repair (seven patients), and concomitant aortocoronary vein bypass graft surgery (eight patients). The only two operative deaths in the total series of 110 patients (operative mortality 1.8%) occurred in two patients who underwent quadruple bypass surgery in the setting of postmyocardial infarction unstable angina. In each instance, postmortem examination revealed vein graft occlusion and acute myocardial infarction. Thus, no deaths have been attributed to the ventriculomyectomy operation per se. There have been three late deaths, one due to cancer, one due to unrepaired aortic regurgitation, and one occurred following a re-operation (biventricular myectomy) 8 years following a successful left-sided myectomy. Eight-year survival was 93% ± 4%. The dramatic symptomatic and hemodynamic benefit of ventriculomyectomy surgery in this center has previously been documented [2–4, 46–48].

Latent Obstructive HCM: As previously indicated (Table 4), although beta-blocker therapy in our hands has been unimpressive in obstructive HCM, it has been very effective in cases with latent obstruction [2, 3]. Indeed, we have treated some 70 patients with latent obstruction with beta-blockers with salutary results and no deaths [3]. We believe these drugs are effective in this group of patients because they prevent provocation of the obstruction by sympathetic influences and sometimes following vasodilatation. In our experience, the majority of these latent obstructive cases have relatively localized subaortic hypertrophy and relatively normal diastolic function. Thus, by preventing the provocation of the outflow obstruction, their symptoms are usually dramatically relieved. We have rarely used disopyramide for latent obstruction because this drug does not prevent catecholamine provocation of the obstruction and the negative inotropic properties of the drug would impair left ventricular relaxation. Similarly, we have not used the calcium antagonists because their vasodilating properties could provoke outflow tract obstruction. A few patients with latent obstruction and extensive hypertrophy have subsequently developed resting obstruction and have required ventriculomyectomy surgery.

Atrial Fibrillation in Obstructive HCM: The deleterious effect of atrial fibrillation in obstructive HCM with impaired relaxation is well recognized [3]. In HCM, as in other types of heart disease, the occurrence of atrial fibrillation is principally related to left atrial size, and we have documented that left atrial enlargement occurs in more than 90% of patients with obstructive HCM and in fewer than 20% of nonobstructive HCM [3]. Thus atrial fibrillation is particularly common in the obstructive form of the disease. Everything possible should be done to restore normal sinus rhythm in these patients [3, 6]. As previously indicated, left atrial size decreases following ventriculomyectomy (Fig. 4), particularly in patients under the age of 45. Thus, the best long-term measure to prevent atrial fibrillation in obstructive HCM is a successful ventriculomyectomy operation. We consider the occurrence of atrial fibrillation in obstructive HCM to be an indication for surgery.

Ventricular Arrhythmias in Obstructive HCM: Ventricular tachycardia on ambulatory monitoring is believed to increase the risk of sudden death in HCM eightfold [49]. There is some evidence, but no proof, that sudden death is less frequent in obstructive HCM following surgery [50]. The annual mortality following surgery is less than that prior to operation [51, 52]. For these reasons, the occurrence of serious ventricular arrhythmias in patients with obstructive HCM is an added indication for ventriculomyectomy.

Midventricular Obstruction

Currently, there is no established medical or surgical therapy for midventricular obstruction (MVO). The same groups of negative inotropic agents that are used in the medical therapy of muscular subaortic stenosis may also be used in this situation, with the same precautions. Intravenous disopyramide can reduce the pressure gradient in MVO. Various surgical procedures have been used, including a midventricular ventriculomyectomy, resection of the papillary muscles and mitral valve replacement, as well as resection of the left ventricular apex in a case of MVO with apical myocardial infarction and aneurysm formation.

Right Ventricular Outflow Tract Obstruction

Although negative inotropic agents may theoretically lessen right ventricular outflow tract obstruction in HCM, if the obstruction is hemodynamically significant, we believe a right-sided myectomy procedure should be carried out.

Severe Mitral Regurgitation in Nonobstructive HCM

Severe mitral regurgitation is occasionally encountered in nonobstructive HCM or following a successful ventriculomyectomy operation. In these instances, the mitral leak may be due to mitral valve prolapse, ruptured chordae tendinae, mitral annular calcification, congenital mitral valve anomalies, or in post-ventriculomyectomy cases, fibrosis of the mitral leaflets due to previous repeated mitral leaflet-septal contact. Although afterload reduction therapy is contraindicated in obstructive HCM, it is very much indicated in non-obstructive HCM with significant mitral regurgitation. If this therapy does not control the situation, mitral valve repair or replacement should be undertaken.

End-Stage HCM

In the late stages of HCM, left ventricular systolic and diastolic function becomes impaired because of progressive interstitial fibrosis and/or myocardial infarction due to small vessel coronary artery disease. At this stage of the disease, there is no outflow tract obstruction, because the early systolic ejection velocity is not sufficient to cause mitral leaflet systolic anterior motion. Instead, congestive heart failure occurs. Although digitalis glycosides, diuretics, and afterload reduction are contraindicated in the presence of outflow tract obstruction, in end-stage HCM they are very much indicated and may result in significant improvement in these seriously ill patients. When medical therapy fails in these patients, they should be considered for cardiac transplantation.

Summary

In this discussion, we have only dealt with those clinical syndromes of HCM in which there is a rational choice between medical and surgical therapy. In the presence of obstruction to left ventricular outflow, medical therapy consists of the use of negative inotropic agents to reduce or abolish the obstruction, and the avoidance of positive inotropic or afterload reducing agents, which could worsen the obstruction. Conversely, in the late stages of the disease when ventricular function is depressed and there is no obstruction to outflow, positive inotropic and afterload reducing agents are very much indicated and negative inotropic agents are to be avoided.

In obstructive HCM, a successful ventriculomyectomy operation provides far more hemodynamic and clinical benefit than any form of medical therapy currently available and can be performed at a very low risk. To deny the significance of obstruction to left ventricular outflow in HCM is to deny these patients appropriate medical and/or surgical therapy.

References

1. Wigle ED, Heimbecker RO, Gunton RW (1962) Idiopathic ventricular septal hypertrophy causing muscular subaortic stenosis. Circulation 26:325–340
2. Wigle ED, Adelman MD, Felderhof CH (1974) Medical and surgical treatment of the cardiomyopathies. Circ Res 34, 35 II-196–207
3. Wigle ED, Sasson Z, Henderson MA, Ruddy TD, Fulop J, Rakowski H, Williams WG (1985) Hypertrophic cardiomyopathy. The importance of the site and the extent of hypertrophy. A review. Prog Cardiovasc Dis 28:1–83
4. Wigle ED (1987) Hypertrophic cardiomyopathy. A 1987 viewpoint. (Editorial) Circulation 75:311–322
5. Wigle ED, Rakowski H (1987) Evidence for true obstruction to left ventricular outflow in obstructive hypertrophic cardiomyopathy (muscular of hypertrophic subaortic stenosis). Z Kardiol 76:61–68
6. Wigle ED (1988) Hypertrophic cardiomyopathy 1988. Mod Concepts Cardiovasc Dis 57:1–6
7. Murgo JP, Alter BR, Dorethy JF, Altobelli SA, McGranahan GM Jr (1980) Dynamics of left ventricular ejection in obstructive and nonobstructive hypertrophic cardiomyopathy. J Clin Invest 66:1369–1382
8. Falicov RE, Resnekov L, Bharati S et al (1976) Midventricular obstruction: a variant of obstructive cardiomyopathy. Am J Cardiol 37:432–437
9. Criley MJ, Lewis KB, White RI, Ross RS (1965) Pressure gradients without obstruction: a new concept of "hypertrophic subaortic stenosis". Circulation 22:881–887
10. Grose RM, Strain JE, Spindola-Franco H (1986) Angiographic and hemodynamic correlations in hypertrophic cardiomyopathy. Am J Cardiol 58:1085–1092
11. Wigle ED, Auger P, Marquis Y (1966) Muscular subaortic stenosis: the initial left ventricular inflow tract pressure as evidence of outflow tract obstruction. Can Med Assoc J 95:793–797

12. Wigle ED, Marquis Y, Auger P (1967) Muscular subaortic stenosis: Initial left ventricular inflow tract pressure in the assessment of intraventricular pressure differences in man. Circulation 35:1100–1117
13. Criley MJ, Seigel RJ (1985) Has 'obstruction' hindered our understanding of hypertrophic cardiomyopathy? Circulation 72:1148–1154
14. Wigle ED, Adelman AG, Silver MD (1971) Pathophysiological considerations in muscular subaortic stenosis. In: Wolstenholme GEW, O'Connor M (eds) Hypertrophic obstructive cardiomyopathy. Ciba Foundation Study Group 47. Ciba Foundation, London, pp 63–76
15. Gilbert BW, Pollick C, Adelman AG, Wigle ED (1980) Hypertrophic cardiomyopathy: subclassification by M-mode echocardiography. Am J Cardiol 45:861
16. Pollick C, Gilbert BW, Rakowski H, Morgan CD, Wigle ED (1982) Muscular subaortic stenosis: the temporal relationship between systolic anterior motion of the anterior mitral leaflet and the pressure gradient. Circulation 66:1087–1093
17. Pollick C, Rakowski H, Wigle ED (1984) Muscular subaortic stenosis: the quantitative relationship between systolic anterior motion and the pressure gradient. Circulation 69-I:43–49
18. Glasgow GA, Gardin JM, Burns CS, Childs WJ, Henry WL (1980) Echocardiographic and Doppler flow observations in idiopathic hypertrophic subaortic stenosis (IHSS) Circulation 62:III-99 (abstr)
19. Bonow RO, Ostrow HG, Rosing DR, Cannon RO, Leon MB, Watson RM, Bacharach SL, Green MV, Epstein SE (1984) Dynamic pressure-volume alterations during left ventricular ejection in hypertrophic cardiomyopathy: evidence for true obstruction to left ventricular outflow. Circulation 70:II-17 (abstr)
20. Hatle L, Angelsen B (1985) (eds) Doppler ultrasound in cardiology. Lea and Febiger, Philadelphia, pp 205–217
21. Bonow RO, Crawford-Green C, Betocci S, Rosing DR, Maron BJ (1985) Left ventricular ejection dynamics in hypertrophic cardiomyopathy: comparison with valvular aortic stenosis. J Am Coll Cardiol 5:395 (abstr)
22. Pouleur H Van Eyll C, Gurne O, Hanet C, Rousseau MF (1985) Regional velocity of shortening in hypertrophic cardiomyopathy: evidence for true impedance to shortening in the presence of outflow gradients. Circulation 72:III-448 (abstr)
23. Rakowski H, Sasson Z, Wigle ED (1988) Echocardiographic and Doppler assessment of hypertrophic cardiomyopathy. J Am Soc Echo 1:31–47
24. Stewart WJ, Schiavone WA, Salcedo EE, Lever HM, Cosgrove DM, Grill CC (1985) Intraoperative Doppler velocity correlates with outflow gradient in HOCM pre- and postmyectomy. Circulation 72:III-447 (abstr)
25. Holt B, Sahn DJ, Dalton N, Smith SC, Yun Y, Dittrich H (1985) Color Doppler flow mapping studies of jet formation in hypertrophic cardiomyopathy (HCM). Circulation 72:III-447 (abstr)
26. Sasson Z, Yock PG, Hatle LK, Alderman EL, Popp R (1986) Noninvasive determination of the pressure gradient in hypertrophic cardiomyopathy. Circulation 74:II-215 (abstr)
27. Wigle ED, Adelman AG, Auger P, Marquis Y (1969) Mitral regurgitation in muscular subaortic stenosis. Am J Cardiol 24:698–706
28. Adelman AG, McLoughlin MJ, Marquis Y, Auger P, Wigle ED (1969) Left ventricular cineangiographic observations in muscular subaortic stenosis. Am J Cardiol 24:689–697
29. Ross J Jr, Braunwald E, Gault JH, Mason DT, Morrow AG (1966) The mechanism of the intraventricular pressure gradient in idiopathic hypertrophic subaortic stenosis. Circulation 34:558–578
30. Wigle ED, Auger P, Marquis Y (1967) Muscular subaortic stenosis: the direct relation between the intraventricular pressure gradient and left ventricular ejection time. Circulation 36:36–44
31. Sasson Z, Henderson M, Wilansky S, Rakowski H, Wigle ED (1989) Causal relation between the pressure gradient and left ventricular ejection time in hypertrophic cardiomyopathy. J Am Coll Cardiol 13:1275–1279

32. Maron BJ, Gottdiener JS, Arce J, Rosing DR, Wesley YE, Epstein SE (1985) Dynamic subaortic obstruction in hypertrophic cardiomyopathy: analysis by pulsed Doppler echocardiography. J Am Coll Cardiol 6:1–15
33. Pierce GE, Morrow AG, Braunwad E (1964) Idiopathic hypertrophic subaortic stenosis III. Intraoperative studies of the mechanism of obstruction and its hemodynamic consequences. Circulation 30:IV, 152–207
34. Bircks W, Bostroem B, Gleichmann U, Kruezer H, Loogen F (1968) Electromagnetic flow measurement in the ascending aorta before and after repair of valvular and subvalvular lesions including IHSS. Proceedings of the Vth European Congress of Cardiology (Athens), pp 13–22
35. Jenni R, Ruffman K, Vieli A, Anlinker M, Krayenbuehl HP (1985) Dynamics of aortic flow in hypertrophic cardiomyopathy. Eur Heart J 6:391–398
36. Hernandez RR, Greenfiled JC Jr, McCall BW (1964) Pressure-flow studies in hypertrophic subaortic stenosis. J Clin Invest 43:401–407
37. Cannon RO, Rosing DR, McIntosh CL, Epstein SE (1985) Hypertrophic cardiomyopathy (HCM): improved hemodynamics, metabolism, and anginal threshold following surgical relief of obstruction. Circulation 72:III-447 (abstr)
38. Frank MJ, Abdulla AM, Watkins O, Prisant L, Stefadouros MA (1983) Long-term medical management of hypertrophic cardiomyopathy: usefulness of propranolol. Eur Heart J 4:155–164
39. Kaltenbach M, Hopf R, Kober G, Bussman WD, Keller M, Petersen Y (1979) Treatment of hypertrophic obstructive cardiomyopathy with verapamil. Br Heart J 42:35–42
40. Kaltenbach M, Hopf R (1985) Treatment of hypertrophic cardiomyopathy: Relation to pathological mechanisms. J Mol Cell Cardiol 17:59–68
41. Rosing DR, Kent KM, Border JS, Seides SF, Maron BJ, Epstein SE (1979) Verapamil therapy: a new approach to the pharmacologic treatment of hypertrophic cardiomyopathy I. Hemodynamic effects. Circulation 60:1201–1207
42. Rosing DR, Condit JR, Maron BJ, Kent KM, Leon MB, Bonow RO, Lipson LC, Epstein SE (1981) Verapamil therapy: A new approach to the pharmacologic treatment of hypertrophic cardiomyopathy: III. Effects of long-term administration. Am J Cardiol 48:545–553
43. Rosing DR, Idanpaan-Heikkila U, Maron BJ, Bonnow RO, Epstein SE (1985) Use of calcium-channel blocking drugs in hypertrophic cardiomyopathy. Am J Cardiol 55 (Suppl) 185B–195B
44. Pollick C (1982) Muscular subaortic stenosis. Hemodynamic and clinical improvement after disopyramide. N Eng J Med 307:997–999
45. Pollick C, Kimball B, Henderson M, Wigle ED (1988) Disopyramide in hypertrophic cardiomyopathy I. Hemodynamic assessment after intravenous administration. Am J Cardiol 62:1248–1251
46. Wigle ED, Chrysohou A, Bigelow W (1963) Results of ventriculomyotomy in muscular subaortic stenosis. Am J Cardiol 11:572–586
47. Bigelow WG, Trimble AS, Wigle ED, Adelman AG, Felderhof C (1974) The treatment of muscular subaortic stenosis. Thorac Cardiovasc Surg 68:384–392
48. Williams WG, Wigle ED, Rakowski H, Smallhorn J, Le Blanc J, Trusler GA (1987) Results of surgery for idiopathic hypertrophic obstructive cardiomyopathy (IHSS). Circulation 76-II:104–108
49. McKenna WJ, England D, Doi YL, Deanfiled JE, Oakley C, Goodwin JF (1981) Arrhythmia in hypertrophic cardiomyopathy I. Influence on prognosis. Br Heart J 46:168–172
50. Shah PM, Adelman AG, Wigle ED et al (1975) The natural (and unnatural) history of hypertrophic obstructive cardiomyopathy. Circ Res 34, 35 (Suppl 2):179–186
51. Maron BJ, Epstein SE, Morrow AG (1983) Symptomatic status and prognosis of patients after operation for hypertrophic obstructive cardiomyopathy and myectomy. Eur Heart J 4 (Suppl F):175–185
52. Beahrs MM, Tajak AJ, Seward JB et al (1983) Hypertrophic obstructive cardiomyopathy: 10–21 year follow-up after partial septal myectomy. Am J Cardiol 51:1160–1166

Changes in Left Ventricular Hemodynamics of Hypertrophic Obstructive Cardiomyopathy (HOCM) Patients Treated with VAT Sequential Pacing

T. Richter, L. Cserhalmi, M. Lengyel, I. Kassai, and J. Ványi

The functional behavior of the left ventricular (LV) outflow obstruction, and its accessibility by artificial pacing in patients suffering from hypertrophic obstructive cardiomyopathy (HOCM) is known from the literature [1, 3, 7, 8]. The basic principle of this attempt, described by Hassenstein et al. [2] and by Johnson and Daily [3] in 1975, is to stimulate the LV in a P-wave-triggered (VAT) mode, but with a much shorter conduction time than the patient's atrioventricular (AV) conduction. Thus, foreign excitation of the ventricles from the right ventricular apex delays the contraction of the obstructive segment of the septum and diminishes the pressure gradient of the outflow tract.

Besides some case reports, Duck et al. [7] had four patients and Jüsgen [8] also had four patients with a specially programmed permanent pacemaker (PM), who were followed for several months. Since their investigational methods were different, we attempt to present a 6-month complete follow-up of four patients treated with VAT sequential pacing.

Patients and Methods

Data of the one male and three female patients are listed in Table 1. They had had symptoms of cardiovascular disease for 2–20 years (mean 10 years) and clinically documented HOCM for 1–12 years (mean 7 years). All but one patient had been treated medically for 3–12 years (mean 9 years). The diagnosis of HOCM was based on cardiac catheterization, two-dimensional echocar-

Table 1. Age and sex distribution; cardiac catheterization and angiography

Patient No.	Age	Sex	Gradient	LVEDP	Ins. Bicusp	Maron classi- fication	VS/LVFW Ratio
1	47	F	95	22	I	III	2.2
2	44	F	90	28	I–II	III	1.8
3	35	F	80	34	I	III	1.4
4	56	M	110	18	III→I	III	1.5

VS, ventricular septum; LVFW, left ventricular free wall.

diography, and Doppler recordings. All patients were in class III according to the two-dimensional echocardiographic criteria of Maron et al. [5]. Electrophysiological investigations were also performed to exclude accessory pathways or any presence of retrograde conduction. Diplos 05 generators from Biotronik were implanted with endocardial leads inserted under local anesthesia via the right subclavian and/or cephalic vein. Doppler echocardiography, phonomechanocardiographic investigation, and radionuclide determination of cardiac index and stroke volume index using the first pass technique were performed within 1 week and also 3 months after the operation. Radionuclide ventriculography with parametric scan phase amplitude analysis was performed to investigate the sequential movement of different parts of the left ventricle. All measurements were taken in the switched-off position of the PM and during artificial pacing.

Cardiac catheterization was repeated within 3–6 months after the PM implantation. At recatheterization, LV outflow pressure gradients were measured at different AV conduction times and in sinus rhythm. The pulsed Doppler technique was used to detect and grade mitral regurgitation. The patients were asked to fill in a questionnaire to determine any changes in their exercise tolerance and physical symptoms.

All but one patient received propranolol and occasionally diuretics. Drug therapy was left unchanged throughout this study. Because of the small number of cases, no statistical significance was calculated.

Results

There was no complication in permanent PM therapy during this 6-month follow-up. In the male patient who had had attacks of atrial fibrillation previously, the upper tracking rate response of the PM was set at 100 bpm. Results of CW Doppler recordings are presented in Table 2. LV outflow pressure gradients decreased in PM rhythm in all cases in the short-term study and in all but one at long-term follow-up. Mitral insufficiency was mild in all cases but one, and it decreased at late follow-up in patient No. 4 from grade III to grade I.

Table 2. CW Doppler recordings of LV outflow gradients (mmHg)

Patient No.	Sinus rhythm[a]	PM rhythm[a]	Pm rhythm 3 months postop.	Difference (mmHg)	Decrease (%)
1	120	100	50	−70	58
2	64	36	64	0	0
3	64	36	36	−28	44
4	100	60	36	−64	64

[a] Within 1 week after PM implantation.

Table 3. LV outflow tract gradients measured by cardiac catheterization (mmHg)

Patient No.	Pre-operatively[a]	Post-operatively[b]	Difference (mmHg)	Decrease (%)
1	95	30	−65	69
2	90	60	−30	33
3	80	30	−50	63
4	110	20	−90	82

[a] Sinus rhythm before PM implantation.
[b] PM rhythm 3–6 months after PM implantation.

Table 4. Phono- and mechanocardiographic pattern changes

| Patient No. | PEP/LVET | | Systolic murmur | | First sound | | Fourth sound | |
			Type	Amplitude				
1	0.171	0.363	Holosyst.	↓	=	↑	–	=
2	0.212	0.406	Holosyst.	↓	=	↑	+	–
3	0.179	0.371	Mesosyst.	↓	=	↑	+	–
4	0.166	0.228	Holo-meso-syst.	↓	=	↑	–	=
	PM switched off	with PM	PM switched off	with PM	PM switched off	with PM	PM switched off	with PM

+, Present; =, unchanged; –, disappeared.

LV outflow gradients measured by cardiac catheterization are listed in Table 3. A remarkable decrease of the gradient was observed in each patient (between 33% and 82%). Recatheterization data are listed in detail later.

Phono- and mechanocardiographic pattern changes show the normalization of the pre–ejection period/left ventricular ejection time (PEP/LVET) ratio from the previously abnormal low values as a result of the shortening of the ejection time (Table 4). The amplitude of the systolic murmur diminished in every patient. The first heart sound became detectable. The fourth heart sound, previously detectable in patients Nos. 2 and 3 disappeared (Fig. 1).

Radionuclide ventriculography demonstrated the relatively delayed contraction of the upper septal region and an increased emptying rate of the left ventricle at pacing. Figure 2 shows the tendency of the stroke volume index (SVI) values towards normal using the radionuclide method in paced patients. The LV outflow gradients at four different AV conduction times, measured at recatheterization are shown in Fig. 3. With regard to the dp/dt max values (not listed in the table) we felt that the optimal AV delay was 40 or 65 ms. At this setting dp/dt max values decreased by about −18% when compared with sinus rhythm. These data suggest that the gradient can be much more favorably influenced by a PM than by, for example verapamil therapy [4]. Figure 4

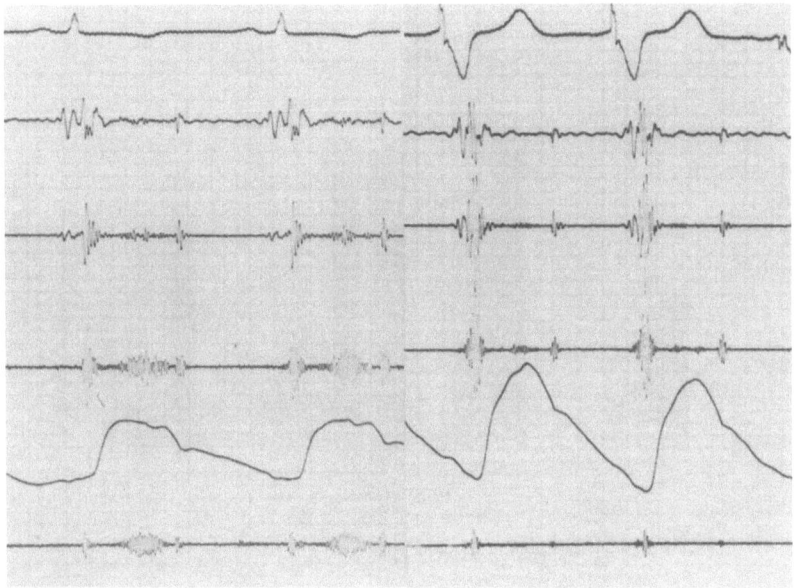

Fig. 1. Sinus rhythm (left panel) and PM rhythm (right panel) in patient No. 3. Note the lower systolic murmur and swift upstroke when paced

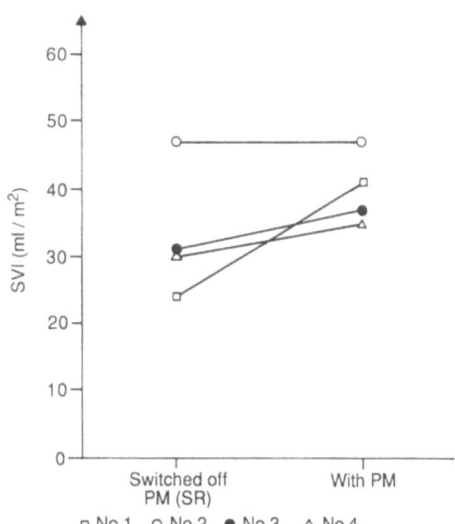

Fig. 2. Tendency of stroke volume index toward normal values

illustrates the changes in the subjective symptoms of the patients. The moderate changes in exercise tolerance cannot be taken into account because all three female patients had a weight gain of 6–10 kg after the operation. Cerebral

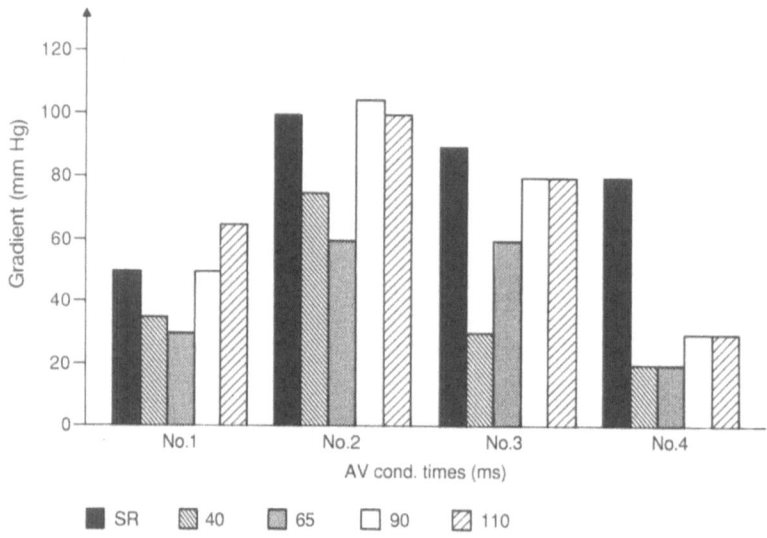

Fig. 3. Left ventricular outflow tract gradients at different AV conduction times

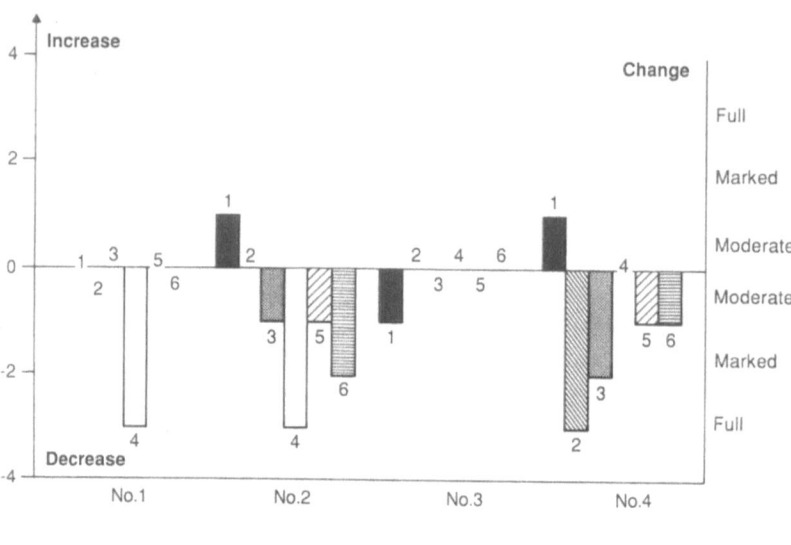

1: Exercise capacity   4: Syncope
2: Dizziness   5: Short. of breath
3: Angina   6: Palpitation

Fig. 4. Changes of exercise capacity and symptoms at 3 months after PM implantation

syncopal attacks, when present previously, disappeared. There were moderate to marked beneficial changes in some other symptoms such as angina, dyspnea, and palpitation.

Discussion

Different investigational methods verified, in our series, the beneficial effects of VAT sequential pacing on left ventricular hemodynamics of HOCM patients. Some questions have, however, to be discussed.

If we consider that, according to Maron et al. [5]. 72% of HCM cases have significant septal hypertrophy and that 92% of the obstructive cases fall into classes II and III, we can speculate that a high number of the obstructive cases may be potentially influenced by VAT sequential pacemaker therapy. The optimum AV delay, between 0 ms and 65 ms, to be programmed into the PM is also not clear. Duck [6] and Jüsgen [8] recommend zero conduction times, but the further drop of the gradient compared to 40 ms is only 10–15 mmHg. Optimal AV conduction times are also dependent on the patients' own antegrade conduction velocity. In our patient No. 4, with a PR time of 0.22 ms, there was no remarkable difference in the gradient between 15- and 110-ms programmed AV conduction times. We believe that the 40- and 65-ms conduction times, calibrated individually at recatheterization, offer more optimal loading conditions in the left ventricle than zero conduction time, which is reflected in myocardial contractility values. However, the changes in diastolic function have not been investigated in detail in this study.

Conclusions

1) Permanent VAT PM therapy with very short AV delay decreases the LV outflow gradient in HOCM patients and has a beneficial effect on LV hemodynamics.
2) This effect is stable and reproducible 3–6 months after PM implantation with different investigational methods.
3) For optimal programming of the PM, cardiac catherization is necessary.
4) PM therapy is an alternative method to myectomy in patients with severe outflow obstruction.

References

1. Hassenstein P, Storch HH, Schmitz W (1975) Results of electrical pacing in patients with hypertrophic obstructive cardiomyopathy. Thoraxchirurgie 23:496–498
2. Hassenstein P, Walther H, Dittrich J (1975) Haemodynamische Veränderungen durch Einfach- oder Gekoppelte Stimulation bei Patienten mit obstruktiver Kardiomyopathie. Verh Dtsch Ges Inn Med 81:17
3. Johnson AD, Daily PO (1975) Hypertrophic subaortic stenosis complicated by a high degree heart block: successful treatment with an atrial synchronous ventricular pacemaker. Chest 67:491–494
4. Hopf R, Stock W, Bussmann W-D, Kunkel B, Kaltenbach N (1981) Die Wirkung vor intravenös und oral verabreichtem Verapamil auf die linksventrikuläre Hämodynamik bei Patienten mit hypertrophischer Kardiomyopathie (HCM). Z Kardiol 70:626

5. Maron BJ, Gottdiener JS, Epstein SE (1982) Echocardiographic identification of patterns of left ventricular hypertrophy in hypertrophic cardiomyopathy. In: Kaltenbach M, Epstein SE (eds) Hypertrophic cardiomyopathy. Springer, Berlin Heidelberg New York
6. Duck HJ, Hutschenreiter W, Pankau H, Trenckmann H (1984) Vorhofsynchrone Ventrikelstimulation mit verkürzter AV-Verzögerungszeit als Therapieprinzip der hypertrophischen obstruktiven Kardiomyopathie. Z Gesamte Inn Med 39:437–447
7. Duck HJ, Hutschenreiter W, Pankau W, Krosse B, Trenckmann H (1984) Applikative Aspekte der Therapie mit vorhofgesteuerten Ventrikelschrittmachern (VAT) mit verkürzter AV-Verzögerungszeit. Z Gesamte Inn Med 39:611–617
8. Jüsgen W (1984) Therapie der hypertroph-obstruktiven Kardiomyopathie mit AV-sequentiellen Herzschrittmachersystemen. In: Weikl A (ed) Physiologische Stimulation des Herzens. Perimed, Erlangen

Future Trends in Research in Hypertrophic Cardiomyopathy

S. E. Epstein

The past three decades have seen major progress in our understanding of the clinical, hemodynamic, and morphologic abnormalities in hypertrophic cardiomyopathy [1]. Major future advances will undoubtedly relate to an elucidation of the basic cellular abnormalities responsible for this fascinating syndrome, and perhaps to the identification of specific genetic defects present in this disease.

Whatever cellular abnormality is hypothesized as being responsible for the development of hypertrophic cardiomyopathy (HCM), it must explain several of the characteristic features of this disease. It must account for the myocardial hypertrophy, the myocardial cellular disarray [2], the myocardial fibrosis [3, 4] and the abnormal small intramural coronary arteries (characterized by marked medial hypertrophy and intimal proliferation, often with resulting narrowing of the vessel lumen) [5].

The range of possible cellular abnormalities producing the syndrome we call hypertrophic cardiomyopathy are myriad. The current discussion is meant to focus on three potential mechanisms that merit particular attention.

Abnormalities in Cardiac Norepinephrine Kinetics

It has frequently been suggested that HCM may be caused by exposure of the heart to excessive catecholamine stimulation [6–8]. One of the key elements to his "catecholamine" hypothesis was the demonstration by Pearse in 1964, that norepinephrine content and sympathetic innervation were increased in myocardium that was removed from the septum of hearts of HCM patients undergoing septal myectomy for relief of left ventricular outflow tract obstruction [8]. Other findings compatible with this hypothesis are the hyperdynamic state of the left ventricle in most patients with HCM, the salutary effect beta adrenergic blocking drugs have in controlling symptoms, and the fact that catecholamines can experimentally induce myocardial hypertrophy [9–13].

It was subsequently demonstrated that the histochemical techniques used by Pearse and coworkers, which identified an abnormality in cardiac norepinephrine stores, were not specific for norepinephrine [14, 15]. This refutation of the original data cast doubt on the norepinephrine hypothesis. Newer studies, however, have rekindled interest in this concept.

We recently demonstrated that the production rate of norepinephrine (arterio-venous difference across the heart times coronary blood flow) was elevated in the hearts of patients with HCM, and that this increased spillover of norepinephrine into the blood appeared to be due to impaired neuronal uptake of cardiac norepinephrine [16]. Such a defect could lead to elevated norepinephrine levels at the neuroeffector junctions of the myocardial and vascular smooth muscle adrenoceptors. If this concept is correct, the resulting abnormality could contribute importantly to the pathophysiologic genesis of HCM, including the myocardial hypertrophy of the hyperdynamic left ventricle and hyperplasia of the media of small coronary arteries [5]. As adrenergic stimulation of the coronary arteries causes coronary vasoconstriction and can thereby precipitate myocardial ischemia (particularly so in the presence of intramural coronary arteries narrowed by intimal and medial hyperplasia), this mechanisms could also explain the often extensive myocardial scar present in many patients at necropsy [3, 4].

Abnormalities in Cardiac Calcium Regulation

Because the hearts of HCM patients are hyperdynamic and exhibit impaired relaxation [17–20], and because these abnormalities and patients' symptoms respond to calcium antagonists [21–22], it would seem reasonable to examine the hypothesis that increased cytosolic calcium levels may account for the pathogenesis of HCM. It is now not possible technically to determine whether cytosolic calcium levels are elevated in HCM patients. However, an intriguing finding relating to this hypothesis has recently been reported. We measured the density of dihydropyridine binding sites present in the hearts of HCM patients undergoing surgery, and found that the density of these binding sites is elevated in HCM patients [23]. Since dihydropyridine is a prototype of one major class of calcium antagonists (into which fall nifedipine, nitrendipine, and nicardipine), the increase in dihydropyridine binding sites probably represents an increase in the density of voltage sensitive calcium channels. That this defect was not a nonspecific finding was indicated by the fact that beta adrenergic receptor density was unchanged. Hence, it would appear reasonable to pursue the hypothesis that abnormalities in cytosolic calcium regulation may play a role in the pathophysiology of HCM.

Evidence Suggesting a Proliferative Disorder

Myocardium from HCM patients exhibits myocardial hypertrophy, excess scar tissue, hyperplasie of the smooth muscle present in small coronary arteries, and apparent neovascularization. Although other explanations are possible, the findings are compatible with the intriguing hypothesis that HCM may be a primary proliferative disorder involving several cardiac cell types. Because of our interest in this and related concepts, we examined cardiac tissue to determine whether it contained growth factors which, if present, would at least provide a mechanism for the "proliferative disorder" concept.

Extensive studies in our laboratories have demonstrated that the normal heart contains acidic and basic fibroblast growth factors (aFGF, and bFGF), which are angiogenic peptides and mitogens for fibroblast, smooth muscle, and endothelial cells [25]. Potent mitogens, presumably aFGF and bFGF, were also found in the hearts of patients with HCM [25]. It ist therefore possible that HCM may be caused by increased production of, or increased sensitivity to, these growth factors.

These speculations only touch the surface of the possible cellular abnormalities that may contribute to or actually cause the clinical syndrome we call hypertrophic cardiomyopathy. It is highly likely that, in the course of future investigations, new findings will suggest other possible pathophysiologic mechanisms. However, on the basis of this very early work attempting to define the cellular biology of HCM, an interesting hypothesis can be formulated; namely, that the basic cellular abnormality in HCM might be due to abnormal activity of growth factors, abnormal intracellular calcium regulation, and/or abnormal cardiac norepinephrine kinetics. It would be of further interest if some link could be found amongst these mechanisms such that, for example, increased levels of growth factors are discovered to cause abnormalities in calcium and norepinephrine kinetics. Whatever the role, if any, of these potential mechanisms, it is clear that one of the major future trends in research in HCM will be to define the cellular disorders that induce the abnormalities in cardiac function and morphology that are characteristic of HCM.

References

1. Maron BJ, Bonow RO, Cannon RO, Leon MB, Epstein SE (1987) Hypertrophic cardiomyopathy: Interrelation of clinical manifestations, pathophysiology, and therapy. N Engl J Med 316:780–789
2. Maron BJ, Roberts WC (1979) Quantitative analysis of cardiac muscle cell disorganization in the ventricular septum of patients with hypertrophic cardiomyopathy. Circulation 59:689–706
3. Tanaka M, Fujiwara H, Onodera T, Wu D-J, Hamashima Y, Kawai C (1986) Quantitative analysis of myocardial fibrosis in normals, hypertensive hearts, and hypertrophic cardiomyopathy. Br Heart J 55:575–581
4. Maron BJ, Epstein SE, Roberts WC (1979) Hypertrophic cardiomyopathy and transmural myocardial infarction without significant atherosclerosis of the extramural coronary arteries. Am J Cardiol 43:1086–1102
5. Maron BJ, Wolfson JK, Epstein SE, Roberts WC (1986) Intramural ("small vessel") coronary artery disease in hypertrophic cardiomyopathy. J Am Coll Cardiol 8:545–557
6. Goodwin JF (1974) Prospects and predictions for the cardiomyopathies. Circulation 560:210
7. Pearse AGE (1964) Histochemistry and electronmicroscopy of obstructive cardiomyopathy. CIBA foundation Symposium, Boston. Little, Brown and Co, p 132
8. Perloff JK (1981) Pathogenesis of hypertrophic cardiomyopathy: hypotheses and speculations. Am Heart J 102:219–226
9. Laks MM, Morady F, Swan HJF (1973) Myocardial hypertrophy produced by chronic infusion of subhypertensive doses of norepinephrine in the dog. Chest 64:75–78
10. Panagia V, Pierce GN, Dhalla KS, Ganguly PK, Beamish RE, Dhalla NS (1985) Adaptive changes in subcellular calcium transport during catecholamine-induced cardiomyopathy. J Mol Cell Cardiol 17:411–420

11. Starksen NF, Bishopric NH, Coughlin SR, Lee WMF, Ordahl CP, Simpson PC, Williams LT (1985) Adrenergic-stimulated hypertrophy is associated with expression of the C-MYC-proto-oncogene in neonatal rat cardiac cells. (Abstract). Circulation 72 (Suppl III) III:26
12. Meidell RS, Sen A, Slahetka MF, Kumar C, Siddiquie MAQ, Chien KR (1985) Stimulation of cultured rat myocardial cells by norepinephrine or phorbol ester increases myofibrillar and non-myofibrillar mRNA content. (Abstract) Circulation 72 (Suppl III) III:27
13. Simpson P (1983) Norepinephrine-stimulated hypertrophy of cultured rat myocardial cells in an alpha$_1$ adrenergic response. J Clin Invest 72:732
14. Van Noorden S, Olsen EG, Pearse AGE (1971) Hypertrophic obstructive cardiomyopathy: a histological, histochemical and ultrastructural study of biopsy material. Cardiovasc Res 5:118
15. Kawai C, Yui Y, Hishino T, Sasayama S, Matsumori A (1983) Myocardial catecholamines in hypertrophic and dilated (congestive) cardiomyopathy: a biopsy study. J Am Coll Cardiol 2:834–840
16. Brush JE, Eisenhofer G, Stull R, Garty M, Maron BJ, Cannon RO, Panza J, Epstein SE, Goldstein DS (1989) Cardiac norepinephrine kinetics in hypertrophic cardiomyopathy. Circulation (in press)
17. Spirito P, Maron BJ, Chiarella F, et al (1985) Diastolic abnormalities in patients with hypertrophic cardiomyopathy: relation to magnitude of left ventricular hypertrophy. Circulation 72:310–316
18. St John Sutton MG, Tajik AJ, Gibson DG, Brown DJ, Seward JB, Giuliani ER (1978) Echocardiographic assessment of left ventricular filling and septal and posterior wall dynamics in idiopathic hypertrophic subaortic stenosis. Circulation 57:512–520
19. Hanrath P, Mathey DG, Siegert R, Bierfield W (1980) Left ventricular relaxation and filling pattern in different forms of left ventricular hypertrophy: an echocardiographic study. Am J Cardiol 45:15–23
20. Bonow RO, Rosing DR, Bacharach SL, et al (1981) Effects of verapamil on left ventricular systolic function and diastolic filling in patients with hypertrophic cardiomyopathy. Circulation 64:787–796
21. Rosing DR, Kent KM, Borer JS, Seides SF, Maron BJ, Epstein SE (1979) Verapamil therapy: a new approach to the pharmacologic treatment of hypertrophic cardiomyopathy. I. Hemodynamic effects. Circulation 60:1201–1207
22. Rosing DR, Kent KM, Maron BJ, Epstein SE (1979) Verapamil therapy: a new approach to the pharmacologic treatment of hypertrophic cardiomyopathy. II: Effects on exercise capacity and symptomatic status. Circulation 60:1208–1213
23. Wagner JA, Sax FL, Weisman HF, Porterfield J, McIntosh C, Weisfeldt ML, Snyder SH, Epstein SE (1989) Calcium-antagonist receptors in the atrial tissue of patients with hypertrophic cardiomyopathy. N Engl Med 320:755–761
24. Casscells W, Speir E (1987) Purification and characterization of heparinbinding mitogens from human left ventricular myocardium. Clin Research 35:255a
25. Karasik P, Lee M, Casscells W, Epstein SE (1989) Identification of heparinbinding growth factors in myocardium of patients with hypertrophic cardiomyopathy (Submitted for publication)

II Dilated Cardiomyopathy

Experimental Viral Myocarditis: Immunopathogenetic Aspects

A. Matsumori, Y. Matoba, N. Tomioka, and C. Kawai

Introduction

Clinically, viral myocarditis manifests a wide variety of features, ranging from a total lack of clinical symptoms to sudden death, which may be caused by a fatal arrhythmia, high-degree atrioventricular block, or circulatory collapse.

In addition to the broad spectrum of clinical presentations of acute viral myocarditis, possible complications and late sequelae are of concern. Myocarditis may be subacute or even chronic, leading to progressive myocardial failure and death. Because of the relative infrequency of this disease and the difficulty in recognizing the lesions, clinical investigation is difficult [8]. Therefore, we have looked towards experimental models of viral myocarditis for systematic investigations. In this review, we will discuss lymphocyte subsets, anti-heart antibody, and atrial natriuretic polypeptide in our model of viral myocarditis [11, 12].

Serial Changes in Lymphocyte Subsets in Myocarditis and the Effect of Prednisolone

Lymphocyte Subset in Viral Myocarditis

Four-week-old BALB/c mice were inoculated intraperitoneally with encephalo-myocarditis (EMC) virus as described previously [11]. Mice were sacrificed 7, 14, 28 and 70 days after virus inoculation. Each lymphocyte subset in the peripheral blood was measured by flow cytometry using monoclonal antibodies to T cells (Thy1.2), helper-inducer T cells (Lyt1), cytotoxic-suppressor T cells (Lyt2), and B cells (goat anti-mouse IgG). Six-week-old BALB/c mice without virus inoculation served as controls.

For immunocytochemical analysis, frozen sections of the myocardium were stained to determine T cell subset using the labeled avidin-biotin technique. Each T cell subset was expressed as a percentage of the total inflammatory cells enumerated by methyl green counter staining.

The percentage of Thy1.2 cells increased on days 14 and 28 (Fig. 1). Lyt1 cells decreased significantly on day 7. However, there was no change in Lyt2 or B cells. Immunocytochemical study of the heart showed that a significant number of infiltrating cells were Thy1.2-positive cells (10%, 11%, 10% on days

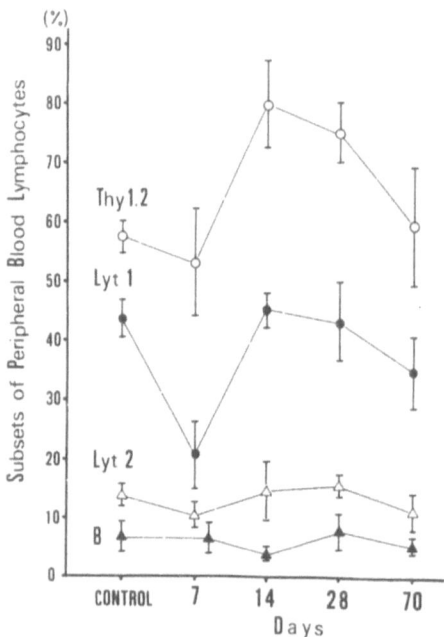

Fig. 1. Lymphocyte subsets in the peripheral blood. Thy1.2 (T cells) increased 2 and 4 weeks after EMC virus inoculation, and Lyt1 (helper-inducer) cells decreased significantly 1 week after infection

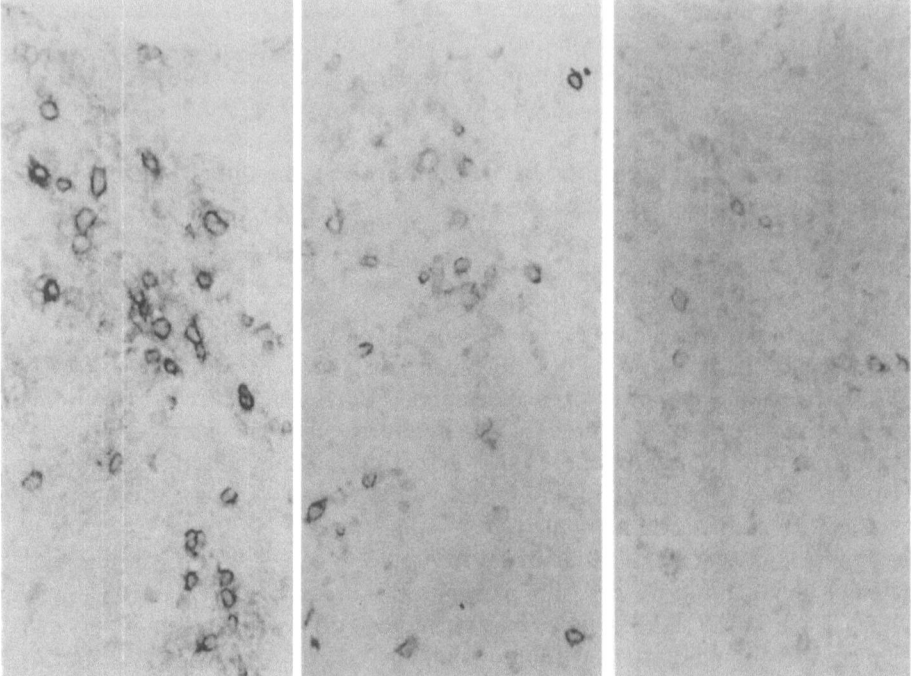

Fig. 2. Lymphocyte subset in the heart in situ. Frozen section was stained by labeled avidin-biotin technique using a monoclonal antibody against Thy1.2 (T cells, *left*), Lyt1 (helper-inducer T cells, *middle*) and Lyt2 (cytotoxic-suppressor T cells, *right*). A significant number of infiltrating cells were Thy1.2-positive cells and Lyt1 cells predominante; × 220

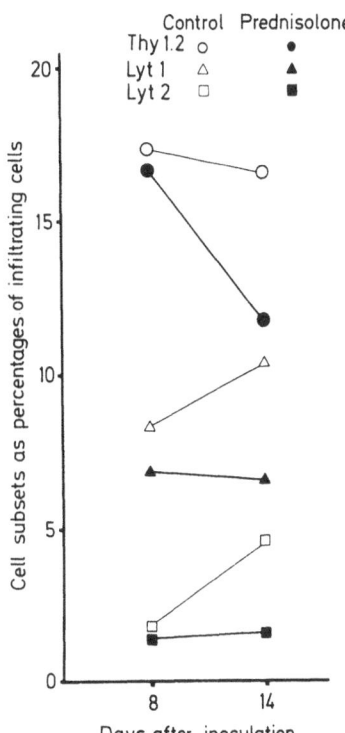

Fig. 3. The effect of prednisolone on lymphocyte subsets. The percentage of Thy1.2-positive cells decreased, and there was no increase in the percentage of Lyt1 and Lyt2 cell subsets as compared with the untreated group

7, 14, and 28, respectively), Lyt1 cells increased on day 14 (8%), but Lyt2 cells did not show a significant change and were in low frequency (Fig. 2) [16]. Thus, helper-inducer T cells showed significant changes during the course of EMC virus myocarditis and suggests that these cells may be involved in the immuno-pathogenesis of this disease.

The effect of prednisolone was studied in BALB/c mice with EMC virus myocarditis [7]. Prednisolone was injected intramuscularly, 10 mg/kg once a day, on days 4–13. On day 14, Lyt1 and Lyt2 cell subsets seemed to have increased slightly in mice without treatment. In animals treated with predniso-lone, infiltrating T cells in the heart on day 14 demonstrated a decrease in Thy1.2-positive T cells with no increase in Lyt1- and Lyt2-positive T cells (Fig. 3).

Anti-heart Antibodies

Anti-heart autoantibodies were found in the sera of DBA/2 mice infected with EMC virus. Positive granular staining was first seen on day 4 and persisted until day 90; the titer was highest on day 21 (Figs. 4, 5) [13]. The demonstration of the presence of anti-heart antibodies in this model of viral myocarditis suggests that they play a pathogenetic role in the subsequent cardiomyopathy, which has been previously demonstrated to occur. The precise pathogenetic function of

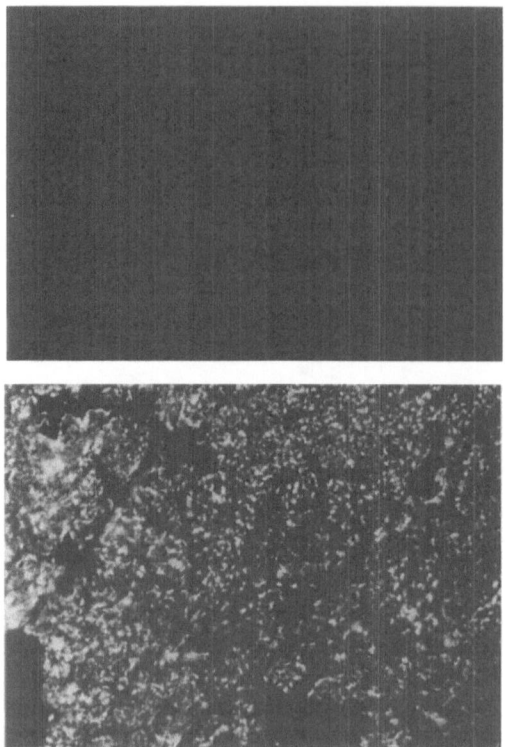

Fig. 4. Anti-heart antibody in DBA/2 mouse on day 21 after EMC virus inoculation. Indirect immunofluorescence

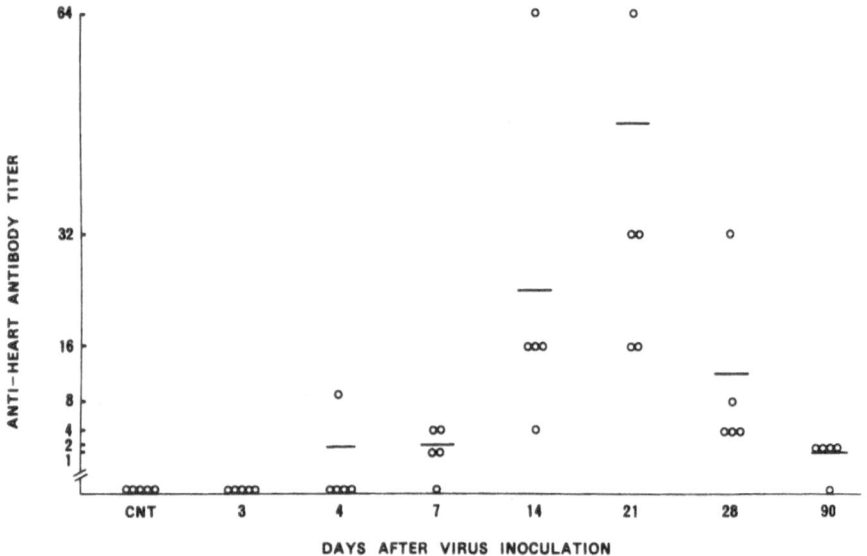

Fig. 5. Anti-heart antibody was first seen on day 4. The titer was highest on day 21 and persisted to day 90

these antibodies in vivo remains to be clarified. Cyclosporine treatment caused higher titers of anti-heart autoantibody in the acute stage, but no significant difference was seen in lymphocyte subsets, neutralizing antibody or virus concentrations in the heart. Thus, cyclosporine may have selective effect on the production of anti-heart autoantibody in the early stages of viral myocarditis in mice, which is associated with a higher mortality rate [10].

Atrial Natriuretic Polypeptide in Experimental Viral Myocarditis: Increased Synthesis and Secretion in the Ventricle and Atrium

Since atrial natriuretic polypeptide (ANP) was isolated from the atria of mammalian species [3, 6], much interest has been focused on its implication in cardiovascular disease. Plasma ANP levels were increased in patients with congestive heart failure [1]. On the other hand, the atrial ANP level in cardiomyopathic hamsters was reported to be decreased [4]. In addition, the ANP level in ventricles was recently shown to be increased in the hypertrophied heart caused by aortic ligation in rats [2], in cardiomyopathic hamsters with congestive heart failure [4, 5], and in patient with dilated cardiomyopathy [20]. These studies suggest that ANP plays a pathophysiological role in heart failure despite its function as a naturally occurring vasodilator and an endogenous diuretic. We recently demonstrated increased synthesis and secretion of ANP in the ventricle and atrium in our model of viral myocarditis [15, 18].

Myocarditis developed in BALB/c mice inoculated with EMC virus. ANP-like immunoreactivity (ANP-LI) in the extracts was measured by a radioimmunoassay that recognizes the common C-terminal sequence of α-human ANP and α-rat ANP (α-rANP), as described previously [19]. As shown by the nucleotide sequence of the mouse ANP gene, the 28 C-terminal amino acid sequence of mouse ANP is identical to α-rANP. The atrial ANP level decreased to 22% of that of the non-inoculated age-matched mice on day 7, increased to the value 1.6 times higher than the control value on day 14, and returned to nearly the same value as that of the control mice on day 28. The ventricles of the control mice contained approximately 1000 times lower concentration of ANP than the atria. The ventricular ANP concentration of the infected mice was three times higher than the control value on day 7, increased to 21 times the control level on day 14 and still remained nine times higher on day 28.

The plasma ANP level of the infected mice was also elevated on all days examined: seven times higher on day 7, 20 times higher on day 14, and seven times higher on day 28 than the control values. Frozen sections were prepared from the atria and ventricles of the control and infected mice and an indirect immunofluorescence was performed. Anti-ANP antibody stained atrial myocytes but did not stain ventricular myocytes in normal hearts. Staining became more prominent in the atrial myocytes near the foci of myocardial lesions on day 7 and was more extensive on day 14 (Fig. 6). Positive staining was seen in the ventricular myocytes after day 7 (Fig. 7). Electron microscopy revealed an increased number of electron-dense granules in atrial myocytes (Fig. 8) 14 days

Fig. 6. Anti-ANP antibody stained atrial myocytes. Staining became more prominent and extensive on day 14. Immunofluorescence; × 180

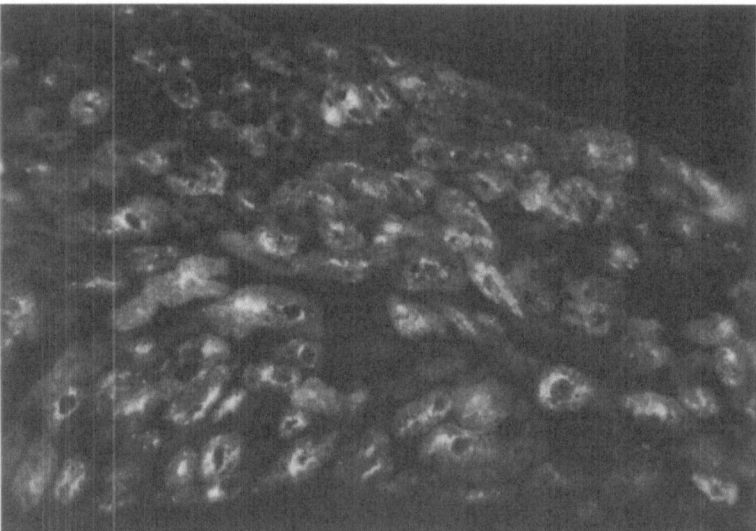

Fig. 7. Anti-ANP antibody did not stain ventricular myocytes in normal hearts. Positive staining was seen in the ventricular myocytes after day 7 of infection; × 180

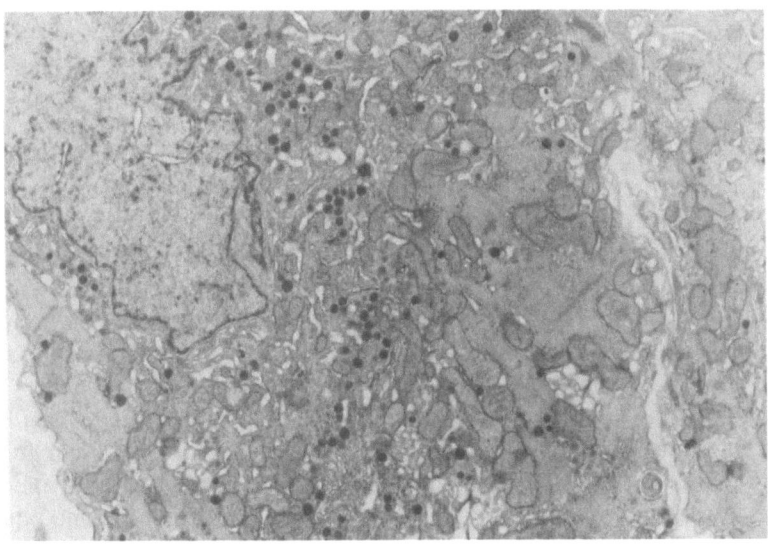

Fig. 8. Electron microscopy of an atrial myocyte on day 14 after EMC virus inoculation. An increased number of electron-dense granules were seen as compared to control mice; × 4000

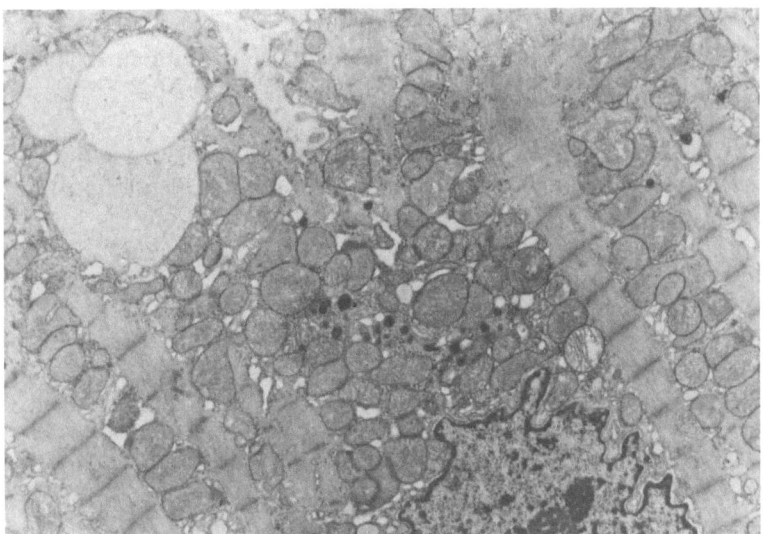

Fig. 9. Electron microscopy of a ventricular myocyte on day 14. Granules were seen in the ventricle on day 14 of EMC virus infected mice, but were not seen in the ventricle of control mice; × 4000

after infection. Electron-dense granules were seen in the ventricles of inoculated mice on day 14 (Fig. 9), although such granules were not present in the ventricles of control mice.

A most striking result in the present study is a marked increase of the ventricular ANP level. Although the ventricular concentration and content of ANP were much lower than those of the atria even in the infected mice, it is noteworthy that the ventricular ANP level elevated to a value 21 times higher than that of the control mice, whereas the atrial ANP level showed only a twofold increase. The present study suggests that an increase in mechanical load during the development of heart failure gives rise to the re-expression of the ANP gene in ventricular myocytes which is suppressed in the normal adult ventricle.

It is known that the gene expression for the ventricular myosin heavy chains composing three types of myosin isoforms is developmentally regulated [9] and that the myosin isoforms expressed in rats with pressure and volume overload states, and in cardiomyopathic hamsters revert to the fetal and perinatal forms presumably so as to mediate myocardial adaptation to imposed cardiac load [17, 21]. Myosin isoforms have been demonstrated to shift to fetal forms in EMC virus induced myocarditis [14].

We propose that ANP gene is re-expressed in the ventricles of a diseased heart corresponding to the increase in mechanical load. In addition, since ANP staining was particularly strong in the areas surrounding lesions in immunofluorescence, local effects stimulating ANP synthesis are suggested to exist. Further studies are necessary to elucidate the possible mechanism responsible for enhanced ANP synthesis in this model.

Acknowledgement: This work was supported, in part, by a research grant from the Ministry of Health and Welfare, Grant-in-Aid for scientific research on priority areas, and for general scientific research from the Ministry of Education, Science and Culture, Japan and Kanazawa Research Fund.

References

1. Burnett JC, Kao PC, Hu DC, Heser DW, Heublein D, Granger JP, Opgenorth TJ, Reeder GS (1986) Atrial natriuretic peptide elevation in congestive heart failure in man. Science 231:1145
2. Day ML, Schwartz D, Wiegand RC, Stockman PT, Brunnert SR, Tolunay GE, Currie MG, Standaert DG (1987) Ventricular atriopeptin unmasking of messenger RNA and peptide synthesis by hypertrophy or dexamethasone. Hypertension 9:485
3. De Bold AJ (1985) Atrial natriuretic factor: a hormone produced by the heart. Science 230:767
4. Ding J, Thibault G, Gutkowska J, Garcia R, Karabatsos T, Jasmin G, Genest J, Cantin M (1987) Cardiac and plasma atrial natriuretic factor in experimental congestive heart failure. Endocrinology 121:248
5. Edwards BS, Ackermann DM, Lee ME, Reeder GS, Wold LE, Burnett JC (1988) Identification of atrial natriuretic factor within ventricular tissue in hamsters and humans with congestive heart failure. J Clin Invest 81:82
6. Kangawa K, Matsuo H (1984) Purification and complete amino acid sequence of α-human atrial natriuretic polypeptide. Biochem Biophys Res Commun 118:131

7. Kawai C, Tomioka N, Matsumori A, Kishimoto C (1987) Steroid treatment in viral myocarditis in mice: with special reference to serial changes in lymphocyte subsets. Eur Heart J 8 [Suppl J]:257

8. Kawai C, Matsumori A, Fujiwara H (1987) Myocarditis and dilated cardiomyopathy. Annu Rev Med 38:221

9. Lompre AM, Nadal-Ginard B, Mahdavi V (1984) Expression of the cardiac ventricular α- and β-myosin heavy chain genes is developmentally and hormonally regulated. J Biol Chem 259:6437

10. Matoba Y, Matsumori A (1987) Cyclosporine accelerates the development of anti-heart antibody in viral myocarditis in mice. Circulation 76 [Suppl IV]:264

11. Matsumori A, Kawai C (1982) An experimental model for congestive heart failure following encephalomyocarditis virus myocarditis in mice. Circulation 65:1230

12. Matsumori A, Kawai C (1982) An animal model of congestive (dilated) cardiomyopathy: dilatation and hypertrophy of the heart in the chronic stage in DBA/2 mice with myocarditis caused by encephalomyocarditis virus. Circulation 66:355

13. Matsumori A, Thorp K, Crumpacker CS, Abelmann WH (1984) Anti-heart antibody in an experimental model of viral myocarditis. Circulation 70 [Suppl II]:140

14. Matsumori A, Thorp K, Khaw BA, Haber E, Abelmann WH (1984) Distribution of cardiac myosin isozymes in the mouse with viral myocarditis as determined by selective monoclonal antibody. Circulation 70 [Suppl II]:402

15. Matsumori A, Morii N, Tomioka N, Nakao K, Imura H (1987) Atrial natriuretic polypeptide in experimental viral myocarditis: increased synthesis and secretion in the ventricle and atrium. Circulation 76 [Suppl IV]:211

16. Matsumori A, Tomioka N, Kawai C (1989) Viral myocarditis: immunopathogenesis and the effect of immunosuppressive treatment in a murine model. Jpn Circ J 53:58

17. Mercadier JJ, Lompre AM, Wisnewsky C, Samuel JL, Bercovici J, Swynghedauw B, Schwartz K (1981) Myosin isoenzymatic change in several models of rat cardiac hypertrophy. Circ Res 49:525

18. Morii N, Nakao K, Matsumori A, Tomioka N, Kawai C, Imura H (1989) Increased synthesis and secretion of atrial natriuretic polypeptide during viral myocarditis. J Cardiovasc Pharmacol 13 [Suppl 6]:S5

19. Nakao K, Sugawara A, Morii N, Sakamoto M, Suda M, Soneda J, Ban T, Kihara M, Yamori Y, Shimokura M, Kiso Y, Imura H (1984) Radioimmunoassay for α-human and rat atrial natriuretic polypeptide. Biochem Biophys Res Commun 124:815

20. Saito Y, Nakao K, Arai H, Nishimura K, Okumura K, Obata K, Takemura G, Fujiwara H, Sugawara A, Yamada T, Itoh H, Mukoyama M, Hosoda K, Kawai C, Ban T, Yasue H, Imura H (1989) Augmented expression of atrial natriuretic polypeptide gene in ventricle of human failing heart. J Clin Invest 83:298

21. Wiegrand V, Stroh E, Henniges A, Lossnitzer K, Kreuzer H (1983) Altered distribution of myosin isoenzymes in the cardiomyopathic syrian hamster (BIO 8, 262). Basic Res Cardiol 78:665

Dichotomous Effects of Cyclophosphamide
in Murine Coxsackievirus B3-Induced Myocarditis*

M. Herzum, S. A. Huber, and B. Maisch

Introduction

Enteroviruses, especially of the Coxsackie group, seem to be major causative agents for myocarditis in humans. Murine Coxsackie B3-induced myocarditis resembles the human disease closely. The immune system plays an essential role in mediating the disease [12]. As in humans, cellular and humoral immune reactions to the myocardium have been described. In BALB/c mice, Huber et al. demonstrated cytotoxic T lymphocytes to virally infected and uninfected cardiac myocytes [5]. Antibodies to cardiac myosin of the IgG isotype and other epitopes have been demonstrated to be responsible especially for the chronic stage of Coxsackie B3-induced murine myocarditis [1]. In humans, antibodies to myocardial cells can be found at a high incidence in the serum of patients with acute myocarditis and postmyocarditic heart muscle disease [9, 10]. Monoclonal antibodies cross-reacting between Coxsackie B3 epitopes and myocardium have recently been described [6].

But there is no general susceptibility to myocarditis, either in human or in mice. Susceptibility and resistance are linked to the major histocompatibility complex [2]. Furthermore, the sex of the infected individual is another determining factor for susceptibility to myocarditis by the action of sex hormones. Whereas testosterone worsens the course and outcome of Coxsackie B3 myocarditis in mice, estrogens – by the induction of suppressor cells – are protective. Adoptively transferring T lymphocytes of female BALB/c mice after Coxsackie B3 inoculation into susceptible male BALB/c mice largely reduces cardiac inflammation in those mice as compared to untreated male BALB/c mice. Suppressor cells generated in female mice during the infection are most likely responsible for this protection [7, 8]. Interestingly, there is a male preponderance for myocarditis in humans compared to females [12].

Administering cyclophosphamide early after virus inoculation inhibits the generation of suppressor cells [3, 11]. In Coxsackie B3 myocarditis, the protection of female BALB/c mice by suppressor cells could be removed by a single administration of the drug. Giving cyclophosphamide on the day of virus inoculation proved to be most effective to stop the resistance [7]. On the other hand, giving the drug at a higher dose or for a longer period of time exerts

---
* Supported by the Deutsche Forschungsgemeinschaft He 1438–1.

cytotoxic effects on a variety of cell types including the cells of the immune system. Lymphopenia and a decrease in antibody production are observed. With respect to the results mentioned above, we studied the effects of cyclophosphamide in strains of mice genetically resistant to Coxsackie B3-induced myocarditis.

Methods

Male CBA and C57B16 mice, 6–7 weeks old, were purchased from the Jackson Laboratory (Bar Harbor, ME). They were inoculated intraperitoneally with 1 × 10⁵ plaque-forming units of Coxsackie B3 (Nancy strain). Cyclophosphamide (Sigma Chemicals) at a dose of 50 mg/kg body weight was administered intra-peritoneally on day 0 to one group of mice, and on day 3–5 relative to the day of virus inoculation to a second group of mice. Animals in the control group received intraperitoneal injections of sterile saline. The mice were sacrificed on day 7 after virus infection. The hearts were divided into two pieces, one half was frozen for virus titration on HeLa cells, the other half fixed in formalin and stained with hematoxylin-eosin for histology. Inflammatory and necrotic lesions were scored blindly by two observers. Statistical analysis was done using the Wilcoxon ranked score test.

Results

Mortality did not change significantly in any groups, except in the group of C57B16 that got cyclophosphamide only once on day 0 relative to the day of virus inoculation. It went up to 56% in this group. Cardiac virus titers increased

Table 1. Mortality, cardiac virus titers (virus), inflammation and necrosis score in C57B16 and CBA mice after Coxsackie B3 inoculation and administration of cyclophosphamide on day 0 and days 3–5 relative to the day of infection

	Mortality (%)	Virus (lgPFU)	Inflammation (Score 1–4)	Necrosis
C57B16 (n=9)				
CB3	11	6.6	0.06 ± 0.06	0.06 ± 0.06
CB3 + Cy0	56	7.9	0.50 ± 0.35	0.38 ± 0.24
CB3 + Cy3–5	22	8.2[a]	1.25 ± 0.37[b]	0.70 ± 0.25[b]
CBA (n = 9)				
CB3	0	5.6	0.06 ± 0.06	0.06 ± 0.06
CB3 + Cy0	0	7.9[a]	0.90 ± 0.27[b]	0.50 ± 0.14[b]
CB3 + Cy3–5	22	7.0[a]	0 ± 0	0 ± 0

[a] $p < 0.01$.
[b] $p < 0.05$.
CB3, Coxsackie B2 virus; Cy0, cyclophosphamide on day 0; Cy3–5, cyclosphosphamide on days 3–5 relative to the day of infection.

in all groups that got cyclophosphamide. As could be expected from previous experiments, the inoculation of C57B16 and CBA mice with virulent Coxsackie B3 virus did not induce significant myocarditis with respect to inflammation and necrosis in the heart. Giving cyclophosphamide once to either strain rendered both of them susceptible to the disease. Inflammatory and necrotic lesions increased considerably but reached statistically significant levels only in CBA mice, where mortality was low at the same time. Multiple administrations of cyclophosphamide had different effects on both strains of mice: whereas it increased myocarditis in C57B16 mice, it abrogated the disease completely in CBA mice. Neither inflammatory cells or necrotic lesions were detectable by light microscopy, although there was a considerable amount of replicating virus in myocardial cells (Table 1).

Discussion

Enteroviruses like Coxsackie viruses are ubiquitously occurring microorganisms. But only in a few individuals do they lead to serious illness of the brain, heart, muscle, pancreas, or intestine [12]. Genetic factors seem to play a role in the natural resistance to these virus infections. For Coxsackie B3-induced myocarditis, Buie et al. demonstrated an association of susceptibility to myocarditis to certain haplotypes of the major histocompatibility complex [2]. Our findings underline these results. Although there are considerable amounts of replicating Coxsackie B3 present in the myocardium on day 7 after virus infection, cardiac pathomorphology is minimal in those mice known to be genetically resistant. Suppressing factors like suppressor T lymphocytes, which have been shown to confer resistance to myocarditis in female BALB/c mice, seem to be responsible for the resistance of C5B16 and CBA mice. There is no lack of functioning and cytolytic immune cells since they could be demasked by a single administration of cyclophosphamide leading to considerable myocarditis in these strains of mice. Huber et al. demonstrated that cyclophosphamide given at the dose used in this experiment will preferably remove suppressor T lymphocytes [7]. This strongly suggests that a similar protective T cell population renders C57B16 and CBA mice resistant to myocarditis.

Multiple administration of cyclophosphamide, however, led to a further increase of myocarditis in C57B16 mice, whereas CBA mice showed benefit from the treatment. Immune effector mechanisms, sensitive to a longer treatment with cyclophosphamide, seem to be responsible for myocarditis in CBA mice, since the drug not only inhibits the generation of suppressor T lymphocytes and antibody production, but also exerts strong cytotoxicity to other white blood cells and other cell types. In contrast to this result, C57B16 mice, genetically different from CBA mice, developed worse myocarditis with longer treatment. The data parallels experience from treatment trials in patients with myocarditis, where the response to various treatment regimens is heterogeneous [4]. Further characterization of immune pathomechanisms is necessary for better prediction of the efficacy of certain treatments in enterovirus-induced myocarditis.

References

1. Alvarez FL, Neu N, Rose NR, Craig SW, Beisel KW (1987) Heart-specific autoantibodies induced by coxsackievirus B3: identification of heart autoantigens. Clin Immunol Immunopathol 43:129–139
2. Buie C, Lodge P, Herzum M, Huber SA (1987) Genetics of coxsackie virus B3 and encephalomyocardits virus-induced myocarditis in mice. Eur Heart J 8 [Suppl J]:399–401
3. Greeley EH, Segre M, Segre D (1982) Suppressor cells in cyclophosphamide-treated autoimmune mice. Immunopharmacology 4:355–363
4. Herum M, Huber SA (1986) Immunosuppressive Therapie der Virusmyokarditis. Schwerpunktmed 9:9–13
5. Huber SA, Lodge PA (1984) Coxsackievirus B3 myocardits in BALB/c mice: evidence for autoimmunity to myocyte antigens. Am J Pathol 116:21–29
6. Huber SA, Simpson K, Weller A, Herzum M (1988) Immunopathogenic mechanisms in experimental myocarditis: evidence for autoimmunity to the virus receptor and antigenic mimicry between virus and cardiocyte. In: Schultheiss HP (ed) New concepts in viral heart disease. Springer, Berlin Heidelberg New York, pp 177–187
7. Job LP, Lyden DC, Huber SA (1986) Demonstration of suppressor cells in coxsackievirus group B, type 3 infected female BALB/c mice which prevent myocarditis. Cell Immunol 98:104–113
8. Lyden DC, Huber SA (1984) Aggravation of coxsackievirus, group B, type 3-induced myocarditis and increase in cellular immunity to myocarditis and increase in cellular immunity to myocyte antigens in pregnant BALB/c mice and animals treated with progesterone. Cell Immunol 87:462–472
9. Maisch B (1986) Immunologic regulator and effector functions in perimyocarditis, post-myocarditic heart muscle disease and dilated cardiomyopathy. Basic Res Cardiol 81 [Suppl 1]:217–242
10. Schultheiss HP, Bolte HD (1985) Immunological analysis of autoantibodies against the adenine nucleotide translocator in dilated cardiomyopathy. J Mol Cell Cardiol 17:603–617
11. Sym SN, Miller SD, Claman HN (1977) Immune suppression with supraoptimal doses of antigen in contact sensitivity: I. Demonstration of suppressor cells and their sensitivity to cyclophosphamide. J Immunol 119:240–244
12. Woodruff JF (1980) Viral myocarditis: a review. Am J Pathol 101:426–484

Enterovirus RNA Sequences in Hearts with Dilated Cardiomyopathy: A Pathogenetic Link Between Virus Infection and Dilated Cardiomyopathy

L. C. Archard, N. E. Bowles, L. Cunningham, C. A. Freeke, P. Morgan-Capner, E. G. J. Olsen, N. R. Banner, M. L. Rose, M. H. Yacoub, B. T. Meany, and P. J. Richardson

Introduction

An association between enterovirus infection of myocardium and heart muscle disease has been established by the use of virus-specific molecular hybridisation probes under circumstances where the isolation of infectious virus or the immunocytochemical demonstration of virus antigens is generally not possible [3]. It is widely accepted that enteroviruses are major aetiological agents of inflammatory heart muscle disease [6, 7], and we have detected enteroviral RNA in endomyocardial biopsy samples from six of ten histologically proven cases of acute myocarditis [2]. However, patients are rarely biopsied at this early stage, and we have been concerned with the persistence of enteroviral RNA in myocardium in the progression from healing myocarditis to so-called idiopathic dilated cardiomyopathy [1] and even end-stage disease requiring cardiac transplantation [3].

The present article summarises our current data relating to the role of enterovirus infection in the development of dilated cardiomyopathy. We describe the significance of virus persistence in the progression to end-stage disease and its implications for prognosis. We also present data which indicate that establishment of virus persistence results from the generation of virus defective in control of RNA synthesis.

Detection of Enterovirus in Myocardium in Histologically Proven Grades of Heart Muscle Disease

Enterovirus RNA sequences were detected in samples of myocardium by molecular hybridisation with an ^{32}P-labelled enterovirus group-specific probe in a quantitative slot blot assay: the cDNA probe was a copy of the conserved 3' region of Coxsackie B2 virus genomic RNA [5].

Tissue from the hearts of 123 patients with either healing myocarditis or dilated cardiomyopathy was compared with tissue from 57 pathologically irrelevant controls (total 180 patients). Of the tissue obtained from 86 patients with dilated cardiomyopathy, 67 were endomyocardial biopsy samples and 19 were tissue samples from the explanted hearts of endstage dilated cardiomyopathy patients who underwent orthotopic cardiac transplantation. Enteroviral RNA

Table 1. Detection of enterovirus RNA in samples of myocardium from 123 patients with healing myocarditis or dilated cardiomyopathy or from 57 patients with other specific heart muscle diseases (total 180 patients)

Enterovirus RNA	Endomyocardial biopsy samples			Explanted hearts	
	Healing myocarditis	Dilated cardio-myopathy	Controls	Dilated cardio-myopathy	Controls
	(n) (%)	(n) (%)	(n) (%)	(n) (%)	(n) (%)
+ve	13 35	28 42	0 0	6 32	1 5
−ve	24	39	38	13	18
total	37	67	38	19	19

sequences were detected in biopsy samples from 13 of 37 (34%) cases of healing myocarditis and 28 of 67 (42%) cases of dilated cardiomyopathy compared with none of 38 samples of tissue from other specific heart muscle diseases without a viral aetiology ($p < 0.0002$). Additionally, enteroviral sequences were detected in tissue samples from six of 19 (32%) explanted hearts from cases of end-stage dilated cardiomyopathy compared with tissue from one of 19 controls comprising cases of ischaemic, congenital or amyloid heart muscle disease ($p < 0.05$). These data are summarised in Table 1.

Prognostic Significance of Enterovirus Persistence

The data presented here demonstrate that enterovirus RNA can persist in myocardium until end-stage disease requiring cardiac transplantation. We have evaluated the prognostic significance of persisting virus infection by a prospective study of 123 patients with myocarditis, dilated cardiomyopathy or other specific heart muscle disease. Routine clinical assesment included duration of symptoms, history of preceding viral illness and other aetiological factors such as ethanol abuse, exposure to other toxins or systemic disease known to be related to heart muscle disease. Cardiac catheterisation with left ventriculography and, where clinically indicated, coronary arteriography was performed to exclude significant coronary artery disease. Percutaneous transfemoral endomyocardial biopsy was performed using a long biopsy sheath and a King's bioptome [9]. Biopsy samples were subjected to histological, histochemical and ultrastructural evaluation and classified according to the Dallas criteria [4]. Portions of the same biopsy samples were probed for enterovirus RNA by molecular hybridisation as described above. Of 123 patients, 41 were positive for the presence of enterovirus RNA sequences in myocardium. Of the patients with myocarditis or dilated cardiomyopathy, those positive or negative for enterovirus RNA in myocardium did not differ significantly in their clinical characteristics at presentation. In particular, there was no statistically significant difference between patient groups with respect to age, duration of symptoms, cardiothoracic ration, left ventricular end diastolic filling pressure or ejection fraction (Table 2).

Table 2. Clinical variables in patients with heart muscle disease and survival rates in enterovirus-positive or enterovirus-negative groups. Average follow-up: 24.5 months

Probe	Positive (n = 41)	Negative (n = 82)	p value
Age (years)	44.6 ± 14	45.2 ± 10	NS
Duration (symptoms) (years)	7.8 ± 9.6	14.9 ± 20.3	NS
CTR	48 ± 0.08	47 ± 0.10	NS
LVEDP	19.9 ± 10	18.2 ± 9.8	NS
EF	34.2 ± 17	38.9 ± 18	NS
Survival	31 (75%)	77 (94%)	0.005

Table 3. Predictors of survival in patients with myocarditis or dilated cardiomyopathy

Multiple regression analysis	F value
Enterovirus positive	0.0229
EF	0.0266
Age	0.6064
Duration	0.2841
LVEDP	0.9596

Significant if $F \leq 0.0376$.

Patients had routine clinical review at 6–12 month intervals (mean follow-up period 24.5 months) to assess clinical status and survival. Patients whose biopsies were positive for enterovirus RNA had a decreased probability of survival compared with patients who were enterovirus negative (virus positive 75%, virus negative 94%; $p < 0.005$: Table 2). Multiple regression analysis indicated that the presence of enterovirus in myocardium was the strongest predictor of outcome, even when compared with ejection fraction at presentation: age, duration of disease and left ventricular end diastolic filling pressure were not significant (Table 3).

Molecular Basis of Virus Persistence

Molecular hybridisation with an enterovirus group-specific probe demonstrates that virus RNA is present in myocardium after the inflammatory state of myocarditis and can persist until end-stage dilated cardiomyopathy (Table 1). This demonstrates that virus can persist in the affected tissue without generating a cellular immune response. In addition, we investigated whether virus persistence was accompanied by a continuing virus-specific IgM response. Sera were examined from 20 patients with dilated cardiomyopathy, nine of whom were positive for enterovirus RNA. Three of these 20 patients had Coxsackie B virus-specific IgM [8] and two of these were positive for enterovirus RNA. Thus, virus can persist in myocardium without gross cytopathology or consistently attracting the attention of either arm of the immune response. As

Table 4. Detection of enterovirus RNA in samples of myocardium: relative abundance of virus genomic and template RNA strands

Sample	Ratio: autoradiographic signal positive strand RNA/negative strand RNA
Productive infection control	> 100
Patient HG2B	1.1
Patient 62	1.1
Patient 64	2.3
Patient 40	3.0
Patient 61	3.3
Patient 6	4.7

infectious virus cannot be isolated nor can viral antigens be detected at this stage of disease, this suggests that a complete cycle of productive virus infection does not take place.

We have used single-stranded riboprobes complementary to either the positive genomic strand of virus RNA or the negative template strand to determine the relative abundance of these two species of viral RNA. Like the cDNA probe described above, these are copied from a conserved region of the Coxsackie B2 virus genome and so are enterovirus group specific. It is well known that during productive cytolytic infection by enteroviruses, synthesis of viral RNA is asymmetric [10]. We have determined that in Coxsackie B2 virus-infected cells in culture, the synthesis of the positive genomic strand of viral RNA predominates over synthesis of negative template RNA by a factor of more than 100-fold (Table 4). By contrast, in samples of myocardium from non-inflammatory heart disease which are positive for the presence of enterovirus RNA, the two polarities of virus RNA are present in near equimolar amounts (Table 4). We have observed the same phenomenon in enterovirus-related non-inflammatory skeletal muscle disease (our unpublished data). This indicates an aberration in the control of virus RNA synthesis and suggests that persistent infection results from the generation of defective virus.

Conclusions

We present data from molecular hybridisation with virus-specific probes which demonstrate a major association between persisting enterovirus infection of myocardium and the development of dilated cardiomyopathy. Despite the sampling error inherent in the endomyocardial biopsy procedure and thus the unknown frequency of false negatives, tissue samples from approximately 40% of patients with histologically confirmed dilated cardiomyopathy were positive for the presence of enterovirus RNA. During the subsequent follow-up period (average 2 years) of 41 enterovirus-positive and 82 enterovirus-negative patients, persisting enterovirus infection was shown to be the most important predictor of survival. The predictive value of detection of enterovirus RNA in myocardium was even greater than that of reduced ejection fraction: no other clinical parameter correlated with survival.

Persistence of virus in dilated cardiomyopathy does not generally elicit either a cellular or humoral immune response. The use of single-stranded riboprobes demonstrates a loss of control of the normally asymmetric synthesis of virus-specific RNA. We propose that dilated cardiomyopathy associated with persisting enterovirus infection results from generation of defective virus during the prior, cytolytic stage of disease.

The mechanism by which persistent virus infection perturbs myocardial function is not yet understood.

References

1. Archard LC, Bowles NE, Olsen EGJ, Richardson PJ (1987) Detection of persistent Coxsackie B virus RNA in dilated cardiomyopathy and myocarditis. Eur Heart J 8 [Suppl J]:437–440
2. Archard LC, Richardson PJ, Olsen EGJ, Dubowitz V, Sewry CA, Bowles NE (1987) The role of Coxsackie B viruses in the pathogenesis of myocarditis, dilated cardiomyopathy and inflammatory muscle disease. Biochem Soc Symp 53:51–62
3. Archard LC, Freeke CA, Richardson PJ et al (1989) Persistence of enterovirus RNA in dilated cardiomyopathy: a progression from myocarditis. In: Schultheiss H-P (ed) New concepts in viral heart disease. Springer, Berlin Heidelberg New York, p 347
4. Aretz HT, Billingham ME, Edwards WD et al (1986) Myocarditis. A histopathologic definition and classification. Am J Cardiovasc Pathol 1:3–14
5. Bowles NE, Richardson PJ, Olsen EGJ, Archard LC (1986) Detection of Coxsackie-B-virus-specific RNA sequences in myocardial biopsy samples from patients with myocarditis and dilated cardiomyopathy. Lancet i:1120–1123
6. El-Hagrassy MMO, Banatvala JE, Coltart DJ (1980) Coxsackie-B-virus-specific IgM responses in patients with cardiac and other diseases. Lancet ii:1160–1162
7. Grist NR, Bell EJ (1974) A six year study of Coxsackie virus B infections in heart disease. J Hyg (Lond) 73:165–172
8. King ML, Shaikh A, Bidwell D, Voller A, Banatvala JE (1983) Coxsackie-B-virus-specific IgM responses in children with insulin-dependent (juvenile-onset; type I) diabetes mellitus. Lancet I:1397–1399
9. Richardson PJ (1974) King's endomyocardial bioptome. Lancet i:660–661
10. Rotbart HA, Abzug MJ, Murray RS, Murphy NL, Levin MJ (1988) Intracellular detection of sense and antisense enteroviral RNA by in situ hybridization. J Virol Methods 22:295–301

HLA Haplotype in Idiopathic Dilated Cardiomyopathy: Genetically Determined Immune Response Factors of Etiologic Importance?

J. L. Anderson, J. F. Carlquist, M. B. Murray, and J. B. O'Connell

Introduction

Idiopathic dilated cardiomyopathy (IDC) is a disease of increasing interest but of uncertain etiology. One postulated mechanism of pathogenesis is that a viral infection triggers a host response with autoimmune features directed at the heart, resulting in an initial myocarditis followed by a dilated cardiomyopathy [1]. The tissue histocompatibility locus antigens (HLA) are known to be associated with immune regulatory functions. Further, many human diseases with autoimmune features have been found to have positive HLA antigen associations [2]. Because IDC may represent an autoimmune disease, we have explored and validated possible associations between IDC and the HLA haplotype patterns.

Of particular interest are the human class II histocompatibility antigens, believed to be expressed products of immune response genes [2]. They are dimeric molecules composed of two noncovalently linked glycoproteins (the alpha and beta chains). The loci for these genes have been mapped to within the major histocompatibility complex (MHC) on the short arm of chromosome 6. Within the class II region, subregions have been identified that include HLA DP, DQ, and DR. All of these subregions contain loci for at least one alpha and one beta chain. Each locus generally has multiple alleles. These class II proteins are some of the most polymorphic gene products yet recognized.

Of functional significance, the class II antigens have been shown to be restriction elements for the interaction of the helper (CD4+) lymphocytes with foreign antigens [4, 5]. Processed foreign antigen must first physically associate with class II molecules on the cell surface in order to be recognized by CD4+ lymphocytes [2–5]. MHC-restricted antigen recognition then enables these helper lymphocytes to perform their spectrum of functional activities, including induction or suppression of antibody synthesis [6–8], assistance in the clonal expansion of cytotoxic (CD8+) lymphocytes, mediation of delayed-type hypersensitivity with production of interleukin-2 (IL-2) and other cytokines [9, 10] and, in some cases, direct cytotoxicity against class II antigen-bearing target cells [11]. Thus, the MHC class II antigens and CD4+ lymphocytes play a key regulatory role in most immune responses.

In keeping with their immune response role, class II antigens have been studied for relationships with diseases associated with immunoregulatory dysfunction or autoimmunity. A recently published review [12] listed those diseases for which strong evidence of linkage to the HLA class II region has been obtained. A few of the notable diseases include: rheumatoid arthritis (associated with DR4), myasthenia gravis (DR3), multiple sclerosis (DR2), systemic lupus erythematosis (DR3), and insulin dependent diabetes mellitus (DR3, DR4) [2, 12].

Studies on insulin-dependent diabetes mellitus (IDDM) have allowed formulation of a model for HLA associated diseases. HLA-DR3 and HLA-DR4 were found in early investigations to be strongly associated with the presence of the disease [13, 14]. Subsequent work employing restriction endonuclease digestion and rehybridization with HLA-D region cDNA probes showed D region restriction fragment length polymorphisms (RFLP) that could distinguish between HLA-DR4 positive diseased subjects and HLA-DR4 positive controls [15]. Recently available D region probes have revealed a DQ beta chain polymorphism showing the highest degree of association with the disease [16, 17]. A comparison of the amino acid sequences of DQ beta chains from all HLA haplotypes known to increase risk for IDDM and all haplotypes previously shown to confer resistance to disease indicated that aspartic acid in position 57 of the DQ beta chain conferred resistance whereas alanine, serine or valine increased disease susceptibility [18]. Position 57 lies in what is believed to be the antigen binding site of the DQ molecule; amino acid substitutions at this site by affecting binding capacity could also affect immune regulatory response [2, 19].

A number of immune regulatory abnormalities have been identified in IDC, including humoral and cellular autoimmune reactivity against myocytes [20, 21] decreased natural killer cell activity [22], and functional deficiency in suppressor cell activity [23–25]. These and other findings potentially implicate regulatory defects in IDC. Because such defects may relate to patterns of MHC expression, we have undertaken a series of investigations of IDC patients to evaluate HLA A, B, DR, and DQ antigen expression. We report here on our initial exploratory [26] and recent validation studies.

Methods

Patient Selection: Patients fulfilling previously established diagnostic criteria for IDC [26, 27] were entered into the study. These criteria included a dilated left ventricular chamber of idiopathic cause with an ejection fraction of <45%. Control subjects consisted of healthy blood bank donors. All subjects were entered into the study after obtaining informed consent.

Lymphocyte Isolation: Lymphocytes for HLA typing were isolated by Ficoll-Hypaque density gradient centrifugation. Approximately 20 ml of heparinized blood was mixed with an equal volume of McCoy's 5A tissue culture medium and layered onto 10–15 ml Ficoll-Hypaque (Pharmacia). Centrifugation was performed at $400 \times g$ for 40 min, and the mononuclear cell layer was recovered from the plasma: Ficoll-Hypaque interface, resuspended in McCoy's medium, and washed three times.

Purified B lymphocytes for DR and DQ typing were obtained by suspending the entire mononuclear cell pellet in 0.5 ml McCoy's medium containing 5% heat-inactivated fetal calf serum (FCS). The cell suspension was then applied to a 0.5×5 cm plastic column containing loosely packed, scrubbed nylon wool (Fenwall Laboratories) and then incubated for 1 h at 37 °C in 5% CO_2. The nonadherent cells were washed from the column by successive washes (20–25 ml total) in McCoy's medium, and the adherent B lymphocytes were recovered by sequentially squeezing and washing the column with McCoy's medium without serum. B lymphocytes have also been isolated employing B-Quick B-lymphocyte isolation reagent (One Lambda, Inc.). The B lymphocytes were adjusted to a final concentration of $1–2 \times 10^6$/ml in serum-free McCoy's.

Cytotoxicity Assay: HLA-DR and -DQ typing was performed using the method of Terasaki [28]. Briefly, a 1 ml lymphocyte suspension was added to each well of a typing tray (One Lambda, Inc.): The tray was incubated at 37 °C for 30 min for HLA-A and -B, or 60 min for HLA-DR and -DQ, after which 5 mcl of rabbit complement was added to each well, and the tray was incubated at room temperature for 1 h for A and B typing, or for 2 h for DR and DQ. Dead cells were stained by adding 2 mcl eosin Y (50%) and fixing in formalin after 3 min. Viability was assessed visually by employing an inverted phase-contrast microscope. Samples testing positive for only one haplotype were assumed to be paired with a blank rather than an identical, double haplotype.

Statistical Analysis: Comparison between patients and control subjects was performed employing 2×2 contingency tables [29]. The strength of an association between an antigen and disease is estimated by the relative incidence ratio or relative risk. This is the calculated ratio of the cross product of the four entries in the 2×2 table (number of antigen-positive patients $\times$ number of antigen-negative controls/antigen-negative patients $\times$ antigen-positive controls). The etiologic fraction (EF) was calculated by the method of Bengtsson [30]. Specific comparisons between patient and control groups used a contingency table with chi-square or Fisher's exact test.

Results

Exploratory Study

In our initial exploratory study, we examined 35 consecutive patients with IDC for HLA-A, -B, and -DR phenotype and compared results to those in local population control subjects (for A and B, control $n = 2,863$; for DR, control $n = 82$) [26]. Patients were of average age 49 ± 14 years (range, 20–75); 24 were men; all but one was Caucasian. Radionuclide ejection fraction averaged 26 ± 10% (range, 11–40), except for two outliers (50% and 54%) who showed marked clinical improvement at the time of evaluation. Although no single HLA type could account for all cases, unequal distributions for patient and control groups were noted for several HLA types. Among the class I antigens,

Table 1. Frequency of HLA-DR haplotype occurrence in patients and controls

HLA type	Exploratory Study				Validation Study				Combined Study			
	IDC (%)	(n)	Control (%)	(n)	IDC (%)	(n)	Control (%)	(n)	IDC (%)	(n)	Control (%)	(n)
1	9	6	15	24	3	2	10	9	6	8	13	33
2	10	7	13	22	15	9	14	13	12	16	14	35
3	19	13	15	25	11	7	10	9	15	20	13	34
4	31[a]	22	18	30	26[b]	16	11	10	29[c]	38	16	40
5	7	5	8	13	19	12	7	7	13	17	8	20
w6	4[a]	3	13	22	5	3	13	12	5[c]	6	13	34
7	17	12	9	15	18	11	14	13	17	23	11	28
w8	3	2	6	7	0	0	10	9	2[c]	2	6	16
9	0	0	2	3	0	0	2	2	0	2	2	5
w10	0	0	1	2	0	0	2	2	0	0	2	4

[a] Nominal $p < 0.05$ (uncorrected).
[b] $p < 0.05$ (prospectively evaluated).
[c] $p < 0.01$ for combined series.

the frequency of HLA-B27 haplotype was increased in patients over that observed for 5726 population control haplotypes (0.145 vs. 0.033; $p < 0.001$). The relative risk of B27 was calculated to be 14 and the etiologic fraction, 0.27. In addition, the HLA-A2 haplotype comprised 0.42 of haplotype frequency in the patient group, versus 0.26 in the controls ($p < 0.02$).

Typing for HLA-DR antigens also revealed differences (Table 1). DR4 was found in 54% of 35 patients compared with 32% of 82 controls ($p < 0.03$). The corresponding DR4 haplotype fraction was 0.31 in patients and 0.18 in controls. The relative risk (RR) for DR4 was calculated to be 2.2, and the etiologic fraction, 0.29. An additional observation was that DRw6 (6Y) was underrepresented in IDC (9% of patients positive vs. 26% of controls, $p < 0.04$; haplotype fractions, 0.04 vs. 0.13, respectively). The relative risk for DRw6 was 0.27 and the preventive fraction 0.19.

It is noteworthy that 68% of patients were positive for DR4 or B27 or both. Of relevance, the DR and B loci lie closest together of any class I and class II loci. Thus, disequilibrium is expected and observed between many DR and B antigens. However, B27 and DR4 do not show evidence of linkage disequilibrium in healthy individuals [31], which possibly indicates the involvement of a novel haplotype in some patients with IDC.

Validation Study for DR and Exploratory Study for DQ Antigen Associations

Despite the apparent association between these antigens and IDC in the exploratory study, there are uncertainties associated with the interpretation of results of an initial exploratory study. First, in a preliminary study in which a number of antigens are studied simultaneously, there is the possibility of finding a significant antigen association by chance (type 1 error) as well as missing other associations when the study groups are relatively small (type 2 error). Type 1 errors are especially likely when multiple comparisons are made, as pointed out by Bonferroni [32]. To minimize these errors, nominal p values are often "corrected" by multiplying by the number of comparisons. However, a second prospective study with an a priori hypothesis regarding relative frequency for a specific antigen(s) of interest is a more definitive approach to validate proposed associations suggested by the pilot study [29].

Because the HLA-DR4 antigen haplotype did not occur in all patients, it is possible that its increased frequency in IDC relates to another gene(s) showing linkage disequilibium with DR4, or that IDC has multiple etiologies, only one of which relates to the HLA-DR4 locus. Moreover, HLA-DR4 is a public specificity that carries a number of more specific haplotype antigens, only one (or some) of which may be linked to IDC. Individuals possessing the DR4 specificity may also express a variety of serologically detectable polypeptide products from the DQ and DP regions [13, 33–36]. At least five DR4-containing haplotypes have been identified by Dw (mixed lymphocyte reaction) typing and/or by serological typing of associated DQ alleles. However, a noteworthy feature of the class II region is the strong linkage disequilibrium between some of the DQ and DR alleles [37]. Thus, typing for additional haplotype markers, e.g., DQ, would be of interest in exploring related subregions close to DR, looking further for evidence of a genetic basis for IDC.

Validation of DR Haplotype Results: We therefore performed a second study with a prospective hypothesis to confirm our preliminary findings. We postulated first, that the relative frequency of HLA-DR4 would be increased, and second, that DRw6 would be reduced in additional consecutive patients with IDC compared with concurrent controls. We also included DQ typing to help identify the chromosomal location of the disease-related genes involved. We studied an additional 47 healthy blood bank donors and 31 consecutive IDC patients (Table 1). Average age of the 31 patients was 47.7 ± 12.9 years (range, 21–74); 21 were men.

This validation study confirmed a relative increase in frequency of HLA-DR4: 52% of patients had at least one DR4 allele vs. 22% of controls ($p <$ 0.01). Corresponding haplotype fractions were 0.26 for IDC and 0.11 for controls. In the validation study, the relative risk of DR4 was 3.95 and the etiologic fraction, 0.39.

A trend toward a decreased frequency of DRw6 was again noted in IDC (10% of patients positive vs. 26% of controls; haplotype fractions 0.05 and 0.13) but this difference did not achieve significance, possibly because of relatively small group sizes. Increased DR5 and reduced DR8 frequencies in IDC patients were noted in this series although the p values were not significant when corrected for multiple comparisons.

DQ Haplotype and IDC: An association between IDC and one DQ allele was also noted (Table 2): DQw4 was found in 26% of patients and 6% of controls

Table 2. Frequency of HLA-DQ haplotype occurrence in patients and controls

HLA type	IDC ($n = 62$)		Population Controls ($n = 94$)		p Value[a]
	(%)	(n)	(%)	(n)	
1	31	19	33	31	NS
2	13	8	20	19	NS
3	29	18	30	28	NS
4	13	8	3	3	<0.03
7	23	14	24	23	NS

[a] Nominal, uncorrected values.

Table 3. Calculated relative risks and etiologic fractions

HLA antigen	Frequency		Relative risk	Etiologic fraction	Preventive fraction
	IDC	Control			
DR4[a]	0.53	0.28	2.7	0.33	–
DRw6[a]	0.09	0.26	0.29	–	0.18
DQ4	0.26	0.06	5.1	0.21	–
DR4/DQ4	0.13	0	∞	0.13	–

[a] Combined series.

(haplotype fractions 0.13 and 0.03), $p < 0.02$, corrected $p < 0.1$. The calculated relative risk for DQw4 is thus 5.1, and the etiologic fraction 0.21.

The combined DR4-DQw4 haplotype was found in four (13%) of 31 IDC patients and in none of the 47 controls ($p < 0.02$) (Table 3). It is of interest that in population studies, the DR4 allele is in linkage disequilibrium with DQw4 in Japanese populations, but DR4 is generally associated with the DQw3 specificity in Caucasian populations, not DQw4, as in our Caucasian IDC patients.

Combined Results for DR Associations with IDC

Because there were no significant differences between DR4 and DRw6 haplotype frequences in IDC and control groups in the initial and validation studies, results of the two studies were combined to give an overall result (Table 1; Fig. 1). Overall, DR4 was found in 53% of 66 IDC patients vs. 28% of 129 control subjects ($p < 0.001$). Conversely, DRw6 was found in 9% of patients vs. 26% of controls ($p < 0.01$). Reduced DR1 and DR8 antigen frequences were also noted in the combined series, but the corrected p values were not significant.

On the basis of the combined experience, the relative risk of DR4 is 2.7 and the etiologic fraction, 0.33. The relative risk of disease in the presence of DRw6 is 0.29 and the preventive fraction, 0.18 (Table 3).

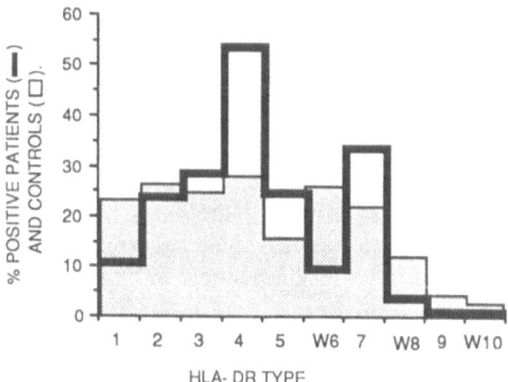

Fig. 1. Percentage of patients *(open bars, bold outline)* and controls *(shaded bars)* positive for each DR antigen in combined experience (exploratory plus validation studies)

Discussion

Idiopathic dilated cardiomyopathy is almost certainly a heterogeneous disease in which multiple factors are contributory, including infectious, toxic, and genetic ones. It is thus not surprising that a single HLA haplotype pattern was not found in all or nearly all cases of IDC examined. However, our findings do indicate that in a certain number cases, suggested by the etiologic fractions obtained to be about one-third to one-half, genetically determined immune regulatory factors associated with MHC antigens may be involved in pathogenesis. Our validation study specifically confirms a positive association of IDC with DR4 and raises the further probability of DQw4 involvement. It also suggests that a milder, negative association with DRw6 may be present.

The etiologic fraction is one estimate used to assess the strength of an association between a particular antigenic specificity and a disease. Theoretically, it represents the fraction of disease occurrences that is etiologically associated with the antigen in question. The etiologic fraction has also been shown, in some conditions, to provide an estimate about the linkage disequilibrium between the antigenic marker and other, closely mapping gene(s) which are actually involved in the pathogenis of the disease [30].

In our studies, consideration of the etiologic fractions, calculated for the specificities studied (DR4 = 0.33; DQw4 = 0.21; B27 = 0.27), does not readily point to a unique site for a putative disease-associated gene, because values are all relatively similar. Several explanations for this result should be considered. First, it is of interest that the combined DR4/DQw4 haplotype was identified in approximately 13% of IDC patients but was not found in any healthy controls. The relative risk for the combined haplotype pattern is very high ("infinite"). (Numbers are small, however, and risk estimates will require further assessment.) This implies that the actual disease "locus" may lie between the DR and DQ loci, and that the particular disease-producing allele is in linkage disequilibrium with both DR4 and DQw4. Another interpretation of our findings is that the "disease gene" is actually associated with a subtype of DR4 that is defined by its linkage with DQw4, e.g., the Dw15 subtype. In this case, the "disease" gene would be linked to DR4, but the calculated relative risk of DR4 would represent an average of all DR4 subtypes, including those linked to the disease and those not associated with it. This would result in an artificially low calculated value for relative risk. Finally, the possibility should be considered that two (or more) genes may contribute to disease pathogenesis; for example, one may associate with DR4 and another with DQw4. This case has been described for insulin dependent diabetes, in which the relative risk associated with each of two alleles was less than 1.0 when they occurred separately, but when they occurred together on a single haplotype, the relative risk jumped to 12.1 [38].

Conclusion

In conclusion, these studies provide evidence for an association between certain genetically determined HLA antigens and a fraction of IDC cases. The association between DR4 and IDC observed in a preliminary study has been validated in a second, prospective study. This study has also suggested the involvement of DQw4 carrying haplotypes in disease predisposition. These associations raise the possibility that immune response determinants in the HLA region may importantly contribute to increased disease susceptibility (and resistance), perhaps by regulating the interaction of host and certain infectious (viral) agents. Although the mechanisms and implications of these associations have not been shown, the evidence obtained is sufficiently compelling to warrant further investigation.

Acknowledgement: This project was supported in whole or in part by BRSG SO7 RR 05804-09 awarded by the Biomedical Research Support Grant Program, Division of Research Resources, National Institutes of Health.

References

1. Robinson JA, O'Connell JB (1983) Myocarditis: precursor of cardiomyopathy. Collamore, Lexington
2. Carpenter CB, David J (1989) Histocompatibility antigens and immune response genes. In: Rubenstein E, Federman D (eds) Scientific American Medicine. Scientific American, New York, ch pt 6-V
3. Biddison WE, Rao PE, Talle MA, Goldstein G, Shaw S (1982) Possible involvement of the OKT4 molecule in T cell recognition of class II antigens. Evidence from studies of cytotoxic T lymphocytes specific for SB antigens. J Exp Med 156:1065–1076
4. Swain SL (1983) T cell subsets and the recognition of MHC class. Immunol Rev 74:129–142
5. Meuer SC, Schlossman SF, Reinherz EL (1982) Clonal analysis of human cytotoxic T lymphocytes: T4+ and T8+ effector T cells recognize products of different major histocompatibility complex regions. Proc Natl Acad Sci USA 14:4395–4399
6. Morimoto C, Letvin NL, Distaso JA, Aldrich WR, Schlossman SF (1985) The isolation and characterization of the human suppressor inducer T cell subsets. J Immunol 134:1508–1515
7. Morimoto C, Letvin NL, Boyd AW, Hagan M, Brown HM, Kornacki MM, Schlossman SF (1985) The isolation and characterization of the human helper inducer T cell subset. J Immunol 134:3762–3769

8. Rich RR, el Masry MN, Fox EJ (1986) Human suppressor T cells: induction differentiation, and regulatory functions. Hum Immunol 17:369–387
9. Raulet DH, Bevan MJ (1982) A differentiation factor required for the expression of
   cytotoxic T-cell function. Nature 296:754–757
10. Wagner H, Hardt C, Rouse BT, Rollinghoff M, Scheurich P, Pfizenmaier K (1982)
    Dissection of the proliferative and differentiative signals controlling murine cytotoxic T
    lymphocyte responses. J Exp Med 155:1876–1881
11. Torpey DJ, Lindsley MD, Rinaldo CR (1989) HLA-restricted lysis of herpes simplex
    virus-infected monocytes and macrophages mediated by CD4+ and CD8+ T lympho-
    cytes. J Immunol 142:1325–1332
12. Svejgaard A, Platz P, Ryder LP (1983) HLA and disease – a survey. Immunol Rev
    70:193–226
13. Nepom GT, Nepom BS, Antonelli P, Mickelson E, Silver J, Goyert SM, Hansen JA
    (1983) The HLA DR4 family of haplotypes consists of a series of distinct DR and DS
    molecules. J Exp Med 159:394–404
14. Reinsmoen NL, Bach FH (1982) Five HLA-D clusters associated with HLA-DR4. Hum
    Immunol 4:249–258
15. Owerbach D, Hagglof B, Lernmark A, Holmgren G (1984) Susceptibility to insulin
    dependent diabetes defined by restriction enzyme polymorphism of HLA-D region geno-
    mic DNA. Diabetes 33:958–965
16. Kim SJ, Holbeck SL, Nisperos B, Hansen JA, Maeda H, Nepom GT (1985) Identifi-
    cation of a polymorphic variant associated with HLA-DQw3 and characterized by
    specific restriction sites within the DQ beta-chain. Proc Natl Acad Sci USA 82:8139–
    8143
17. Nepom BS, Palmer J, Kim SJ, Hansen JA, Holbeck SL, Nepom GT (1986) Specific
    genomic markers for the HLA-DQ subregion discriminate between DR4+ insulin depen-
    dent diabetes mellitus and DR4+ seropositive juvenile rheumatoid arthritis. J Exp Med
    164:345–350
18. Todd JA, Bell JI, McDevitt HO (1987) HLA-DQ beta gene contributes to susceptibility
    and resistance to insulin-dependent diabetes mellitus. Nature 329:599–604
19. Todd JA, Acha-Orbea H, Bell JI, Chao N, Fronek Z, Jacob CO, McDermott M, Sinha
    AA, Timmerman L, Steinman L, McDevitt HO (1988) A molecular basis for MHC class
    II associated autoimmunity. Science 240:1003–1009
20. Kawai C, Takatsu T (1975) Clinical and experimental studies on cardiomyopathy. N Engl
    J Med 293:592–597
21. Bolte HD, Grothe K (1977) Cardiomyopathies related to immunological processes. In:
    Reiker G, Weber A, Goodwin J (eds) Myocardial failure. Springer, Berlin Heidelberg
    New York
22. Anderson JL, Carlquist JF, Hammond EH (1982) Deficient natural killer cell activity in
    patients with idiopathic dilated cardiomyopathy. Lancet 2:1124–1127
23. Fowles RE, Bieber CP, Stinson EB (1979) Defective in vitro suppressor cell function in
    idiopathic congestive cardiomyopathy. Circulation 59:483–491
24. Anderson JL, Fowles RE, Bieber CP, Stinson EB (1978) Idiopathic cardiomyopathy, age
    and suppressor cell dysfunction as risk determinants of lymphoma after cardiac trans-
    plantation. Lancet 2:1174–1177
25. Gerli R, Rambotti P, Spinozzi F, Bertotto A, Chiodini V, Solinas P, Gernini I, Davis S
    (1986) Immunologic studies of peripheral blood from patients with idiopathic dilated
    cardiomyopathy. Am Heart J 112:350–355
26. Anderson JL, Carlquist JF, Lutz JR, DeWitt CW, Hammond EH (1984) HLA A, B, and
    DR typing in idipopathic dilated cardiomyopathy: a search for immune response factors.
    Am J Cardiol 53:1326–1330
27. Goodwin J, Oakley C (1972) The cardiomyopathies. Br Heart J 34:545–552
28. Terasaki PI, McClelland JD, Park MS, McCurdy B (1973) Microdroplet lymphocyte
    cytotoxicity test. In: Manual of tissue typing techniques. US Government Printing
    Office, Washington DC, pp 54–61 (DHEW Publ No NIH 74–545)
29. Svejgaard A (1976) HLA and disease. In: Rose NR, Friedman H (eds) Manual of clinical
    immunology. American Society for Microbiology. Washington DC, pp 841–850

30. Bengtsson BO, Thompson G (1981) Measuring the strength of associations between HLA antigens and diseases. Tissue Antigens 17:356–363
31. Bauer MP, Neugebauer M, Albert ED (1984) Reference tables of two-locus haplotype frequencies for all MHC marker loci. In: Albert ED et al (eds) Histocompatibility testing 1984. Springer, Berlin Heidelberg New York, p 677
32. Snedecor GW, Cochran WG (1980) Statistical methods, 7th edn. Iowa State University Press, Ames, p 116
33. Nepom BS, Nepom GT, Mickelson E, Antonelli P, Hansen JA (1983) Electrophoretic analysis of human HLA-DR antigens from HLA-DR4 homozygous cell lines: correlation between beta chain diversity and HLA-D. Proc Natl Acad Sci USA 80:6962–6966
34. Groner JP, Watson AJ, Bach FH (1983) Dw/LD related molecular polymorphisms of DR-4 beta chains. J Exp Med 157:1687–1691
35. Suzuki M, Yabe T, Satake M, Juji T, Hamaguchi H (1984) Two-dimensional gel electrophoretic analysis of the MT3 and DR4 molecules from the different D typed cells. J Exp Med 160:751–758
36. Holbeck SL, Kim SJ, Silver J, Hansen JA, Nepom GT (1985) HLA-DR4 associated haplotypes are genotypically diverse within HLA. J Immunol 135:637–641
37. Kao H-T, Gregerson PK, Tang JC, Takahashi T, Wang CY, Silver J (1989) Molecular analysis of the HLA class II genes in two DRw6-related haplotypes, DRw13 DQw1 and DRw14 DQw3. J Immunol 142:1743–1747
38. Sheehy MJ, Scharf SJ, Rowe JR, Neme de Gimenez MH, Meske LM, Erlich HA, Nepom BS (1989) A diabetes-susceptible HLA haplotype is best defined by a combination of HLA-DR and -DQ alleles. J Clin Invest 83:830–835

Humoral and Cell-Mediated Immunity: Pathogenetic Mechanisms in Dilated Cardiomyopathy

B. Maisch, E. Bauer, M. Herzum, G. Hufnagel, T. Izumi, S. Nunoda, and U. Schönian

Introduction

Dilated cardiomyopathy (DCM) according to the definition of the WHO/ISCF task force as "heart disease of unknown cause" [47] is a feasible working definition for the clinician. On hemodynamic grounds it defines DCM as systolic pump failure, which – as we know better today – may also have features of a diastolic compliance disturbance and severe dysrhythmias. For the cardiologist interested in pathogenetic mechanisms of this form of heart failure and its etiology, it is, however, not a satisfying explanation. Instead, it more likely describes our lack of knowledge than a disease entity. Recent evidence has pointed to viral etiology and the persistence of the enteroviral genome in a proportion of patients. Similarly, also the presence of cytomegalovirus DNA in active myocarditis could be ascertained (own unpublished results) in about 15% of patients. In addition, the investigation of immunologic regulator [1, 10, 11, 27, 28, 39, 54, 57], humoral [3, 5, 15, 19, 22–38, 40–47, 49–51, 55, 56], and cellular effector mechanisms in humans [2, 8, 9, 12, 13, 20, 27, 28, 34, 35, 41, 43, 55, 56] has broadened both our understanding of the primary etiology and secondary immunopathogenesis in DCM.

From animal and our own human studies in myocarditis [27–44] and DCM [35], it can be deduced that autoreactivity to cardiac structures by antibody- and cell-mediated immune reactions is not only an in vitro phenomena but bears diagnostic and pathogenetic implications in vivo. After an initial triggering attack, e.g., by a virus that may or may not persist, polyclonal or highly selective autoreactivity which could initially be directed to the triggering virus and to different cardiac epitopes or to both (molecular mimicry) follow. This host response appears to be also determined by genetic factors although direct evidence for this largely comes from animal data. What we may observe in end-stage dilated cardiomyopathy are, from an immunological point of view, mostly the footprints of a former viral infection or autoreactivity that may still go on or persist on a "chronic" inflammatory level. It may also be that the antibodies that we can demonstrate are primarily biographic markers as are IgG antibodies after a measles infection many years ago. The relevance of humoral and cellular phenomena must therefore be judged by their functional capacity in vivo and in vitro to attribute to them additional pathophysiologic relevance for the present state of the heart disease.

Table 1. Lymphocyte subpopulations in dilated heart muscle disease

	DCM ($n = 50$)	Postmyocarditic HMD ($n = 24$)	Controls ($n = 56$)
Pan T cells (CD3)	72.1 ± 1.3	74.5 ± 3.7	72.6 ± 7.0
T helper/inducer cells (CD4)	50.3 ± 1.8	50.4 ± 2.9	48.7 ± 7.3
T suppressor/cytotoxic cells (CD8)	21.1 ± 1.7	17.5 ± 2.9[a]	22.9 ± 5.7
B cells (DR)	22.4 ± 1.8	20.1 ± 3.1	23.6 ± 7.6
Monocytes (OKMI)	18.6 ± 1.9	10.7 ± 2.3	13.2 ± 5.6

[a] $p < 0.05$ by chi-square analysis.
DCM, dilated cardiomyopathy; *HMD*, heart muscle disease.

T Cell Subsets and T Suppressor Cell Activity

The methods have been described previously [1, 7, 10, 11, 27, 39]. Enumerations of peripheral T cells in our patients with DCM revealed no alteration when compared to healthy controls, only OKMI-positive monocytes [and natural killer cells (NK cells)] were increased (Table 1). In myocarditis patients an increase in OKIa1-positive B cells or activated T cells could be observed [28, 39]. Whereas Fowles et al. [11] and Eckstein et al. [10] demonstrated decreased T suppressor cell activity in dilated cardiomyopathy, in our studies [27, 39] T suppressor cell activity, carried out according to established methods [14, 39] in patients with myocarditis [39], postmyocarditic heart muscle disease, and DCM was no different from daily, age-matched controls.

Cellular Effector Mechanisms in Dilated Cardiomyopathy

Various studies have been presented on the effector mechanisms of peripheral blood lymphocytes [2, 13, 26, 27, 33, 41, 55, 56]. Using these, either the first-line defense mechanism of NK cells or target cell-specific cardiocytolysis, which is not MHC restricted, can be analyzed.

NK Cell Activity

Methods for the assessment of NK cells were first described by Perlmann and Perlmann [46] using K562 cells, an erythroblast cell line, as the appropriate target. NK cell activity (Fig. 1) in DCM and postmyocarditic cardiomegaly was found reduced in our patients [27, 28], as had been previously shown by Anderson et al. [1, 2]. Others supplement the in vitro shown by Anderson et al. [1, 2]. Others supplemented the in vitro assays with interferon gamma [8] or interleukin 2 (IL-2) [56] in patients with DCM and could then reconstitute NK cell activity to normal. All data concerning NK cell activity have to take into account, however, that frozen lymphocytes may give inconsistent and reduced NK cell activity. Thus stringent controls of normal cells frozen in exactly the

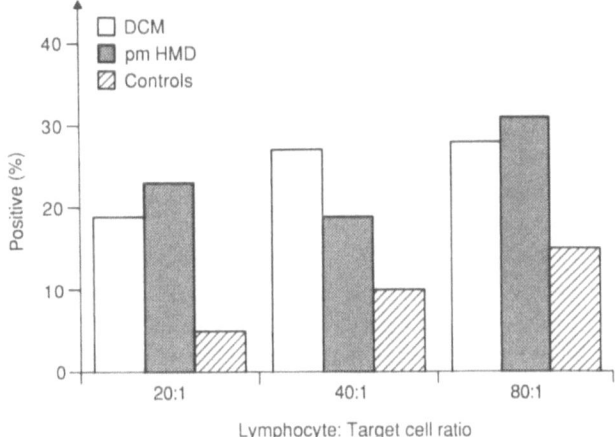

Fig. 1. NK cell activity measured by a [51]chromium release assay in different lymphocytes to target cell ratio is reduced significantly in DCM and slightly diminished in postmyocarditic heart muscle disease with cardiomegaly

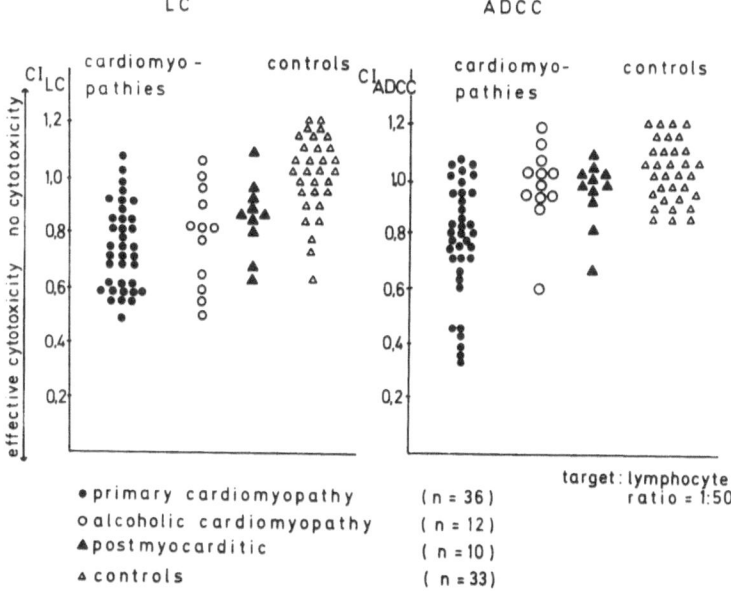

Fig. 2. *Left,* lymphocytotoxicity to isolated heart muscle cells is demonstrable in 30% of patients with an index of cardiocytolysis of < 0.75 being an indicator of effective cardiocytotoxicity. The index is calculated according to the following formula: [half-life (t_{50p}) of cardiocytes in the presence of patient's lymphocytes]; [half-life of cardiocytes (t_{50c}) in presence of control lymphocytes of a HLA-typed panel] (from [35]). *Right,* antibody-dependent cellular cytotoxicity (homologous test) of the DCM patients' lymphocytes when incubated with heterologous heart cells and the patients' serum. The index is calculated according to the cardiocytolytic index mentioned above

same way, or even better, immediate assays with freshly isolated effector cells are mandatory [27, 28] before making definite conclusions. It should be noted that reduced NK cell activity is by no means a cardiospecific finding but may explain in part the present or constitutional immunologic state of patient.

Target Cell-Specific Non-MHC-Restricted Lymphocytotoxicity in DCM

Methods for target cell-specific non-MHC-restricted lymphocytotoxicity to heterologous cardiocytes have been published previously [27, 34, 35]. Although the true activity of cytolytic T cells can be assessed only in experimental animals which have autologous myocytes as target cell with an identical MHC determinant available, we could recently present evidence that a heart cell-specific, non-MHC-restricted cytotoxicity of peripheral blood lymphocytes can be assayed by using heterologous myocytes [27, 34, 35, 45]. This lymphocyto-toxicity is clearly different from mere NK cell activity; it is directed against vital rat heart cells, and we found it enhanced in DCM (Fig. 2), in postmyocarditic heart muscle disease [35] and in some patients with myocarditis [34].

Antibody-Dependent Cellular Cytotoxicity

Antibody-dependent cellular cytotoxicity (ADCC) can be analyzed either with autologous lymphocytes ($ADCC_{auto}$) or homologous lymphocytes from a healthy donor ($ADCC_{homo}$); the latter system is the most widely used assay. We used both systems: an increased cardiocytotoxicity was present in assays of ADCC in DCM [35] and postmyocarditic heart muscle disease [35] (Fig. 2, right) as well as in some patients with myocarditis [27, 28, 34]. When compared to the heart cell-specific lymphocytotoxicity, enhancement of this was seen by the addition of the patient's serum in one-third of cases, indicating that ADCC is truly operative in vitro in this subgroup of DCM patients.

At present only little is known about the function of neutrophils and macro-phages in DCM.

Humoral Immune Reactions

A wide variety of different circulating antibodies directed against cardiac struc-tures, e.g., the membrane [5, 9, 15, 25–36, 40–43], the membrane-associated calcium channel [55], the beta-receptor [25], contractile proteins (see [26–28, 35] for overview in literature), and to mitochondrial proteins [22–24, 49–51] have recently been published. Klein et al. [22] could demonstrate in our patients a cardioselective antimitochondrial antibody directed against the M7 fraction of a mitochondrial preparation (Fig. 3). This finding was loosely asso-ciated with the presence of anti-interfibrillary antibodies (IFA; Fig. 4a) in the serum of the patients. Anti-M7 antibodies are not restricted to DCM and are also found in hypertrophic cardiomyopathy and to a smaller extent in myo-

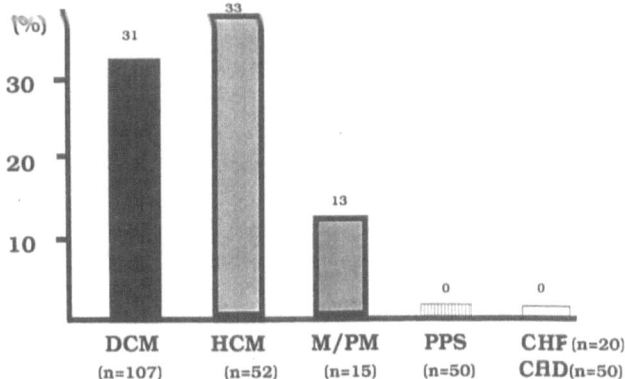

Fig. 3. Anti-M7 antibodies in cardiomyopathies (modified from [22]). Anti-M7 antibodies are found in almost one-third of patients with dilated cardiomyopathy *(DCM)* and hypertrophic cardiomyopathy *(HCM)*. They are not present in postpericardiotomy syndrome *(PPS)*, congestive heart failure *(CHF)* independent of DCM, or in coronary artery disease *(CAD)*

carditis, but not in controls and in coronary artery disease. Therefore it is clearly distinguishable from the antibody to the ANT-carrier [24, 49–51] which has homologies with the calcium channel and was proposed to be cross-reactive with it [55].

IFA as well as antifibrillary antibodies of the anti-myosin type (Fig. 4b) or the anti-actin type (Fig. 4c) occur with increasing frequency the more severe the heart disease is (Fig. 5): patients with DCM of NYHA classes III and IV are twice as often carriers of antibodies to contractile proteins or the interfibrillary substance than are patients of NYHA classes I and II. This does not apply, however, to important antimyolemmal antibodies [AMLA].

Circulating Antimembrane Antibodies

In 1982 we first described cytolytic antimembrane antibodies that could be demonstrated in active myocarditis. They were complement dependent [34]. These AMLAs directed against the inner sarcolemmal membrane (myolemma) are of particular interest because they are diagnostic markers of myocarditis (incidence > 85%; Fig. 4d). In myocarditis they belong to the IgG, IgM, IgA classes and may fix complement. In 1983 we could also demonstrate cytolytic antibodies in some patients with DCM and a larger proportion of patients with postmyocarditic heart muscle disease [35].

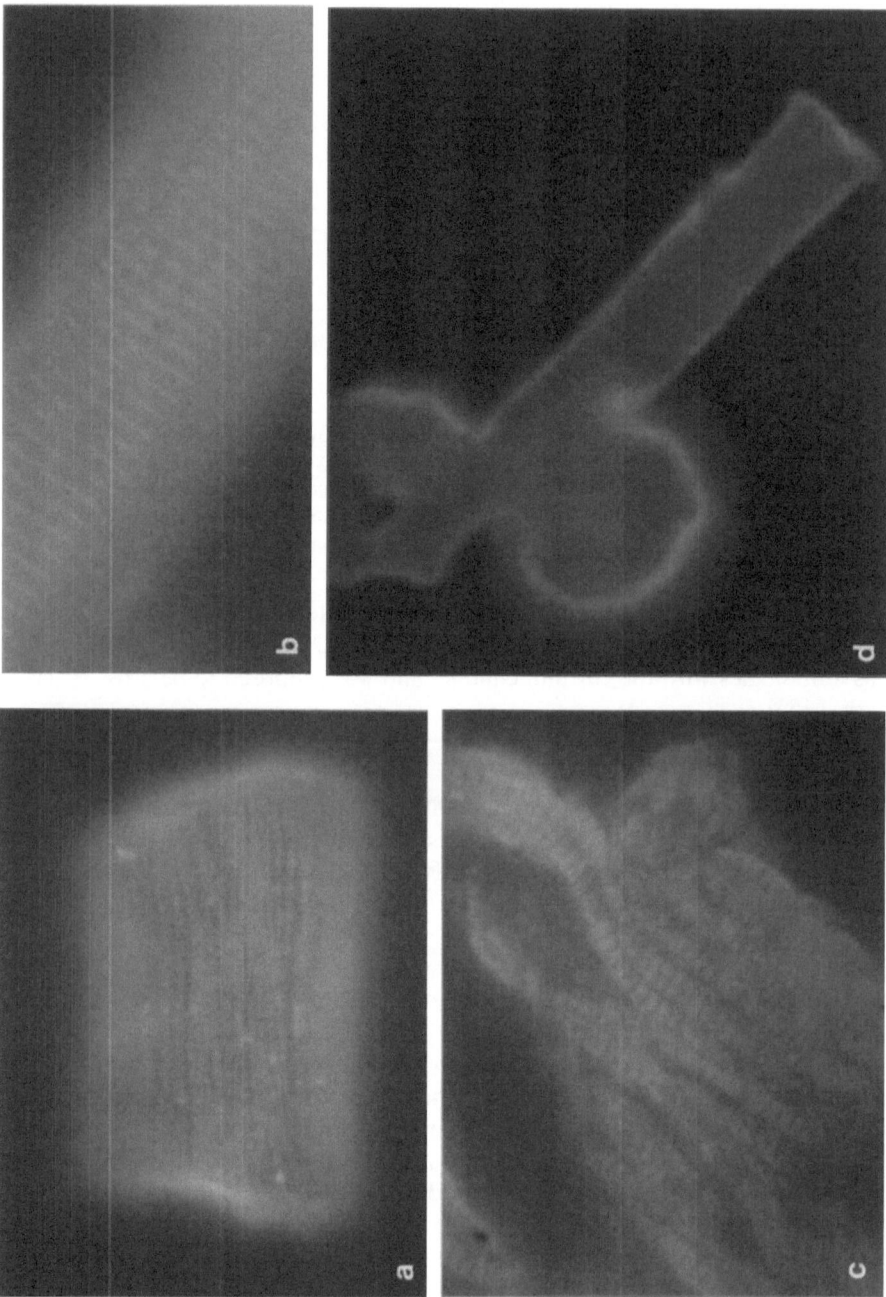

Fig. 4. a Demonstration of anti-interfibrillary antibodies with an isolated rat heart cell from a patient with dilated cardiomyopathy, NYHA class IV (titer 1 : 80). The patient's serum was also positive for high-titer (1 : 320) anti-M7 antibodies. **b** Demonstration of anti-myosin antibodies (titer 1 : 80) in a 39-year-old female patient with secondary postmyocarditic heart muscle disease (demonstrated with isolated myocytes). **c** Anti-actin antibodies (titer 1 : 80) in a 48-year-old patient with DCM. **d** Antimyolemmal antibodies in a 27-year-old patient with postmyocarditic heart muscle disease as demonstrated with an isolated intact human atrial myocyte (titer 1 : 320)

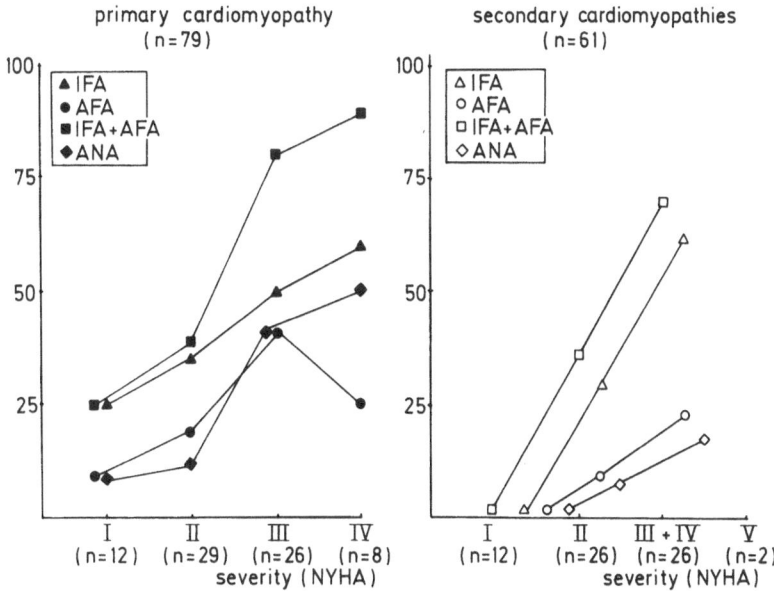

Fig. 5. The incidence of anti-interfibrillary antibodies *(IFA)*, antifibrillary antibodies *(AFA)* and antinuclear antibodies *(ANA)* in patients with DCM increased with the degree of cardiac impairment and NYHA classification. (Modified from [35])

Bound Antibodies in the Endomyocardial Biopsy of Patients with DCM

Correspondingly bound antisarcolemmal antibodies (Fig. 6a) were detected in the same biopsy specimen as were the circulating antibodies (Fig. 6b) after incubation of the autologous biopsy specimen with the patient's serum. These antimembrane antibodies were detected in more than 90% of cases in the biopsies of patients with histologically proven myocarditis and in more than 65% of patients with postmyocarditic heart muscle disease [27–30, 35, 36, 43], and about 50% of patients with DCM. They may be diagnostic markers of an autoreactive process. They are often associated with bound antibodies to com-

Table 2. Immunohistologic findings in dilated heart muscle disease (multicenter study 1980–1989)

Clinical diagnosis	n	Trivalent	IgG	IgM	IgA	C_3	C_3/IgM
Dilated cardiomyopathy	55	60[a]	56[a]	48[a, b]	12	48	
Postmyocarditic	28	79[a]	75[a]	18	36	61[a, b]	75[a, b]
Dilated HMD with increased alcohol intake	20	60[a]	60[a]	15	25[a]	35	40[a, b]
Noncardiac controls	17	12	12	12	0	0	0
Coronary artery disease	100	43[a]	41[a]	11	20[a]	3	14

[a] $p < 0.05$, when compared to noncardiac controls by chi-square analysis.
[b] $p < 0.05$, when compared to coronary artery disease by chi-square analysis.
HMD, heart muscle disease.

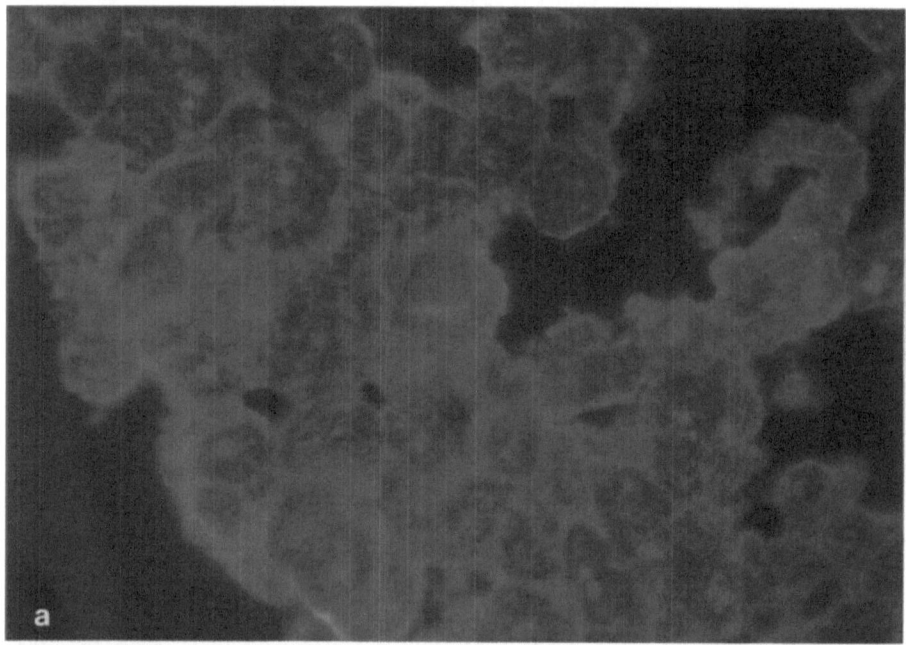

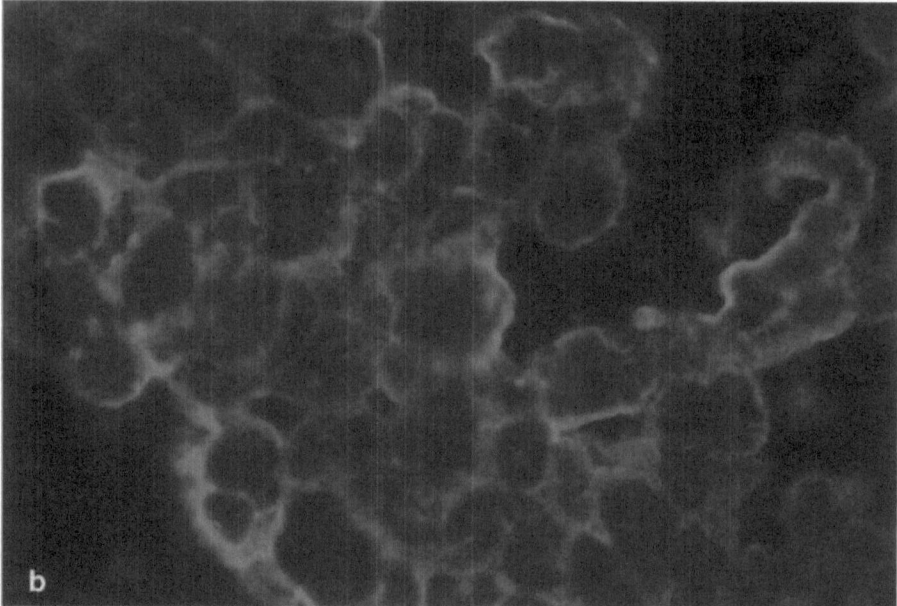

Fig. 6. a Demonstration of bound IgG in a 37-year-old patient with DCM. Immunoglobulin binding is present on sarcolemma, interstitial space and vascular endothelium. Demonstration by a rhodamin-labeled antihuman IgG [F(ab)$_2$ fragments, Medac; dilutions of TRITC-labeled antibody 1 : 100]. **b** Using a double sandwich technique, the identity of circulating and already bound immunoglobulin can be demonstrated (same patient as in *a*, same section). Demonstration by an FITC-labeled antihuman IgG [F(ab)$_2$ fragments, Medac; dilution of serum 1 : 40; dilution of FITC-labeled antibody 1 : 100]. (From [27] with permission)

pounds of the interstitial space (collagen, extracellular matrix) or capillaries and vascular endothelium. If they play a role in the disturbed alignment or impaired myocardial ultrastructure and cytoskeleton in cardiomyopathy hearts [48] remains an attractive but speculative hypothesis. Their, exact percentage can be derived from (Table 2).

Fine Specificity of the AMLAs in DCM

Preliminary data [31] using the Western blot technique of electrophoretically separated sarcolemmal preparations [29] indicate that the AMLAs in DCM are part of a microheterogeneity of antimembrane antibodies. If their cytolytic (with complement) or cytotoxic (without complement) properties are analyzed in vitro, the cytolytic/cytotoxic antibody-containing serum shows predominant binding to a membrane protein in the 70-kD range; it is mostly of the IgG type. The noncytolytic AMLA-positive sera have a predominant binding to a 43 kD protein instead and are primarily of the IgM type. It appears that the cytolytic-/cytotoxic IgG antibody is found particularly often in DCM patients with severe heart failure (NYHA classes III and IV), and the noncytolytic IgM antibody in DCM patients without overt signs of congestive heart failure [31]. Although this is still indirect evidence, the association of possible pathogenetic autoreactive mechanisms to function become apparent. AMLAs are therefore more than innocent bystanders or a mere biographic epiphenomenon. Of course, many of the antibodies detected in myocardial diseases are probably "natural" antibodies. They may be directed against the extracellular matrix (collagen, structural proteins, laminin, microfilaments, intracellular proteins, etc.) and seem to possess little pathogenetic relevance. One has become more and more aware of the fact that in many healthy normals natural antibodies may be remnants of former infections without being true markers of disease [4, 6, 52, 53]. Their suggested regulatory or pathogenetic relevance is still poorly defined, however. At present natural antibodies are thought to belong primarily to the IgM class. This may be true for the 43-kD IgM AMLAs as well. We have separated them from the pathogenetically relevant AMLAs by their in vitro function: cytolytic and/or cytotoxic properties decide their pathogenetic relevance.

Acknowledgements: The excellent technical assistance of M. Cirsi, M. Crombach, C. Dienesch, A. Peter, P. Thometzek, R. Weller, and I. Wendl is gratefully acknowledged. The histological investigations of endomyocardial biopsies were performed by Prof. U. Pfeiffer MD, Department of Pathology, Würzburg Medical School or by A. Bittinger MD, Department of Pathology, Philipps University, Marburg, or in selected cases by E. G. J. Olsen MD (London). We gratefully acknowledge all contributing centers: the university hospitals of internal medicine in Würzburg, Marburg (Department of Cardiology), Hannover, Department of Pediatric Cardiology, Tübingen in collaboration with Prof. A. A. Schmaltz MD, the German Heart Center, Munich in collaboration with V. Regitz MD, the Departments for Heart, Thoracic, and Cardiovascular Surgery in Würzburg, Gießen, Hannover in collaboration with Prof. A. Haverich MD, and Prof. P. Deeg MD of the Deegenberg Sanatorium, Bad Kissingen, and the Südklinik Straubing.

References

1. Anderson JL, Greenwood JH, Kawanishi H (1981) Evaluation of suppressor immune regulatory function in idiopathic congestive cardiomyopathy and rheumatic heart disease. Br Heart J 4:410–414
2. Anderson JL, Carlquist JF, Hammond FH (1982) Deficient natural killer cell activity in patients with idiopathic dilated cardiomyopathy. Lancet 2:1124–1127
3. Aretz HT, Southern JF, Palacios IF, Dec GW Jr, Howard CA, Fallon JT (1987) Morphological and immunnological findings in heart biopsies of patients with suspectecd or treated myocarditis. Eur Heart J 8 [Suppl J]:187–190
4. Avremeas S (1986) Natural autoreactive B cells and autoantibodies: the know thyself of the immune system. Ann Inst Pasteur Immunol [Suppl D] 137:150–156
5. Bolte HD, Schultheiss P, Cyran J, Goss F (1980) Binding of immunoglobulins in the myocardium (biopsy). In: Bolte HD (ed) Myocardial biopsy. Springer, Berlin Heidelberg New York, pp 85–92
6. Boyden SV (1963) Natural antibodies and the immune response. Adv Immunol 5:1–28
7. Breshnihan B, Jasin ME (1977) Suppressor function of peripheral blood mononuclear cells in normal individuals and patients with systemic lupus erythematosus. J Clin Invest 59:106–116
8. Cambridge G, Campbell-Blay G, Wilmhurst P, Coltan DJ, Stern CMM (1983) Deficient "natural" cytotoxicity in patients with congestive cardiomyopathy (Abstr). Br Heart J 49:623
9. Das SK, Petty RE, Meengs WA, Tubergen DG (1980) Studies of cell-mediated immunity in cardiomyopathy. In: Sekiguchi M, Olsen EGJ (eds) Cardiomyopathy. University of Tokyo Press, Tokyo, pp 375–377
10. Eckstein R, Mempel W, Bolte HD (1982) Reduced suppressor cell activity in congestive cardiomyopathy and in myocarditis. Circulation 59:1224–1229
11. Fowles RE, Bieber CP, Stinson EB (1978) Defective in vitro suppressor of cell function in idiopathic congestive cardiomyopathy. Circulation 59:483–491
12. Frencesini R, Petillo A, Corazza M, Nizzo MC, Azzolini A, Gianrossi R (1983) Lymphocyte response in dilated cardiomyopathy. IRCS Med Sci 11:1019
13. Gentle TA, Baynham MID, Gammage MD, Lowry PJ, Thompson RA, Littler WA (1987) T cell function in idiopathic congestive cardiomyopathy. Eur Heart J [Suppl J] 8:145–146
14. Hallgren HM, Yunis EJ (1977) Suppressor lymphocytes in young and aged humans. J Immunol 118:2004–2008
15. Hammond EG, Menlove RL, Anderson JL (1988) Immunofluorescence microscopy in the diagnosis and follow-up of patients suspected of having inflammatory heart disease. In: Schultheiss HP (ed) New concepts in viral heart disease – virology, immunology and clinical management. Springer, Berlin Heidelberg New York, pp 303–311
16. Herzum M, Maisch B (1988) Humoral and cellular immune response in human myocarditis and dilated cardiomyopathy. Pathol Immunopathol Res 7:240–250
17. Herzum M, Maisch B (1989) Anti-viral and anti-myocyte antibodies in experimental myocarditis. Springer Sem Immunopathol 11:69–76
18. Herzum M, Maisch B, Kochsiek K (1987) Circulating immune complexes in perimyocarditis and infective endocarditis. Eur Heart J [Suppl J] 8:323–325
19. Izumi T, Maisch B, Kochsiek K (1987) Experimental murine myocarditis after immunization with cardiac membranous proteins. Eur Heart J [Suppl J] 8:419–424
20. Jacobs B, Matsuda Y, Daeodhar S, Shirey S (1979) Cell-mediated cytotoxicity to cardiac cells of lymphocytes from patients with primary myocardial disease. Am J Clin Pathol 72:1–4

21. Jerne NK (1955) The natural selection theory of antibody formation. Proc Natl Acad Sci USA 41:849–857
22. Klein R, Maisch B, Kochsiek K, Berg PA (1984) Demonstration of organ specific antibodies against heart mitochondria (anti-M/) in sera from patients with some forms of heart disease. Clin Exp Immunol 58:283–292
23. Klein R, Spiel L, Klemann U, Hassenstein P, Berg PA (1987) Relevance of antimitochondrial antibodies (anti-M7) in cardiac disease. Eur Heart J [Suppl J] 8:223–226
24. Kühl U, Ulrich G, Schultheiss HP (1987) Cross-reactivity of antibodies to the ADP/ATP translocator of the inner mitochondrial membrane with the cell surface of cardiac myocytes. Eur Heart J [Suppl J] 8:219–222
25. Limas CJ, Limas C (1988) Beta-adrenocepter autoantibody in idiopathic dilated cardiomyopathy. In: Schultheiss HP (ed) New concepts in viral heart disease – virology, immunology and clinical management. Springer, Berlin Heidelberg New York, pp 217–224
26. Lowry PJ, Thompson RA, Littler WA (1983) Humoral immunity in cardiomyopathy. Br Heart J 50:390–394
27. Maisch B (1986) Immunologic regulator and effector functions in perimyocarditis, post-myocarditis heart muscle disease and dilated cardiomyopathy. Basic Res Cardiol [Suppl 1] 81:217–242
28. Maisch B (1987) Immunological mechanism in human cardiac injury. In: Spry CJF (ed) Immunology and molecular biology of cardiovascular disease. MTP, London, pp 225–252 (Current status of clinical cardiology)
29. Maisch B (1987) The sarcolemma as antigen in the secondary immunopathogenesis of myopericarditis. Eur Heart J [Suppl J] 8:155–165
30. Maisch B (1988) These use of myocardial biopsy in heart failure. Eur Heart J [Suppl H] 9:59–71
31. Maisch B, Bauer E (1987) Diagnostic and pathogenetic relevance of cytolytic, cross-reactive antibodies against the cardiac membrane of adult human myocytes in coxsackie B and in etiologically undefined myocarditis (Abstr). European Society against Virus Diseases, Davos
32. Maisch B, Kochsiek K (1983) Humoral immune reactions in uremic pericarditis. Am J Nephrol 3:264–271
33. Maisch B, Maisch S, Kochsiek K (1982) Immune reactions in tuberculous and chronic constrictive pericarditis. Am J Cardiol 50:1007–1013
34. Maisch B, Trostel-Soeder R, Stechmesser E, Berg PA, Kochsiek K (1982) Diagnostic relevance of humoral and cell-mediated immune reactions in patients with acute viral myocarditis. Clin Exp Immunol 48:533–545
35. Maisch B, Deeg P, Liebau G, Kochsiek K (1983) Diagnostic relevance of humoral and cytotoxic immune reactions in primary and secondary dilated cardiomyopathy. Am J Cardiol 52:1071–1078
36. Maisch B, Büschel G, Izumi T, Eigel P, Regitz V, Deeg P, Pfeifer U et al (1985) Four years of experience in endomyocardial biopsy – an immunohistologic approach. In: Segikuchi M, Olsen EGJ, Goodwin JF (eds) Myocarditis and related disorders. Springer, Berlin Heidelberg New York, pp 59–67
37. Maisch B, Cirsi M, Gehrke J, Kirschner A (1987) Lectin binding sites of the sarcolemma and the surrounding interstitial tissue. Eur Heart J [Suppl J] 8:175–180
38. Maisch B, Dienesch C, Wendl I (1987) Effect of leucotrienes on isolated vital cardiac cells – an in vitro model of cardiocytotoxic mediators in inflammation? Eur Heart J [Suppl J] 8:463–465
39. Maisch B, Hauck H, Köninger U, Endter S, Klopf D, Schmier U, Schmier K (1987) T-suppressor cell activity in (peri)myocarditis and infective endocarditis. Eur Heart J [Suppl J] 8:147–153
40. Maisch B, Schwab D, Bauer E, Sandhage K, Schmaltz AA (1987) Antimyolemmal antibodies in myocarditis in children. Eur Heart J [Suppl J] 8:167–173
41. Maisch B, Selmayer N, Brugger E, Ertl G, Eilles C, Heinrich J, Gerhards W et al (1987) Cardiac sarcoidosis – a clinical and immunoserologic study. Eur Heart [Suppl J] 8:63–71
42. Maisch B, Wedeking U, Kochsiek K (1987) Quantitative assessment of antilaminin antibodies in myocarditis and perimyocarditis. Eur Heart J [Suppl J] 8:233–235

43. Maisch B, Herzum M, Izumi T, Nunoda S (1988) Importance of humoral and cellular immunological parameters for the pathogenesis of viral myocarditis. In: Schultheiss HP (ed) New concepts in viral heart disease – virology, immunology and clinical management. Springer, Berlin Heidelberg New York, pp 259–273
44. Obermayer U, Scheidler J, Maisch B (1987) Antibodies against micro- and intermediate filaments in carditis and dilated cardiomyopathy – are they a diagnostic marker? Eur Heart J [Suppl J] 8:181–186
45. Paris S, Fosset M, Samuel D, Ailhaud G (1977) Chick embryo plasma membrane from cardiac muscle and cultured heart cells: isolation procedures and absence of fatty acid-activating enzymes. J Mol Cell Cardiol 9:161–173
46. Perlmann P, Perlmann H (1971) Cytotoxic lymphocytes, mechanisms of activation and target cell destruction. Int Arch Allergy Appl Immunol 41:36–39
47. Ragosta M, Crabtree J, Sturner WQ, Thompson PD (1980) Report of the WHO-ISFC task force on the definition and classification of cardiomyopathies. Br Heart J 44:672
48. Schaper J, Froede R, Bucho A, Bleese N (1988) Impaired myocardial ultra-structure and cytoskeleton in cardiopathic human myocardium. In: Schultheiss HP (ed) New concepts in viral heart disease – virology, immunology and clinical management. Springer, Berlin Heidelberg New York, pp 295–302
49. Schultheiss HP (1987) The mitochondrium as antigen in inflammatory heart disease. Eur Heart J [Suppl J] 8:203–210
50. Schultheiss HP, Bolte HD (1985) Immunological analysis of auto-antibodies against the adenine nucleotide translocator in dilated cardiomyopathy. J Mol Cell Cardiol 17:601–617
51. Schultheiss HP, Kühl U, Schauer R, Schulze K, Kemkes B, Becker BF (1988) Antibodies against the ADP/ATP carrier after myocardial function by disturbing cellular energy metabolism. In: Schultheiss HP (ed) New concepts in viral heart disease – virology, immunology and clinical management. Springer, Berlin Heidelberg New York, pp 243–251
52. Schwarz RS (1986) Are natural autoantibodies real? Ann Inst Pasteur Immunol [Suppl D] 137:156–159
53. Seligman M (1986) The origin and nature of autoantibodies. Introduction. Ann Inst Pasteur Immunol [Suppl D] 137:149–150
54. Shervish E, O'Connel JB, Kowalczyk D, Robinson JA (1987) Suppressor cell function in dilated cardiomyopathy. Eur Heart J [Suppl J] 8:141–143
55. Ulrich K, Kühl U, Metzner J, Jander J, Schäfer B, Schultheiss HP (1988) In: Schultheiss HP (ed) New concepts in viral heart disease – virology, immunology, clinical management. Springer, Berlin Heidelberg New York, pp 225–235
56. Yamakawa K, Fukuta S, Yoshinaga T, Umemeto S, Itagaki T, Kusukawa R (1987) Study of immunological mechanisms in dilated cardiomyopathy. Jpn Circ J 51:665–675
57. Yokoyama A, Aoki S, Aizawa Y, Shibata A (1985) Analysis of peripheral lymphocyte subpopulation in patients with dilated cardiomyopathy. J Dev Med 133(3):187–188

Biomolecular Changes in Dilated Cardiomyopathy

H. P. Schultheiss, U. Kühl, K. Schulze, P. Schwimmbeck, and B. E. Strauer

Introduction

Based on circumstantial evidence from clinical, serological, epidemiological, and histological studies, a causal relationship between myocarditis and dilated cardiomyopathy (DCM) has long been suspected [1–5]. The basis of this association were observations during epidemics of Coxsackie B virus infection. Although the majority of affected individuals recovered without evidence of subsequent myocardial dysfunction, a few of these patients subsequently developed DCM. Similarly, serological studies of patients with DCM implicated a viral infection in the etiology of DCM. This has been confirmed by recent findings of Bowles and Kandolf and their coworkers demonstrating the presence of enteroviral RNA in the myocardium of patients with myocarditis and DCM [6–9]. These findings suggest the possibility that Coxsackie B virus persists in the myocardium of patients with myocarditis and may in some way be responsible for the subsequent development of DCM. Thus, the viral infection may act as a trigger initiating the autoimmunological process by altering the host's immune system, by causing the release or expression of sequestered antigens or through antigenic determinants shared by the virus and the host cell [10, 11].

Immunocytochemical studies have shown that many of the infiltrating cells in biopsies are activated T-lymphocytes having cytotoxic activity in vitro. Furthermore, the cultured T-cells are often oligoclonal, as shown by restriction fragment length polymorphism analysis of the beta chain of the T-cell receptor [5]. However, it is still unknown whether the infiltrating lymphocytes are due to persistent virus that is still replicating or to an ongoing autoimmune disease. Moreover, biopsy specimen from patients with clinically suspected myocarditis often show no inflammation. One possible explanation is that the transvenous technique does not sample enough myocardial sites to detect each case of disease. Another possibility is that the functional abnormality in myocarditis is caused by some non-cell-mediated process, whereas the inflammatory-cell response is a separate phenomenon that may not correlate closely, either temporally or topographically, with the functional impairment of the myocardium. The role and significance of humoral immune reactions in the development of DCM is also still unresolved. Anti-myocardium specific autoreactivity has been shown to occur in most of the patients suffering from myocarditis or

DCM [12–14]. Although it is quite likely that most of the autoantibodies reflect a nonspecific response to myocardial injury, a subset of antibodies has been shown to be immunopathogenic. These autoantibodies are directed against critical enzymes necessary for the pump function of the heart, for example, against ion channel proteins, gap junctions, or intracellular transport proteins [15–18].

Characterization of the Autoantibodies

Recently, we identified an antibody population showing cross-reactivity between two cell surface proteins, the Ca^{2+} channel and connexion, and a mitochondrial protein, the adenine nucleotide translocator [15].

To characterize the targets of the antibodies, different immunochemical methods such as enzyme-linked immunosorbent assay (ELISA), immunoprecipitation, and Western blotting were used. To test the possible effect of the antibodies on nucleotide transport in vitro, the exchange rate of mitochondria was determined by the inhibitor-stop method combined with the back exchange [19]. The interaction of the antibodies with the Ca^{2+} channel could be demonstrated by the whole-cell patch-clamp method and by measuring the contraction velocity of isolated cardiac myocytes [17, 18].

The Adenine Nucleotide Translocator as an Autoantigen

When the sera of patients with clinically suspected myocarditis were tested in the enzyme-linked immunosorbent assay (ELISA) against the ADP/ATP carrier from heart, a significant antibody titer was seen in 20 of 22 patients with acute/healing myocarditis and in 26 of 44 patients with histologically diagnosed "healed myocarditis." In 28 of 49 patients with DCM, the autoantibody titer against ADP/ATP carrier was significantly elevated. In comparison to the controls, the sera from patients with coronary heart disease did not contain autoantibodies against the ADP/ATP carrier (Fig. 1).

Further studies have shown that the antibodies against the ADP/ATP carrier are organ and confirmation specific (13–15). Functionally, these organ-specific antibodies inhibit nucleotide transport from heart mitochondria in vitro by specific binding to the substrate/ligand binding site of the carrier protein [15]. This remarkable organ specificity of the autoantibodies and the ADP/ATP carrier was previously seen to reflect isoenzyme distribution of the carrier in different organs. Although the concept of isoenzymes seemed at first bold and premature, it has meanwhile been extended to several other instances. The organ specifity of the ADP/ATP carrier, which has been confirmed by peptide maps [20] and studies of the cDNA sequence [21], may reflect tissue-specific regulation of nucleotide transport. This regulation may be adapted according to the specific requirements in different tissues by the expression of specific isoenzymes.

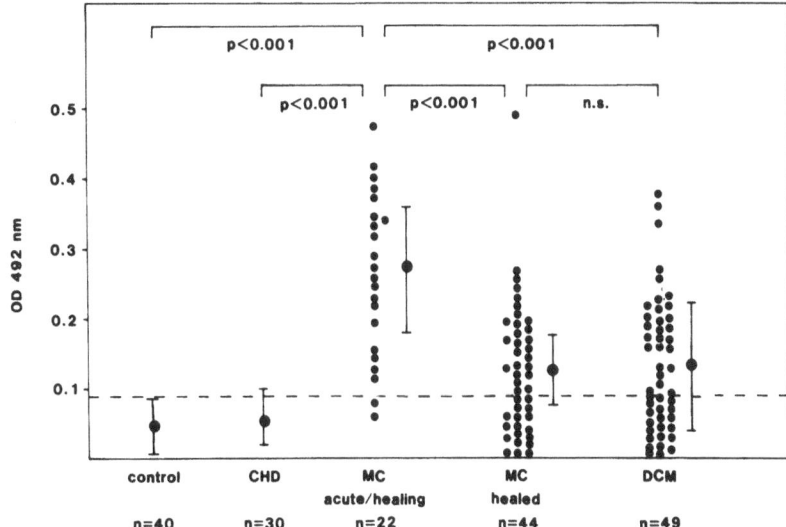

Fig. 1. The binding of autoantibodies in ELISA to the ADP/ATP carrier from hearts from patients with myocarditis (*MC;* acute healing, healed), dilated cardiomyopathy (*DCM*), coronary heart disease (*CHD*) and healthy blood donors (controls)

Besides the principal importance of the organ specificity of the protein for understanding the basic regulatory mechanism for differentiated organisms, this aspect has also become particularly significant for the characterization of autoimmune processes. In relation to the pathogenetic etiology of the disease, it seems certain that the inciting cause for the production of these highly specific autoantibodies should be limited to the local milieu. However, this observation is not in agreement with previous theories, suggesting that the immunologic abnormalities in myocarditis and DCM result from a generalized defect in immune regulation. In particular, the high concentration and restricted specificities of the anti-ADP/ATP autoantibodies argue strongly against a random polyclonal activation of lymphocytes.

Molecular Mimicry: Reactivity Between Coxsackie B₃ and the Adenine Nucleotide Translocator

One mechanism by which a virus could trigger an autoimmune response is molecular mimicry. Different molecules share similar structures either in their amino acid sequence or in their conformational shape. Structural similarities have frequently been noted between a number of both RNA and DNA viruses and "self"-proteins. In addition, antiviral antibodies which cross-react with host tissues have been found in several studies and may play a role in the pathogenesis of autoimmune disease.

Since Coxsackie B_3 virus (CB_3) has been shown to induce myocarditis in mice and man [22, 23], we searched for homologous determinants shared between the recently determined sequence of CB_3 and the adenine nucleotide translocator, a main autoantigen in viral heart disease. Utilizing the Dayhoff Data Bank, computer search, and computer predictions of the secondary structure of this protein, a homology was found between the adenine nucleotide translocator and CB_3 [24, 25].

Further experiments demonstrated that this homology translated into immunological cross-reactivity [26]. These results show that the sharing of cross-reacting antigenic determinants between CB_3 and the adenine nucleotide translocator may play a role in the pathogenesis of viral heart disease. However, these cross-reacting autoantibodies need not always be deleterious. Nevertheless, molecular mimicry may, in part, account for the enigma of persistent immunity in the absence of continued exposure to the virus!

Cross-reactivity Between the Adenine Nucleotide Translocator and the Ca^{2+} Channel

Evidence for cross-reactivity between the ADP/ATP carrier and a cell surface protein was first obtained by indirect immunofluorescence. Incubation of frozen sections of heart tissue with the above-characterized anti-ADP/ATP carrier antibodies showed, besides intracellular staining, antibodies binding to the plasma membrane. This was confirmed by positive staining of isolated cardiac myocytes showing a sarcolemmal immunofluorescence (Fig. 2). After neutralization of anti-ADP/ATP carrier antibodies by preadsorption with the isolated ADP/ATP carrier, intracellular staining and staining of the cell surface disappeared. Preimmune sera did not react with the cell surface at all.

This cross-reactivity between antibodies and the cell surface was also demonstrated by radioimmunobinding assay, showing a time-dependent binding of antibodies to myocytes. After 60 min most of the antibodies were bound to the cell. Prolonged incubation for up to 180 min could not increase antibody binding significantly. Preimmune serum IgG (control) did not bind to myocytes. Antibody dilution from 1:1000 to 1:6000 resulted in a reduction of antibody binding up to 1:5000, where no significant binding could be detected any more. The specificity of the antigen-antibody reaction was demonstrated by inhibition of the binding to myocytes by immunoadsorption. Preincubation of the antibody with increasing amounts of the isolated ADP/ATP carrier (1–1500 ng) resulted in a concentration-dependent decrease of antibody binding.

Incubation of cardiac myocytes with anti-ADP/ATP carrier antibodies (affinity-purified IgG) in a concentration higher than 1:1000 resulted in a concentration-dependent decrease of cell viability. Deterioration of myocytes, monitored visually, involved in sequence: rhythmic contraction, bleb formation, contracture to an almost cuboid shape, cell rounding, and finally cell death, demonstrated by rapid uptake of trypan blue (Fig. 3).

This antibody-mediated cytotoxic effect was strictly calcium dependent. Using an antibody concentration of 1:100 and a calcium concentration of 1 mM, 20% of myocytes died after 30 min, 40% after 1 h, and about 80% after 3 h. In contrast, only 10% of myocytes incubated with preimmune serum IgG

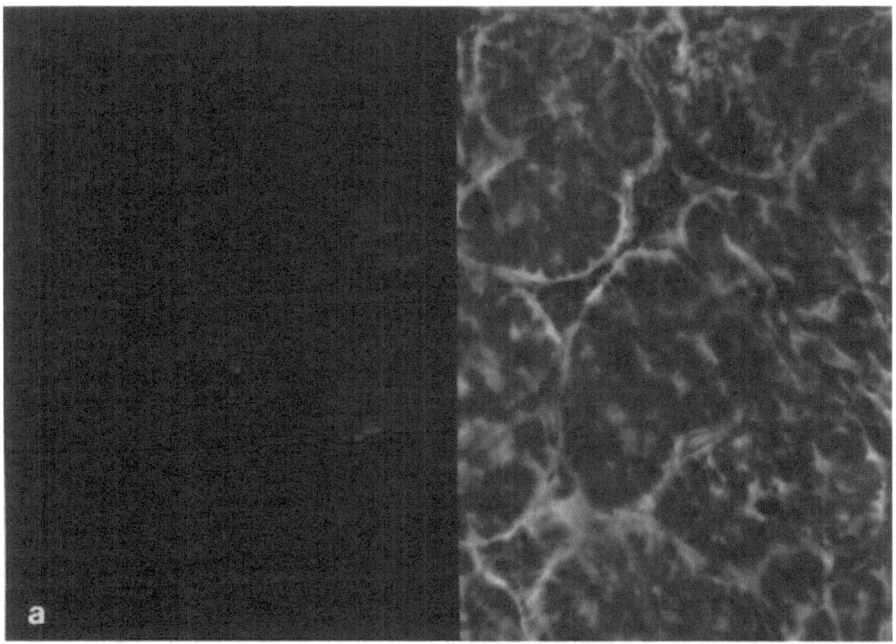

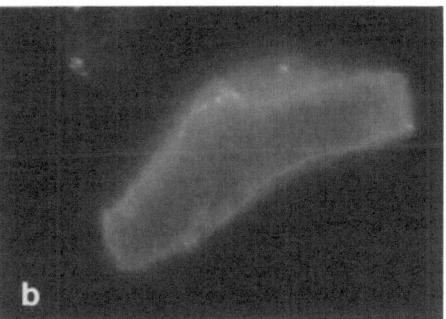

Fig. 2a, b. Immunofluorescence on heart tissue sections and on isolated living cardiac myocytes. **a** Disappearance of cell-surface reaction after neutralization of antibodies with purified ADP/ATP carrier. **b** Cell-surface staining of isolated adult rat cardiac myocytes with anti-ADP/ATP carrier antibodies

(control) survived for less than 3 h. With decreasing concentrations of calcium the effect of antibody-mediated cytotoxicity is gradually suppressed. With an antibody concentration of 1:100 and essentially no calcium, only 10% of cells died within 3 h. The corresponding control showed a mortality of 5% during the first 3 h.

The use of calcium-channel antagonist together with anti-ADP/ATP carrier antibodies (IgG 1:100) in myocyte suspension (1 mM Ca^{2+}) reduced the cytotoxic effect of antibodies dramatically. Nifedipine and nitrendipine (both 10^{-6} M) seemed to be more potent in protecting the cells than did verapamil (10^{-6} M). Without antibodies, none of the calcium-channel antagonists had a significant influence on cell viability. The use of β-receptor antagonist propranolol (10^{-7} M) together with anti-ADP/ATP carrier antibodies had no effect on cell viability (Fig. 4).

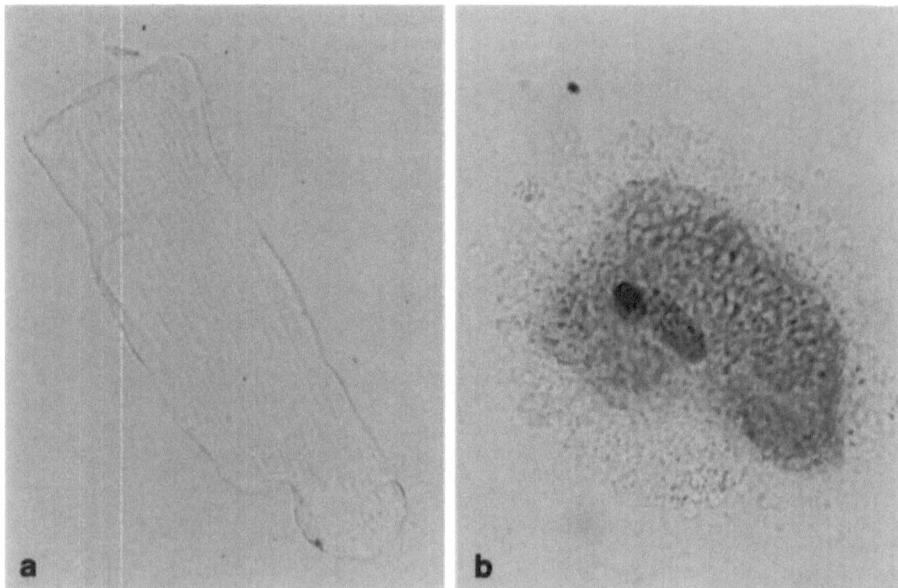

Fig. 3a, b. Appearance of isolated cardiac myocytes during incubation with anti-ADP/ATP carrier antibodies (dilution 1:100, 1 mM, 1 mM Ca^{2+}). **a** Normal rod-shaped cell. **b** Final cell death (plus trypan blue)

The results thus far suggest that antibodies against the ADP/ATP carrier bind specifically to the cell surface of cardiac myocytes and enhance their calcium permeability. To obtain further support for this idea, we measured the effect of antibodies on the calcium current of isolated rat myocytes, using a previously described enzymatic isolation technique.

Whole-cell clamp experiments showed that exposure of myocytes from guinea pig or rat hearts to antibodies against the adenine nucleotide translocator caused a marked potentiation of the transmembrane calcium current (I_{Ca}). The onset of the enhancement of I_{Ca} was rapid, and generally 20–30 s were sufficient for the full effect of the antibodies to take place (Fig. 5). This enhancement of I_{Ca} was only slowly reversible. The enhancing effect of antibodies on I_{Ca} was blocked by addition of nifedipine (10^{-6} to 5×10^{-5} M). The enhancing effect of the antibodies on I_{Ca} was quite similar to that measured upon addition of Bay K 8644, a new calcium-blocking agent. In contrast, β-blockers (propranolol 10^{-6} M) had no effect on the antibody-induced enhancement of I_{Ca}, ruling out a possible role of β-receptors in the enhancement of I_{Ca}. Parallel to the enhancement of I_{Ca}, the antibodies prolonged the action potential and potentiated twitch tension.

We conclude from our results that the antibodies against the ADP/ATP carrier cross-react with the cardiac Ca^{2+} channel and enhance I_{Ca}. In intact tissue this effect causes a prolongation of the action potential and potentiation of tension. The enhanced calcium inward current may lead to Ca^{2+} overload and subsequently, to cell death.

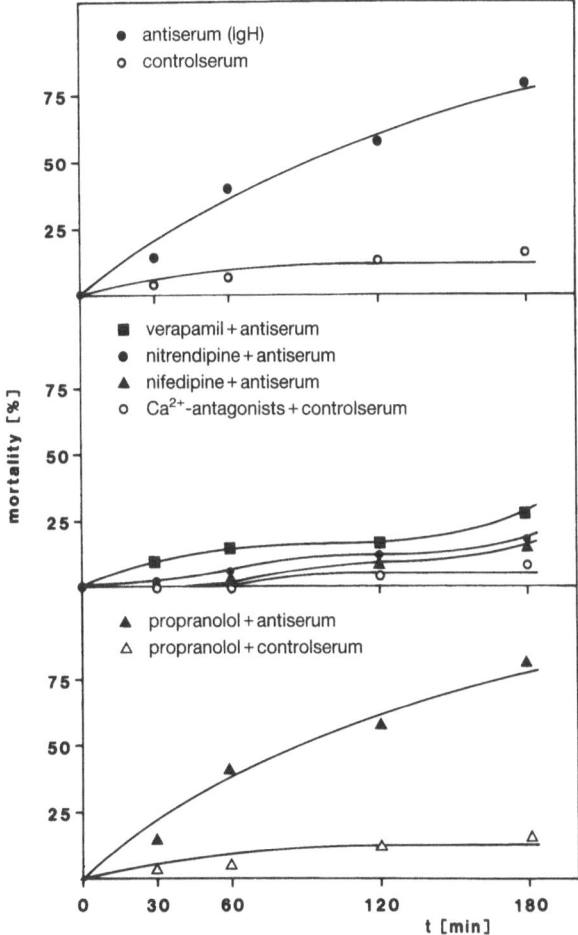

Fig. 4. Mortality of cardiac myocytes after addition of Ca^{2+} channel blockers (10^{-6} M) or β-blockers in the presence of preimmune serum (control) and of antibodies to the ADP/ATP carrier (antiserum)

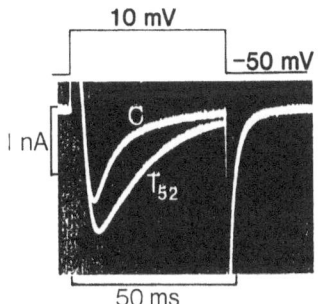

Fig. 5. Effect of antibody on I_{Ca} of rat ventricular myocytes, activated at + 10 mV from a holding potential of –50 mV, upon addition of antibodies (IgG, T52). External solutions contained 2 mM Ca^{+2} and 10^{-5} M TTX. Internal solutions contained 100 mM CsCl, 20 mM TEA, 20 mM glucose, 5 mg ATP, 10 mM EGTA, 1 mM HEPEs, at pH 2.3 buffered with CsOH at room temperature

Antibody-Mediated Myocardial Dysfunction

In order to demonstrate a pathophysiological significance of autoantibodies, one has to show that a given autoantibody is an essential component of a pathological mechanism which leads to organ dysfunction. Following this line, autoantibodies to cell membrane receptors have been documented in a number of disease states in man, and there is good evidence for a pathogenic role of at least some of these autoantibodies. In order to answer the question whether the antibodies against the adenine nucleotide translocator which cross-react with the Ca^{2+} channel alter myocardial function, we measured the hemodynamic data from guinea pigs immunized with the isolated carrier protein.

The hearts were isolated and perfused as working heart preparations as described previously [16, 27]. A preload of 12 cmH$_2$O and the mean developed afterload determined the pressure-volume work of the left ventricle. External heart work was calculated as the sum of pressure-volume work and acceleration work (1/2 ejected volume mean velocity of flow^2) during ejection. Working-heart preparations from guinea pigs immunized with the ADP/ATP carrier showed a marked decrease in cardiac function compared to controls of hearts from nonimmunized animals (Table 1), [35]. Mean aortic pressure, stroke volume, stroke work, and external heart work of the left ventricle were found to be lowered by 40%–80%, with external heart work diminished from 375 mJ/g per min to 62 mJ/g per min. In parallel, myocardial oxygen extraction, calculated as the difference of oxygen saturation from the affluent perfusate and the coronary effluent, was found to be lowered, while myocardial lactate production, measured as lactate release in the coronary effluent, was found to be significantly increased in the immunized animals.

These functional data support the hypothesis that the antibodies reacting with the adenine nucleotide translocator and/or the Ca^{2+} channel cause a dysfunction of the heart. Our findings suggest that these antibodies might be an essential component of the pathological mechanism involved in viral heart disease [15].

There are several ways in which the antibodies against the ADP/ATP carrier could alter the function of the heart. First, the antibodies might inhibit carrier

Table 1. Hemodynamic and metabolic parameters of isolated working guinea pig hearts from control animals ($n = 5$) and immunized animals ($n = 6$). External heart work was calculated as the sum of pressure-volume work and acceleration work (1/2 $\times$ ejected volume $\times$ mean velocity of flow$^{2)}$) during ejection

	Controls ($n = 5$)	Immunized animals ($n = 6$)
Mean aortic pressure (mmHg)	93	53
Stroke volume (μl/g)	138	54
Stroke work (mJ/g)	1.74	0.42
External heart work (mg/g · min)	375	62
Lactate release (μmol/min · g)	1.84	4.36
Oxygen consumption (μmol/min · g)	16.3	6.8

function by an antibody binding to the carrier protein. This inhibition may be due to direct binding of the antibody to or near the active site of the translocator, thereby sterically hindering the translocation process. A second possibility to be considered is that the antibodies react with the primary translocation product, hindering the incorporation of the carrier protein into the inner mitochondrial membrane. Both possibilities are supported by immunohistological and immunoelectron microscopical results which show immunoglobulin binding to the mitochondrial membrane of the immunized animals. A further possibility would be that the antibodies interact with the cross-reacting cell-surface protein, the Ca^{2+} channel, thereby indirectly influencing the carrier function.

Since it is known that an elevated intracellular Ca^{2+} concentration (Ca^{2+} overload) affects the rate at which the carrier functions, due to a collapse of the mitochondrial membrane potential, it may well be that the antibodies against the ADP/ATP carrier/Ca^{2+} channel indirectly disturb cellular energy metabolism.

If the energy metabolism of the cell is altered in such a way as to limit the supply of ATP to the organelles responsible for the maintenance of cellular homeostasis, then this should lead to an alteration in the overall myocardial function, as was shown in the experiments described above. Since there are no methods available to determine the function of the ADP/ATP carrier in the living organ, we measured the cytosolic-mitochondrial difference of the phosphorylation potential of ATP ($\Delta b_{\text{cyt-mit}}$) by nonaqueous fractionation of myocardium [28] to show whether the transport activity of the ADP/ATP carrier is influenced in the immunized animals. Based on the functional characteristics of the adenine nucleotide translocator, it was shown by Klingenberg and co-workers [29–31] that the force for the regulation of this transport protein is derived from the potential difference between the cytosolic and mitochondrial phosphorylation state of ATP. Since the energization of the mitochondrial membrane, expressed by $\Delta G_{\text{cyt-mit}}$, modulates the ADP/ATP carrier activity so as to operate in the manner required for the energy needs of the cell, a decreased phosphorylation potential difference of ATP can be taken as an indicator for a reduced total transport capacity of the carrier [31]. Under normal conditions, the nucleotide exchange capacity of the carrier is high enough to guarantee a stable intracellular nucleotide distribution. A decrease of the cytosolic-mitochondrial difference of $\Delta G'_{\text{ATP}}$ stimulates the ADP/ATP carrier to a higher asymmetry in nucleotide transport, so as to supply more ATP to the cytosol. Thus, asymmetric ADP-ATP transport continues until the energy balance between the transmembrane potential and $\Delta G_{\text{(cyt-mit)}}$ is restored.

In the hearts of the immunized guinea pigs, the concentration of ATP was slightly lowered in the cytosol, while being increased in the mitochondria (Table 2). The ATP/ADP ratio as well as the phosphorylation state of ATP, expressed as the ratio [ATP]/[ADP] $\times$ [P_i], were significantly lower in the cytosol, whereas in the mitochondria a substantial increase was observed. The cytosolic phosphorylation potential ($\Delta G'_{\text{ATP}}$) decreased from 22.2 $\pm$ 0.4 kJ/mol ATP (controls) to 21.4 $\pm$ 0.3 kJ/mol ATP ($p < 0.005$). The parallel

Table 2. Subcellular distribution of myocardial high energy phosphates in isolated perfused guinea pig hearts. Fractionation of tissue into cytosolic (cyt) and mitochondrial (mit) fractions was accomplished by density gradient centrifugation in nonaqueous media. Ratios of free cytosolic ATP/ADP were calculated from mass action ratio of creatine kinase reaction. Values are mean ± standard deviation

| | Controls ($n = 5$) | | Immunized animals ($n = 6$) | |
	Cyt	Mit	Cyt	Mit
ATP (mM)	13.2 ± 2.0	8.1 ± 2.3	11.3 ± 2.9	18.3 ± 5.9
ADP (mM)	1.9 ± 0.4	1.6 ± 0.3	2.5 ± 0.5	1.1 ± 0.2
ATP/ADP P_{free} (μM)	61.8 ± 7.9	5.1 ± 0.5	50.2 ± 8.8	17.1 ± 4.9
[ATP]/[ADP] × [P_i] (mM)	5487 ± 644	926 ± 215	4105 ± 624	3349 ± 1445
$\Delta G'$ (kJ/mol ATP)	22.2 ± 0.3	17.6 ± 0.6	21.4 ± 0.4	20.7 ± 1.2
$\Delta G'_{cyt\text{-}mit}$ (kJ/mol ATP)	4.6 ± 0.5		0.7 ± 1.2	

increase of the mitochondrial phosphorylation potential, which rose from 17.6 ± 0.6 kJ/mol ADP to 20.7 ± 1.2 kJ/mol ATP ($p < 0.005$), was much more pronounced. Consequently, the cytosolic/mitochondrial difference of ΔG_{ATP}, which expresses best the state of energy metabolism of the myocardial cell and combines all of the variables evaluated, decreased from 4.6 kJ/mol ATP in the controls to 0.7 kJ/mol ATP in the hearts of the immunized animals. These data indicate that the immunoreaction against the adenine nucleotide translocator and/or the Ca^{2+} channel alter myocardial function by an imbalance between energy delivery and demand [15, 16].

Conclusion

A number of investigators have suggested that immunopathologic mechanisms, both humoral and cellular, may contribute, at least in part, to the pathogenesis of myocarditis and DCM [2]. Recent data demonstrating persistence of viral RNA in the myocardium from patients with myocarditis and dilated cardiomyopathy make a persistent viral infection in these diseases quite likely [6, 9]. Interest is now focused on the link between persistent viral infection, the induction of autoimmunity and the alteration of differentiated functions of the myocardium in myocarditis and DCM. One hypothesis to explain virus-induced autoimmunity is that immunogenic determinants of a virus can induce the formation of antibodies during an infection which in turn may react with homologous but not identical epitopes on a host protein. The immune response initiated against the foreign virus material may therefore not only react with the virus but also with the "self" protein. Depending on the biological function of the host protein which is recognized, the outcome of the interaction may be disease. The data presented here show, for the first time, molecular mimicry between Coxsackie B3 virus and an autoantigen in myocarditis and DCM, the adenine nucleotide translocator, as a possible mechanism for the development of autoimmunity in viral heart disease [24–26].

Further investigations will have to prove whether the immunologic reaction against the virus epitope can cause pathologic lesions characteristic for myocarditis and DCM. In principle, the clinical and experimental data presented give evidence that the antibodies against the adenine nucleotide translocator, cross-reacting with the Ca^{2+} channel (or vice versa), can influence myocardial function by altering the energy metabolism of the cell [15, 16, 18].

Although cross-reactivity between these proteins seems, at first glance, surprising, it has recently been suggested that there may be a common structural similarity between various membrane channels [32]. For example, a high degree of structural similarity between gap junction polypeptides, the sodium channel, and the nicotinic acetylcholine receptor has already been described. Furthermore, similarities have been reported between several voltage-gated channels (K, Na, Ca).

It has been postulated that membrane channels, although functionally related, nevertheless individually quite distinct, are simple variations of a common structural theme: The α-helical bundle is a structural motif common to the bilayer portion, the hydrophobicity plots are similar, the corresponding secondary and tertiary configurations are largely the same, and the channels apparently posses cyclic symmetry, or a very good approximation to it, with the symmetry axis delineating the pore through the membrane. These similar structural patterns might indicate that the channels respond to chemical or electrical stimuli by related mechanisms. Thus, the universal multisubunit structures of the membrane proteins hint at the possibility that these proteins not only have a similar mode of function but also have a common evolutionary origin. Considering the aspects discussed above, the observed cross-reactivity between the ADP/ATP carrier and the calcium channel seems quite plausible. The observed influence of the antibodies upon the function of the two channel proteins, the ADP/ATP carrier and the calcium channel, might indicate a similar mode of function for both proteins. Abnormalities in calcium metabolism of the myocardium from patients with DCM are thought to be involved in the pathogenesis of this disease [33, 34]. So far, the mechanism underlying disturbed calcium metabolism is not clear. Limas et al. [33] suspected a lower calcium-uptake rate by the sarcoplasmic reticulum; Gwathmey et al. [34], an increased calcium entry through voltage-dependent sarcolemmal channels and a diminished capacity to restore resting calcium levels during diastole. Since we can show the existence of antibodies against the Ca^{2+} channel in patients with myocarditis and DCM, these antibodies enhancing the Ca^{2+} channel activity may in fact contribute to the pathogenesis of these diseases by inducing chronic Ca^{2+} overload [17, 18]. An increase in the intracellular Ca^{2+} concentration well induce a collapse of the mitochondrial membrane potential, which subsequently will lead to decreased activity of the adenine nucleotide translocator. Since the activity of the adenine nucleotide translocator apparently represents the rate-limiting step in energy supply to the cytosol, this inhibition of the carrier protein must lead to an imbalance between energy need and supply in the cytosol with the consequence of a diminished myocardial function.

Regardless of the mechanism of action of the antibodies, either directly through antibody-mediated inhibition of the carrier protein or indirectly

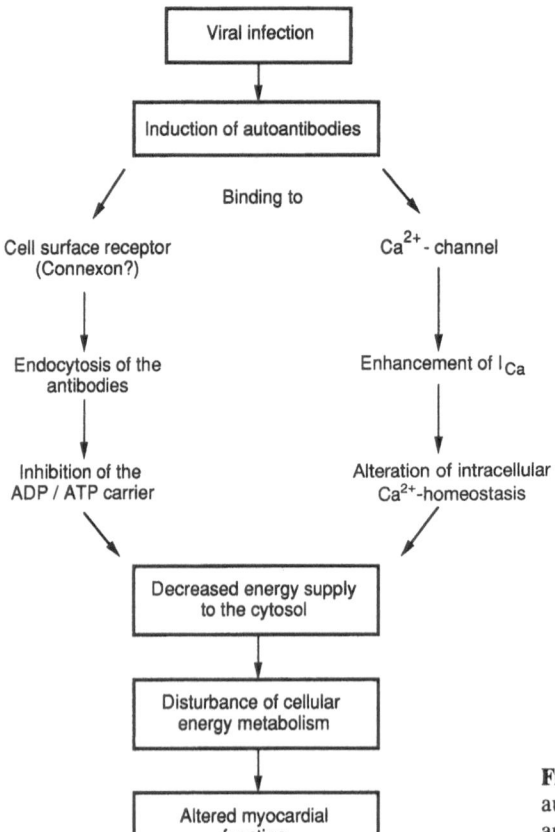

Fig. 6. Possible role of autoantibodies in the development and pathogenesis of viral heart disease

through antibody-mediated disturbance of intracellular Ca^{2+} homeostasis, our data indicate a new mechanism for an antibody-mediated dysfunction of the myocardium (Fig. 6). These results may be of major importance for the understanding of the pathomechanisms, underlying myocarditis and dilated cardiomyopathy and subsequently, may result in new therapeutical regimens for these diseases.

References

1. Gravanis MB, Ansari AA (1987) Idiopathic cardiomyopathies. Arch Pathol Lab Med 111:915–929
2. Kereiakes DJ, Parmley WW (1984) Myocarditis and cardiomyopathy. Am Heart J 108:1318–1326
3. Kawai C, Matsumori A, Fujiwara H (1987) Myocarditis and dilated cardiomyopathy. Ann Rev Med 38:221–239
4. Dec GW, Palacios IF, Fallon JT, Aretz T, Mills J, Lee DCS, Johnson RA (1985) Active myocarditis in the spectrum of acute dilated cardiomyopathy. N Engl J Med 312:885–890

5. Fallon JT (1987) Myocarditis and dilated cardiomyopathy: different stages of the same disease? Contemp Issues cardiovasc Clin 18:155–162
6. Bowles NE, Richardson PJ, Olsen EGJ, Archard LC (1986) Detection of Coxsackie B virus specific RNA sequences in myocardial biopsy samples from patients with myocarditis and dilated cardiomyopathy. Lancet 1:1120–1122
7. Archard LC, Freeke CA; Richardson PJ, Meany B, Olsen EGJ, Morgan-Capner P, Rose ML, Taylor P, Banner NR, Yacoub MH, Bowles NE (1988) Persistence of enterovirus RNA in dilated cardiomyopathy: a progression from myocarditis. In: Schultheiss HP (ed) New concepts in viral heart disease. Springer, Berlin Heidelberg New York, pp 349–362
8. Kandolf R, Ameis D, Kirschner P, Canu A, Hofschneider PH (1987) In situ detection of enteroviral genomes in myocardial cells by nucleic acid hybridization: an approach to the diagnosis of viral heart disease. Proc Natl Acad Sci USA 84:6272–6276
9. Kandolf R, Kirschner P, Ameis D, Canu A, Erdmann E, Schultheiss HP, Kemkes B, Hofschneider PH (1988) Enteroviral heart disease: diagnosis by in situ hybridization. In: Schultheiss HP (ed) New concepts in viral heart disease. Springer, Berlin Heidelberg New York, pp 337–348
10. Southern P, Oldstone MBA (1986) Medical consequences of persistent viral infection. N Engl J Med 314:359–366
11. Shoenfeld Y, Schwartz RS (1984) Immunologic and genetic factors in autoimmune diseases. N Engl J Med 311:1019–1029
12. Maisch B, Deeg P, Liebau G, Kochsiek K (1983) Diagnostic relevance of humoral and cytotoxic immune reactions in primary and secondary dilated cardiomyopathy. Am J Cardiol 52:1072–1078
13. Schultheiss HP (1987) The mitochondrium as antigen in inflammatory heart disease. Eur Heart J 8 [Suppl J]:203–210
14. Schultheiss HP, Bolte HD (1985) The immunochemical analysis of autoantibodies against the adenine nucleotide translocator in dilated cardiomyopathy. J Mol Cell Cardiol 17:603–617
15. Schultheiss HP (1989) The significance of autoantibodies against the ADP/ATP carrier for the pathogenesis of myocarditis and dilated cardiomyopathy – clinical and experimental data. Springer Semin Immunopathol 11:15–30
16. Schulze K, Becker B, Schultheiss HP (1989) Autoimmunity to an intracellular protein: antibodies to the ADP/ATP carrier penetrate into myocardial cells and disturb energy metabolism in vivo. Circ Res 64:179–192
17. Morad M, Davies N, Ulrich G, Schultheiss HP (1988) Antibodies against ADP/ATP carrier enhance the calcium current in isolated cardiac myocytes. Am J Physiol 24:H960–H964
18. Schultheiss HP, Ulrich G, Janda I, Kühl U, Morad M (1988) Antibody-mediated enhancement of calcium permeability in cardiac myocytes. J Exp Med 168:2105–2119
19. Schultheiss HP, Klingenberg M (1984) Immunochemical characterization of the adenine nulceotide translocator: organ and conformation specificity. Eur J Biochem 143:599–605
20. Rasmussen UB, Wohlrab H (1986) Conserved structural domains among species and tissues-specific differences in the mitochondrial phosphate-transport protein and the ADP/ATP carrier. Biochem Biophys Acta 852:306–314
21. Neckelmann L, Li K, Wade RP, Shuster R, Wallace DC (1987) cDNA sequence of a human skeletal muscle ADP/ATP translocator: lack of a leader peptide, divergence form a fibroblast translocator cDNA, and coevolution with mitochondrial DNA genes. Proc Natl Acad Sci USA 84:7580–7584
22. Neu N, Beisel KW, Traystman MD, Rose NR, Craig SW (1987) Autoantibodies specific for the cardiac myosin isoform are found in mice susceptible to coxsackievirus B3-induced myocarditis. J Immunol 138:2488–2492
23. Wolfgram LJ, Beisel KW, Rose NR (1985) Heart-specific autoantibodies following murine Coxsackie B3 myocarditis. J Exp Med 161:1112–1121
24. Schwimmbeck PL, Schultheiss HP, Strauer BE, Oldstone MBA (1989) Sharing of antigenic determinants between Coxsackie B3 virus and autoantigens in viral myocarditis and dilative cardiomyopathy. J Am Coll Cardiol 13:253A

25. Schwimmbeck PL, Schultheiss HP, Strauer BE, Oldstone MBA (1989) Antigenic mimicry between Coxsackie B3 virus and myocardial autoantigens: autoimmune pathogenesis of myocarditis and dilative cardiomyopathy. Proceedings of the 7th international congress of immunology, Berlin, pp 789

26. Schwimmbeck PL, Schultheiss HP, Strauer BE, Oldstone MBA (1989) The use of synthetic peptides in the study and diagnosis of myocarditis and dilative cardiomyopathy. Proceedings of the 7th international congress of immunology, Berlin, pp 818

27. Bünger R, Sommer O, Walter G, Stiegler H, Gerlach E (1979) Functional and metabolic features of an isolated perfused guinea pig heart performing pressure-volume work. Pflugers Arch 380:259–266

28. Soboll S, Bünger R (1981) Compartimentation of adenine nucleotides in working guinea pig heart stimulated by noradrenaline. Hoppe Seylers Z Physiol Chem 362:125–132

29. Klingenberg M (1985) The ADP/ATP carrier in mitochondrial membranes. In: Martonosi A (ed) The enzymes of biological membranes. Plenum, New York, pp 511–553

30. Klingenberg M, Appel M (1980) Is there a common binding center in the ADP/ATP carrier for substrate and inhibitors? FEBS Lett 119:195–199

31. Klingenberg M, Heldt HW (1982) The ADP/ATP translocation in mitochondria and its role in intracellular compartmentation. In: Sies H (ed) Metabolic compartmentation. Academic, London, pp 101–122

32. Unwin N (1986) Is there a common design for cell membrane channels? Nature 323:12–13

33. Limas CJ, Olivari MT, Goldenberg IF, Levine TB, Benditt DG, Simon A (1987) Calcium uptake by cardiac sarcoplasmatic reticulum in human dilated cardiomyopathy. Cardiovasc Res 21:601–605

34. Gwathmey JK, Copelas L, MacKinnon R, Schoen FJ, Feldman MD, Grossman W, Morgan JP (1987) Abnormal intracellular calcium handling in myocardium from patients with end-stage heart failure. Circ Res 61:70–76

35. Schulze K, Becker BF, Schauer R, Schultheiss HP (1990) Antibodies to ADP/ATP carrier – an autoantigen in myocarditis and dilated cardiomyopathy – impair cardiac function. Circulation 81:959–969

The β-Adrenergic Receptor-G Protein-Adenylate Cyclase Complex in Idiopathic Dilated Cardiomyopathy

E. M. Gilbert and M. R. Bristow

Introduction

Significant alterations in both the receptor-G protein-adenylate cyclase (RGC) complex and cardiac adrenergic neurons occur in subjects with idiopathic dilated cardiomyopathy and heart failure. These alterations result in subsensitivity of the failing heart to β-adrenergic stimulation. These changes may also have an important influence on the natural history of heart failure. Certain therapeutic interventions such as β-blockade or angiotensin converting enzyme inhibition may alter key components of the RGC complex and partially restore the sensitivity of the β-adrenergic pathway. This paper will review the current information about the myocardial RGC complex in both nonfailing and failing human hearts and summarize recent findings about the effects of therapy of heart failure on the myocardial RGC complex.

β-Adrenergic Pathways in Nonfailing Ventricular Myocardium

The development of techniques to directly identify receptors through radiolabeling [1, 2] and the availability of human cardiac tissue from surgically explanted transplant recipients and donors has lead to a great expansion of our knowledge regarding the pharmacology and biochemistry of the human β-adrenergic receptor. Endomyocardial biopsy tissue can now be used to measure β-receptor density [3], enabling us to extend these findings to the intact human heart. β_2-adrenergic receptors found on circulating lymphocytes are also altered in heart failure [4, 5], suggesting that lymphocyte β-receptor density could be used to assess the β-adrenergic pathway in heart failure. Unfortunately, only a poor correlation exists between lymphocyte β-receptor density and total cardiac β-receptor density in patients with heart failure, and there is no correlation between lymphocyte β-receptor density and cardiac β_1-receptor density [6, 7].

There are marked interspecies differences in cardiac receptor pharmacology. The human heart relies on β_1-adrenergic inotropic support as the primary mechanism to increase myocardial performance [8, 9]. However, in many commonly studied laboratory species, other receptor pathways support myocardial performance. For example, in the rat both α- and β_1-adrenergic pathways support myocardial performance [10, 11], while in the guinea pig the H_2-histamine pathway is more prominent than the β_1-adrenergic pathway [12]. Human ventricular myocardium also differs from all known laboratory animals by having a significant proportion of β_2-receptors coupled to adenylate cyclase [13–15] and muscle contraction [16–20]. Because of these interspecies differences, it is important to study human myocardial tissue when studying adrenergic mechanisms in human heart failure.

The RGC complex is depicted schematically in Fig. 1. Stimulation of thre RGC complex results in the formation of cyclic adenosine monophosphate (cAMP) from adenosine triphosphate (ATP) [9, 21]. The most proximal component of this system are the cell surface membrane receptors. Membrane receptors interact with extracellular "first messengers" including neurotransmitters, autacoids, and hormones [9, 21]. This interaction results in receptor coupling to numerous guanine nucleotide regulatory (G) proteins including the stimulatory (G_s) and the inhibitory (g_i) G proteins [9, 21 22]. Among the receptors coupled to the G_s protein are the β_1, β_2, H_2-histamine, and vasoactive intestinal protein (VIP) receptors [9, 21]. The G_s protein transduces and amplifies signals from the receptors to adenylate cyclase, which is the the catalytic subunit for generating cAMP from ATP [9, 21, 22]. Thus, stimulation of these four receptors activates adenylate cyclase and increases cAMP production. Signals transduced via the G_i protein inhibit activation of adenylate cyclase. The A_1 adenosine, somatostatin, and M_2 muscarinic receptors are examples of receptors coupled to the G_i protein and stimulation of these receptors inhibits adenylate cyclase activity. The "second messenger" cAMP activates protein kinase A, which leads to phosphorylation of various proteins (including calcium channels and phospholamban) and ultimately increased intracellular calcium and myocardial contractility [9, 21, 22].

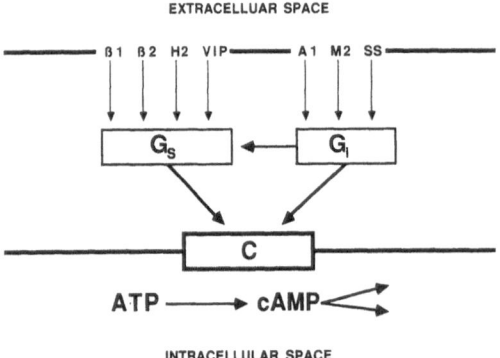

Fig. 1. Schematic representation of the receptor-G protein-adenylate cyclase complex in the human myocardial cell surface membrane. The direction of biologic signaling are given by the *arrows*; note that the G_i signal is inhibitory, while all other signals are stimulatory. β_1, β_1-receptor; β_2, β_2-receptor; H_2, H_2-histamine receptor; *VIP*, vasoactive intestinal protein receptor; A_1, A_1 adenosine receptor; M_2, M_2-muscarinic receptor; SS, somatostatin receptor; G_s, G_s protein; G_i, G_i protein; C, adenylate cyclase. See text for further details

There are considerable differences in the magnitude of contractile response mediated by maximal receptor occupancy of the various receptors coupled to the G_s protein in the RGC complex. Activation of β_1- and β_2-adrenergic receptors yields the largest contractile response [8, 9, 21]. In in vitro tissue bath experiments, VIP receptor activation results in approximately 40% of the contractile response observed with stimulation of β-adrenergic receptors [23, 24]. However, VIP receptor stimulation does not appear to be a significant mechanism for supporting contractile response in the intact human heart since ventricular myocardium contains only a very small quantity of VIP and VIP probably does not act as a circulating hormone [25]. Only a relatively minor inotropic effect is observed with H_2-histamine receptor activation [26, 27].

In nonfailing left and right ventricular myocardium, β_1-receptors comprise 80% and β_2-receptors comprise approximately 20% of the total β-receptor population [28, 29]. Although β_1- and β_2-receptors are qualitatively similar in their coupling to G_s, the degree of coupling to adenylate cyclase is four to five times greater for β_2-receptors [20, 30, 31]. However, the degree of inotropic stimulation produced by β_1-receptor versus β_2-receptor stimulation is proportional to the numbers of receptors present [28]. There are also marked differences in the affinity of norepinephrine, the most important cardiac neurotransmitter, for the β_1- and β_2-receptors. The affinity of norepinephrine for the β_1-receptor is 30–50 times greater than its affinity for the β_2-receptor [32]. Because of the differences in receptor population and agonist affinity, the β_1-receptor is the predominante adrenergic subtype regulating contractility in nonfailing human myocardium.

β-Adrenergic Pathways in Heart Failure

Significant alterations in the RGC complex occur in the failing human heart and are summarized in Table 1. As shown in Fig. 2, major change occurs in the β_1-receptor population. In severe heart failure, there is a 60%–70% reduction in β_1-receptor density [19, 33, 34]. In contrast, β_2-receptor density is not changed in heart failure, but β_2-agonist responsiveness is mildly reduced (approximately 30%) due to β_2-receptor "uncoupling" [15, 20]. A 30%–40% increase in the activity of the G_i protein is also present in heart failure [35, 36]. Preliminary observations suggest that β_2-receptor uncoupling may be related to this increase in G_i activity [35, 36].

Table 1. Summary of receptor pathway abnormalities in the failing human heart

Constituent	Abnormality
β_1-Receptor	Decreased density
β_2-Receptor	Uncoupled
G_i protein	Increased activity
VIP receptor	Decreased density, increased affinity

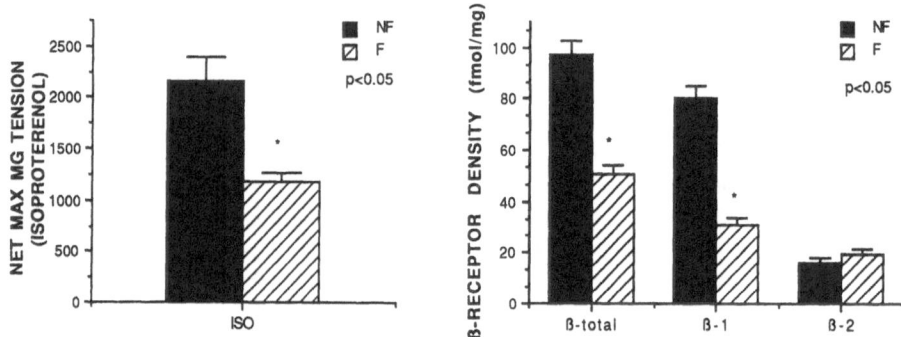

Fig. 2. Maximal isoproterenol tension response in isolated RV trabeculae compared with β-receptor densities in membranes derived from right ventricular free wall of nonfailing hearts *(NF)* and failing hearts in patients with idiopathic dilated cardiomyopathy *(F)*. For muscle contraction, nonfailing subjects $n = 24$ and idiopathic dilated cardiomyopathy subjects $n = 30$. For β-receptor densities, nonfailing subjects $n = 34$ and idiopathic dilated cardiomyopathy subjects $n = 41$. (From [91])

Changes also occur in other components of the RGC complex in the failing human heart. The VIP receptor density is decreased by approximately 60% in the failing human heart, but it also exhibits an increased affinity for VIP which tends to counteract the effects of receptor down-regulation [24]. G_s protein function has been reported to be decreased in some studies [37, 38], but unchanged in others [35]. The H_2-histamine receptor [26, 27], M_2-muscarinic receptor (unpublished observation), α-receptor [33, 39], and adenylate cyclase [22] are not significantly altered in the failing human heart.

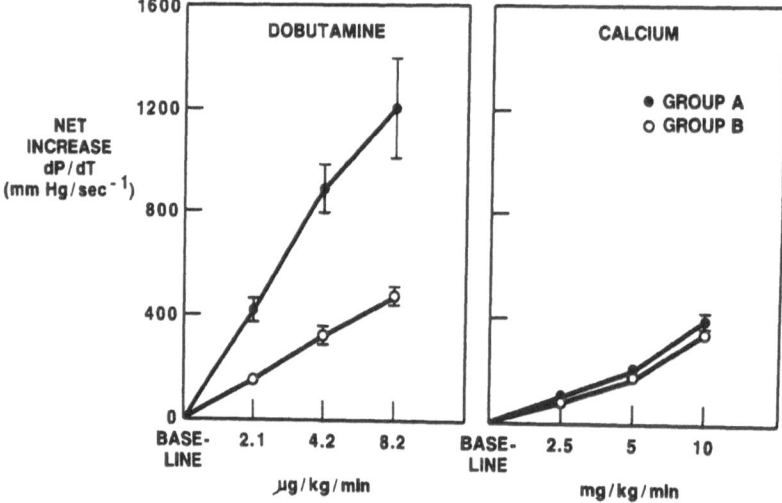

Fig. 3. Peak dP/dt responses to dobutamine and calcium in control subjects with left ventricular ejection fraction > 40% (group A) and patients with idiopathic dilated cardiomyopathy and left ventricular ejection fraction < 20% and a 50% reduction in β-receptor density (group B). (From [3])

Since the human heart does not appear to have "spare" β-adrenergic receptors [40–42], the reductions in β_1-receptor density and β_2-receptor affinity in heart failure result in a 50% decrease in the response to exogenously administered β-agonists [3, 40, 42]. In contrast, the inotropic response to calcium administration is unchanged in heart failure when administered either in vitro [5, 9, 43] or in vivo [3, 9] (see Figs. 2 and 3). While these changes may theoretically serve a "cardioprotective" function, they compromise the ability of the RGC system to support cardiac function in times when increased contractility is desirable.

Etiology of RGC Complex Abnormalities in Heart Failure

In chronic heart failure, the adrenergic nervous system is activated both systemically [47, 48] and regionally in the heart [48] and kidney [48], but not in the lung or skeletal muscle [48]. As a result, the heart becomes a net producer of norepinephrine in heart failure [49]. The signal for this activation of cardiac adrenergic activity in heart failure is unknown. We have found the coronary sinus norepinephrine concentration, a crude measure of cardiac adrenergic activation, can be correlated with elevated ventricular filling pressures, but not with other measures of cardiac performance including cardiac index, system arterial pressure, vascular resistance, or left ventricular ejection fraction.

The increase in cardiac derived norepinephrine may be due to a decrease in norepinephrine uptake [50–52] and/or an increased release [48] from cardiac adrenergic neurons. Using the isotopic methods of Rose et al. [52], we have directly measured norepinephrine uptake and release in six subjects with idiopathic dilated cardiomyopathy and mild to moderate heart failure. In comparison to control subjects with normal ventricular function, norepinephrine uptake and release were reduced by 78% and 61%, respectively (unpublished observation). Since norepinephrine uptake is reduced to a greater degree than norepinephrine release, coronary sinus, interstitial and presumably synaptic cleft norepinephrine can be expected to be increased.

The factors responsible for the changes which occur in the RGC complex in heart failure have not been completely identified. However, there is a considerably body of evidence that increased cardiac norepinephrine concentration contributes to the decrease in β_1-receptor density in the failing human heart. For example, chronic exposure to norepinephrine is a powerful down-regulating stimulus in model systems [53]. In addition, the degree of decrease in β-receptor density can be inversely correlated with coronary sinus norepinephrine concentration [54, 55]. The human β_1-receptor has a higher affinity for norepinephrine than either the β_2- or α_1-receptors, which do not decrease in density in heart failure [52]. Finally, decreasing the norepinephrine occupancy of β_1-receptor with competitive β_1-blocking agents increases β-adrenergic receptor density in subjects with heart failure [56].

However, there is evidence that norepinephrine exposure is not the only factor responsible for β-receptor down-regulation. The inverse relationship between coronary sinus norepinephrine concentration and β-receptor density is only fair [55]. A fraction of the myocardial β-receptors appear to be resistant to catecholamine-induced down-regulation in cell culture [53] and intact failing human heart [15, 20, 54]. Other membrane receptors coupled to the G_s protein are abnormal in heart failure, apparently in the absence of an increase in endogenous agonist [24]. These observations suggest that other factors may also be important in regulating β-adrenergic receptors in heart failure.

The RGC Complex as a Target for Therapeutic Intervention in Heart Failure

Effect of Phosphodiesterase Inhibition

Endogenous cyclic nucleotide phosphodiesterases (PDE) degrade cAMP and thereby reduce the intensity of β-adrenergic receptor mediated inotropic stimulation [57]. Drugs which inhibit PDE increase cAMP and subsequently increase myocardial contractility [58]. Pharmacologically, stimulation of adenylate cyclase combined with PDE inhibition should have at least an additive positive inotropic effect, since both actions will increase cAMP concentration [9].

To study this hypothesis, we measured the effects of the β-agonist dobutamine combined with the PDE inhibitor enoximone on adenylate cyclase activity and contractility in vitro, and on hemodynamic parameters in patients with severe heart failure [59, 60]. As shown in Fig. 4a, enoximone and dobutamine had additive effects on adenylate cyclase activity in cardiac homogenates from failing human ventricles. In ventricular trabeculae from failing human hearts, enoximone significantly shifted the dobutamine inotropic dose response curve upwards and to the left (Fig. 4b).

Since the hemodynamic effects of enoximone are due to its combined inotropic and vasodilatory effects [61], we compared the additivity of dobutamine with enoximone to dobutamine with nitroprusside, a pure vasodilator [60]. Administration of enoximone and nitroprusside resulted in similar effects on systemic and pulmonic pressures. However, as shown in Fig. 5, the effects of dobutamine and enoximone on cardiac index were additive, while the effects of dobutamine and nitroprusside were subadditive. Similar additivity of a PDE inhibitor combined with a β-agonist have been reported for amrinone with dobutamine [62]. Thus, therapy with PDE inhibitors can pharmacologically at least partially restore β-adrenergic receptor responsiveness to β-receptor agonists.

It is possible that administration of PDE inhibitors could results in receptor desensitization or changes in cardiac adrenergic drive in subjects with heart failure [42]. Maisel et al. [63] have reported that a 72-h infusion of the PDE inhibitor amrinone results in an increase in venous catecholamine concentrations and down-regulation of lymphocyte $β_2$-receptors. However, as discussed above, values for lymphocyte β-receptor density correlate poorly with cardiac β-receptors density. Because of this, it is not clear what effects amrinone therapy had on cardiac adrenergic pathways. We studied the effects of PDE inhibition on cardiac adrenergic receptors using surgically explanted hearts

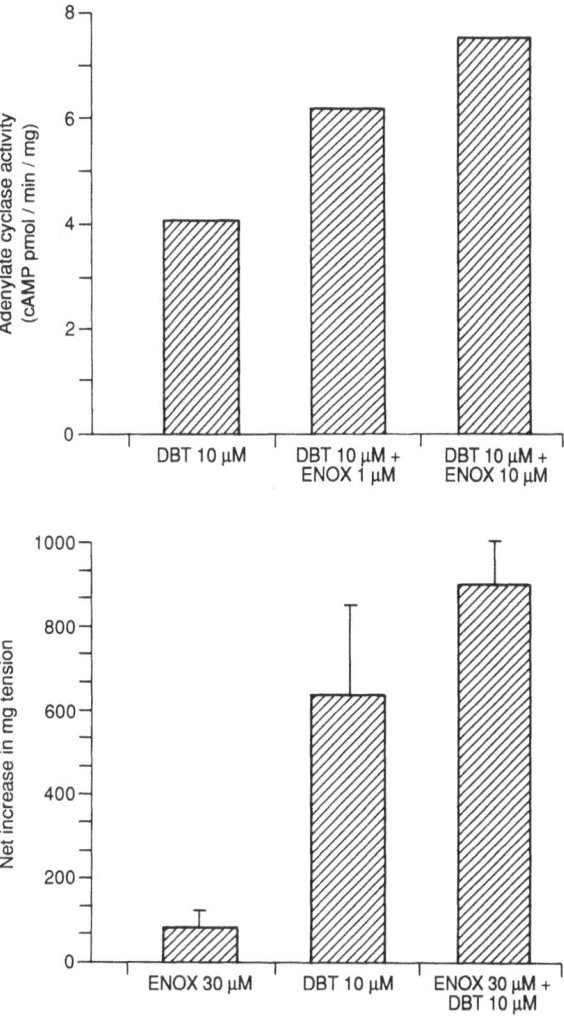

Fig. 4. a Potentiation of cAMP generation in particulate fractions of ventricular myocardium from a subject with severe heart failure by dobutamine alone (10 μ*M*) and dobutamine with enoximone (1 μ*M* and 10 μ*M*). Enoximone produces a dose-dependent additive effect on dobutamine stimulation of human adenylate cyclase. **b** Contractile response of isolated right ventricular trabeculae from ten subjects with severe heart failure by enoximone alone (30 μ*M*), dobutamine alone (10 μ*M*), and the combination of these doses of enoximone and dobutamine. The inotropic effects of dobutamine and enoximone are additive. (From [92])

from subjects treated with enoximone as a bridge to heart transplantation [64, 65]. The total β-adrenergic receptor population was unchanged, but a shift in receptor subtypes was observed with a reduction in β_1-receptor and an increase in β_2-receptors. The reason for these enoximone-associated changes in receptor subtypes is not presently known.

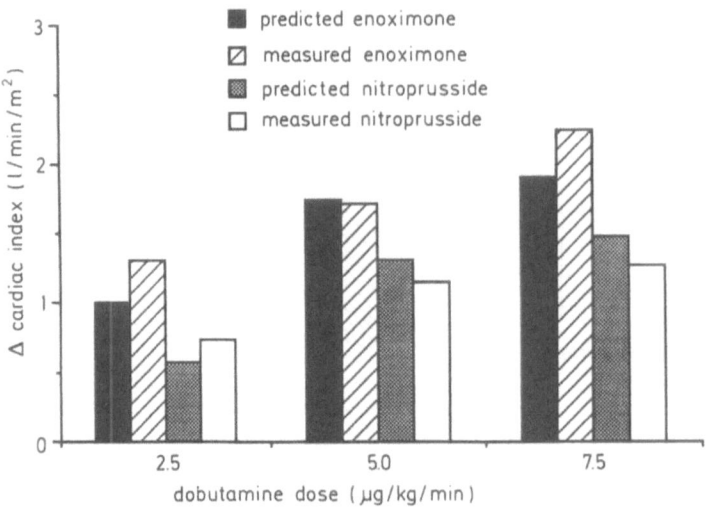

Fig. 5. Shown are the predicted and measured additive effects of enoximone with dobutamine and nitroprusside with dobutamine for eight patients with severe heart failure. To predict the additive effects of dobutamine with nitroprusside or dobutamine, the changes in cardiac index with dobutamine alone were added to the changes in cardiac index with enoximone alone or nitroprusside alone. For the combination of dobutamine with enoximone, the actual measured Δ cardiac index was greater than or equal to the predicted value at all doses of dobutamine. For the combination of dobutamine with nitroprusside, measured Δ cardiac index was lower than predicted at dobutamine doses of 5.0 and 7.5 µg/kg/min. (From [92])

Effect of β-Adrenergic Agonists

Alteration of β-adrenergic responsiveness has been observed with both short-term [66, 67] and long-term [5, 68] therapy with β-agonists. The degree of desensitization produced by individual β-agonists appears to be highly variable. For example, a decrease in the therapeutic response to dopamine can be observed after a 48-h continuous infusion, while no change in efficacy is observed with a 48-h infusion of dobutamine [66, 67, 69]. However, tolerance to dobutamine administration does develop after longer periods of time [67]. Tolerance also develops with long-term therapy with the β_2-agonist pirbuterol [5] and the selective β_1-partial agonist prenalterol [68], the indirect agonist dopexamine [69], but not with the β_1-partial agonist xamoterol [70]. Different β-agonists may also produce different degrees of β-adrenergic receptor down-regulation [71, 72].

We have studied the effects of dobutamine administration in heart failure. Ventricular tissue was obtained at the time of transplantation from patients who were treated with dobutamine for at least 48h. In these hearts we observed a slight decrease in both β_1- and β_2-receptor density when compared to failing controls who did not receive dobutamine [54]. This finding is not surprising, since dobutamine is a nonselective β-agonist [73]. However, subjects treated with high-dose dobutamine for long periods of time were found to have higher β_1-adrenergic receptor density than subjects treated with low dose dobutamine for shorter periods of time [54]. Thus, treatment with dobutamine may have variable effects on β-adrenergic receptor density. Dobutamine administration is associated with a reduction in adrenergic activity [42, 69], perhaps as a response to improved hemodynamics. This reduction of myocardial exposure to endogenous norepinephrine may offset the down-regulating effects of exogenous dobutamine administration and lead to the paradoxical effect of β-receptor up-regulation. Thus, the development of desensitization to β-adrenergic agonists is variable and is probably dependent on multiple factors including the individual β-agonist administered, the method of its administration, the baseline state of the RGC complex and the effect of agonist administration on myocardial exposure to endogenous catecholamines.

Effect of Angiotensin Converting Inhibition

Therapy with angiotensin converting enzyme inhibitors is associated with sustained hemodynamic improvements and decreases in venous norepinephrine concentration [74, 75]. Angiotensin II receptor stimulation may facilitate adrenergic neurotransmission [76, 77]. Thus, angiotensin converting enzyme inhibition may reduce circulating norepinephrine either directly by inhibition of angiotensin II facilitated norepinephrine release or indirectly by improvement in hemodynamics resulting in reduction of adrenergic activity. In contrast, the direct acting vasodilator hydralazine and the calcium channel blocker nifedipine increase venous norepinephrine concentration in heart failure [78, 79].

We recently investigated the effects of the angiotensin converting enzyme inhibitor lisinopril on systemic and myocardial adrenergic activity in a placebo-controlled randomized clinical trial [80]. In subjects with increased adrenergic drive, lisinopril therapy significantly decreased coronary sinus and central venous norepinephrine concentration and increased cardiac β-adrenergic receptor density. No changes were observed with lisinopril therapy in subjects without increased adrenergic drive, or in either subset with placebo therapy. The beneficial long-term effects of angiotensin converting enzyme inhibitor therapy may be in part due to this reduction in cardiac adrenergic activity and myocardial β-adrenergic receptor up-regulation.

Effect of β-Blocker Therapy

Several reports have suggested that chronic β-blockade may improve hemodynamic and clinical function in patients with idiopathic dilated cardiomyopathy [81–84]. Several factors have been postulated to contribute to the β-blocker-related improvements including protection from the cardiotoxic effects of increased catecholamines [85, 86], up-regulation of myocardial β_1-adrenergic receptors which would improve myocardial responsiveness to β-stimulation during times of stress [56, 83], improved myocardial energetics, favorable alterations of coronary blood flow, improved ventricular diastolic function and perhaps peripheral effects such as reduced renin release [87].

As discussed above, β_1-adrenergic receptor down-regulation in the failing human heart is probably caused by exposure to increased levels of cardiac-derived norepinephrine. In theory, prevention of β_1-adrenergic receptor occupancy by norepinephrine with a β-blocker would remove this down-regulating stimulus and lead to receptor up-regulation. A recent clinical trial [56] demonstrated that treatment with the β_1-selective blocking agent metoprolol is associated with an increase in β-adrenergic receptor density and an increased responsiveness to β-agonist stimulation (Fig. 6).

These changes also explain the increased exercise tolerance in subjects treated with low to moderate doses of metoprolol [82, 83]. During exercise there is an increase in cardiac norepinephrine release [48] which elevates myocardial interstitial norepinephrine concentration sufficiently to displace metoprolol from β_1-adrenergic receptor site. Since β-adrenergic responsiveness to exogenous norepinephrine has been increased by β_1-receptor up-regulation, there is an increase in exercise performance.

Protection of the myocardium from damage by catecholamines may also be one of the mechanisms responsible for β-blocker-related improvement [85, 86]. Since β_2-adrenergic receptors comprise as much as 40% of the total β-adrenergic receptor population in heart failure [2, 3], a nonselective β-blocking agent should have a theoretical advantage over a selective β_1 antagonist for optimal cardiac protection from catecholamine injury.

We evaluated this hypothesis using bucindolol, which is a potent nonselective β-blocking agent with direct acting vasodilatory properties [88] in a randomized, double-blind, placebo-controlled trial [89]. As shown in Table 2, chronic bucindolol therapy significantly improved resting cardiac function, symptoms of

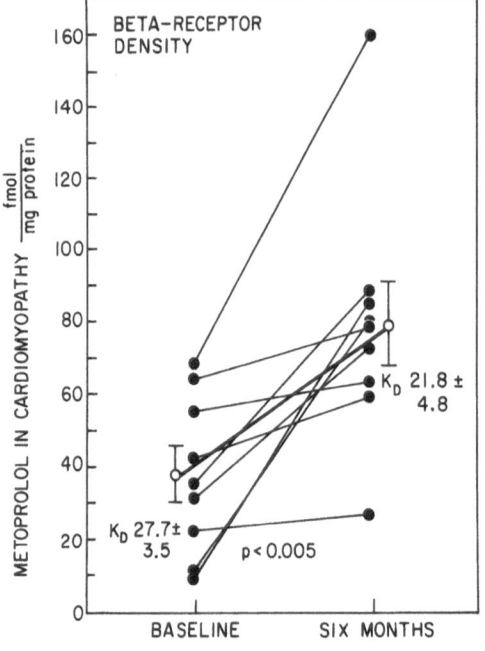

Fig. 6. β-Receptor density in nine subjects with idiopathic dilated cardiomyopathy at baseline and after six months therapy with metoprolol. (From [56])

Table 2. Bucindolol vs. placebo: mean percentage change from baseline of selected functional measures

Functional parameter	Bucindolol ($n = 13$) (%)	Placebo ($n = 9$) (%)
Heart rate	−13	− 3
Left ventricular ejection fraction	+35	+ 5[a]
Pulmonary artery wedge pressure	−41	+21[a]
Cardiac index	+14	−13[a]
Left ventricular stroke work index	+40	− 8[a]
Symptom score	−40	+ 6[a]
Venous norepinephrine concentration	−50	+26[a]

[a] $p < 0.05$ for bucindolol vs. placebo.

congestive heart failure, and also resulted in a significant fall in systemic venous norepinephrine concentration. The observed fall in norepinephrine concentration indicates a treatment-induced reduction of generalized adrenergic activity that occurred in conjunction with improvement of cardiac function. Since plasma venous norepinephrine is an indicator of prognosis [90], it might be speculated that this reduction of generalized sympathetic activity would result in a favorable effect on the natural history of heart failure.

Summary and Conclusions

Significant alterations in the RGC complex occur in the failing human heart including marked down-regulation of β_1-receptors, mild uncoupling of β_2-receptors from the G_s protein, and mild up-regulation of the G_i protein. These changes may play a direct role in the pathophysiology of heart failure be decreasing myocardial responsiveness to positive inotropic stimulation in times of stress. Therapeutic interventions in heart failure which lower cardiac adrenergic activity such as β-blockade, angiotensin converting enczyme inhibition and certain inotropes tend to partially restore the sensitivity of β-adrenergic pathways. Further study will be necessary to define the optimal methods of modulating receptor pathways and the clinical settings in which such changes will be beneficial.

References

1. Lefkowitz RJ, Mukherjee C, Coverstone M, Caron M (1974) Stereospecific [³H](-)-alprenolol binding sites, β-adrenergic receptors and adenylate cyclase. Biochem Biophys Res Commun 60:703–709
2. Aurbach GD, Fedak SA, Woodard CJ, Palmer J, Hauser D, Troxler F (1974) β-adrenergic receptor: stereospecific interaction of iodinated β-blocking agent with high affinity site. Science 186:1223–1224

3. Fowler MB, Laser JA, Hopkins GL, Minobe W, Bristow MR (1986) Assessment of the β-adrenergic receptor pathway in the intact failing human heart: progressive receptor down-regulation and subsensitivity to agonist response. Circulation 74:1290–1302

4. Gordon EP, Bristow MR, Laser JA, Monobe WA, Fowler MB, Savian WM (1983) Correlation between β-adrenergic receptors in human lymphocytes and heart. Circulation 68:III-99 (abstr)

5. Colucci WS, Alexander RW, Williams GH, Rude RE, Holman BL, Konstam MA, Wynee J, Mudge GH, Braunwald E (1981) Decreased lymphocyte beta-adrenergic-receptor density in patients with heart failure and tolerance to the beta-adrenergic agonist pirbuterol. N Engl J Med 305:185–190

6. Brodde OE, Kretsch R, Ikezono K, Zerkowski HR, Reidemeister JC (1986) Human β-adrenoceptors: relation between myocardial and lymphocyte β-adrenoceptor density. Science 231:1584–1585

7. Brodde EO, Michel MC, Gordon EP, Sandoval A, Gilbert EM, Bristow MR (1989) β-adrenoceptor regulation in the human heart: can it be monitored in circulating lymphocytes. Eur Heart J (in press)

8. Bristow MR (1988) The β-adrenergic receptor: configuration, regulation, mechanism of action. Postgraduate medicine: a special report. February 29, 1988, pp 19–26

9. Hershberger RE, Bristow MR (1988) Receptor alterations in failing human heart. Heart Failure 3:230–238

10. Bristow MR, Sandoval AB, Gilbert EM, Deisher T, Minobe W, Rasmussen R (1988) Myocardial alpha and beta-adrenergic receptors in heart failure: is cardiac derived norepinephrine the regulatory signal? Eur Heart J 9:35–40

11. Hayes JS, Wyss VL, Schenck KS, Cohen ML (1986) Effects of prolonged isoproterenol infusion on cardiac and vascular responses to adrenoceptor agonist. J Pharmacol Exp Ther 237:757–763

12. McNeill JH, Muschek LD (1972) Histamine effects on cardiac contractility, phosphorylase and adenyl cyclase. J Mol Cell Cardiol 4:611–624

13. Bristow MR, Laser JA, Ginsburg R, Minobe W (1985) β_1 and β_2 receptors are coupled to adenylate cyclase in human ventricular myocardium. Clin Res 33:171A

14. Gille E, Lemoine H, Ehle B, Kaumann AJ (1985) The affinity of (-)-propranolol for β_1- and β_2-adrenoceptors of human heart. Naunyn-Schmiedeberg's Arch Pharmacol 331:60–70

15. Bristow MR, Hershberger RE, Port JD, Rasmussen R (1989) β_1 and β_2 adrenergic receptor mediated adenylate cyclase stimulation in nonfailing and failing human ventricular myocardium. Mol Pharmacol 35:293–303

16. Ginsburg R, Bristow MR, Zera P (1984) β_2 receptors are coupled to muscle contraction in human ventricular myocardium. Circulation 70:II-67 (abstr)

17. Ask JA, Stene-Larsen G, Helle KB, Resch F (1985) Functional β_1- and β_2-adrenoceptors in the human myocardium. Acta Physiol Scand 123:81–88

18. Mugge A, Posselt D, Reimer U, Schmitz W, Scholz H (1985) Effects of the β_2-adrenoceptors agonists fenoterol and salbutamol on force of contraction in isolated human ventricular myocardium. Klin Wochenschr 63:26–31

19. Bristow MR, Ginsburg R (1986) β_2 receptors are present on myocardial cells in human ventricular myocardium. Am J Cardiol 57:3F–6F

20. Bristow MR, Ginsburg R, Fowler M, Minobe W, Rasmussen R, Zera P, Menlove R, Shah P, Stinson E (1986) β_1 and β_2-adrenergic receptor subpopulations in normal and failing human ventricular myocardium: coupling of both receptor subtypes to muscle contraction and selective β_1 receptor down-regulation in heart failure. Circ Res 59:297–309

21. Bristow MR (1989) Myocardial cell surface membrane receptors in heart failure. Heart Failure 5:47–50

22. Kessler PD, Van Dop C, Feldman AM (1988) G proteins: transmembrane signal processors in the heart. Heart Failure 3:239–247

23. Hershberger RE, Anderson FL, Bristow MR (1988) The vasoactive intestinal peptide receptor in failing and nonfailing human ventricular myocardium: supersensitivity of failing heart due to increased receptor affinity; diminished maximal inotropic response from decreased receptor density. J Am Coll Cardiol 11:1

24. Hershberger RE, Anderson FL, Bristow MR (1989) The vasoactive intestinal peptide receptor in failing human ventricular myocardium exhibits increased affinity and decreased density. Circ Res (in press)
25. Hershberger RE, Anderson FL, Bristow MR (1989) Vasoactive intestinal peptide receptor pharmacology in nonfailing and failing human heart. Heart Failure 5:51–61
26. Bristow MR, Cubicciotti R, Ginsburg R, Stinson EB, Johnson C (1982) Histaminemediated adenylate cyclase stimulation in human myocardium. Mol Pharmacol 21:671–679
27. Baumann G, Mercader D, Busch U, Felix SB, Loher U, Ludwig L, Sebening H, Heidecke CD, Hagl S, Sebening F, Blomer H (1983) Effects of the H_2-receptor agonist impromidine in human myocardium from patients with heart failure due to mitral and aortic valve disease. J Cardiovasc Pharmacol 5:618–625
28. Bristow MR, Ginsburg R, Umans V, Fowler M, Minobe W, Rasmussen R, Zera P, Menlove R, Shah P, Jamieson S, Stinson EB (1986) β_1- and β_2-adrenergic-receptor subpopulations in nonfailing and failing human ventricular myocardium: coupling of both receptor subtypes to muscle contraction and selective β_1-receptor down-regulation in heart failure. Circ Res 59:297–309
29. Stiles GL, Taylor S, Lefkowitz RJ (1983) Human cardiac β-adrenergic receptors: subtype heterogeneity delineated by direct radioligand binding. Life Sci 33:467–473
30. Brodde EO, O'Hara N, Zerkowski HR, Rohm N (1984) Human cardiac β-adrenoceptors: both β_1- and β_2-adrenoceptors are functionally coupled to the adenylate cyclase in right atrium. J Cardiovasc Pharmacol 6:1184–1191
31. Kaumann AJ, Lemoine H (1987) β_2-adrenoceptors-mediated positive inotropic effect of adrenaline in human ventricular myocardium. Naunyn-Schmiedeberg's Arch Pharmacol 225:403–411
32. Bristow MR, Minobe W, Rasmussen R, Hershberger RE, Hoffmann BB (1988) Alpha-1-adrenergic receptors in the nonfailing and failing human heart. J Pharmacol Exp Ther 247:1039–1045
33. Brodde OE, Schuler S, Kretsch R, Brinkmann M, Borst HG, Hetzer R, Reidemeister JC, Warnecke H, Zerkowski HR (1986) Regional distribution of β-adrenoceptors in the human heart: coexistence of functional β_1- and β_2-adrenoceptors in both atria and ventricles in severe congestive cardiomyopathy. J Cardiovasc Pharmacol 8:1235–1242
34. Denniss AR, Marsh JD, Quigg RJ, Gordon JB, Colucci WS (1989) β-adrenergic receptor number and adenylate cyclase function in denervated transplanted and cardiomyopathic human hearts. Circulation 79:1028–1034
35. Feldman AM, Cates AE, Veazey WB, Hershberger RE, Bristow MR, Baughman KL, Baumgartner WA, Van Dop C (1988) Increase of the 40,000-mol wt pertussis toxin substrate (G protein) in the failing human heart. J Clin Invest 82:189–197
36. Neumann J, Schmitz W, Scholz H, Meyerinck LV, Doring V, Kalmar P (1988) Increase in myocardial G_i-proteins in heart failure. Lancet 2:936–937
37. Horn EM, Corwin SJ, Steinberg SF, Chow YK, Neuberg GW, Cannon PJ, Powers ER, Bilezikian JP (1988) Reduced lymphocyte stimulatory guanine nucleotide regulatory protein and β-adrenergic receptors in congestive heart failure and reversal with angiotensin converting enzyme inhibitor therapy. Circulation 78:1373–1379
38. Ransnas LA, Hjalmarson A, Insel PA (1988) Dilated cardiomyopathy is associated with an impaired activation of the stimulatory G-protein, G_s, by GTP in heart membranes. Circulation 78:II-178 (abstr)
39. Bohm M, Diet F, Feiler G, Kemkes B, Erdmann E (1988) α-adrenoceptors and α-adrenoceptors-mediated positive inotropic effects in failing human myocardium. J Cardiovasc Pharmacol 12:357–364
40. Bristow MR, Ginsburg R, Minobe WA, Cubicciotti RS, Sageman WS, Lurie K, Billingham ME, Harrison DC, Stinson EB (1982) Decreased catecholamine sensitivity and β-adrenergic receptor density in failing human hearts. N Engl J Med 307:205–211
41. Port JD, Bristow MR (1988) Lack of spare β-adrenergic receptors in the human heart. FASEB J 2:A602 (abstr)
42. Colucci WS, Denniss Ar, Leatherman GF, Quigg RJ, Ludmer PL, Marsh JD, Gauthier DF (1988) Intracoronary infusion of dobutamine to patients with and without severe congestive heart failure. J Clin Invest 81:1103–1110

43. Ginsburg R, Bristow MR, Billingham ME, Stinson EB, Schroeder JS, Harrison DC (1983) Study of the normal and failing isolated human heart: decreased response of failing heart to isoproterenol. Am Heart J 106:535–540

44. Chidsey CA, Braunwald E, Morrow AG (1965) Catecholamine excretion and cardiac stores of norepinephrine in congestive heart failure. Am J Med 39:442–451

45. Thomas JA, Marks BH (1978) Plasma norepinephrine in congestive heart failure. Am J Cardiol 41:233–243

46. Cohn JN, Levine TB, Olivari MT, Garberg V, Lura D, Francis GS, Simon AB, Rector T (1984) Plasma norepinephrine as a guide to prognosis in patients with chronic congestive heart failure. N Engl J Med 311:819–823

47. Swedberg K, Viquerat C, Rouleau JL, Roizen M, Atherton B, Parmley WW, Chatterjee K (1984) Comparison of myocardial catecholamine balance in chronic congestive heart failure and in angina pectoris without failure. Am J Cardiol 54:783–786

48. Hasking GJ, Esler MD, Jennings GL, Burton D, Johns AJ, Korner PI (1986) Norepinephrine spillover to plasma in patients with congestive heart failure: evidence of increased overall and cardiorenal sympathetic nervous activity. Circulation 73:615–621

49. Braunwald E, Harrison DC, Chidsey CA (1964) The heart as an endocrine organ. Am J Med 36:1–3

50. Petch MC, Nayler WG (1979) Uptake of catecholamines by human cardiac muscle in vitro. Br Heart J 41:336–339

51. Rose CP, Burgess JH, Cousineau D (1983) Reduced aortocoronary sinus extraction of epinephrine in patients with left ventricular failure secondary to long-term pressure or volume overload. Circulation 68:241–244

52. Rose CP, Burgess JH, Cousineau D (1985) Tracer norepinephrine kinetics in coronary circulation of patients with heart failure secondary to chronic pressure and volume overload. J Clin Invest 76:1740–1747 (abstr)

53. Port JD, DeBellis CC, Wiederin J, Peeters GA, Hershberger RE, Barry WH, Bristow MR (1988) Long-term β-adrenergic receptor desensitization in cultured chick myocardial cells. Pharmacologist:A96 (abstr)

54. Rasmussen R, Shah P, Larrabee P, Murray J, Ginsburg R, Renlund DG, O'Connell JB, Bristow MR (1987) β_1 and β_2 receptor down-regulation associated with β agonist administration in the failing human heart. Circulation 76:IV-307 (abstr)

55. Sandoval A, Gilbert EM, Ginsburg R, Rasmussen R, Minobe W, Larrabee P, Bristow MR (1988) Is β_1 receptor down-regulation in the failing human heart the result of exposure to cardiac-derived norepinephrine? J Am Coll Cardiol 11:117A (abstr)

56. Heilbrunn SM, Shah P, Bristow MR, Valantine HA, Ginsburg R, Fowler MB (1989) Increased beta-receptor density and improved hemodynamic response to catecholamine stimulation during chronic metoprolol therapy. Circulation 79:483–490

57. Wells JN, Harman JC (1977) Cyclic nucleotide phosphodiesterase. Adv Cyclic Nucleotide Res 8:119–143

58. Scholz H (1984) Inotropic drugs and their mechanisms of action. J Am Coll Cardiol 4:309–397

59. Gilbert EM, Hershberger Re, Watson F, O'Connell JB, Renlund DG, Bristow MR (1987) Additivity of the effects of enoximone and dobutamine in the failing human heart. Circulation 76:IV-255 (abstr)

60. Gilbert EM, Mealey P, Volkman K, Eastburn T, O'Connell JB, Renlund DG, Bristow MR (1988) Combination therapy with enoximone and dobutamine is superior to nitroprusside and dobutamine in heart failure. Circulation 78:II-28

61. Roebel LE, Dage RC, Chang HC, Woodward JK (1982) Characterization of a new cardiotonic agent, MDL-17043. J Cardiovasc Pharmacol 4:721–729

62. Gage J, Rutman H, Lucido D, LeJemtel TH (1986) Additive effects of dobutamine and amrinone on myocardial contractility and ventricular performance in patients with severe heart failure. Circulation 74:367–373

63. Maisel As, Wright CM, Carter SM, Ziegler M, Motulsky HJ (1989) Tachyphylaxis with amrinone therapy: association with sequestration and down-regulation of lymphocyte beta-adrenergic receptors. Ann Intern Med 110:195–201

64. Lee HR, O'Connell JB, Renlund DG, Gilbert EM, Mealey PC, Volkman K, Larrabee PA, Bristow MR (1989) Use of enoximone in cardiac transplant candidates; effect on β adrenergic receptors. J Am Coll Cardiol 13:248A (abstr)
65. Bristow MR, Lee HE, Gilbert EM, Renlund DG, Hegewald MG, Hershberger RE, O'Connell JB and the UTAH Cardiac Transplant Program (1989) Use of enoximone in patients awaiting cardial transplant. Br J Clin Pract 42:69–72
66. Leier CV, Heban PT, Huss P, Bush CA, Lewis RP (1978) Comparative systemic and regional hemodynamic effects of dopamine and dobutamine in patients with cardiomyopathic heart failure. Circulation 58:466–475
67. Unverferth DV, Blanford M, Kates RE, Leier CV (1980) Tolerance to dobutamine after a 72 hour continuous infusion. Am J Med 69:262–266
68. Lambertz H, Meyer J, Erbel R (1984) Long-term hemodynamic effects of prenalterol in patients with severe congestive heart failure. Circulation 69:298–305
69. Gilbert EM, Volkman K, Mealey PC, Bristow MR (1989) Tachyphylaxis associated with dopexamine administration in severe heart failure. J Am Coll Cardiol 13:247A (abstr)
70. The German and Austrian Xamoterol Study Group (1988) Double-blind placebo-controlled comparison of digoxin and xamoterol in chronic heart failure. Lancet 2:489–493
71. Reynolds EE, Molinoff PB (1986) Down regulation of beta adrenergic receptors in S49 lymphoma cells induced by atypical agonists. J Pharmacol Exp Ther 239:654–660
72. Maccarrone C, Malta E, Raper C (1984) β-adrenoceptor selectivity in dobutamine: in vivo and in vitro studies. J Cardiovasc Pharmacol 6:132–141
73. Giles TD, Katz R, Sullivan JM, Wolfson P, Haugland M, Kirlin P, Powers E, Rich S, Hackshaw B, Chiaramida A, Rouleau JL, Fisher MB, Pigeon J, Rush JE, for the Multicenter Lisinopril-Captopril Congestive Heart Failure Study Group (1989) Short- and long-acting angiotensin-converting enzyme inhibitors: a randomized trial of lisinopril versus captopril in the treatment of congestive heart failure. J Am Coll Cardiol 13:1240–1247
74. Levine TB, Cohn JN (1982) Determinants of acute and long-term response to converting enzyme inhibitors in congestive heart failure. Am Heart J 104:1159–1164
75. Cleland JGF, Dargie HJ, Ball SG, Gillen G, Hodsman GP, Morton JJ, East BW, Robertson I, Ford I, Robertson JIS (1985) Effects of enalapril in heart failure: a double blind study of effects on exercise performance, renal function, hormones, and metabolic state. Br Heart J 54:305–312
76. Kiran BK, Khairallah PA (1969) Angiotensin and norepinephrine efflux. Eur J Pharmacol 6:102–108
77. De Jonge A, Knape JTA, Van Meel JCA, Kalkman HO, Wilffert B, Thoolen MJMC, Van Brummelen P, Timmermans PBMWM, Van Zwieten PA (1983) Effect of captopril on sympathetic neurotransmission in pithed normotensive rats. Eur J Pharmacol 88:231–240
78. Elkayam U, Roth A, Hsueh W, Weber L, Freidenberger L, Rahimtoola SH (1986) Neurohumoral consequences of vasodilator therapy with hydralazine and nifedipine in severe congestive heart failure. Am Heart J 111:1130
79. Lin MS, McNay JL, Shepherd AMM, Musgrave GE, Keeton TK (1983) Increased plasma norepinephrine accompanies persistent tachycardia after hydralazine. Hypertension 5:257–263
80. Gilbert EM, Sandoval A, Larrabee P, Renlund DG, O'Connell JB, Bristow MR (1988) Effect of lisinopril on cardiac adrenergic drive and myocardial β-receptor density in heart failure. Circulation 78:II-576 (abstr)
81. Waagstein F, Hjalmarson A, Swedberg K, Wallentin I (1983) Beta-blockers in dilated cardiomyopathies: they work. Eur Heart J 4:173–178
82. Engelmeier RS, O'Connell JB, Walsh R, Rad N, Scanlon PJ, Gunnar RM (1985) Improvement in symptoms and exercise tolerance by metoprolol in patients with dilated cardiomyopathy: a double-blind, randomized, placebo-controlled trial. Circulation 72:536–546
83. Heilbrunn SM, Valantine HV, Mullin AV, Fowler MB (1987) Improvement in exercise parameters of myocardial performance with metoprolol therapy in dilated cardiomyopathy. Circulation 76:1222

84. Anderson JL, Lutz JR, Gilbert EM, Sorensen SG, Yanowitz FG, Menlove RL, Bartholomew M (1985) A randomized trial of low-dose beta-blockade therapy for idiopathic dilated cardiomyopathy. Am J Cardiol 55:471–475
85. Bristow MR (1984) The adrenergic nervous system in heart failure. N Engl J Med 311:850–851
86. Reichenbach DD, Bendilt EP (1979) Catecholamines and cardiomyopathy: the pathogenesis and potential importance of myofibrillar degeneration. Hum Pathol 1:125–150
87. Alderman J, Grossman W (1985) Are β-adrenergic blocking drugs useful in the treatment of dilated cardiomyopathy? Circulation 71:834–857
88. Deitchman D, LaBudde JA, Seidehaml RJ (1983) Bucindolol. In: Scriabine A (ed) New drugs annual: cardiovascular drugs. Raven, New York, pp 1–18
89. Gilbert EM, Anderson JL, Deitchman D, Bartholomew M, Mealey P, Yanowitz FG, Bristow MR (1987) Chronic β-blockade with bucindolol improves resting cardiac function in dilated cardiomyopathy. Circulation 76:1423
90. Cohn JN, Levine TB, Olivaire MT (1984) Plasma norepinephrine as a guide to prognosis in patients with chronic congestive heart failure. N Engl J Med 311:819–823
91. Bristow MR, Port TF, Sandoval AB, Rasmussen R, Ginsburg R, Feldman AM (1989) β-adrenergic receptor pathways in the failing human heart. Heart Failure 5:77–90
92. Gilbert EM, Port TD, Hershberger RE, Bristow MR (1989) Clinical significance of alterations in the β-adrenergic receptor-adenylate cyclase complex in heart failure. Heart Failure 5:91–98

Immune-Genetic Control of Anti-β-Receptor Antibodies in Human Idiopathic Dilated Cardiomyopathy

C. J. Limas and C. Limas

There is growing recognition that changes in β-adrenoceptor function play an important role in determining myocardial dysfunction in the syndrome of clinical heart failure [1, 2]. β-Adrenergic pathways are involved in several pathways regulating inotropism, including sarcolemmal calcium channels, the sarcoplasmic reticulum calcium pump and the affinity of contractile proteins for Ca^{2+}. Diminished ability to modulate these pathways through stimulation of the β-adrenergic receptors in heart failure may not only contribute to the impaired pump performance but, also, limit the usefulness of β-agonists as therapeutic agents.

The biochemical basis for reduced inotropic responsiveness of the failing myocardium to β-agonists is the observed loss of membrane-bound β-adrenoceptors and consequent decline in the activity of isoproterenol-sensitive adenylate cyclase [1, 2]. Modification of the guanine nucleotide binding proteins may also play a role but the data are not yet conclusive [3]. In any case, the pathogenesis of the β-receptor changes is likely to be multifactorial. Within the context of end-stage heart failure, loss of cell membrane β-receptors is usually associated with a substantial activation of the sympathetic nervous system [4] and it is possible that agonist-induced "down" regulation of the receptors plays an important role. This mechanism, however, is less likely to participate in earlier stages or milder degrees of heart failure in which activation of the sympathetic nervous system is modest or absent. Furthermore, the contribution of the disease processes leading to heart failure has not been systematically evaluated.

We have recently reported [5] that a substantial subset of patients with dilated cardiomyopathy have serum autoantibodies reacting with cardiac β-adrenoceptors as judged by a ligand binding inhibition assay. The autoantibodies appear to react preferentially with $β_1$-receptors and modulate the activity of isoproterenol-sensitive adenylate cyclase. There is a quantitative difference in the ability of sera from dilated cardiomyopathy (DCM) or ischemic/valvular heart disease (IVD) patients to inhibit binding of [^{3}H]dihydroalprenolol to cardiac β-receptors; i.e., about 40% of IDC but only 15% of IVD patients are positive at a 100-fold serum dilution (Fig. 1). It should be noted that, although rat cardiac membranes were routinely used for the ligand binding assay in these experiments, a strong correlation with results obtained using human myocardial tissue (Fig. 2) validates the appropriateness of this approach.

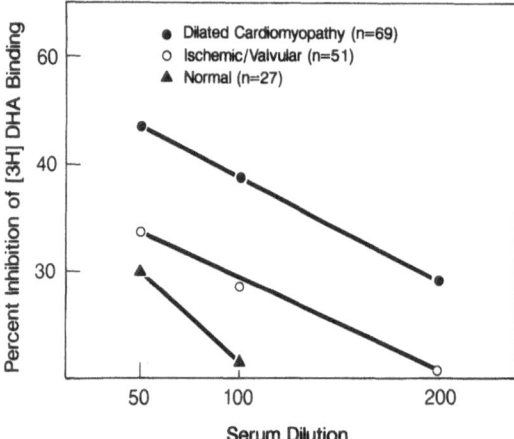

Fig. 1. Comparison of the effects of sera from dilated cardiomyopathy or ischemic/valvular heart disease patients and normal controls on [³H]dihydroalprenolol binding to rat cardiac membranes. Reactions were carried out as previously described and the results are expressed as percent inhibition of binding to control membranes (in the absence of serum)

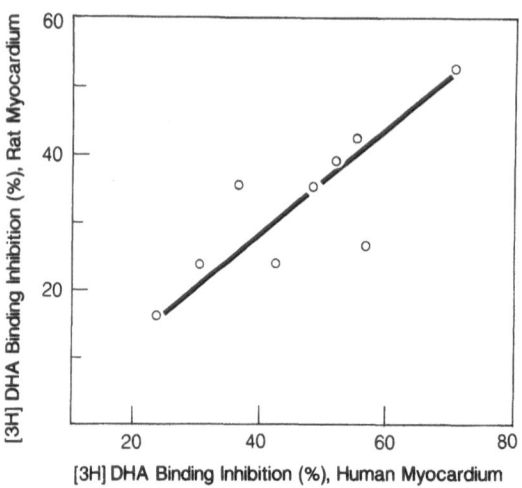

Fig. 2. Comparison of the results of ligand-binding inhibition assays using either rat or human cardiac membranes for nine patients with dilated cardiomyopathy who underwent cardiac transplantation. Serum (100-fold dilution) and left ventricular tissue from the same patient were used for each assay

It is not clear what distinguishes the subgroup of patients with DCM who present with anti-receptor antibodies from those who do not. It is quite possible that the nosologic heterogeneity of dilated cardiomyopathy is a partial explanation. Since this disease is defined by the presence of systolic dysfunction and ventricular dilatation in the absence of identifiable etiology, it may represent the morphologic expression of different pathogenetic pathways. It would be useful, therefore, to examine the possible association of anti-receptor antibodies with specific pathophysiologic mechanisms.

We have obtained initial evidence that immunogenetic factors may play a role both in the genesis of dilated cardiomyopathy and the presence of anti-receptor antibodies. First, as the data in Tables 1 and 2 demonstrate, there is a statistically significant increase in the prevalance of HLA-DR4 phenotype in DCM patients (40% compared to 24% in normals or patients with ischemic heart disease). This would correspond to a relative risk of 2.2 and an etiologic factor of 0.24. Similar results have been reported [6] by Komajda et al. In contrast, no difference exists in the distribution of Class I HLA antigens. Although this association is not as high as that reported for other diseases of presumed autoimmune origin [7], this may simply reflect the heterogeneity of dilated cardiomyopathy. This hypothesis is supported when the distribution of HLA antigens among anti-receptor antibody-positive and -negative patients is compared (Fig. 3).

Although the distribution of Class I HLA antigens is similar in the two groups (data not shown), two important differences are apparent in the distribution of HLA-DR antigens. First, there is a sixfold difference in the prevalence of

Table 1. Distribution of Class I HLA antigens in dilated cardiomyopathy (DCM, $n = 120$) and normal controls (N, $n = 617$)

	HLA-A DCM		N		HLA-B DCM		N		HLA-C DCM		N
	(n)	(%)	(%)		(n)	(%)	(%)		(n)	(%)	(%)
A_1	42	35.0	27.4	B_7	29	24.2	24.8	Cw_1	3	2.0	7.5
A_2	69	57.5	49.3	B_8	22	18.3	19.6	Cw_2	7	5.8	9.7
A_3	32	27.0	25.0	B_{13}	7	5.8	3.9	Cw_3	19	15.8	20.1
A_{11}	13	10.8	11.5	B_{14}	7	5.8	7.9	Cw_4	13	10.8	22.1
Aw_{24}	25	20.8	19.4	B_{27}	13	10.8	7.6	Cw_5	7	5.8	11.7
A_{28}	11	9.2	8.3	Bw_{35}	10	8.3	16.4				
Aw_{30}	10	8.3	4.0	Bw_{39}	4	3.3	4.2				
Aw_{32}	7	5.8	7.8	Bw_{44}	42	35.0	23.2				
				Bw_{51}	10	8.3	9.9				
				Bw_{62}	25	20.8	10.9				

Table 2. Distribution of HLA-DR antigens in dilated cardiomyopathy patients and normal controls

HLA-DR	DCM (n)	(%)	N (%)
DR_1	20	17.0	20.0
DR_2	31	25.8	31.5
DR_3	34	28.3	23.1
DR_4	49	40.8[a]	24.0
DR_5	31	25.8	18.4
DRw_6	29	24.2	20.0
DR_7	27	17.0	22.5
DRw_8	7	5.8	3.4

[a] $p_c < 0.001$.

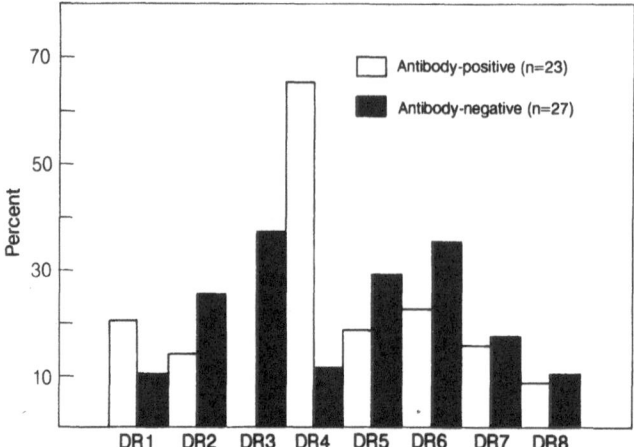

Fig. 3. Percentage distribution of Class II HLA antigens (*DR*) in anti-β-receptor antibody-positive (*n* = 23) or -negative (*n* = 27) patients with dilated cardiomyopathy

HLA-DR4 antigen between antibody-positive and -negative patients (65% vs. 11%). Secondly, there is a striking difference in the distribution of HLA-DR3 between the two groups: none of the 23 antibody-positive compared to ten of the 27 (37%) antibody-negative patients typed for HLA-DR3. These findings have two important implications: first, they confirm the predominant association of the presence of anti-receptor antibodies with the HLA-DR4 phenotype in dilated cardiomyopathy. The presence of such antibodies is, therefore, limited to a subgroup of dilated cardiomyopathy patients in which immunogenetic factors appear to play a major role. Secondly, they raise the possibility that factors protecting against the development of autoimmune responses may also exist and be linked to the presence of HLA-DR3 phenotype.

The nature of the association between HLA-DR4 and anti-receptor antibodies was further examined. As shown in Fig. 4, the presence of antibodies in HLA-DR4(+) patients was considerably higher than in HLA-DR4(–) patients; in the latter, it was mostly limited to those with HLA-DR1 phenotype. This

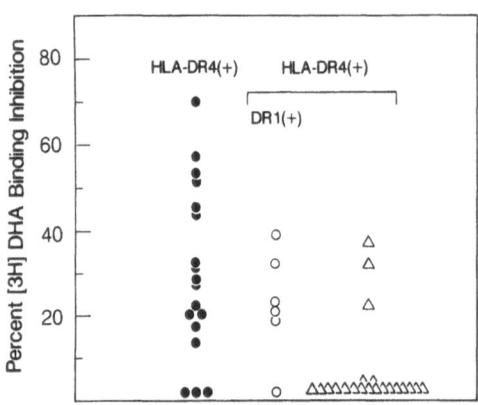

Fig. 4. Comparison of the ligand-binding inhibition assays using 100-fold serum dilutions from HLA-DR4 (+) and -DR4 (–) negative patients with dilated cardiomyopathy

may have pathogenetic implications because of the reported [8] homology between the β-chain of HLA-DR1 and the Dw14 subtype of HLA-DR4. Indeed, in preliminary experiments, we have found that about 80% of the HLA-DR4(+) patients type as Dw14. If confirmed by a larger series, this would indicate that the predominant association of anti-receptor antibodies is with the Dw14 subtype of HLA-DR4.

The second question addressed is whether the presence of anti-receptor antibodies in ischemic heart disease also shows an association with HLA-DR4 phentoype. As Table 3 shows, however, no such association was found in this series, indicating that different mechanisms operated in cardiomyopathy and noncardiomyopathy patients. The higher prevalence of the HLA-DRw6 antigen in ischemic cardiomyopathy increases in accord with our recent observation [9]. Interestingly, none of the HLA-DR4 patients with ischemic/valvular heart disease belonged to the Dw14 subtype.

There has been longstanding speculation about the role of immunological dysfunction in the etiology of dilated cardiomyopathy and, indeed, several humoral and cellular immune defects have been described [10–13]. These, however, are usually present in the established stage of the disease and their relationship to the initiation of myocardial damage is uncertain. Morphologic evidence of acute myocarditis is the exception rather than the rule in cases of dilated cardiomyopathy. It is likely that immunologic factors are involved in only a subset of dilated cardiomyopathy, and identification of this subset may help not only in the pathophysiologic subclassification of dilated cardiomyopathy, but also in designing better therapeutic strategies. Our results suggest that development of anti-receptor antibodies and, possibly other autoimmune responses, is linked to the presence of the HLA-DR4 phenotype. Whether this association is limited to specific DR4 subtypes is not established, but is currently under investigation in our laboratory. Since β-receptor autoantibodies can modify cardiac adenylate cyclase activity [5], their presence may have important functional implications in the failing human myocardium. There may be considerable heterogeneity in the interactions of anti-receptor antibodies with the cardiac β-receptor-adenylate cyclase system. For example, we have found both stimulatory and inhibitory effects of sera from dilated cardiomyo-

Table 3. Distribution of HLA-DR antigens in antireceptor antibody-positive and -negative patients with ischemic or valvular heart disease

| | Antibody-positive ($n = 15$) | | Antibody-negative ($n = 54$) | |
	(n)	(%)	(n)	(%)
DR_1	5	30	11	20
DR_2	3	20	10	18
DR_3	3	20	12	22
DR_4	4	25	12	22
DR_5	2	13	13	25
DRw6	6	40	22	41
DR_7	1	7	6	11
DRw8	–	–	3	7

pathy patients on the cardiac adenylate cyclase. It is also possible that, in some cases, the predominant interaction takes place with post-receptor components; e.g., the G proteins or the catalytic subunit component of the enzyme. These issues remain to be systematically studies.

Our recent observation [14] that the titer of anti-receptor antibodies declines following cardiac transplantation underscores the dynamic interaction between abnormal immune responses and the presence of exposed autoantigens. Since immunosuppressant are routinely used following cardiac transplantation, the decline in autoantibody titers may be a consequence of such therapy. The implication of this interpretation would be that demonstration of anti-receptor antibodies may identify a subgroup of dilated cardiomyopathy patients in whom immunosuppressive therapy might be effective. This hypothesis has yet to be directly tested.

References

1. Bristow MR, Ginsburg R, Minobe W, Cubicciotti RS, Sageman NS, Lurie K, Billingham ME, Harrison DC, Stinson EG (1982) Decreased catecholamine sensitivity and β-adrenergic receptor density in failing human hearts. N Engl J Med 307:205–211
2. Goff SA, Andersen D, Hansson V (1986) Beta-adrenoceptor density and adenylate cyclase response in right atrial and left ventricular myocardium of patients with mitral valve disease. Cardiovasc Res 20:331–336
3. Insel PH, Ransnas LA (1988) G proteins and cardiovascular disease. Circulation 78:1511–1513
4. Francis GS (1988) Neuroendocrine manifestations of congestive heart failure. Am J Cardiol 62:9A–14A
5. Limas CJ, Goldenberg IF, Limas C (1989) Autoantibodies against β-adrenoceptors in human idiopathic dilated cardiomyopathy. Circ Res 64:97–103
6. Komajda M, Raffoux C, Salame E (1987) Antigenes HLA A, B et DR dans les myocardiopathies dilatées. Arch Mal Coeur 80:1233–1237
7. Svejgaard A, Platz P, Ryder LP (1983) HLA and disease, 1982. Immunol Rev 70:193–218
8. Todd JA, Bell JI, McDevitt HO (1987) HLA-DQ$_\beta$ gene contributes to susceptibility and resistance to insulin-dependent diabetes mellitus. Nature 329:599–604
9. Limas CJ, Limas C (1988) HLA-DRw6 antigen linkage in chronic congestive heart failure secondary to coronary artery disease (ischemic cardiomyopathy). Am J Cardiol 62:816–818
10. Franceschini R, Petillo A, Corrazza M, Nizzo MC, Azzolini A, Gianrossi R (1983) Lymphocyte blastogenic response in dilated cardiomyopathy. IRCS Med Sci 11:1019–1023
11. Anderson JL, Carlquist IF, Hammond EH (1982) Deficient natural killer cell activity in patients with idiopathic dilated cardiomyopathy. Lancet 2:1124–1127
12. Sanders V, Ritts RE Jr (1965) Ventricular localization of bound gammaglobulins in idiopathic disease of the myocardium. JAMA 196:171–174
13. Takamoto T, Hory Y, Takenaga M (1987) Surface marker studies on activated peripheral blood lymphocytes in idiopathic dilated cardiomyopathy. J Clin Lab Immunol 22:157–162
14. Limas CJ, Goldenberg IF, Limas C (1989) Effect of cardiac transplantation on anti-beta-receptor antibodies in idiopathic dilated cardiomyopathy. Am J Cardiol 63:1134–1137

Catecholamines, β-Receptors and Morphology in Dilated Cardiomyopathy: A Preliminary Report

R. De Maria, R. Accinni, G. Baroldi, A. Repossini, G. Garino-Canina, A. Caroli, T. Vago, M. Bevilacqua, and A. Pellegrini

Introduction

In experimental and human congestive heart failure marked reduction in myocardial catecholamine concentration and increased plasma catecholamine levels have been observed. This adrenergic activation appears independent of underlying heart disease and correlates to severity of failure [1–8].

The mechanisms leading to tissue catecholamine depletion are still unclear. Norepinephrine turnover seems unchanged [2] and an increase in norepinephrine release [9] is partly due to reduced cardiac uptake [10]. Reduction in tyrosine-hydroxylase in experimental right heart failure [11] and increase in dopamine concentration associated with norepinephrine depletion in the cardiomyopathic Syrian hamster [12, 13] suggested a block in norepinephrine synthesis, due to loss of dopamine-beta-hydroxylase from nerve terminals in response to sympathetic overstimulation. Dopamine accumulation should induce a negative feedback on norepinephrine synthesis, a concept apparently supported by the findings in small human series [14, 15], but not confirmed in a larger one, in which variable myocardial catecholamine patterns were observed [7].

Other studies in failing hearts excised at transplantation [18] and in biopsies from patients with heart failure [19] have shown a decrease in beta-adrenergic receptor density, related to the degree of contractile dysfunction. This decrease seems prevalently due to a selective beta$_1$-down-regulation, while the beta$_2$-subpopulation is apparently preserved [20].

The lack of a correlative study on myocardial catecholamine concentration, beta-adrenergic receptor density, contractile status, and morphology suggested the present investigation.

Materials

Our study population includes 40 consecutive patients undergoing heart transplantation for end-stage heart failure. They were subdivided as follows: 18 with dilated cardiomyopathy (DC), eight with a prosthetic valve (mitral in seven, aortic in one) for valvular heart disease (VHD), and 14 with ischemic heart disease (IHD with previous myocardial infarction in 12, anterior in eight,

Table 1. Clinical, histologic, and hemodynamic findings in heart failure patients. Values are mean ± standard deviation

Variable	All cases	DC	IHD	VHD
Age (years)	41 ± 15	38 ± 12	41 ± 19	47 ± 10
Male/female ratio	4.7	5	6	3
Duration of disease (months)	65 ± 53	51 ± 34	81 ± 72	74 ± 52
Duration of failure (months)	13 ± 16	11 ± 16	15 ± 16	15 ± 18
			b	
Heart weight (g)	504 ± 138	501 ± 114[a]	[a]407 ± 72[b]	[b]656 ± 134
LV fibrosis (%)	14.8 ± 23	2 ± 4[a]	[a]37 ± 28[b]	[b]4 ± 5
RV fibrosis (%)	0.5 ± 0.9	0.3 ± 0.5	0.6 ± 1.3	0.6 ± 0.9
LV thickness (mm)	15.2 ± 4	16.5 ± 2[b]	[b]12.2 ± 5[b]	[b]17.5 ± 4
IVS thickness (mm)	13.6 ± 4	14.3 ± 3[c]	[c]10.9 ± 4[c]	[c]15.8 ± 3
RV thickness (mm)	8.4 ± 3	8.2 ± 3	8.3 ± 3	8.8 ± 4
Mean right atrial press (mmHg)	10 ± 13	9 ± 7	14 ± 22	8 ± 6
Mean wedge pressure (mmHg)	24 ± 9	25 ± 10	23 ± 10	23 ± 7
Pulmonary vascular res. (Wu)	2.7 ± 1.6	3.1 ± 1.6	2.4 ± 1.7	2.2 ± 1.3
Cardiac index (l/min/sm)	2.2 ± 0.6	2.1 ± 0.5	2.2 ± 0.7	2.3 ± 0.5
Ejection fraction (%)	21 ± 11	16 ± 15[c]	[c]27 ± 15	20 ± 6

[a] $p < 0.001$.
[b] $p < 0.01$.
[c] $p < 0.05$.

inferior or posterior in four). Mean age, duration of disease and duration of overt heart failure were not different in the three groups (Table 1). Fifteen DC, ten IHD, and eight VHD patients had right heart catheterization prior to transplantation. Ejection fraction was obtained at angiography in five and at echocardiography in 20 patients (Table 1).

The heart of a 46-year-old male donor was used as normal control. This heart was not transplanted because of the recipient's death just prior to surgery. The donor had been treated with low dose dopamine (< 10 mcg/kg/min) during observation. Time interval between brain death and excision was 12 h and from excision to sampling four hours, during which the heart was preserved in cold saline at +4 °C.

Methods

The heart excised at transplantation was weighed. Myocardial thickness was measured at the basal and apical level of the anterior and posterior right and left ventricular wall and interventricular septum. Transmural myocardial samples were obtained by a manual cork bore (1 cm cross-section) from ten sites at different levels of both ventricular chambers; a sample was also obtained from the anterior papillary muscle (except for VHD patients with mitral prosthesis, in whom it had been previously removed at surgery) and apex.

Each transmural sample was then longitudinally divided in two halves, frozen in liquid nitrogen and stored at −80 °C for subsequent analysis. One-half was assayed with high-performance liquid chromatography with electrochemical detection for norepinephrine, epinephrine, and dopamine concentration. In the other half, beta-adrenergic receptor density and dissociation constant were measured by radioligand binding assay using H_3-dihydroalprenolol (DHA, specific activity 90–92 Ci/mole).

In eleven cases (six DC, five IHD) an additional sample obtained from the apical portion of the left ventricular posterior wall was subdivided in three parts (epicardium, endocardium, and middle zone) for catecholamine assay.

Coronary arteries were sequentially cross sectioned at 3-mm intervals. The heart was then cut into five slices and fixed in 10% buffered formalin. Myocardial tissue surrounding each transmural sample for biochemistry was coded. Samples for histology were embedded in paraffin. Each section was stained with hematoxylin-eosin, Masson's trichrome and van Gieson stain for elastin. The area of each histologic section was calculated by computer analysis. A semiquantitative evaluation in percent fibrosis per total section area was performed on each slide. The normal donor heart was processed according to the same protocol.

Statistical Analysis

Intergroup and intragroup differences between means were tested by Student's t test on paired and unpaired data. Differences between sites were tested by the method of Friedman (analysis of variance for paired data). Correlation coefficients were calculated to determine the relationship between two variables. Standard deviations of the means are given. Stepwise multiple regression was used to identify independent variables capable of influencing norepinephrine and beta-receptor concentrations in the myocardium. All statistical computations were performed using the Statistical Package for the Social Sciences Program (SPSS by SPSS Inc. Chicago, Ill).

Results

Biochemical Data

For this analysis 27 cases in whom all sites gave reproducible results were included (Tables 2, 3).

Similar significant right to left and base to apex gradients were demonstrated for myocardial norepinephrine in all the three groups. In the 11 cases in whom the epi-endocardial gradient was tested, no difference in norepinephrine content in the three layers was noted. As regards dopamine distribution, only in DC cases a right to left gradient was shown. No gradients were evident for beta-adrenergic receptors and dissociation constant, except in IHD patients, in whom RV showed a higher density and higher dissociation constant than LV.

Norepinephrine concentration (expressed in pg/mg) was similar in all cases without significant differences (DC 671 ± 296, IHD 792 ± 644, VDH 605 ± 874).

Table 2. Myocardial catecholamine concentration in heart failure patients

Site	RV	LV		Basal	Apical		Total
	mean ± SD n%	mean ± SD n%	p	mean ± SD n%	mean ± SD n%	p	
Norepinephrine (pg/mg)							
Normal	2312	1573		2266	1618		1942
Dilated CMP 13	882 ± 416 38	459 ± 239 29	0.001	770 ± 365 34	571 ± 272 35	0.14	671 ± 296
Ischemic HD 5	1190±1018 51	396 ± 298 25	0.034	878 ± 683 39	708 ± 650 44	0.000	792 ± 644
Valvular HD 6	774 ± 517 33	437 ± 272 28	0.044	502 ± 295 31	502 ± 295 31	0.022	605 ± 874
24	934 ± 638 40	427 ± 250 27	0.000	782 ± 456 35	589 ± 397 36	0.000	685 ± 406
Dopamine (pg/mg)							
Normal	2173	1606		1998	1781		1889
Dilated CMP 13	241 ± 198 11	128 ± 119 8	0.009	169 ± 109 8	201 ± 227 11	0.563	185 ± 150
Ischemic HD 5	394 ± 190 18	216 ± 264 13	0.230	270 ± 107 14	340 ± 216 19	0.588	305 ± 108
Valvular HD 6	93 ± 70 4	78 ± 88 5	0.319	99 ± 95 5	72 ± 61 4	0.127	86 ± 78
24	236 ± 196 11	134 ± 126 8	0.005	173 ± 117 9	198 ± 221 11	0.509	186 ± 144

LV, Anterior basal + anterior apical + posterior basal + posterior apical LV samples; *RV,* Anterior basal + anterior apical + posterior basal + posterior apical RV samples; *Basal,* LV anterior and posterior basal + RV anterior and posterior basal samples; *Apical,* LV anterior and posterior apical + RV anterior and posterior apical samples; *SD,* standard deviation; *n%,* percentage of normal values.

RV dopamine was significantly lower in VHD vs. DC (93 ± 70 vs. 291 ± 198, p 0.03) and vs. IHD (93 ± 70 vs. 394 ± 190 p 0.02). VHD and IHD patients showed a lower beta-receptor density (expressed in μmol/mg of wet tissue) vs. DC (49 ± 18 vs. 74 ± 13, p 0.001 and 44 ± 21 vs. 74 ± 13, p 0.01). However when right and left ventricular samples were seperately analyzed, differences were significant in DC vs. VHD for the right ventricle only (RV DC 75 ± 14 vs. VHD 40 ± 21, $p < 0.01$) and in DC vs. IHD for the left ventricle only (LV DC 73 ± 17 vs. IHD 32 ± 17, $p < 0.01$). Dissociation constant was lower in IHD vs. DC (.67 ± .14 vs. .84 ± .17, p 0.04) and vs. VHD (.67 ± .14 vs. 1.04 ± .21, p 0.01).

To evaluate the effects of differing degrees of pump dysfunction on biochemical variables, two groups according to ejection fraction values (EF < 0.20 and EF > 0.20) were examined. A significantly greater beta-receptors density was present in patients with lower ejection fraction (71 ± 17 vs. 43 ± 23, p 0.01 for whole heart, 70 ± 21 vs. 36 ± 15, p 0.01 for LV).

Morphopathology

In DC and VHD patients coronary arteries were practically normal, whereas in all IHD patients severe obstructive atherosclerotic lesions were observed. VHD hearts were significantly more hypertrophic than DC hearts, while both

Table 3. Myocardial beta-adrenergic receptor density and dissociation constant in heart failure patients

Site	RV			LV				Basal			Apical				Total	
	mean ± SD	n%		mean ± SD	n%	p		mean ± SD	n%		mean ± SD	n%	p		mean ± SD	
Beta-adrenergic receptors (f. mol/mg)																
Normal	184			157				182			159				170	
Dilated CMP	14	75 ± 14	41	73 ± 18	46	0.78		75 ± 15	41		73 ± 13	46	0.25		741 ± 13	
Ischemic HD	6	56 ± 26	30	32 ± 17	20	0.004		45 ± 22	24		43 ± 20	28	0.056		44 ± 21	
Valvular HD	3	40 ± 21	22	58 ± 17	37	0.11		50 ± 16	27		49 ± 20	31	0.90		49 ± 18	
	23	65 ± 22	35	61 ± 24	39	0.78		64 ± 22	35		63 ± 21	40	0.51		63 ± 21	
Dissociation constant (nM)																
Normal	1.57			1.46				1.58			1.45				1.51	
Dilated CMP	13	0.80 ± 0.17	51	0.84 ± 0.17	58	0.41		0.86 ± 0.21	54		0.78 ± 0.14	54	0.17		0.82 ± 0.15	
Ischemic HD	6	1.0 ± 0.24	64	0.67 ± 0.14	46	0.001		0.83 ± 0.20	53		0.84 ± 0.18	28	0.91		0.83 ± 0.19	
Valvular HD	3	0.92 ± 0.20	59	1.04 ± 0.21	71	0.66		1.04 ± 0.04	66		0.92 ± 0.04	31	0.10		1.98 ± 0.01	
	22	0.87 ± 0.15	55	0.82 ± 0.04	56	0.35		0.82 ± 0.03	52		0.88 ± .04	40	0.087		0.82 ± 0.15	

LV, Anterior basal + anterior apical + posterior basal + posterior apical LV samples; *RV*, Anterior basal + anterior apical + posterior basal + posterior apical RV samples; *Basal*, LV anterior and posterior basal + RV anterior and posterior basal samples; *Apical*, LV anterior and posterior apical + RV anterior and posterior apical samples; *SD*, standard deviation; *n%*, percentage of normal values.

DC and VHD were significantly more hypertrophic than IHD hearts as expressed by heart weight and LV wall and septal thickness. The LV anterior wall was significantly more fibrous in IHD vs. DC and VHD (37% ± 28 vs. 2 ± 4, $p < 0.001$ and vs. 4 ± 5, $p < 0.01$). RV wall thickness was mildly increased, with minimal fibrosis in the three groups (Table 1).

Linear Regression Analysis

For this analysis all cases in whom catecholamines and beta-receptors were assayed in the RV and LV anterior wall were included (18 DC, 14 IHD, and eight VHD). A p value < 0.01 was considered significant. In all cases a significant correlation was found, independently of underlying heart disease, between norepinephrine and dopamine concentration in the right ventricle ($r\,0.44$, $p\,0.003$).

All clinical, histologic, hemodynamic and biochemical variables listed in Tables 1–3 were analyzed by linear regression analysis. Only the following significant correlations were found:
- In IHD an inverse relationship between septal thickness and LV fibrosis ($r\,0.68$, $p\,0.007$).
- In VHD and inverse relationship between LV norepinephrine and LV wall thickness ($r\,0.81$, $p\,0.007$).

Stepwise Multiple Regression Analysis

A multivariate analysis was performed to select variables influencing myocardial catecholamines content and beta-adrenergic receptor density. The following variables were considered: underlying heart disease, NYHA class at surgery, duration of disease, duration of heart failure, the histologic and hemodynamic variables listed in Table 1. In 20 cases the major independent variable inversely related to norepinephrine concentration was NYHA class at the time of transplantation (r 0.33, $p < 0.01$). In respect of dopamine concentration, no relation with any variable was found. In 17 cases, the major independent variables linked with beta-adrenergic receptor density were the percentage of myocardial fibrosis and underlying heart disease. Beta-receptor density was progressively more reduced in valvular heart disease than in ischemic heart disease and dilated cardiomyopathy (r^2 0.52, $p < 0.01$). In 13 of these 17 cases, in whom ejection fraction was available, the multivariate analysis showed a direct relationship between beta-receptor density and pulmonary vascular resistance and an inverse relationship between beta-rezeptor density and ejection fraction. Dissociation constant was inversely related to wedge pressure only (r 0.42, p 0.01).

Discussion

In heart failure, the adrenergic nervous system exerts a critical function in supporting contractility. However, chronic stimulation of the beta-adrenergic pathway, through increased circulating levels of catecholamines and increased turn over rate of norepinephrine at myocardial nerve endings, results in beta-receptors down-regulation. Consequently decresed cardiac contractility activates a vicious circle of depressed inotropism and increased catecholamine stimulation with further depression of inotropism [21, 22]. Based on these theoretical principles, clinical studies using beta-blockers in heart failure [16, 17] represent an attempt to break this vicious circle. The long-term administration of beta-blockers seems to provide effective cardioprotection with associated beta-receptor up-regulation [22, 17].

The present study confirms the existence of myocardial right to left and base to apex gradients for catecholamines [6, 7, 23, 24]. Furthermore, it shows the absence of an epi-endocardial gradient; this finding validates the data obtained on tissue sampled at endomyocardial biopsy. In disagreement with others [25], no myocardial gradient for beta-receptors was seen. Thus, in contrast to norepinephrine, the sampling site seems to have no particular relevance in respect of beta-receptor distribution.

One limiting factor in any biochemical tissue study of the myocardium is the difficulty to have normal control values. In respect of catecholamine content in normal myocardium, we only refer to a single autopsy heart obtained at four hours after death from a 58-year-old patient dying from lymphocytic lymphoma of the brain [24], or to small amounts of tissue sampled from specific sites during surgery from nonfailing but diseased hearts [14]. The present material was compared with a single normal donor heart. However, in agreement with others [6, 18], we found a 65% reduction in myocardial norepinephrine and 56% reduction in beta-receptor density with parallel behavior of dissociation constant. The lack of information on the normal content of dopamine in human myocardium may question the 90% reduction in dopamine found in all the three groups. The high concentration in the donor heart might partly be due to treatment. The low content of myocardial dopamine in healthy monkeys [24] may support this view. Nevertheless, the supposed marked elevation of myocardial dopamine in heart failure [14, 15] contrasts with these reference values. In VHD dopamine concentration and beta-receptor density in the right ventricle were significantly more reduced than in DC and IHD. One might speculate that in VHD a greater impairment of right ventricular function is responsible for lower RV dopamine and beta-receptor concentration, despite any evidence of specific clinical and hemodynamic abnormalities. However, most of the tests were obtained at entry into the waiting list (an average of 3.5 months before transplantation) and some change in the hemodynamic asset might have occurred in this interval. Multivariate analysis did not show any relation between all variables and catecholamine concentration. Only a clinical index of failure, i.e., NYHA class at the time of surgery, was linked to norepinephrine reduction.

In IHD left ventricular beta-receptor density and dissociation constant were significantly more reduced than in DC. By multiple regression analysis beta-receptor concentration appeared to be significantly influenced by both percentage of fibrosis and underlying heart disease. This finding may question beta-blocker treatment in failing hearts with ischemic heart disease, in which other factors (myocardial fibrosis, etc.) might impair the up-regulation response to therapy.

In contrast to other reports [19], this study fails to confirm a direct relationship between pump function and beta-receptor density. In fact, in the group of DC patients a significantly lower EF value corresponded to a greater receptors content, a finding also observed when all cases were studied in relation to ejection fraction only (EF < or > 0.20), thus showing that the inverse relationship (confirmed by multivariate analysis) is not specific to DC patients.

Conclusions

In this series of patients with heart failure, the aim was to correlate myocardial catecholamine pattern to beta-receptor density, clinical and morphological variables. Correlation between plasma and myocardial catecholamines was not attempted, because of the extreme variability in time elapsing from clinical evaluation to transplantation and the unreliability of data obtained just prior to surgery, in a highly stressful setting. In previous studies increased plasma and coronary sinus levels of norepinephrine were observed, suggesting decreased uptake and increased nerve-terminal secretion of this amine [9, 26]. The results of this study demonstrated a lack of correlation between myocardial catecholamine content and beta-receptors density, suggesting that humoral pattern or turnover rate changes are more important in beta-receptors down-regulation.

References

1. Sole MJ, Lo CM, Laird CW, Sonnenblick EH, Wurtman RJ (1975) Norepinephrine turnover in the heart and spleen of the cardiomyopathic sirian hamster. Circ Res 37:855–863
2. Spann JF, Chidsey CA, Pool PE, Braunwald E (1965) Mechanism of norepinephrine depletion in experimental heart failure produced by aortic constriction in the guinea pig. Circ Res 17:312–321
3. Vogel JHK, Jacobowitz D, Chidsey CA (1969) Distribution of norepinephrine in the failing bovine heart. Circ Res 24:71–84
4. Chidsey CA, Braunwald E, Morrow AG (1965) Catecholamine excretion and cardiac stores of norepinephrine in congestive heart failure. Am J Med 39:442–451
5. Kramer RS, Mason T, Braunwald E (1968) Augmented sympathetic neurotransmitter activity in the peripheral vascular bed of patients with congestive heart failure and cardiac norepinephrine depletion. Circulation 38:629–633
6. Kawai C, Yui Y, Hoshino T, Sasayama S, Matsumori A (1983) Myocardial catecholamines in hypertrophic and dilated (congestive) cardiomyopathy: a biopsy study. J Am Coll Cardiol 2:834–840
7. Pierpont GL, Francis GS, DeMaster EG, Olivari MT, Ring WS, Goldenberg IF, Reynolds S, Cohn JN (1987) Heterogeneous myocardial catecholamine concentrations in patients with congestive heart failure. Am J Cardiol 60:316–321
8. Cohn JN, Levine TB, Olivari MT, Garberg V, Lura D, Francis GS, Simon AB, Rector T (1984) Plasma norepinephrine as a guide to prognosis in patients with chronic congestive heart failure. N Engl J Med 311:819–823
9. Rose CP, Burgess JH, Coustineau D (1983) Reduced aortocoronary sinus extraction of epinephrine in patients with left ventricular failure secondary to long term pressure or volume overload. Circulation 68:241–244
10. Petch MC, Nayler WG (1979) Uptake of catecholamines by cardiac muscle in vitro. Br Heart J 41:336–339
11. Pool PE, Covell JW, Levitt M, Gibb J, Braunwald E (1967) Reduction of tyrosine hydroxylase activity in experimental congestive heart failure. Circ Res 20:349–353
12. Sole MJ, Kamble AB, Hussain MN (1977) A possible change in the rate-limiting step for cardiac norepinephrine synthesis in the cardiomyopathic syrian hamster. Circ Res 41:815–817
13. Sole MJ, Helke CJ, Jacobowitz DM (1982) Increased dopamine in the failing hamster heart: transvescicular transport of dopamine limits the rate of norepinephrine synthesis. Am J Cardiol 49:1682–1690
14. De Quattro V, Nagatsu T, Mendez A, Verska J (1973) Determinants of cardiac noradrenaline depletion in human congestive failure. Cardiovasc Res 7:344–350
15. Pierpont GL, Francis GS, DeMaster EG, Levine TB, Bolman RM, Cohn JV (1983) Elevated left ventricular myocardial dopamine in preterminal idiopathic dilated cardiomyopathy. Am J Cardiol 52:1033–1035
16. Swedberg K, Hjolwarson A, Holmberg S (1979) Effects of work and acute beta-receptor blockade on myocardial norepinephrine release in congestive cardiomyopathy. Clin Cardiol 2:424–430
17. Swedberg K, Hjalmarson A, Waagstein F, Wallentin I (1980) Beneficial effects of long term beta-blockade in congestive cardiomyopathy. Br Heart J 44:117–133
18. Bristow MR, Ginsburg R, Minobe W, Cubicciotti RS, Sageman WS, Lurie K, Billingham ME, Harrison DC, Stinson EB (1982) Decreased catecholamine sensitivity and beta-adrenergic-receptor density in failing human hearts. N Engl J Med 307:205–211

19. Fowler MB, Laser JA, Hopkins GL, Minobe W, Bristow MR (1986) Assessment of the beta-adrenergic receptor pathway in the intact failing human heart: progressive receptor down-regulation and subsensitivity to agonist response. Circulation 74:1290–1302
20. Bristow MR, Ginsburg R, Umans V, Fowler M, Minobe W, Rasmussen R, Zera P, Menlove R, Shah P, Jamieson S, Stinson EB (1986) Beta-1 and beta-2-adrenergic-receptor subpopulations in nonfailing and failing human ventricular myocardium: coupling of both receptor subtypes to muscle contraction and selective beta-1-receptor down-regulation in heart failure. Circ Res 59:297–309
21. Bristow MR (1984) The adrenergic nervous system in heart failure. N Engl J Med 311:850–851
22. Bristow MR, Kantrowitz NE, Ginsburg R, Fowler MB (1985) Beta-adrenergic function in heart muscle disease and heart failure. J Mol Cell Cardiol 17(2):41–52
23. Pierpont GL, DeMaster EG, Reynolds S, Pederson J (1985) Ventricular myocardial catecholamines in primates. J Lab Clin Med 106:205–210
24. Pierpont GL, DeMaster EG, Cohn J (1984) Regional differences in adrenergic function within the left ventricle. Am J Physiol 246 (Heart Circ Physiol 15):H824–H829
25. Baker SP, Boyd HM, Potter LT (1980) Distribution and function of beta-adrenoceptors in different chambers of the canine heart. Br J Pharmacol 68:57–63
26. Swedberg K, Chatterje K, Roizen M, Ports T, Parmley W (1982) Myocardial norepinephrine release in congestive heart failure. Circulation 66 [Suppl II]:23 (abstr)

2 Morphology of Dilated Cardiomyopathy

Histopathological Diagnosis of Acute Myocarditis and Dilated Cardiomyopathy

M. E. Billingham

Introduction

The histopathological diagnosis of acute fulminant myocarditis or endstage idiopathic cardiomyopathy at autopsy does not usually present a diagnostic problem. Clinically, however, it is difficult, if not impossible, to diagnose acute myocarditis because the presenting history and clinical features, as well as hemodynamic and electrophysiologic changes, are often similar to those of idiopathic dilated cardiomyopathy for which it is often mistaken and vice versa. The widespread use of the endomyocardial biopsy raised hopes that it would be possible to diagnose acute myocarditis more accurately by demonstrating a definite inflammatory infiltrate in the myocardium. It has been well documented in the literature that the presence of inflammatory infiltrates, including lymphocytes, in the myocardium are not always due to acute myocarditis and it has also been shown that lymphocytes themselves may be present in idiopathic dilated cardiomyopathy [1, 2]. This has led to confusion and, in some cases, over-diagnosis of acute myocarditis with a resulting diagnostic dilemma [3]. The purpose of this paper, therefore, is to attempt to define the histopathological changes of acute myocarditis in such a way that will allow, or at least help, to differentiate acute myocarditis from idiopathic dilated cardiomyopathy particularly on endomyocardial biopsy.

Patient Study Groups

The experience for this paper was obtained from several patient population groups.

1) Two hundred and fifty-one freshly explanted hearts from patients with endstage dilated cardiomyopathy;
2) Approximately 600 endomyocardial biopsies a year for the last 3 years from patients studied for idiopathic dilated cardiomyopathy prior to cardiac transplantation or on a consultation basis;
3) Approximately 300 endomyocardial biopsies a year over the last 2 years from patients suspected of having acute myocarditis and examined prior to entry into the multicenter myocarditis trial.

In addition, we studied the biopsies from three groups of patients studied particularly by ultrastructural studies: there were ten patients in each of the following groups:

Group 1:   Idiopathic dilated cardiomyopathy (IDCM). These were well-defined, classic cases based on clinical hemodynamic and biopsy criteria. The mean age was 44 ± 14 (SD).

Group 2:   Anthracycline-induced cardiotoxicity (AC). These patients all had grade III scores from their biopsies which is the most severe grade of toxicity and which leads to heart failure and ventricular dilatation. The mean age was 52 ± 19 (SD).

Group 3:   Control (C). These were young heart disease-free cardiac transplant donor hearts from accident victims. The mean age was 25 ± 9 (SD).

Tissue Collection and Processing

Endomyocardial biopsies were all taken from the right ventricular side of the interventricular septum using a Stanford-Caves-Schultz bioptome (9 French) including most of the control hearts although a few were taken with a TRU-cut biopsy needle during the transplant operation. All biopsy tissue was processed for electron microscopy by the same routine method of fixation in 2.5% glutaraldehyde and 2% formaldehyde in $0.1 M$ sodium cacodylate hydrochloride buffer, pH 7.4. All tissue was then post-fixed in 2% osmium tetroxide, stained on block in 2% uranyl acetate, dehydrated in ethanol and propylene oxide and embedded in epoxy resin. Sections for electron microscopy were cut with a diamond knife and an LKB ultratome-3, stained with lead citrate, and examined in a Phillips EM201 electron microscope.

Results   (The results are shown in Table 1)

Idiopathic Dilated Cardiomyopathy in Explanted Hearts

Random sections from 108 idiopathic dilated cardiomyopathy hearts fixed immediately and, in some cases, while still beating showed marked myocyte hypertrophy with some attenuation (thinning of the width by myofibrillar dropout). In every case the sections showed large bizarre-shaped myocyte nuclei in nearly all of the sections. The nuclei were not only much bigger but had more irregular outlines with the lowest form factor when compared with nuclei. These sections from most of the hearts included interstitial parenchymal and sometimes perivascular focal infiltrates of small lymphocytes. Only 13% of the 108 hearts did not contain lymphocytic infiltrates. Eighty-seven percent of the 108 cardiomyopathic hearts examined contained up to 30 foci or aggregates of lymphocytes in the six random sections studied from each heart. Details of this study were described in a previously published paper in much greater detail [1,

Table 1. Histopathology of primary acute myocarditis versus idiopathic dilated cardiomyopathy

Histopathological changes	Acute myocarditis	Dilated cardiomyopathy	Distinguishing features
1. Inflammatory infiltrate	+	+	−
→ Pattern of focal	+	+	−
→ Sparse	+	+	−
→ Diffuse	+	−	Yes
→ Mixed	+	−	Yes
→ Pyroninophilic lymphocytes	+	−	Yes
→ Lymphocyte subsets (T suppressor)	+	±	Possible
→ Endocarditis	+	−	Yes
→ Pericarditis	+	−	Yes
→ Vasculitis	+	−	Yes
2. Myocytes → Hypertrophy (global)	−	+	Yes
→ Hypertrophy (focal)	+	±	Possible
→ Nuclear enlargement (global)	−	+	Yes
→ Nuclear enlargement (focal)	+	−	Yes
→ Nuclear bizarre shape	−	+	Yes
→ Myofibrillar loss	−	+	Yes
→ Necrosis	+	−	Yes
3. Fibrosis → Focal	+	+	−
→ Global	− (unless healing)	+	Possible
4. Endocardium−width < 20 μm	+	−	Yes
> 20 μm	−	+	Yes

2]. It should be emphasized that the lymphocytic infiltrates did not correlate with adjacent myocyte damage. Most of the random sections showed a marked increase in fibrosis from normal; in some cases the right ventricular free wall showed less fibrosis than in the other sections.

Inflammatory Infiltrates in Endomyocardial Biopsies Studied

Myocarditis: The patterns of inflammatory infiltrate are enumerated in Table 1. It can be seen that the pattern of infiltrate in acute myocarditis is usually interstitial and diffuse with adjacent myocyte damage (Fig. 1). The infiltrate may be perivascular or focal however (Fig. 2). In fulminant myocarditis the infiltrate may also affect the endocardium and the pericardium as well as the myocardium. In severe cases the infiltrate is often mixed (with neutrophils, plasma cells and occasional eosinophils) and this is more commonly seen in children or in patients actually dying of acute myocarditis. In the more usual type the infiltrate consists of large activated lymphocytes with pyroninophilic cytoplasm. Lymphocyte subsets were not done in every case but our experience has been that the subsets are often mixed and are unreliable as a means of separating myocarditis from idiopathic dilated cardiomyopathy. In a previous paper we stated that the enumeration of T lymphocyte subpopulations had not yielded identical results by different investigators [4]. Maisch [5], however,

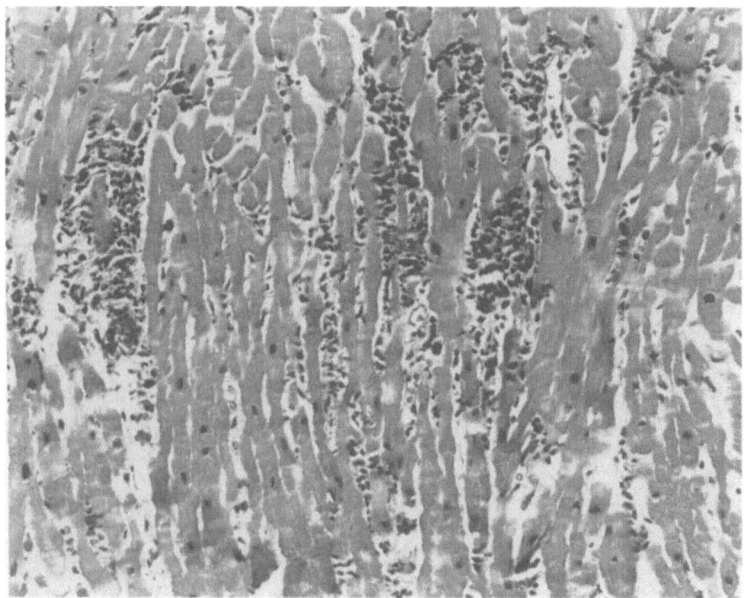

Fig. 1. Endomyocardial biopsy showing acute myocarditis with a diffuse pattern. Note normal background and lack of fibrosis. Hematoxylin and eosin; × 200

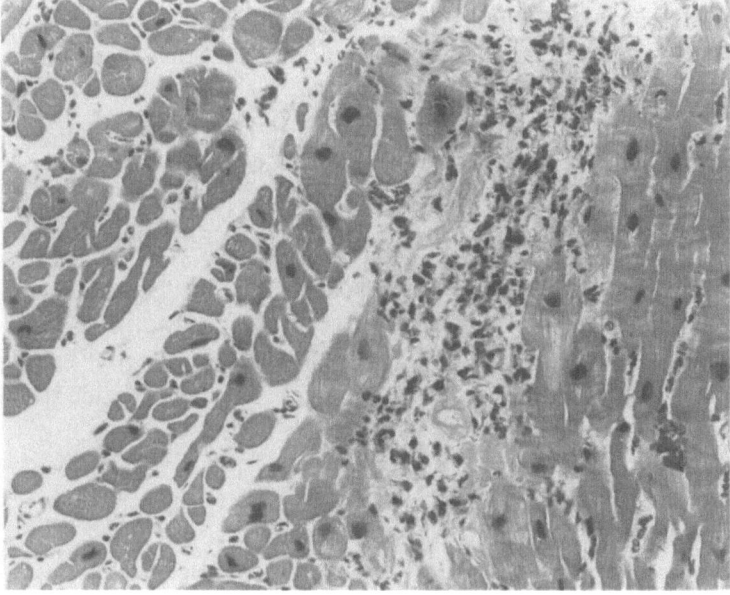

Fig. 2. Endomyocardial biopsy of acute myocarditis with myocyte damage. Note adjacent compensatory hypertrophy only and no interstitial fibrosis. Hematoxylin and eosin; × 200

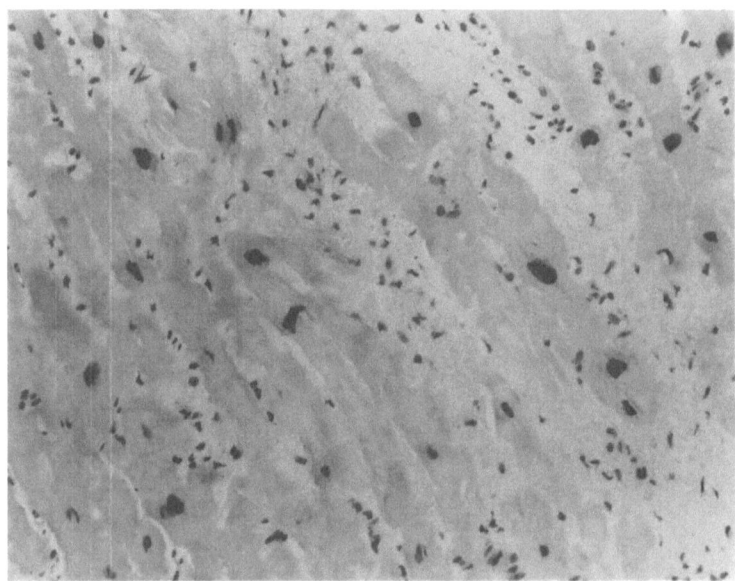

Fig. 3. Endomyocardial biopsy of dilated cardiomyopathy showing marked hypertrophy, interstitial fibrosis with infiltrate which is not myocarditis. Hematoxylin and eosin; × 200

could demonstrate a significant difference in pan-T, T helper, or T suppressor, natural killer cells and monocytes in the peripheral blood of patients with myocarditis. He found that B cells and activated T lymphocytes were significantly increased in acute perimyocarditis, and that there was a tendency for a decrease in T suppressor cells in postmyocarditic dilated heart disease.

Idiopathic Dilated Cardiomyopathy: The lymphocytic infiltrate in IDCM tends to be interstitial and is often within fibrosis (Fig. 3) but occasionally is in a perivascular location although, without vasculitis [1]. The infiltrates are never diffuse in IDCM and are usually only sparse or in small focal aggregates. Mixed infiltrates are not seen and the lymphocytes which are present tend to be composed of small, nonpyroninophilic cells. Occasional small aggregates can be seen in the epicardium but not reflecting a true pericarditis. Lymphocytic subsets in IDCM show a predilection for diminished T suppressor cells compared with acute myocarditis but these data have yielded variable results in different hands as already stated.

Myocyte Morphology

Myocarditis: In severe acute myocarditis the background myocyte morphology is often quite normal (see Fig. 1). When there is hypertrophy present it is usually focal rather than "global" and is usually compensatory to focal myocyte damage or fibrosis. Myocyte nuclei may also be within normal limits in size and shape. Electron microscopy may show myocyte degenerative changes but total myofibrillar loss as in cardiomyopathy (IDCM) is not usually seen (Fig. 4).

Table 2. Morphometric comparison (EM) of normal and dilated cardiomyopathy (IDCM) myocardium

	Control	IDCM	p
Myocyte (µm)	16.8 ± 2.2	29.3 ± 7.2	<0.01
Nuclear area (µm²)	45.0 ± 9.2	88.7 ± 27.1	<0.01
Nuclear form factor	0.43 ± 0.06	0.28 ± 0.09	<0.05

Idiopathic Dilated Cardiomyopathy: Myocyte morphology on light or electron microscopy in dilated cardiomyopathy characteristically shows marked myocyte hypertrophy with concomitant very large, bizarre-shaped nuclei [6]. As seen in Table 2, myocyte width was significantly greater in IDCM than the control ($p < 0.00$) and that the nuclear form factor (indicating a more irregular nuclear

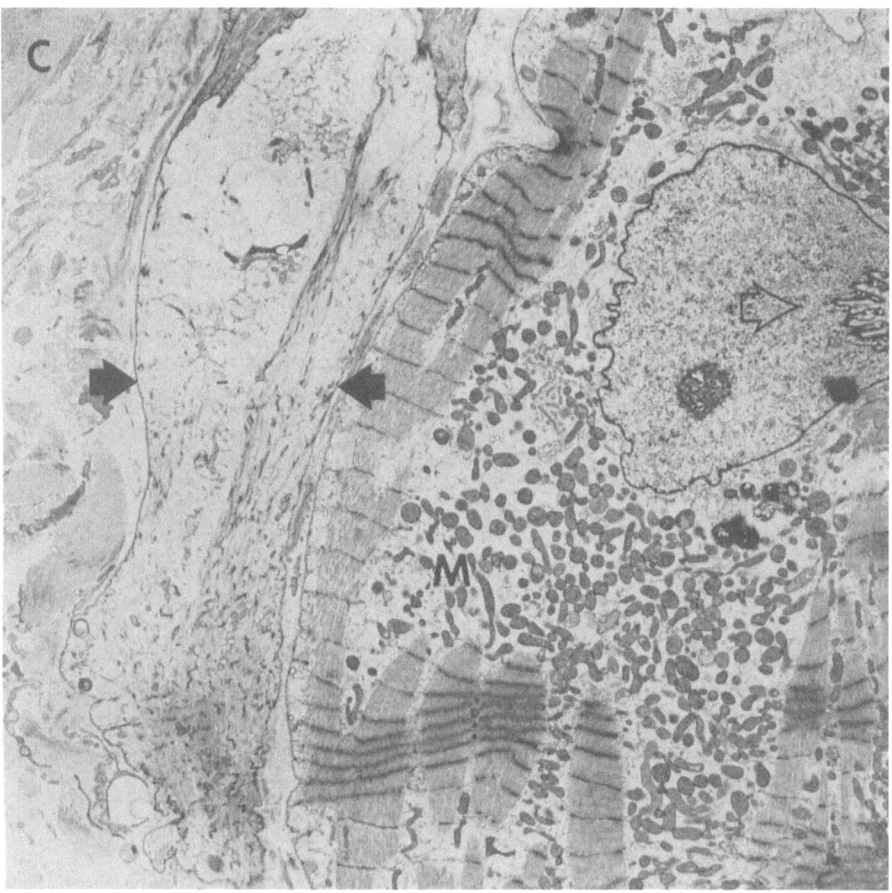

Fig. 4. Electron micrograph of dilated cardiomyopathy showing interstitial collagen (c), total myofibrillar loss in a myocyte (between two black arrows), characteristic small elongated mitochondria (M) and bizarre-shaped myocyte nucleus (*open arrow*). × 4000

outline) was significantly lower in IDCM than in controls corrected for sarcomere length ($p < 0.05$). Sometimes on light microscopy but more clearly on electron microscopy myofibrillar loss can also be seen (Fig. 4).

Fibrosis

Acute Myocarditis: Fibrosis may be entirely absent in an acute episode of myocarditis (see Fig. 1). During "ongoing" myocarditis reparative changes of focal newly formed fibrosis containing fibroblasts may be seen. Small stellate scars or fine immature newly formed fibrous tissue staining a pale blue with trichrome may be present in the interstitium. Large patchy scars of coarse fibrosis are not usually seen.

Idiopathic Dilated Cardiomyopathy: Fibrosis is nearly always present even on biopsies in IDCM. The fibrosis is usually quite mature and coarse, staining a dark blue with Masson's trichrome. The pattern of fibrosis is quite variable from a fine perimyocytic to coarse scars indistinguishable from those in chronic ischemia.

Discussion

From the findings above and Table 1 it can be seen that in certain circumstances a definite distinction between acute myocarditis and idiopathic cardiomyopathy can be made. In some cases the changes are equivocal and a distinction may only be suggestive and in other cases it may not be possible at all to distinguish acute myocarditis from IDCM within the confines of an endomyocardial biopsy. It can be seen from Table 1, however, that in 12 situations out of a possible 20, it is possible to distinguish acute myocarditis from idiopathic dilated cardiomyopathy. And finally, it can be seen that in some aspects the differences in histopathological patterns of acute myocarditis versus IDCM merge imperceptibly due to different time sequences or due to prior treatment with steroids.

The question of focal infiltrates with myocyte damage although fitting the Dallas [7] definition is nevertheless not always unequivocal myocarditis. As pointed out before, this may be due to drug effects or "pressor-catecholamine" effect, "tip of the iceberg" effect of granulomatous disease of the myocardium or it may be due to secondary myocarditis such as Chaga's without the presence of organisms. These pitfalls (Table 3) including sampling error, should be constantly borne in mind while reading endomyocardial biopsies in these disease states.

The question of presentation of the patient in heart failure is also a challenging one. As pointed out by Abelman [8] "remarkably diffuse interstitial infiltrates may be found incidentally in patients dying of extra cardiac causes without clinical heart disease having been evident." It is also our experience in over 10,000 endomyocardial biopsies in cardiac transplant recipients that heart

Table 3. Acute myocarditis: morphologic caveats for endomyocardial biopsies

1. Adequate, well-processed tissue
2. Number of lymphocytes: what is normal?
3. Morphology of lymphocytes
4. Drug-related myocarditis
5. Secondary myocarditis
6. "Tip of iceberg" effect in granulomas
7. Lymphocytes in dilated cardiomyopathy

failure from acute rejection, which is indistinguishable morphologically from acute myocarditis, does not occur with focal infiltrates but only with diffuse infiltrates associated with diffuse loss of myocytes. To these observations may be added the fact that in most cases viral infectious involvement of the heart is quite rare, and overt clinical myocarditis is the exception. Also pointed out by Abelman [8], the incidence of death from acute myocarditis in the United States is only 0.4 per 100000 of the population and that 2%–9% of normal people dying in accident are found to have lymphocytes in the heart, so one must deal with the fact that focal myocarditis even if is results in focal myocyte injury may be a fortuitous finding in patients in heart failure for other reasons than viral myocarditis. Small focal collections of acute or chronic inflammatory cells in isolated microscopic fields should not be over emphasized. Also the presence of focal infiltrates does not always correlate with the history of an arrhythmogenic presentation. It is to be hoped that some of the more difficult questions posed in the last paragraph may be answered by the ongoing myocarditis trial but, until then, the conservative approach to endomyocardial biopsy diagnosis of acute myocarditis is recommended.

Acknowledgement: This work was supported in part by grant no. HL-13108-19, NHL 81, National Institutes of Health, Bethesda, Maryland, USA.

References

1. Tazelaar HD, Billingham ME (1986) Leukocytic infiltrates in idiopathic dilated cardiomyopathy: a source of confusion with active myocarditis. Am J Surg Pathol 10(6):405–412
2. Tazelaar HD, Billingham ME (1986) Myocardial lymphocytes: fact, fancy or myocarditis? Am J Cardiovasc Pathol 1:47–50
3. Billingham ME (1987) Acute myocarditis: a diagnostic dilemma. Br Heart J 58:608
4. Billingham ME (1987) Is acute cardiac rejection a model for myocarditis in humans? Eur Heart J 8(J):19–23
5. Maisch B (1985) Immunologic regulator and effector mechanisms in myocarditis and perimyocarditis. Heart Vessels 1:209–217
6. Rowan R, Masek MA, Billingham ME (1988) Ultrastructural morphometric analysis of endomyocardial biopsies. Am J Cardiovasc Pathol 2:137–144
7. Aretz HT, Billingham ME, Edwards WD, Factor SM, Fallon JT, Fenoglio JJ, Olsen EGJ, Schoen FJ (1986) Myocarditis: a histopathologic definition and classification. Am J Cardiovasc Pathol 1(1):3–14
8. Abelmann WH (1973) Clinical aspects of viral cardiomyopathy. In: Fowler NO (ed) Myocardial diseases. Grune and Stratton, New York, pp 253–275

Ultrastructural Changes in Myocarditis and Dilated Cardiomyopathy

E. Arbustini, A. Pucci, R. Pozzi, M. Grasso, G. Graziano, C. Campana,
A. Gavazzi, and M. Vigano

Introduction

Since its introduction in the study of cardiomyopathies, the clinical application of endomyocardial biopsy has been finalized to supporting the clinical diagnosis of idiopathic forms, to grading anthracycline cardiotoxicity, and to diagnosing myocarditis and specific heart muscle diseases [1, 2]. Electron microscopy (EM) has been used to determine whether further information can be added to that provided by light microscopy. Detailed information on the contractile, nuclear, tubular, mitochondrial, and glycogenic structures can be achieved [3–6]. Although much effort has so far been made in order to reach some specific diagnostic and prognostic index on the basis of the ultrastructural changes [4, 7, 8], controversies still exist, and the inconclusive results obtained have limited a more extensive clinical application of EM.

The aim of our study was:

1) to define whether EM could add useful information for the diagnosis of dilated cardiomyopathy (DCM) and myocarditis;
2) to investigate the role of morphometric assessment of myocardial structures in characterizing DCM; and
3) to ascertain if the morphometric data correlate with indexes of the functional status of the patients.

Materials and Methods

Population Samples

Donor Group: Endomyocardial biopsies taken from ten nonbeating hearts immediately before being transplanted were used as the normal control group. They were chosen among a larger number of biopsies in order to avoid samples with evident ischemic damage (i.e., myofibrillar lysis, mitochondrial damage and T-tubular system dilatation) possibly accounting for a large percentage of empty spaces which could negatively affect ultrastructural morphometric evaluation. The donors were nine males and one female, with a mean age of 23 ± 9

years (range 14–39). Death had occurred due to cerebral trauma in seven, and to cerebral hemorrage in three. Total ischemic time ranged from 59 to 107 min (mean 74 ± 26).

Valvular Heart Disease: Samples from papillary muscles of the left ventricle were taken during cardiac valve replacement in 11 patients with mitroaortic disease. They were used as a control model of myocardial hypertrophy. There were seven females and four males with a mean age of 53 ± 14 years (range 40–64). Angiographic ejection fraction was always <0.45%.

DCM Biopsy Group: From January 1985 to December 1988, DCM was clinically diagnosed in a consecutive series of 290 patients in the Cardiology Department of the Policlinico S. Matteo, Pavia, Italy. They all fulfilled the criteria of the World Health Organization for the diagnosis of idiopathic DCM. In 105 cases, more than one sample was available for EM. These last cases constituted our DCM biopsy study population. The length of disease, from the onset of symptoms or from the first clinical detection to our observation, ranged from 1 to 180 months (mean 21 ± 26). There were 26 females and 79 males, and their mean age was 42 ± 12 years (range 12–62). When they entered the study, 12 patients were in New York Heart Association (NYHA) functional class I, 33 were in class II, 41 in class III, and 19 in class IV. Mean angiographic ejection fraction was 0.32 ± 0.16.

DCM Explanted Hearts: Samples from the middle layer of the right ventricular wall were taken in ten DCM patients who had undergone cardiac transplantation. There were nine males and one female, and their mean age was 31 ± 7 years. All patients were in NYHA class IV. Mean angiographic ejection fraction was 0.18 ± 0.04. The length of the disease ranged from 10 to 120 months (mean 27 ± 31).

Myocarditis: From January 1985 to December 1988, a biopsy-proven diagnosis of myocarditis was formulated according to the Dallas criteria [9] in nine out of 290 biopsies. There were four males and five females, with a mean age of 36 ± 10 years. One patient was in NYHA class I, three patients were in class II, four in class III, and one patient was in class IV. The length of the disease ranged from a few weeks to 13 months (mean 7 ± 8 months).

Biopsy Procedure

Right ventricular endomyocardial biopsy was performed via the right internal jugular vein, using the Caves-Schultz bioptome, according to the Stanford technique. The same bioptome was also used for donor hearts and introduced into the right ventricle via the exposed right atrium immediately before positioning the heart into the chest of the recipient. The sampling was performed in the apical portion of the right ventricular septum.

Ultrastructural Examination

All samples were fixed in glutaraldehyde-formaldehyde 1% solution (Karnowsky liquid) in 0.1 M cacodilate buffer, pH 7.3. They were then postfixed with cool 1% osmium tetroxide in 0.1 M cacodylate buffer, dehydrated in ethanol and propylene-oxide, and embedded in epon-araldite. Ultrathin sections were stained with lead citrate and uranyl acetate, and examined with a Zeiss EM9 electron microscope.

Morphometric Study

Morphometry was carried out on EM using a frame of 100 points [10]. According to the basic principles of morphometry [11], counting points overlying a certain structure results in a quantitative determination of the entire tissue volume under the square grid. The count was performed on ten test areas in myocites free from contraction bands, using a total number of 1000 test points (magnification × 4800). Total test area was 7900 μm^2. Myofibril and mitochondrial volume fractions were evaluated excluding the nuclei, whereas nuclei were evaluated in the entire cell. At least 200 points were counted for each structure investigated. The values obtained were considered representative when the coefficient of error was ≤ 5% [10]. Myocyte width, nuclear diameter, and nuclear/sarcoplasmic ratio were calculated in the same test areas used for the volume fractions.

Atrial Natriuretic Peptide

Immunocytochemical study of atrial natriuretic peptide (ANP) was performed in the 14 cases in which granules were found. Ultrathin sections were deosmicated in an aqueous saturated solution of sodium metaperiodate [12]. The sections were incubated for 12–18 h with 1:100 – 1:400 diluted antiserum to ANP [13]. After washing in Tris-buffered NaCl, the sections were incubated with protein A-gold complex [14]. The grids were finally stained with uranyl acetate and Reynolds' lead citrate.

Qualitative Evaluation

The occurrence of the following aspects was carefully searched and analyzed:
1) Huge nuclei;
2) Lysis of contractile material, with Z band remnants;
3) Hypertrophy of the myocytes;
4) Variation of mitochondrial size and shape, increase in their number (mitochondriosis) and cristolysis (i.e. dissolution of the mitochondrial cristae);
5) T-tubular system dilatation;

 6) Endocrine, ANP-containing granules;
 7) Cellular necrosis or damage and related changes;
 8) Lipid droplets in the myocytes;
 9) Lipid droplets in the interstitium;
10) Adipose cells in the interstitium;
11) Interstitial fibrosis, which was semiquantitatively scored as mild, moderate, and severe, according to its amount and its relationship with myocyte boundaries in the fields examined:
     Mild: myocytes not separated by fibrosis, small foci of fibrous tissue interrupting contiguity of the cells, i.e., fibrosis slightly exceeding the normal myocardial network;
     Moderate: myocytes partially surrounded by fibrosis but preserving contiguity with other cells;
     Severe: myocytes completely surrounded by dense fibrosis with elastic fibers;
12) Interstitial cells (smooth muscle cells, myofibroblasts, fibroblasts, macrophages, mast cells, inflammatory cells);
13) Endocardial fibrosis, elastosis, or thrombosis;
14) Vessels: capillary or small intramural arterial vessel changes and thrombosis.

Statistical Analysis

Data are presented as mean values ± standard deviation. Two-sample t test for unpaired data was used to evaluate statistical significance. Numeric data were processed using the NH Analytical Software Program "Statistix" for personal computers.

Results

Cardiomyopathy

Morphometric Analysis: The mean data for all groups are summarized in Table 1, and group comparisons in Table 2. Myocyte width was significantly higher both in DCM and valvular groups than in the normal group, and it did not vary between DCM and valvular groups. Nuclear diameter was also increased but to a significantly greater extent in the DCM group than in the valvular heart disease group. Accordingly, the nuclear/sarcoplasmic ratio was preserved in the valvular group but significantly increased in the DCM group. Myocyte diameter did not correlate with ejection fraction ($r = 0.2243$, $p =$ NS).

The volume fraction of myofibrils was higher in valvular and DCM groups than in the normal group, but the difference reached statistical significance only in the valvular group. The DCM explanted group showed significantly lower volume fraction of myofibrils than all the other groups, as well as a significantly

Table 1. Quantitative morphometric evaluation

	Mean	SD	Range	(n)
Myocite diameter (μm)				
DCM biopsies	28.70	8.501	13–47	105
DCM explants	28.90	8.517	18–41	10
Valvular	26.09	4.805	19–32	11
Donors	19.50	3.837	13–36	10
Nuclear diameter (μm)				
DCM biopsies	11.11	5.05	4–25	105
DCM explants	12.00	5.33	5–20	10
Valvular	7.54	2.25	4–12	11
Donors	5.40	1.26	4– 8	10
Nuclear-sarcoplasmic ratio				
DCM biopsies	0.373	0.0873	0.238–0.595	105
DCM explants	0.4009	0.0837	0.278–0.528	10
Valvular	0.285	0.0478	0.210–3.750	11
Donors	0.276	0.0301	0.222–0.315	10
Volume fraction of myofibrils (%)				
DCM biopsies	53.98	6.72	35–66	88
DCM explants	46.51	5.21	41–55	10
Valvular	57.27	4.33	52–74	11
Donors	52.40	2.87	47–56	10
Volume fraction of mitochondria (%)				
DCM biopsies	26.78	5.15	17–39	88
DCM explants	23.00	3.39	18–30	10
Valvular	26.36	3.29	19–31	11
Donors	25.30	2.62	21–29	10
Volume fraction of nuclei (%)				
DCM biopsies	13.87	2.70	8–21	88
DCM explants	14.00	2.00	11–18	10
Valvular	10.91	1.58	9–14	11
Donors	11.40	1.26	10–13	10

lower volume fraction of mitochondria. The volume fraction of nuclei was significantly higher in the DCM group than in the other ones. However, it must be pointed out that the error coefficient for mitochondria and nuclei in DCM was slightly higher than the maximum value considered representative (Table 3) [10].

Since the volume fraction of myofibrils reached the lowest value in the DCM explant group, in which all patients belonged to NYHA functional class IV, this could suggest an inverse relationship between functional class and volume fraction of myofibrils. However, no correlation was found in the entire DCM biopsy group between volume fraction of myofibrils and functional class ($r = 0.1137$, $p = $ NS), and between ejection fraction and volume fraction of myofibrils ($r = 0.2244$, $p = $ NS). This was also true when we compared patients in functional class I with patients in class IV (Table 4).

Table 2. Statistical significance

Myocyte diameter

DCM biopsies	vs	donors	$p < 0.0001$
DCM biopsies	vs.	DCM explants	$p = NS$
DCM biopsies	vs	valvular	$p = NS$
Valvular	vs.	donors	$p < 0.0001$

Nuclear diameter

DCM biopsies	vs	donors	$p < 0.0001$
DCM biopsies	vs.	DCM explants	$p = NS$
DCM biopsies	vs	valvular	$p = 0.0003$
Valvular	vs.	donors	$p = 0.0151$

Nuclear-sarcoplasmic ratio

DCM biopsies	vs	donors	$p < 0.0001$
DCM biopsies	vs.	DCM explants	$p = NS$
DCM biopsies	vs	valvular	$p = 0.0001$
Valvular	vs.	donors	$p = NS$

Volume fraction of myofibrils

DCM biopsies	vs	donors	$p = NS$
DCM biopsies	vs.	DCM explants	$p = 0.0014$
DCM biopsies	vs	valvular	$p = 0.041$
Valvular	vs.	donors	$p = 0.0069$

Volume fraction of mitochondria

DCM biopsies	vs	donors	$p = NS$
DCM biopsies	vs.	DCM explants	$p = 0.0072$
DCM biopsies	vs	valvular	$p = NS$
Valvular	vs.	donors	$p = NS$

Volume fraction of nuclei

DCM biopsies	vs	donors	$p < 0.0001$
DCM biopsies	vs.	DCM explants	$p = NS$
DCM biopsies	vs	valvular	$p < 0.0001$
Valvular	vs.	donors	$p = NS$

Table 3. Morphometric evaluation – coefficient of error (%)

	DCM biopsies	DCM explants	Valvular	Donors
Vf myofibrils	3.9	3.5	2.4	1.7
Vf mitochondria	6.08[a]	4.6	3.9	3.3
Vf nuclei	6.1[a]	4.5	4.6	3.5

[a] Coefficient of error slightly over the maximum value ($\leq 5\%$) for evaluation to be representative.

Vf, volume fraction.

Table 4. Morphometric and clinical correlates in DCM biopsy group

	NYHA I	(n)	NYHA IV	(n)	P
Ejection fraction (%)	47 ± 13	11	21 ± 6	20	0.0001
Length of disease (months)	8 ± 5	11	27 ± 25	20	0.002
Myocyte diameter (μm)	26 ± 10	11	29 ± 8	20	NS
Nuclear size (μm)	10 ± 5	11	12 ± 5	20	NS
Vf myofibrils (%)	55 ± 5	10	53 ± 9	16	NS
Vf mitochondria (%)	28 ± 4	10	26 ± 7	16	NS
Vf nuclei (%)	12 ± 3	10	14 ± 3	16	NS

Vf, volume fraction.

Table 5. Qualitative morphologic analysis (data are presented as percentage of the total cases)

n	DCM biopsies 105	DCM explants 10	Valvular 11	Donors 10
Myocyte				
Lysis	82	80	18	—[a]
Huge and bizarre nuclei	63	100	0	0
Hypertrophy	78	100	100	30
– Mild	50	20	45	30
– Moderate	28	50	36	0
– Severe	22	30	18	0
Necrosis/damage	22	30	18	—[a]
Mitochondrial changes	84	90	63	20[a]
T-tubular dilatation	19	20	9	—[a]
Intracellular lipid droplets	80	9	18	30
ANP granules	13	0	0	0
Interstitium				
Fibrosis	91	40	100	40
– Absent	9	60	0	60
– Mild	40	30	18	30
– Moderate	38	10	64	10
– Severe	13	0	18	0
Cells				
– Smooth muscle cells, fibroblasts, myofibroblasts	100	30	100	40
– Lymphocytes	38	10	18	20
– Mast cells	34	20	27	20
– Macrophages	44	20	36	10
Lipid droplets	13	20	0	0
Adipous tissue	18	0	0	10
Vessel: hyperplasia/thrombosis	5/2	0	0	0
Endocardium				
Fibrosis	90	—	100	25
Elastosis	10	—	28	0
Smooth muscle cells	79	—	100	12
Thrombosis	5	—	0	0

[a] Ischemia-related changes are excluded.

Qualitative Evaluation: Results are summarized in Table 5. Qualitative morphologic analysis of myocytes showed a prevalence of filament lysis (Fig. 1), and of huge nuclei (Fig. 2) in the DCM group with respect to the others. Hypertrophy, mitochondrial changes and all other features evaluated did not differ among the groups. ANP granules were found in 14 out of 105 DCM biopsy cases (Fig. 3). No granules were found in normal, valvular, and DCM explant groups. In the interstitium, fibrosis was the most remarkable finding of the evaluated features. Interstitial fibrosis seemed to be more frequent in subendocardial layers (DCM biopsy group: 91%) than in deeper layers (DCM explanted hearts: 40%).

Rare and scattered lymphocytes were seen in all groups, as well as macrophages and mast cells. Capillary thrombosis (Fig. 4) and small vessel hyperplasia were seen in a very low percentage of cases in the DCM biopsy group. Endocardial fibrosis and elastosis were found in the valvular and DCM groups. Endocardial thrombosis was observed in a very few cases of the DCM biopsy group (5%).

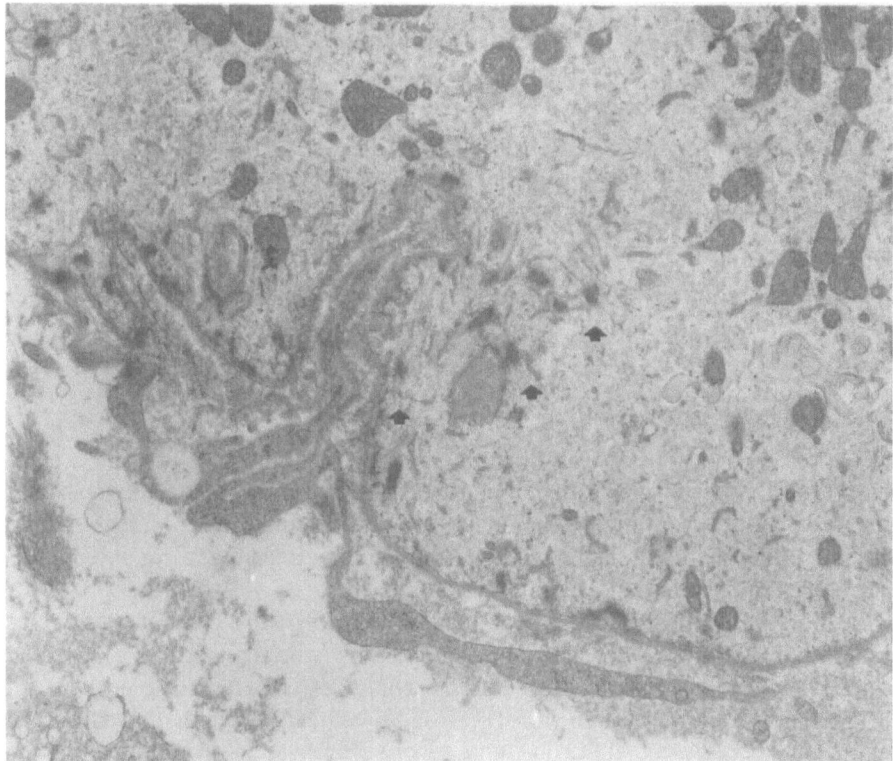

Fig. 1. DCM biopsy case: myofibrillar loss with Z remnants (*arrows*). Uranyl acetate and lead citrate; × 13 700

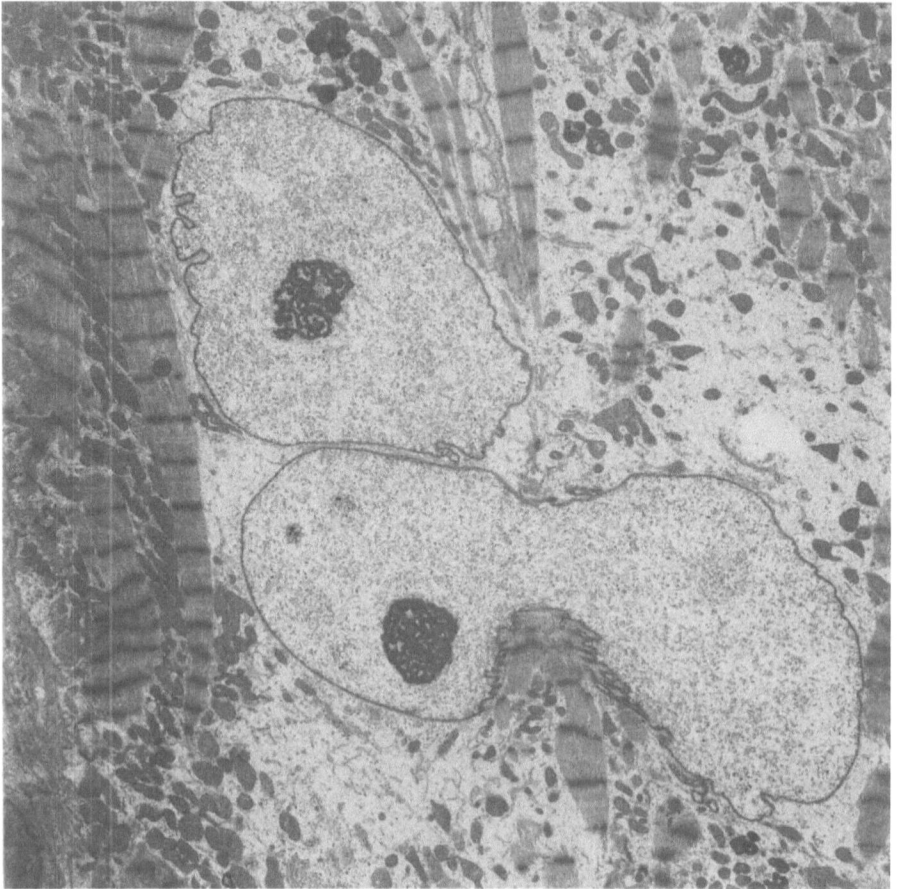

Fig. 2. DCM biopsy case: huge, bizarre-shaped nucleus with prominent nucleoli. Uranyl acetate and lead citrate; × 5300

Myocarditis

Our experience concerns only nine cases of myocarditis. The diagnosis was reached with conventional light microscopy study in all cases. The immuno-phenotype of the inflammatory infiltrates was defined using specific monoclonal antibodies on paraffin and frozen sections.

In the EM samples, some inflammatory infiltrates were present in all cases; in three of them, they were few and scanty. They were constituted by granulo-cytes, lymphocytes, histiocytes, and macrophages, located in a perivascular (Fig. 5) and perimyocyte position (Fig. 6). Myocytes exhibited various degrees of damage, consisting of edema and myofibrillar lysis. Sarcolemma was not sharply discontinued even in those cases which showed adjacent infiltrates. Interstitial changes consisted of variously associated edema and fibrosis. Focal loose fibrosis was seen in six out of the nine cases.

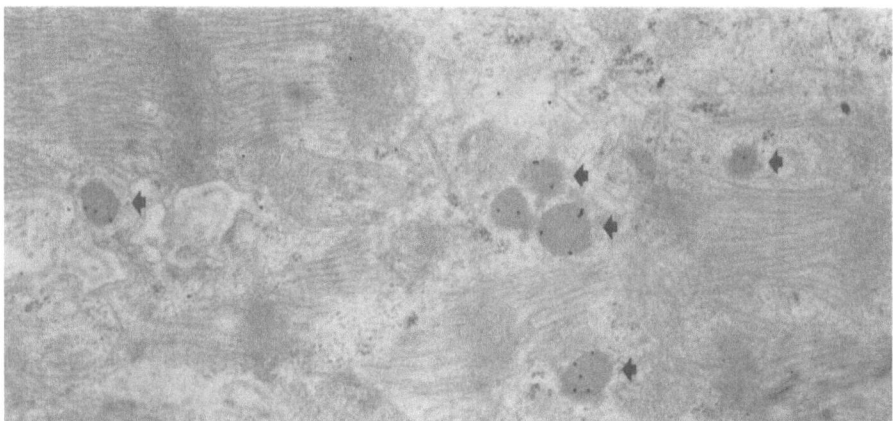

Fig. 3. DCM biopsy case: ANP immunoreactivity selectively localized over the membrane-bound granules (*arrows*). Protein A-gold particles, uranyl acetate and lead citrate; ×23000

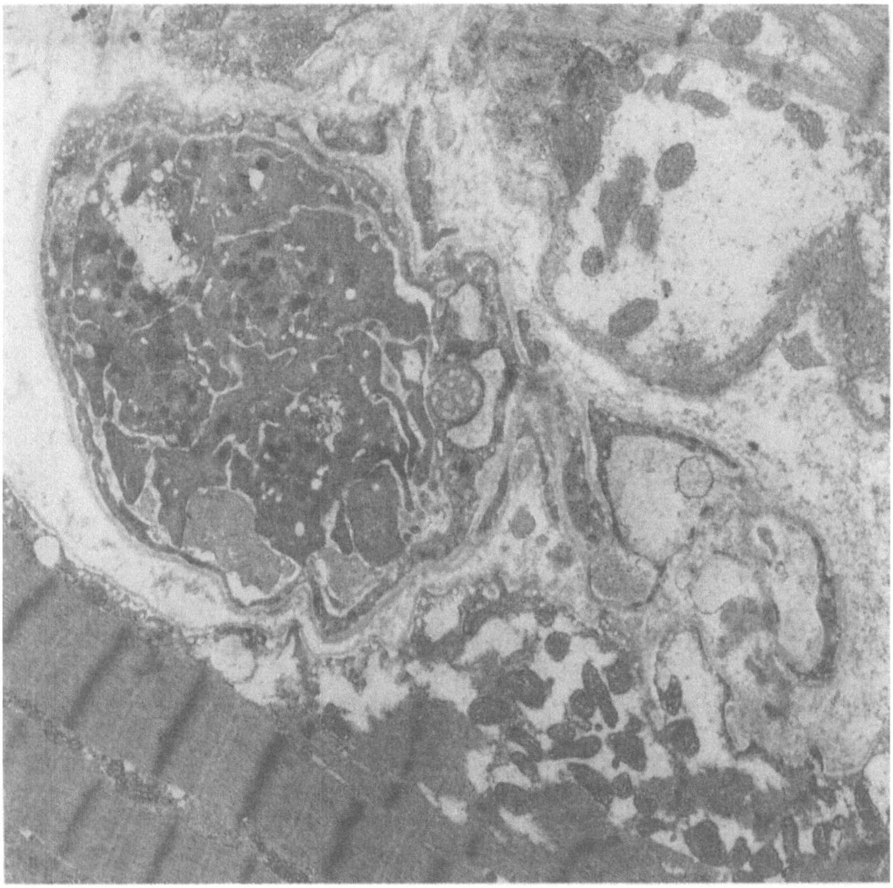

Fig. 4. Capillary thrombosis in a biopsy sample from DCM group. Uranyl acetate and lead citrate; ×13700

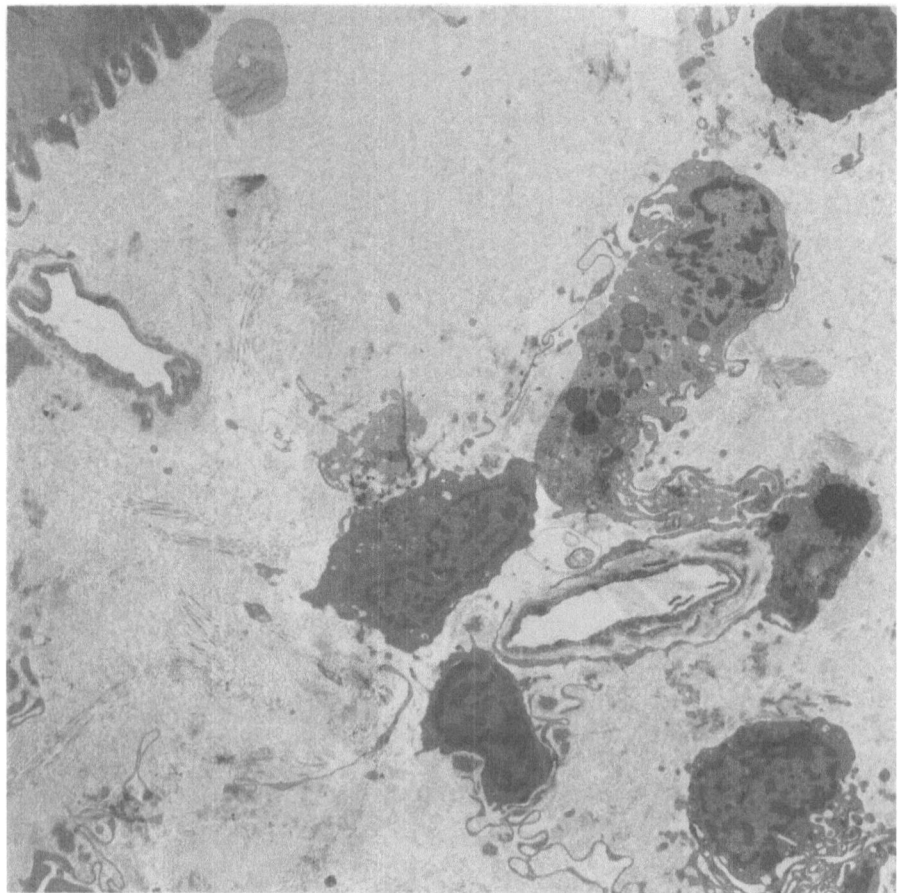

Fig. 5. Myocarditis: perivascular inflammatory infiltrate. Uranyl acetate and lead citrate; × 5300

Discussion

Our study showed that conventional EM can add useful information for a better morphologic characterization of DCM. When combined with immunocytochemical techniques, it also represents a valuable research tool for the study of peculiar metabolic and morphologic patterns.

Methods

We compared ultrastructural morphometric and morphologic data of a large series of DCM with clinically normal hearts. The technique and the sampling site were the same for both groups. Furthermore, we studied surgical samples

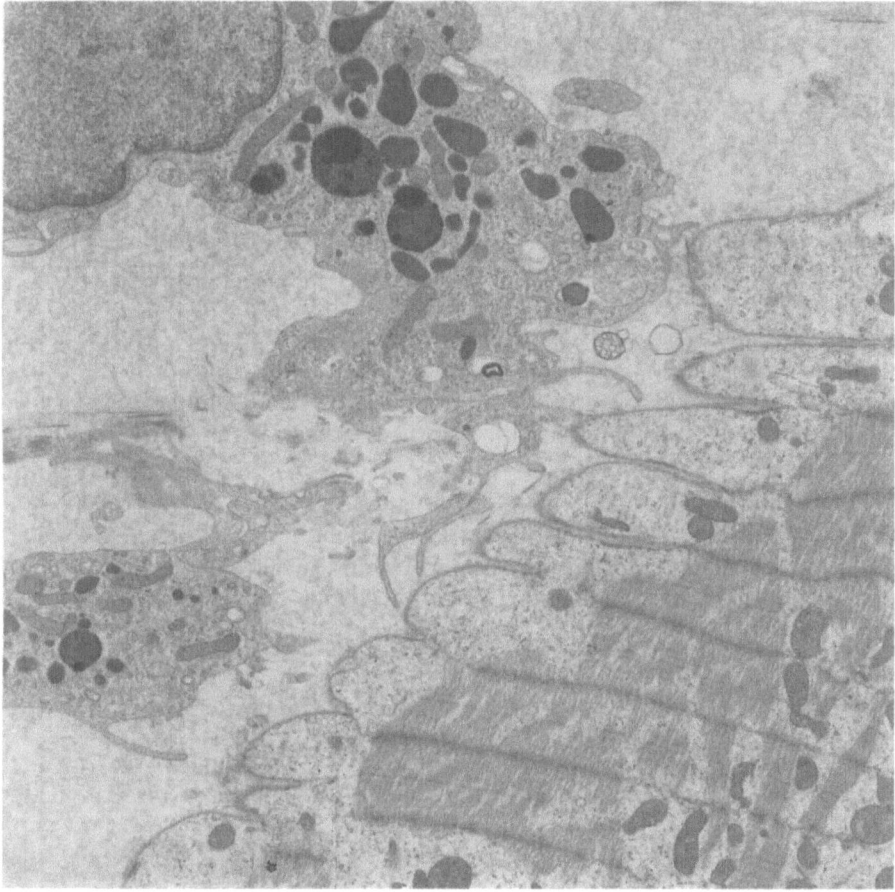

Fig. 6. Myocarditis: granulocytes with pseudopodia close to a myocyte which shows loss of myofibrils but sarcolemma integrity. Uranyl acetate and lead citrate; × 13 700

of left ventricular papillary muscles from valvular heart disease cases in order to assess whether morphologic abnormalities differ in various types of hypertrophy.

We are aware of the problems that can derive from studying and comparing different areas of the right and left ventricles [15], even though such differences are not universally agreed upon [16]. A low but significant correlation between the histologic findings of right and left ventricular biopsy samples was established by Noda [17]. Figulla et al. [18] have recently reported a significant correlation between morphometric indexes and prognosis. This result was derived by pooling biopsy samples from the right and left ventricles, thus considering irrelevant the differences in sampling site.

Some limitations in ultrastructural studies can also derive from the sampling variability due to the very small area explored with respect to light microscopy.

However, when fiber diameters and volume fraction of myofibrils are taken into account, the sampling variability is low [19, 20]. Vice versa, the volume fraction of fibrosis was found to be affected by an excessively high sampling variability [19]. This last result was also confirmed by Baandrup et al. [20], who also reported a coefficient of variance of up to 80% for volume fraction of collagen. Accordingly, we made no attempt to correlate our ultrastructural data on fibrosis with any clinical parameters.

Some considerations should be made regarding our valvular heart disease group. A more precise distinction between pressure and volume overload conditions could be useful in a better histopathologic characterization and comparative analysis. However, practical reasons limited an extensive and rigorous biopsy study of selected patients with valvular heart disease. Therefore, we intended to compare DCM cases with a group of hearts in which dilatation and hypertrophy were primarily caused by pure hemodynamic abnormalities.

Finally, we evaluated the middle layer of the right ventricular wall of DCM explanted hearts separately. This approach was chosen to investigate whether topographic histopathologic differences between the mid-myocardial layer and the endomyocardium usually taken in biopsy samples, do occur.

Quantitative Results

We have shown that myocyte width is similarly increased in DCM and valvular heart disease groups, while nuclear diameter is also increased but to a major extent in DCM. Accordingly, the nuclear/sarcoplasmic ratio is significantly higher only in the DCM group. We tried to label this peculiar pattern that seemed distinctively suggestive of DCM and called it "nuclear/sarcoplasmic mismatch." We use this index to formulate the diagnosis of "consistent with DCM." Oversized and bizarre nuclei were almost invariably associated with the other histopathologic features of DCM. However, it should be pointed out that, within the DCM biopsy group, a certain number of cases showed normal nuclear and sarcoplasmic diameter with preserved ratio.

Our mean myocyte diameter (28.7 μm) in DCM biopsies is in agreement with that reported by Rowan et al. [21] who found 29.3 μm on average. It differs from those reported by other authors on light microscopy studies: 17 μm by Baandrup and Olsen [15], and 18 μm by Noda [17]. Such a wide range of values can be explained as a result of different methods or different pathologic forms of DCM.

Another important contribution of EM derives from the measurement of myofibril volume fraction, which has been proposed as a reliable prognostic index in DCM. In our study, the highest mean value of the myofibril volume fraction was observed in the valvular group, and the lowest in the mid-myocardial layers of DCM explanted hearts. In the DCM biopsy group, the volume fraction of myofibrils was similar to normal. Our normal value is roughly similar to the 52% reported by Fleischer et al. [22], but differs from the 59% found by Schwarz et al. [23]. Some underestimation could have occurred in our normal group due to edema and ischemia-related changes. Moreover, some difference can be explained by the fact that our samples were from the right ventricle, while the above authors examined samples from the left ventricle. An inverse relationship between functional class and volume fraction of myofibrils was suggested by the minor myofibrillar percentage found in the DCM explant group. This result was not confirmed when the DCM biopsy class I subgroup was compared to the DCM biopsy class IV subgroup. Therefore, our results showing a lack of correlation between the clinical status of the patients and volume fraction of myofibrils are in agreement with previously reported studies [6, 18].

Qualitative Results

Huge and bizarre-shaped nuclei and lysis of myofilaments were only found in part of the DCM cases, and these features were quite suggestive of the disease. Nuclear changes have been recently reported to be quite distinctive for different forms of DCM [24]. Hypertrophy of the myocytes was not a discriminating feature for DCM, such as mitochondrial changes and myocyte degenerative patterns, as already described [6].

ANP-containing granules were an interesting feature because no sample in the normal and valvular group showed similar granules. The physiopathologic meaning of their presence in ventricular myocytes remains to be elucidated.

Ultrastructural evaluation of interstitial fibrosis does not represent a reliable index of myocardial disease state due to its sampling variability [19, 20]. However, in DCM groups, interstitial fibrosis seemed to affect subendocardial layers more than deeper myocardium areas. In fact, some fibrosis was almost invariably present in our biopsy cases but it was minimal or absent in most of the deeper myocardial layers studied in DCM explanted hearts.

Finally, the diagnosis of myocarditis did not take much benefit from ultrastructural studies. Viral particles have never been found in our series of myocarditis, and the nature of inflammatory infiltrates was defined by immunohistochemical techniques. A better definition of myocyte damage can be obtained from EM, as suggested by Hammond et al. [8]. Owing to the low number of myocarditis cases in our series, no functional-morphologic correlates were investigated.

Conclusions

1) From a pathologic point of view, DCM can be defined more accurately by ultrastructural morphometric indexes.
2) Nuclear changes, more than sarcoplasmic and interstitial ones, help in histopathologically characterizing DCM biopsies: high nuclear/sarcoplasmic ratio (nuclear/sarcoplasmic mismatch) seems to be a distinguishing feature of DCM.
3) No correlation has been found between the morphometric data and the clinical and functional status of DCM patients.

Acknowledgement: This study was supported in part by grant no. 858 "Diagnosi e Terapia" from Regione Lombardia, and by grant "Cardiomiopatie e Miocardite" from the Ministry of Health to IRCCS Policlinico S. Matteo, Pavia, Ricerche Finalizzate 1988–1989.

References

1. Unverferth DV, Baker PB (1986) Value of endomyocardial biopsy. Am J Med 80 [Suppl 2B]:22–32.
2. Mason JW, O'Connell JB (1989) Clinical merit of endomyocardial biopsy. Circulation 70:923–938.
3. Knieriem HJ (1978) Electron microscopy findings in congestive cardiomyopathy. In: Kaltenbach M, Loogen F, Olsen EGJ (eds) Cardiomyopathy and myocardial biopsy. Springer, Berlin Heidelberg New York, p 2
4. Künkel B, Lapp H, Kober G, Kaltenbach M (1978) Ultrastructural evaluation in early and advanced congestive cardiomyopathies. In: Kaltenbach M, Loogen F, Olsen EGJ (eds) Cardiomyopathy and myocardial biopsy. Springer, Berlin Heidelberg New York, p 87
5. Ferrans VJ (1978) Myocardial ultrastructure in human cardiac hypertrophy. In: Kaltenbach M, Loogen F, Olsen EGJ (eds) Cardiomyopathy and myocardial biopsy. Springer, Berlin Heidelberg New York, p 100
6. Baandrup U, Florio RA, Roters F, Olsen EGJ (1981) Electron microscopic investigation of endomyocardial biopsy samples in hypertrophy and cardiomyopathy. A semiquantitative study in 48 patients. Circulation 63:1289–1298
7. Schwarz F, Mall G, Zebe H, Schmitzer E, Manthey F, Schenrlen H, Kübler W (1984) Determinants of survival in patients with congestive cardiomyopathy: quantitative morphologic findings and left ventricular haemodynamics. Circulation 70:923–938
8. Hammond EH, Menlove RL, Anderson JL (1987) Predictive value of immunofluorescence and electron microscopy evaluation of endomyocardial biopsies in the diagnosis and prognosis of myocarditis and idiopathic dilated cardiomyopathy. Am Heart J 114:1055–1065
9. Aretz HT, Billingham ME, Edwards WD, Factor SM, Fallon JT, Fenoglio JJ, Olsen EGJ, Schoen FJ (1987) Myocarditis: a histopathologic definition and classification. Am J Cardiovasc Pathol 1:3–14
10. Gundersen HJG, Bendtsen TF, Korbo L, Marcussen N, Maller A, Nielsen K, Nyengaard JR, Pakkenberg B, Sokensen FB, Vesterby A, West MJ (1988) Some new, simple and efficient stereological methods and their use in pathological research and diagnosis. APMIS 96:379–394
11. Weibel ER (1969) Stereological principles for morphometry in electron microscopic cytology. Int Rev Cytol 26:235–302
12. Bendayan M, Zollinger U (1983) Ultrastructural localization of antigenic sites on osmium-fixed tissues applaying the protein A-gold technique. J Histochem Cytochem 31:101–109
13. Reinecke M, Nehls M, Forssmann WG (1985) Philogenetic aspects of cardiac hormones as revealed by immunocytochemistry, electron microscopy, and bioassay. Peptides 6 [Suppl 3]:321–331
14. Roths J, Bendayan M, Orci L (1978) Ultrastructural localization of intracellular antigens by the use of protein A-gold complex. J Histochem Cytochem 26:1074–1081
15. Baandrup U, Olsen EGJ (1981) Critical analysis of endomyocardial biopsies from patients suspected of having cardiomyopathy. I. Morphological and morphometric aspects. Br Heart J 45:475–486
16. Dick MR, Unverferth DV, Baba N (1982) The pattern of myocardial degeneration in nonischemic congestive cardiomyopathy. Hum Pathol 13:740–744
17. Noda S (1980) Histopathology of endomyocardial biopsies from patients with idiopathic cardiomyopathy; quantitative evaluation based on multivariate statistical analysis. Jpn Circulation J 44:95–116

18. Figulla HR, Rahlf G, Nieger M, Luig H, Krenzer H (1985) Spontaneous hemodynamics improvement or stabilization and associated biopsy findings in patients with congestive cardiomyopathy. Circulation 71:1095–1104
19. Mall G, Schwarz F, Derks H (1982) Clinicopathologic correlations in congestive heart failure. A study on endomyocardial biopsies. Virchows Arch. Pathol Anat 397:67–82
20. Baandrup U, Florio RA, Olsen EGJ (1982) Do endomyocardial biopsies represent the morphology of the rest of the myocardium? A quantitative light microscopy study of single v. multiple biopsies within the King's bioptome. Eur Heart J 3:171–178
21. Rowan RA, Masek MA, Billingam ME (1988) Ultrastructural morphometric analysis of endomyocardial biopsies. Idiopathic dilated cardiomyopathy, antracycline cardiotoxicity and normal myocardium. Am J Cardiovasc Pathol 2:137–144
22. Fleischer M, Wippo W, Themam H, Achatzy RS (1980) Ultrastructural morphometric analysis of human myocardial left ventricles with mitral insufficiency. Virchows Arch (Pathol Anat) 389:205–210
23. Schwarz F, Kittstein D, Winkler B, Shaper J (1980) Quantitative ultrastructure of the myocardium in chronic aortic valve disease. Basic Res Cardiol 75:109–111
24. Unverferth BJ, Leier CV, Magorien RD, Unverferth DV (1983) Differentiating characteristics of myocardial nuclei in cardiomyopathy. Hum Pathol 14:974–983

Diagnostic and Prognostic Value of Immunofluorescence and Electron-Microscopic Findings in Idiopathic Dilated Cardiomyopathy

E. H. Hammond, J. L. Anderson, and R. L. Menlove

Introduction

Idiopathic dilated cardiomyopathy (IDC) is a disease that is becoming of increasing medical interest, both as a clinical and pathologic entity [1, 2]. Both inflammatory (myocarditis) and noninflammatory forms of IDC are recognized, and it is believed that both may appear as stages at different times in the same patient [2]. However, the pathophysiology of IDC remains unknown, and diagnostic, prognostic, and therapeutic approaches continue to be suboptimal.

In recent years, endomyocardial biopsy has been increasingly applied to patients with IDC in an effort to obtain more specific diagnostic and prognostic information. However, problems with information obtained from biopsy are recognized [3]. One problem relates to the diagnosis of myocarditis. Cellular infiltrates in adults with myocarditis are often focal and sporadic, both in time and type, and may be missed due to sampling error. In addition, there has been a lack of consensus on the microscopic criteria for diagnosis. Recently, leading cardiac pathologists met in Dallas, Texas, to establish uniform criteria. The resulting "Dallas criteria" for light-microscopic diagnosis of myocarditis required that an abnormal inflammatory component be present and associated with "cellular injury" of adjacent myocytes [4]. Even with these criteria, the diagnosis of myocarditis by light microscopy (LM) has limitations. Interobserver variability in the interpretation of biopsy samples among pathologists remains high [5, 6]. Differentiation of infiltrating mononuclear inflammatory cells and plump fibroblasts or pericytes may be difficult. Also, LM is insensitive to the distinction between myocyte degeneration and necrosis unless the latter is florid (an uncommon occurrence). Finally, although inflammatory responses include both cellular and humoral components, the latter is not assessed by the LM method.

Another major problem in the biopsy evaluation of IDC has been the non-specific nature of LM findings and the lack of prognostically important features that would add independently to such functional indexes as ejection fraction in predicting mortality [3, 7, 8].

In a previous report, we proposed that immunofluorescence (IF) microscopy may help in the evaluation of a possible inflammatory component in primary heart muscle diseases, based on an initial experience in 79 patients [9]. Here we review our updated experience for 286 biopsy procedures evaluated by IF in

208 patients (also reported elsewhere [10]). We also review the utility of routine electron microscopy (EM) in IDC diagnosis, including the basis for our proposed use of EM criteria for assessing prognosis.

Methods

Patient Selection for Endomyocardial Biopsy: This review represents our collective initial and expanded experience in consecutively processed endomyocardial biopsy (EMB) samples. Patients selected for EMB generally presented with dilated hearts and systolic dysfunction of variable duration causing heart failure in the absence of coronary artery or valvular heart disease. Tissue samples included in this study were initial transvenous EMB samples sufficient qualitatively and quantitatively to be submitted for light (LM), immunofluorescence (IF), and electron microscopy (EM). EMB samples were obtained from the right ventricle by transvenous sampling from either the internal jugular [11] or the femoral venous approach [12, 13]. EMB submitted for assessment of restrictive or hypertrophic cardiomyopathy, transplant rejection, anthracycline cardiotoxicity, or alcoholic cardiomyopathy were excluded from this study of IDC.

Preparation of EMB Samples: Two to five (median three) EMB samples were submitted to pathology on a saline-soaked filter paper. Sample diameter generally measured 2–3 mm. For IF processing, a fragment of at least two pieces was removed, snap frozen in a cryostat, and immediately sectioned, using ornithine carbamoyltransferase (OCT) as the embedding medium. The remaining major portions of the specimens were prepared for LM by routine processing utilizing formalin as a fixative and paraffin as an embedment. Sections were cut at 6 microns and stained with hematoxylin and eosin. A small fragment was prepared for EM by processing at room temperature in Karnovsky's fixative and embedding in Epon 812. One micron-thick sections were stained in toluidine blue to select areas for EM. Selected areas were then evaluated by EM, performed by standard techniques [14].

LM Evaluation: Myocarditis was diagnosed on LM based on the presence of infiltrating interstitial mononuclear cells (lymphocytes and histiocytes) associated with evidence for myocardial injury using the Dallas criteria [4]. In addition, the number of cells in the entire specimen was tabulated under high power ($\times 400$). Patients showing a mean number of mononuclear inflammatory cells greater than five per high-power field, associated with myocyte injury, were considered to have definite myocarditis [15]. Vasculitis was defined as the presence of infiltrating mononuclear cells in the walls of small arterioles or capillaries (capillaritis) associated with endothelial cell swelling, necrosis of the vessel wall, or microvascular thrombosis. Fibrosis was evaluated in sections stained with trichrome. Inflammatory cells found in regions of fibrosis were ignored [6]. Data were recorded prospectively in computer files.

Immunofluorescence Evaluation of EMB Samples: Frozen sections for IF microscopy were incubated with polyclonal fluorescein-conjugated rabbit antibodies directed against IgG, IgM, IgA, C3, C1q, fibrinogen (BCA-Cappel Laboratories, Westchester, PA) and monoclonal mouse antibodies directed against HLA-DR (Ia-like) (Hybritech), pan-B antigen (B-4, Coulter, Hialeah, FL), pan-T antigen (T-1 lytic, Coulter), and pan-monocyte (M-1, Coulter). T lymphocyte-positive samples were incubated with monoclonal antibodies to CD4 (helper) and CD8 (suppressor/cytotoxic) (Ortho, Raritan, NJ). Frozen sections were air dried, washed in PBS, and incubated with conjugated (IgG, IgM, IgA, C3, C1q, fribrinogen) or unconjugated (HLA-DR, pan-B, pan-T, pan-monocyte) antibodies at optimal dilutions for 30 min at 25°C. After a PBS wash, sections were coverslipped in polyvinyl alcohol (for conjugated antibodies) or incubated with fluorescein-labeled IgG fractions of rabbit-antimouse (BCA-Cappel or Coulter) for 30 min at 25°C. After final incubation, slides were washed, then coverslipped in polyvinyl alcohol. Positive and negative control slides were run with each batch.

IF staining was graded on a scale of 0–3+ based on the amount of antibody deposited in either interstitial or vascular distributions. Staining was considered significant (1+) if it was brighter in intensity than or different in distribution from staining with albumin. HLA-DR staining of blood vessels was graded as strong (bright, generalized), weak (pale, focal), or absent. Stains of inflammatory cells were graded in a similar fashion, and relative intensity of staining for various cell types expressed as a ratio of one to another. Immunofluorescence results were recorded before examination by LM and entered prospectively in computer files. IF was performed using a Zeiss immunofluorescence microscope.

The presence of circulating (species-nonspecific) serum heart-reactive antibody (HRA) was evaluated by incubation of serial dilutions of the patient's serum with sections of normal dog heart and graded by comparison with similar dilutions of normal control serum. HRA was considered positive if present in a dilution of > 1:16. Location of HRA staining was noted as sarcolemmal, myofibrillary, or nuclear.

Electron Microscopy: Areas from the 1-μm toluidine blue sections selected for EM review were those considered to be most abnormal by LM. Where possible, both longitudinal and cross-sectional areas of myocardium were examined. Diagnostic classification was based on a list of 50 ultrastructural parameters, including those relating to interstitial regions, blood vessels, myocytes, and endocardium. Twelve features were ultimately selected for indepth evaluation (Table 1). As for immunofluorescence, EM evaluation was performed by one of us (EHH) prospectively and in a blinded fashion with respect to patients' clinical characteristics and eventual outcome. Each ultrastructural feature was graded 0 (none) to 3+ (extensive). Data were prospectively recorded in computer files. EM was performed on a Jeol 100S microscope.

Data Analysis: Results of LM, immunofluorescence, and EM were entered into the LDS Hospital TANDEM computer database using a classification scheme

Table 1. Selected electron-microscopic features

Actin disorganization
Cellular debris
Collagen
Endothelial cell swelling
Glycogen (increased or pooled)
Intercalated discs (abnormally frequent, tortuous)
Mitochondrial degeneration
Mitochondrial calcification
Myofilament loss
Reduplicated vascular basal lamina
Subsarcolemmal z-bands
Z-band streaming

which recorded the presence and quantity of each feature. Important clinical characteristics were also recorded. Subsequently the data were down-loaded to an IBM PC/XT microcomputer for manipulation and statistical analysis.

The general strategy of data analysis was to perform a preliminary (retrospective) multiple regression analysis to see which variables could be used to identify patients that met the two primary endpoints of interest:

1) cellular infiltration (myocarditis); and
2) survival.

Once a preliminary data set of variables was identified, a decision analysis (receiver-operating characteristics curve analysis) was performed on a simple scale constructed from the appropriate variable sets to see how well these scales could identify patients meeting the two endpoints. A p of less than 0.05 (two-tailed test) was considered significant.

Results

Clinical Characteristics

Characteristics of the initial 79 patients are representative of our patient series [9]: age averaged 51 ± 14 years (range 18–79); 52 were men (two-thirds) and 27 women (one-third). The range of prior symptom duration was broad (1-360 months, mean 22). Ejection fraction was depressed, averaging 30% ± 13%, and was associated with an average functional class of 2.7 ± 0.6. Standard heart failure therapy was given to 77 patients (97%), beta-blockers (experimental) to an additional 32, and immunosuppressants to 12. These clinical features were not shown to correlate significantly with presence or absence of myocarditis or mortality and were not reevaluated for the expanded patient series.

The initial follow-up evaluation period averaged 18.3 months (range 1–48), during which 16 patients died, for a total mortality rate of 20% (annual mortality, 13%). All deaths were cardiovascular and caused by progression of heart failure or cardiac arrest (sudden, presumed arrhythmic).

Results of LM

Eighteen (8.7%) of 208 patients were found to have "active myocarditis" by LM, according to the Dallas criteria [4]. Sixteen patients (7.7%) showed "borderline myocarditis," defined as inflammation present in quantities insufficient to diagnose active myocarditis or not associated with myocyte injury. Additional findings included cardiac hypertrophy in 122 patients (58%) and fibrosis in 62 patients (30%).

Immunofluorescence Findings

Correlation of Immunofluorescence and LM Diagnosis of Myocarditis: Immunofluorescence variables that identified patients with cellular infiltrates included IgG and C3. In our initial experience [9], receiver operating characteristics curve (ROC) analysis suggested that IgG was about twice as closely associated with cellular infiltration as was C3, and that a total immunofluorescence scale score would be optimized by the formula 2 (IgG) + (C3). This formula, modified to require an overall immunofluorescence score >2 and the presence of C3, was then prospectively applied to the expanded patient series.

A 2 × 3 association table was then constructed (Table 2). To construct this table, patients were classified according to the immunofluorescence scale score and the presence or absence of myocarditis on LM by the Dallas criteria. The frequency of patients in each contingent category was then tabulated. Of the 208 patients, 33 (16%) were found to have an immunofluorescence score >2. Of these, 18 (55%) showed active myocarditis; 13 (39%), borderline myocarditis; and two (6%) IDC alone ($p < 0.00001$ for the contingency table). Of those with an immunofluorescence score ≤ 2, only three (2%) had borderline myocarditis, and the rest IDC. HRA was shown in our previous study not to correlate with myocarditis [9] and was not routinely sought in our expanded patient group.

Table 2. Predictive value of immunofluorescence (IF) for LM diagnosis of myocarditis (MC)

	LM diagnosis		
IF score	Active MC (*n*)	Borderline MC (*n*)	IDC (*n*)
IF > 2 (*n* = 33)	18	13	2
IF ≤ 2 (*n* = 175)	0	3	172

Overall $p \ll 0.00001$.
$p \leq 0.055$, active versus borderline MC.
$p < 0.00001$, MC versus IDC.

Immunofluorescence Pattern of Vascular Localization of IgG+C Suggesting Vasculitis: Ten patients (5%) were found to have IgG+C in a vascular distribution. LM showed active myocarditis in three of these, borderline myocarditis in two, but vasculitis in none. The five with myocarditis by LM showed prominent endothelial cell swelling but no infiltration in blood vessels of lymphocytes or polymorphonuclear leukocytes. The remaining five patients showed only IDC by LM. All ten patients also showed vascular HLA-DR staining (see below).

Immunofluorescence Patterns Associated with Other Autoimmune Diseases: In our patient series, several presented with concurrent diagnoses of other autoimmune diseases and were found to have unusual immunofluorescence staining patterns which are of interest. In one, features of mixed connective disease were found, consisting of a speckled pattern of nuclear staining with IgG, and interstitial IgG+C3. Two patients with systemic lupus erythematosus were studied; both showed homogeneous nuclear staining of IgG, suggestive of antinuclear antibody (ANA) activity. Both also showed large amounts of interstitial IgG+C3. One patient with scleroderma was studied and showed strong vascular staining with fibrinogen and marked thickening of blood vessels by LM. Three patients with acute rheumatic fever and associated heart disease were examined. In all three, LM showed and interstitial histiocytic infiltrate, and immunofluorescence showed coarse, granular deposits of C3 and, to a lesser extent, IgG.

Immunofluorescence Identification of Infiltrating Cells: The identity of infiltrating cells was determined by semiquantitative immunofluorescence grading with monoclonal antibodies. Approximately one-half of infiltrating cells in patients with myocarditis were histiocytes. Of the one-half of cells which were lymphocytes, the majority were T cells, which were about equally divided between T helper and T suppressor/cytotoxic cells. Individual patterns varied, however: three patients showed only T lymphocytes; two of these showed persistence of myocarditis on repeat biopsy. Patients with acute rheumatic heart disease showed histiocytes only, and those with connective tissue disease showed a predominance of B over T lymphocytes (Table 3).

Table 3. Lymphocyte subtypes in inflammatory heart disease

Disease type	T only	T+B+H	B> T	Histiocytes only
Myocarditis	3	15	1	2
Acute rheumatic	0	0	0	3
Systemic lupus	0	0	2	0
Mixed connective tissue disease	0	0	1	0

Number of patients given for each category. *H*, histiocytes; *B*, B lymphocytes; *T*, T lymphocytes.

Table 4. Vascular HLA-DR in heart muscle disease

	Myocarditis	Autoimmune heart disease	IDC
HLA-DR +	35	17	2
HLA-DR −	0	0	78

$p \ll 0.00001$.
Number of patients given for each category.

Endothelial Cell Activation with Expression of Vascular HLA-DR: Attention has been drawn recently to endothelial cell activation with expression of vascular HLA-DR (Ia-like antigen) in other active disease with autoimmune mechanisms (e.g., diabetes, thyroid diseases, etc.) [16, 17]. Burger has suggested that the endothelium may act as an antigen-presenting cell, and endothelial DR expression as an early sign of immune activation [18, 19]. In our series, all patients with inflammatory heart disease of all types were positive for HLA-DR (Table 4). In contrast, only two of 80 (3%) of patients with IDC demonstrated vascular HLA-DR staining, and in both of these, staining was weak.

In addition, the five patients noted above with vascular IgG+C staining and IDC showed strong HLA-DR staining, suggesting a distinctive subgroup of patients with evidence of vascular immune complex disease (see "Discussion").

It is apparent that the appearance of vascular HLA-DR is a highly sensitive and discriminating marker for inflammatory heart disease. The contingency table (Table 4) shows a chi-square value of 124, $p \ll 0.0001$. Thus, such staining should prove particular useful for screening for diseases associated with immune activation involving the heart.

Evaluation of Immunofluorescence Findings in Serially Studied Patients: Among patients with inflammatory heart disease followed serially, nine showed resolution of myocarditis and two relapsed. Three had persistent myocarditis, and seven showed progression to advanced IDC. HLA-DR associated with myocarditis became negative within 2–6 months in association with resolution of myocarditis by LM and immunofluorescence.

EM Findings

EM proved useful for: (1) confirming the identity of inflammatory cells; (2) distinguishing cell degeneration and cell necrosis; and (3) providing prognostic information.

EM Confirmation of the Identity of Infiltrating Inflammatory Cells: Ultrastructural features were not found which reliably selected out patients who had histologically confirmed inflammatory infiltrates by LM diagnosed as myocarditis. However, EM did provide a useful function in confirming the identity of infiltrating cells. By LM, such cells are easily confused with swollen perivascular fibroblasts (pericytes) and swollen endothelial cells, which may have nuclear configurations very similar to those of lymphocytes or histiocytes. EM readily distinguishes between vascular and inflammatory cells. Vascular cells are surrounded by basal lamina and contain pinocytotic vesicles, features lacking in lymphocytes and histiocytes. Conversely, lymphocytes and histiocytes may be identified by recognized ultrastructural features [20].

EM was also useful in identifying and differentiating myocyte degeneration from necrosis. Myocyte injury is required as part of the definition of myocarditis by the Dallas criteria [4]. Myocyte degeneration was defined as EM evidence of cellular damage, including myofilament loss, replacement of myofilament volume with increased numbers of mitochondria and/or glycogen, dilation of sarcoplasmic reticulum, accumulation of fat droplets and phagolysosomes, and loss of normal myofilament banding pattern [21, 22]. Myocyte necrosis was determined to be present by EM if plasma and/or nuclear membranes showed discontinuity or disintegration and mitochondria showed lysis of cristae, loss of matrix, and/or dense body formation [21, 22].

By EM, myocyte degeneration was present in virtually all patients examined, whereas myocyte necrosis was present in only 16 (20%) of the 79 patients. In addition, evidence of cardiac hypertrophy by EM was found in 33 (42%) of patients. This was evidenced by tortuous intercalated discs, nuclear irregularities, glycogen-filled subsarcolemmal cytoplasmic aggregates, and increased cellular size [21, 22].

Myofilament Loss by EM and Mortality: Myofilament loss (decreased cellular myofilament volume fraction) proved to be the only significant predictor of survivor outcome of the 12 EM features thought to be potentially useful prognostically (Table 1). A progressive increase in mortality (from 0% to 50%) was observed with increasing grades of myofilament loss ($r = 0.336$, $p < 0.03$) (Table 5). Myofilament loss graded as $>1+$ appeared to be a reasonable single criterion for prediction of mortality. Mortality was 37% for 2–3+ loss, versus 10% for 0–1+ loss, giving a risk ratio of 3.7 (chi-square $= 6.51$, $p < 0.09$). The sensitivity for this determination was 0.69, the specificity 0.70, positive predictive value 0.37, and negative predictive value 0.90. Overall predictive accuracy

Table 5. Myofilament loss by EM and prognosis in ICD

Myofilament loss (grade)	Outcome[a]		Mortality (%)
	Patients alive	Patients dead	
0	20	1	5
1+	24	4	14
2+	17	9	35
3+	2	2	50

$P \leq 0.026$.
[a] Mean follow-up 18.3 months (range to 48 months).

Table 6. Logistic model of clinical data and myofilament loss by EM to predict mortality

Variable	Coefficient	Standard error	p value
Symptom duration	− 0.58121	0.3398	<0.0918
Functional class	− 0.21303	0.5290	<0.6884
Ejection fraction	0.0435	0.0319	<0.1774
Myofilament loss	− 1.1587	0.4333	<0.0094
Constant	2.2590		

was 0.70. The prognostic utility of myofilament loss was similar in those with or without inflammatory infiltration (overall mortality was 28% [4/14] in patients with myocarditis and 18% [12/65] among those without, $p =$ NS).

Further analysis showed the presence of myofilament loss to provide independent prognostic information. In order to evaluate this, a stepwise logistic regression was performed. In the first model, traditional clinical data were forced into the first step to see if myofilament loss would add significantly to the prediction of mortality in the second step. The clinical data used in this analysis included symptom duration ≤1 versus >1 year, ejection fraction, and functional class. Myofilament loss added significantly to these clinical features (improvement chi-square $= 9.02$, $p \leq 0.003$). The variables used in the final (second step) logistic model are shown in Table 6. The contribution of myofilament loss was substantially greater (by a factor of 10, with a $p <0.009$) than that of the clinical variables.

Discussion

The present review of our initial and expanded experience suggests the utility and complementary value of routinely adding immunofluorescence and EM to the LM evaluation of endomyocardial biopsy samples in patients undergoing diagnostic evaluation for heart muscle diseases.

Complementary Role of Immunofluorescence: We have shown that immunofluorescence allows the demonstration of IgG and C3 deposition in the heart, indicators of humoral immune activity which are otherwise not assessed. Staining for IgG and C3 most likely indicates deposition of immune complexes. Their interstitial distribution may result from endothelial injury and consequent vascular permeability, which is an integral part of the inflammatory response in other organs [23] and likely also in the heart. The universal demonstration of HLA-DR appearance in endothelium from patients with inflammatory heart disease provides further evidence of the importance of the endothelium in the inflammatory response in the heart and is consistent with the hypothesis that the endothelium is acting as an antigen-presenting cell [18, 19].

The most important contribution of immunofluorescence to the examination of EMB samples is the complementary and confirmatory role served in the diagnosis of myocarditis and other autoimmune disorders affecting the heart.

Our expanded series confirms the predictive value of IgG and C3 by immunofluorescence of cellular myocarditis present on LM. This information is important, because cellular infiltrates are often focal and sporadic by LM, and could be missed, due to sampling error. The finding of IgG and C3 staining in such biopsies may raise the suspicion of myocarditis, prompting more careful, or repeat, biopsy evaluation. On the other hand, the absence of immunofluorescence staining may raise the question of a false-positive diagnosis, perhaps caused by the misclassification of noninflammatory cells. EM can then be used for definitive identification of these cells. Immunofluorescence also makes possible the subclassification of myocarditis into cellular, humoral, and mixed (the majority) types. Each of these may carry a distinctive prognostic and therapeutic profile; however, our experience to date is insufficient to define these features for each subclass. Finally, immunofluorescence also allows accurate assessment of humoral immune reactions in the heart in the presence of other autoimmune disorders, such as acute rheumatic fever, lupus erythematosus, mixed connective tissue disease, and scleroderma. A distinct subset of patients also showed vascular localization of immune complexes, either with or without associated myocarditis, but without classic features of vasculitis by LM. It is likely that LM evidence of vasculitis may occur at a later or different stage than demonstration of immune complex deposition by immunofluorescence. One recent patient with heart failure and vascular localization of immune complexes without myocarditis was eventually shown to have post-streptococcal glomerulonephritis, an immune complex disease, which responded to therapy. Additional experience with this subgroup of patients will be of interest.

Complementary Role of EM: In our hands, EM proved useful in evaluation of EMB samples for:
1) distinguishing presumed inflammatory cells, observed by LM, from cells of other types, such as swollen pericytes or fibroblasts;
2) subclassifying "myocyte injury" into myocyte degeneration and necrosis, which may appear identical by LM [21, 22]; and, most importantly,
3) predicting clinical outcome. The EM finding of myofilament loss (decreased myofibril volume fraction) appears to represent a feature of unique prognostic importance.

Ultrastructural Features and Prognosis: LM evaluation of EMB generally results in nonspecific findings of debatable prognostic utility. Schwarz et al. found that LM features did not add independent prognostic information to hemodynamic variables [24]. In contrast to LM, EM is suggested by our study to have substantial prognostic potential. The degree of myofilament loss (reduction in myofilament volume fraction) was a strong predictor of mortality in IDC (risk ratio 3.7), whether or not patients had associated myocarditis. Patients could be dichotomized into those with low (10%) and high (37%) 18-month mortality, based on the EM finding of minimal (0–1+) versus significant (2–3+) myofilament loss. Further, mortality risk associated with EM loss was indepedent of the duration of disease, clinical class, and ejection fraction, all of which were poor predictors of individual survival in our group of IDC patients.

Myofilament loss on EM was the single strongest statistical predictor of mortality, emerging over the clinical variables by a factor of 10.

Currently, we are in the process of attempting to validate the predictive value of myofilament loss in a prospectively studied expanded patient series. However, the study of Figulla et al. [25] supports our findings. These authors evaluated myofibril loss by high-resolution LM and correlated findings with subsequent disease course. A cellular myofibril volume fraction of less than 60% was used as the prognostic variable. Reduced myofibril volume fraction was found in 23 of 24 patients who deteriorated or died (sensitivity, 96%), whereas a more normal myofibril volume fraction ($\geq 60\%$) was observed in 14 of 15 whose condition improved or stabilized (specificity, 93%) ($p < 0.002$). Thus, we believe that the ultrastructural assessment of myofibril or myofilament volume is a promising prognostic variable that may add independent predictive value to the usual clinical and hemodynamic variables assessed in IDC.

Conclusion

IDC and myocarditis form a multifaceted disease spectrum that is not well understood. Although endomyocardial biopsy is being increasingly applied in this setting, its utility continues to be reasonably questioned [3, 6, 7]. LM findings are often nonspecific and of little prognostic utility. LM diagnosis of myocarditis is subject to substantial interobserver variability. Our initial and expanded experience suggests that immunofluorescence and EM assessment may provide important additional and complementary diagnostic and prognostic information, both in inflammatory and noninflammatory forms of heart muscle disease. On the basis of these observations, we propose an integrated approach to the use of these three tools in routine EMB evaluation.

In the future, prospective and expanded studies in many centers will be important to confirm and extend these observations and to determine their precise clinical importance. Such additional studies may contribute important additional insights into IDC pathogenesis and therapy, so that more rational diagnostic, prognostic, and therapeutic categories can be formulated.

References

1. Gillum RG (1986) Idiopathic cardiomyopathy in the United States. 1970–82. Am Heart J 111:752–755
2. Robinson JA, O'Connell JB (1983) (eds) Myocarditis: precursor of cardiomyopathy. Collamore, Lexington
3. Mason JW, O'Connell JB (1989) Clinical merit of endomyocardial biopsy. Circulation 79:971–979
4. Aretz HT, Billingham ME, Edwards WD et al (1986) Myocarditis: a histopathologic definition and classification. Am J Cardiovasc Pathol 1:3–14
5. Shanes JG, Ghali J, Billingham ME et al (1987) Interobserver variability in the pathologic interpretation of endomyocardial biopsy results. Circulation 75:401–405

6. Tazelaar HD, Billingham ME (1986) Leukocytic infiltrates in idiopathic dilated cardio-myopathy. A source of confusion with active myocarditis. Am J Surg Pathol 10:405–412
7. MacKay EH, Littler WA, Sleight P (1978) Critical assessment of diagnostic value of endomyocardial biopsy. Br Heart J 40:69–78
8. Ferrans VJ, Roberts WC (1978) Myocardial biopsy: a useful diagnostic procedure or only a research tool? Am J Cardiol 41:965–967
9. Hammond EH, Menlove RL, Anderson JG (1987) Predictive value of immunofluores-cence and electron microscopic evaluation of endomyocardial biopsies in the diagnosis and prognosis of myocarditis and idiopathic dilated cardiomyopathy. Am Heart J 114:1055–1065
10. Hammond EH, Menlove RL, Anderson JL (1988) Immunofluorescence microscopy in the diagnosis and follow-up of patients suspected of having inflammatory heart disease. In: Schultheiss HP (ed) New concepts in viral heart disease. Springer, Berlin Heidelberg New York, pp 303–311
11. Mason JW (1978) Techniques for right and left ventricular endomyocardial biopsy. Am J Cardiol 41:887–892
12. Anderson JL, Marshall HW, Allison SB (1984) The femoral venous approach to endo-myocardial biopsy: comparison with internal jugular and transarterial approaches. Am J Cardiol 53:833–837
13. Anastasiou-Nana MI (1988), Sorensen SG, Fowles RE, Allison SB, Nanas JN, Anderson JL (1988) Validation of a new femoral venous method of endomyocardial biopsy. J Interven Cardiol (4):263–271.
14. Dvorak AM, Hammond EM, Dvorak HF, Karnovsky MJ (1972) Loss of cell surface material from peritoneal exudate cells associated with lymphocyte-mediated inhibition of macrophage migration from capillary tubes. Lab Invest 27:561–574
15. Edwards WD, Holmes DR, Reeder GS (1982) Diagnosis of active lymphocytic myocar-ditis by endomyocardial biopsy. Mayo Clin Proc 57:419–425
16. Jansson K, Karlsson A, Forsum U (1984) Intrathyroidal HLA-DR expression and T lymphocyte phenotypes in Graves' thyrotoxicosis, Hashimoto's thyroiditis, and nodular colloid goitre. Clin Exp Immunol 58:264–272
17. Bottazzo GF, Dean BM, McNally JM, Mackay EH, Swift PGF, Gamble DR (1985) In situ characterization of autoimmune phenomena and expression of HLA molecules in the pancreas in diabetic insulitis. N Engl J Med 313:353–360
18. Burger DR, Vetto RM (1982) Vascular endothelium as a major participant in T-lympho-cyte immunity. Cell Immunol 70:357–361
19. Wagner CR, Vetto RM, Burger DR (1985) Subcultured human endothelial cells can function independently as fully competent antigen presenting cells. Hum Immunol 13:33–48
20. Bessis M (1973) Living blood cells and their ultrastructure. Springer, Berlin Heidelberg New York
21. Knieriem HJ (1978) Electron-microscopic findings in congestive cardiomyopathy. In: Kaltenbach M, Loogen F, Olsen ECJ (eds) Cardiomyopathy and myocardial biopsy. Springer, Berlin Heidelberg New York, pp 71–86
22. Ferrans VJ (1978) Ultrastructure in human cardiac hypertrophy. In: Kaltenbach M, Loogen F, Olsen ECJ (eds) Cardiomyopathy and myocardial biopsy. Springer, Berlin Heidelberg New York, pp 100–121
23. Clark RAF, Dvorak HF, Colvin RB (1981) Fibronectin in delayed type hypersensitivity reactions. Association with vessel permeability and endothelial cell activation. J Immunol 126:787–791
24. Schwarz F, Mall G, Zebe H, Schnitzer E, Manthey J, Scheurlen H, Kubler W (1984) Determinants of survival in patients with congestive cardiomyopathy: quantitative mor-phologic findings and left ventricular hemodynamics. Circulation 70:923–928
25. Figulla HR, Rahlf G, Nieger M, Luig H, Kreuzer H (1985) Spontaneous hemodynamic improvement or stabilization and associated biopsy findings in patients with congestive cardiomyopathy. Circulation 71:1095–1104

3 Clinical Aspects and Treatment of Myocarditis

Natural History of Viral Myocarditis: Critical Viewpoints

M. Sekiguchi, M. Hiroe, S. Nunoda, M. Hongo, and T. Misawa

Introduction

Viral myocarditis is regarded as the most important element in the development of dilated cardiomyopathy (DCM) [1–4]. Also, our analysis of biopsy samples from the myocardium [5–22] in patients with idiopathic DCM and with arrythmias and/or conduction disturbance of an idiopathic nature showed findings highly suggestive of myocarditis in 15% of the DCM cases and in 8.7% of the cases with arrythmias and/or conduction disturbances [17].

In a study in Stanford, biopsy analysis in cases of unexplained congestive heart failure revealed active myocarditis [23]. The authors therefore treated patients with immunosuppressive agents and reported that this seemed effective.

By contrast, Japanese investigators, including us, have reported that patients who showed evidence of myocarditis at the acute stage, i.e. acute myocarditis, recovered very well without programmed immunosuppressive therapy [5, 21]. Therefore, the value of immunosuppressive therapy requires further evaluation. Our aim is to clarify the natural history of patients in whom biopsies were performed and make suggestions on whether or not immunosuppressive therapy is necessary in myocarditis.

Clinical Diagnostic Criteria

The diagnosis should be based on symptomatology, data from clinical laboratory examinations, and definitive autopsy or biopsy findings. We made proposal for clinical diagnosis based on the above constituents; this is presented in Table 1. The criteria were derived from the experience of analyzing four autopsied and 12 biopsied cases in which there were definitive histopathological findings. Programmed immunosuppressive therapies were not given in these cases.

Table 1. Diagnostic criteria of acute viral or idiopathic myocarditis: the criteria were derived from our clinical analysis of patients who had undergone endomyocardial biopsy at the acute stage (from [8])

Major manifestations
1. Cardiac symptoms[a] which appear within 10 days after onset of the preceding symptoms[b]
2. Electrocardiographic abnormalities (severe arrhythmias such as atrioventricular block, ST-T changes, low R wave, abnormal Q wave, and intraventricular conduction disturbances) and an associated rise in cardiac sarcoplasmic enzymes in the serum

Minor manifestations
1. Positive results in neutralizing antibody, complement fixation, or hemagglutination inhibition tests
2. Positive histopathologic diagnosis employing endomyocardial biopsy[c]
3. No significant stenosis revealed by coronary angiography

The diagnosis is justified if both of the major manifestations plus two of the minor manifestations are present.

[a] Cardiac symptoms: Adams-Stokes attack, congestive heart failure, cardiogenic shock.

[b] Preceding symptoms: fever, influenza-like symptoms (cough, sore throat, general malaise, myalgia, arthralgia), gastrointestinal symptoms (nausea, vomiting, anorexia, abdominal pain), chest pain or discomfort.

[c] Endomyocardial biopsy findings: interstitial cellular infiltration consisting of small round cells and large mononuclear cells with or without basophilic cytoplasm, degeneration and lysis of myocytes, and fragmentation of muscle bundles.

Histopathological Diagnostic Criteria

Definition of Myocarditis

Myocarditis has been defined by two distinguished authorities as being "characterized by an inflammatory infiltrate and by injury to the adjacent myocardial cells that is not typical of infarction" [1, 2, 24]. In view of the relatively recent introduction of treatment by corticosteroids or immunosuppressive agents, a sequential biopsy examination is now necessary for classification of myocarditis.

Olsens's descriptions of the essential features of myocarditis [24] are incorporated in the Dallas Pathology Panel's recommendation.

Dallas Pathology Panel Recommendation [25]

The Dallas Panel has set forth useful criteria and guidelines in an attempt to classify the morphologic diagnosis of myocarditis. Billingham [25] listed the requirements for the biopsy diagnosis of myocarditis and the common problems which may be encountered. Diagnostic categories of myocarditis are presented in Table 2.

Table 2. Diagnostic categories of myocarditis (from [25])

First biopsy
- Active myocarditis (with or without fibrosis)
- Borderline myocarditis (not diagnostic and requiring further biopsy)
- No evidence of myocarditis

Subsequent biopsies
- Ongoing (persistent) myocarditis
- Resolving (healing) myocarditis
- Resolved (healed) myocarditis – this group may have the feature of end-stage dilated cardiomyopathy

Analysis of Histopathological Findings

Serial endomyocardial biopsy findings in cases with acute viral or idiopathic myocarditis were analyzed at our laboratory [11, 17, 18]. The histopathological findings were analyzed during the acute stage (10-days after the onset: 8.3 ± 1.9 days) in 6 cases, the subacute stage (11–21 days: 18.2 ± 2.2 days) in 6 cases, and the convalescent stage (22–167 days: 54.5 ± 45.4 days) in 8 cases. The incidence and severity of various changes of the cardiac myocytes and interstitium were analyzed and compared at each stage of the disease. In the acute stage, interstitial cell infiltration was composed of fibroblasts, macrophages, and lymphocytes, in descending order. In the convalescent stage, interstitial cell infiltration showed a marked decrease and was replaced by fibrocytes. In the subacute stage, transitional changes between the acute and convalescent stages were observable. Myocardial samples from 21 control cases with myocardial infarction which were compared at various stages with the myocarditis specimens revealed that in the acute stage, neutrophils were the most prominent, and that in the subacute and convalescent stages, macrophages were most frequent and plasma cells were the least frequent (Tables 3–5).

Table 3. Histopathological characteristics of acute myocarditis obtained using endomyocardial biopsy (from [11, 14])

1. Interstitial cell infiltrate composed of polymorphous fibroblasts, macrophages, and lymphocytes with close contact with adjacent myocytes
2. Fragmentation of the muscle bundles
3. Various forms of myocardial degeneration which are characterized by progressive myocytolysis and disappearance
4. Swelling of the sarcoplasm and nuclei as well as scarcity of myofibrils of myocytes
5. Variation in size of myocytes
6. Dissarrangement of the muscle bundles
7. Interstitial edema
8. Increase in glycogen deposition in myocytes
9. Increase of myocyte branching
10. Interstitial fibrosis
11. Endocarditic changes

Table 4. Histopathological characteristics of postmyocarditic changes obtained using endomyocardial biopsy (from [11, 14])

1. Various changes which are observed in acute myocarditis still exist; however, myocytolysis, swelling of sarcoplasm of myocytes and interstitial edema are no longer evident
2. Decrease in large mononuclear cell infiltration in the interstitium and replacement by fibrocytes increases
3. Myocytes increase in size and show hypertrophy associated with pyknosis, enlargement, and deformities of the nuclei
4. Increase in incidence of double nuclei in myocytes
5. Increase of abnormal branching of myocytes
6. Increase in interstitial fibrosis
7. Endocardial thickening and subendocardial fibrosis
8. Increase of fatty tissue in the myocardium

Table 5. Histopathological characteristics of healed myocarditis (from [14])

1. Increase in interstitial fibrosis showing fibrous replacement
2. Fatty tissue replacement may be present
3. Fragmentation and disarrangement of muscle bundles
4. Less or absence of interstitial mononuclear cell infiltration

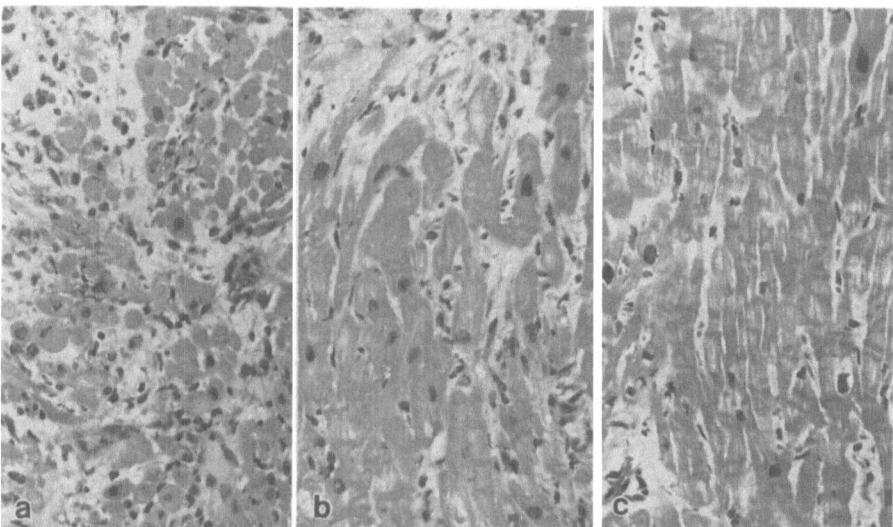

Fig. 1 a–c. Three sequential biopsies on the 9th (**a**), 17th (**b**), and 29th day (**c**) after the onset of acute myocarditis in a 50-year-old man who was admitted to our CCU because of fainting attacks due to slow cardiac ryhthm disturbance (case 9 of ref. [6]). ECG revealed complete atrioventricular (A–V) block. As a result of conventional intensive care without immunosuppressive therapy, he was able to return home 40 days after the onset. The ECG showed recovery of the A–V block but residual intraventricular conduction abnormalities with complete right bundle branch block were seen. **a** Numerous interstitial cell infiltrations are seen. **b** A decrease in cell infiltration and a lessening of the destructive changes of the myocardium are seen. **c** Apparently healed myocardium. (From [6])

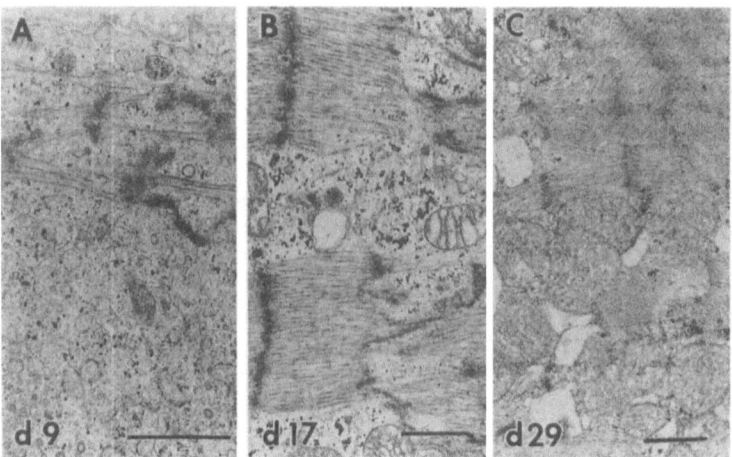

Fig. 2 A–C. Changes of the ultrastructure of the cardiac myocyte over sequential biopsies. The pictures were from the same patient as those in Fig. 1. **A** Extreme reduction of myofibrils and mitochondrial damage at the acute stage (day 9 after the onset of illnes); **B** regenerating process at the subacute stage (day 17) showing increased Z-band architecture; **C** at convalescence (day 29) there is criss-cross interfibrillar disorganization of myofibrils

A further control study of 58 cases comparing the changes in the convalescent stage of myocarditis and the myocardial changes in chronic right ventricular overload revealed that in the former, fragmentation of the muscle bundles, abnormal branching, size variation, glycogen deposition, and large mononuclear cell infiltrations were significantly more frequent.

An example is shown in Figs. 1 and 2.

Natural History of Myocarditis: Profile of Patients Without Immunosuppressive Therapy

A review of 30 patients in whom the diagnosis of acute myocarditis was made at autopsy or biopsy (including serial biopsy) was presented by us [21]. In our initial experience, five autopsied patients revealed cardiogenic shock, congestive heart failure, and grave arrhythmias or conduction disturbances. Twenty-five patients (83%) showed a fairly good recovery (NYHA I–II) even though they had grave clinical features at the onset. Only conventional medical treatment without programmed immunosuppressive therapy was given in our cases. A serial biopsy analysis revealed a resolving or healing course of the myocarditis. A clinical follow-up for 1–14 years (mean 4.1 ± 4.4) was done in 20 patients who left hospital after recovery. Seven patients (35%) showed residual conduction abnormalities, such as advanced atrioventricular block, complete right bundle branch block, and/or left axis deviation. Three of them were on permanent pacemaker. Seven patients (35%) showed normal ECG findings after recovery. It is worthy of note that only two patients (10%) showed clinical evidence of dilated cardiomyopathy.

Kawai [26] recently reviewed the outcome of 31 patients, aged 11–68 years, with myocarditis of unknown etiology who had been treated symptomatically. Diagnosis of myocarditis was mainly based on endomyocardial biopsy or autopsy findings as well as clinical signs and symptoms. A "flu-like" syndrome preceded the illness in 21 (68%) of the 31 patients. In his prognostic survey, 21 patients (68%) improved with only symptomatic or supportive treatment. Two patients died of fulminating myocarditis. Three patients were alive with permanent pacemakers and two died despite implantation of a permanent pacemaker. Three patients with severe myocarditis and circulatory collapse survived the acute phase with the aid of intraaortic balloon pumping and temporary pacemakers, and eventually completely recovered from the illness.

In order to study the clinical status of viral and idiopathic myocarditis in Japan, Kawamura et al. [27], conducted a questionnaire survey and collected data for 218 cases from 62 institutions. The diagnosis was based on clinical and laboratory findings alone in 45% of the cases, and it included endomyocardial biopsy in 24% and autopsy in 9% of the patients. Endomyocardial biopsies were available in 40% of the patients; definite cellular infiltrations were identified in half of them. Males predominated in the patient population; the age range was 30–39 years for both sexes. Cardiac symptoms and signs were common in addition to "common cold" or flu-like symptoms; electrocardiographic abnormalities, leukocytosis, increased erythrocyte sedimentation rate, positive CRP, and increased cardiac enzyme levels were also very common in the acute phase of the disease. Serologic tests for virus titers, performed in 80% of the cases, were positive in 21% only. There was no apparent correlation between serologic results and endomyocardial biopsy findings. In this survey, complete recovery occurred in 43%, incomplete recovery in 40%, recurrences in 3%, and death in 13% of the total patient population (Table 6).

In a subsequent study [28] of the cases with incomplete recovery, it was found that further recovery occurred in 19%, recovery remained incomplete in 73%, and death occurred in 6% (Table 7). Among the cases with incomplete recovery, there were DCM-like states in 15%, hypertrophic cardiomyopathy (HCM)-like ventricular thickening in 2%, and non-DCM, non-HCM states in 49%. In this last group, there were many cases where intraventricular conduction disturbances existed.

Table 6. Initial outcome of myocarditis (7 days to 16 years; $n = 218$) (from [27])

	n	%
1. Complete recovery	93	42.7
2. Incomplete recovery	87[a]	39.9
3. Recurrence	7	3.2
4. Death	29	13.3
5. Unknown	2	0.9

[a] See Table 7.

Table 7. Later outcome in 67 of the 87 patients (77%) with incomplete recovery (7 days to 17 years, mean 2.8 years) (from [28])

	n	%
1. Complete recovery	13	19.4
2. Incomplete recovery[a]	49	73.1
3. Death[a]	4	6.0
4. Others	1	1.5
DCM-like state	8/53	15.1
HCM-like state	1/53	1.9
Non-DCM non-HCM state	26/53	49.1

[a] Incomplete recovery/death.

Role of Biopsy in Postmyocarditic State and in DCM

Controversy exists over the role of endomyocardial biopsy in evaluating patients with DCM, particularly in detecting myocarditis and in assessing prognosis. Interobserver variability, if high, could explain conflicting reports. To assess this possibility, Shanes et al. [29] submitted biopsy specimens from 16 patients with dilated cardiomyopathy to seven cardiac pathologists. The same slides were independently reviewed by each and assessed for fibrosis, hypertrophy, nuclear changes on a 0 to 3+ scale, mean lymphocyte count per high-power field, and myocarditis. The prevalence of significant fibrosis ranged from 25% to 69%, hypertrophy from 19% to 88%, nuclear changes from 31% to 94%, and abnormal lymphocyte count from 0 to 38%. One or more pathologists diagnosed definite or possible myocarditis in 11 of the 16 patients. Of these 11 patients, three pathologists agreed about three and two pathologists agreed about five. Myocarditis was diagnosed by a single pathologist in three cases. Through this study, they concluded that interobserver variability in interpreting biopsy specimens from patients with DCM is high and that quantitative and standardized methods are needed to increase diagnostic consistency.

Practical Guide for Making Histopathological Diagnoses of Myocarditis and Postmyocarditis

It is difficult to make a precise histopathological diagnosis of myocarditis at the convalescent or healed stage of the disease [14, 15, 19, 20]. It is something like seeing a burned-out shell of a building and trying to assess the cause of the fire. Our diagnostic guidelines were made in order to solve this problem and to standardize the interpretation of myocarditic and postmyocarditis changes (Tables 3–5) [14, 20].

The principle of the diagnosis is similar to that of the Dallas criteria [25]. However, the interpretation is more detailed and is applicable even when biopsy is performed only once.

1) A diagnosis of acute or active myocarditis can be made when the findings listed in Table 3 are observed. If the findings are resolving in nature, a diagnosis of subacute or resolving myocarditis can be made.
2) A diagnosis of convalescent or healing myocarditis can be made when the findings listed in Table 4 are observed. A large number of fibrocytes as well as fibroblasts and a lower incidence of lymphocytes may be characteristic.
3) A diagnosis of healed myocarditis should be made only when previous biopsies have been performed. Characteristic findings are listed in Table 5.
4) Diagnostic categorization of myocarditis or postmyocarditis can be done.

It is advisable to interpret the biopsy findings without any clinical information and then to place them into one of the following categories after receiving the information:

(a) Definitely present;
(b) Highly suggestive;
(c) Slightly suggestive;
(d) Doubtful;
(e) Not suggestive.

Stages of disease may also be determined.

Using this system, we were able to classify biopsy findings from specimens taken during a single rather than a serial biopsy. We were also able to divide the disease into acute, subacute, and convalescent stages.

Our analysis [17] revealed that highly suggestive postmyocarditic changes were found in 22 of 145 cases with DCM (15%), 21 of 241 cases with arrhythmias and/or conduction disturbances (8.7%), and 3 of 174 cases with HCM (1.7%).

In order to assess the feasibility of biopsy diagnosis of myocarditis, a histopathological diagnosis was made without any clinical information by three investigators at our cardiac biopsy laboratory who are well experienced and the results were evaluated by receiver operating characteristics (ROC) analysis [22]. The outcome was that observers A, B, and C had true-positive rates of 100%, 100%, and 93% and false-negative rates of 26%, 31%, and 24%, respectively. So, we have to reconcile the false-positive and false-negative rates.

An English group [32] recently reported that enterovirus RNA detected in myocardial biopsies was related to Coxsackie B virus IgM and B_1-B_5 neutralizing antibody (NAT). One hundred patients with heart muscle disease were studied. Virus RNA was detected in 60% with active myocarditis, 47% with healing myocarditis and 55% with healed myocarditis or dilated cardiomyopathy. Whereas NAT did not correlate with muscle virus RNA, in all patients with Coxsackie-specific IgM enterovirus RNA was detected in biopsy tissue.

They stated than the virus RNA is present in more than 50% of patients with myocarditis. Detection of Coxsackie B-specific IgM further implicates this virus in the pathogenesis of human myocarditis.

On the Existence of Chronic Myocarditis

The term "chronic myocarditis" causes confusion whether it is based only on clinical features alone or on histopathological evaluation [30]. We believe that this term should be applied in those cases where the biopsy findings showed the features compatible with presence of the disease. Such a case is illustrated in Fig. 3. This biopsy picture was taken 3 weeks after the onset of flu-like symptoms as the second biopsy in a sequence. This patient was the only one where a sustained DCM-like state was observed. This type of observation was rarely ever made by us, i.e., 2 out of 100 patients with DCM. At the time of the pacemaker replacement for the sustained atrioventricular block after the onset of acute myocarditis, this patient underwent the third biopsy, which was 8 years after onset of the illness. The biopsy showed no signs of active myocarditis but instead interstitial fibrosis of moderate degree and loose myofibrils of the cardiac myocytes. The term "healed myocarditis" can suitably be applied in this case. We have observed a similar case where the diagnosis was made 9 years after the onset of fully documented acute myocarditis. No immunosuppressive therapy was given in the above two cases.

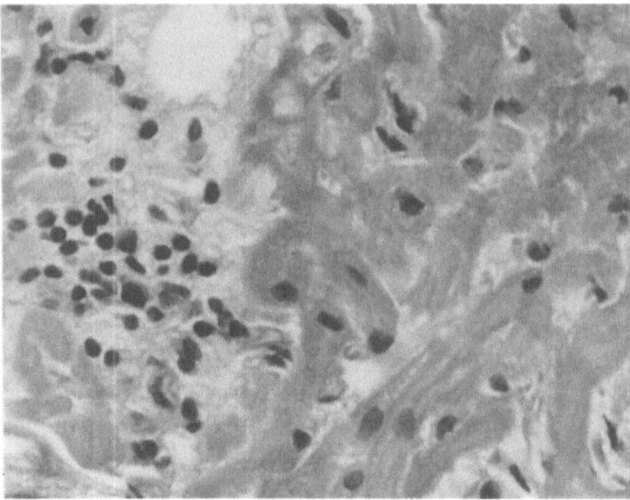

Fig. 3. An endomyocardial biopsy picture suggesting active or chronic myocarditis in a 55-year-old male patient who showed clinical evidence of acute myocarditis (case 7 of ref. [6]). A right ventricular endomyocardial biopsy was performed 3 weeks after the onset of the illness. Note the focal lymphocytic and plasma cell infiltration in the interstitium and disarrangement of the muscle bundles

The Usefulness of Immunosuppressive Therapy

There are differences of opinion regarding the use of anti-inflammatory agents such as steroids and other immunosuppressive agents [33–35]. Generally, the use of corticosteroids appears to be controversial in myocarditis of viral etiology because of their suppressive effect on systemic defense and myocardial regeneration, as well as the suppression of interferon [33, 34]. Mason et al. [23] showed, on the basis of endomyocardial biopsy findings, that immunosuppressive therapy using prednisone and/or azathioprine was effective in eliminating myocardial inflammation and improving myocardial performance in ten patients with acute myocarditis. These patients, however, had suffered from congestive heart failure for over 4–18 months following the onset of myocarditis, and therefore one should consider that an immune reaction may be progressing in this type of patient from the start. Our experience of employing sequential endomyocardial biopsy in cases of acute myocarditis has shown that healing of myocarditis can occur without the use of immunosuppressive agents [5–21].

Steroids may be beneficial in the prevention of cardiogenic shock, but not in the healing process of myocarditis. Therefore, the question of whether or not immunosuppressive therapy is necessary and effective during the acute stage of myocarditis remains unanswered.

Camerini's group [36] reported that active myocarditis was diagnosed in 17 out of 295 patients who underwent endomyocardial biopsy. To evaluate the effects of prednisone (50 mg m^{-2} day^{-1}, then tapered) and azathioprine (75 mg m^{-2} day^{-1}), patients underwent endomyocardial biopsy and ejection fraction measurement during the minimum treatment period of 6 months. After 2 months of treatment, persistent myocarditis was present in only three patients, while healing or healed myocarditis was present in eight and six patients, respectively. Continuos treatment was associated with the disappearance of the histological signs of myocarditis in 14 patients. Subsequent reduction or interruption of treatment was associated with a worsening histology in ten patients. Ejection fraction estimated at the end of the treatment period (six patients) or at the latest follow-up (11 patients) improved from 37.8 ± 14% to 44.8 ± 17.6%, $p = 0.031$. They concluded that the immunosuppressive treatment was associated with a reduction of the histological signs of myocarditis in most patients and, concomitantly, significant improvement of ejection fraction was observed.

However, their results do not seem to differ from those of Japanese studies in which immunosuppressive therapy was not given. Richardson's group [37] gave immunosuppressive therapy in their biopsy-proven acute myocarditis cases ($n = 23$) and reported results of a long-term follow-up of up to 4–5 years. They observed that characteristic features of DCM developed in 12 patients (52%), 4 of whom died. They then showed that left ventricular function 6–8 months following acute myocarditis predicts outcome; the late follow-up has shown progression to DCM in 50% of cases and most patients have persistent impairment of cardiac reserve.

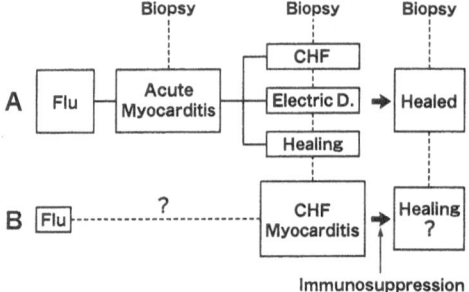

Fig. 4. Controversial points in diagnosing and treating myocarditis with regards to immunosuppressive therapy (see text for explanation)

Differentiating Acute and Active Myocarditis and Immunosuppressive Therapy

We believe that lymphocytic infiltration is not always indicative of acute myocarditis. In our sequential biopsy study with acute myocarditis, infiltrated lymphocytes were not the most frequent interstitial cell constituents but fibroblasts or macrophages [11, 18]. One can thus say that the lymphocytic criteria for the diagnosis are not fulfilled even in cases of "acute" myocarditis [20]. In the biopsy cases of Mason et al. [23] or Edwards et al. [31] the biopsies were not performed immediately after the onset of myocarditis, and lymphocytic cells were the most frequent infiltrating cells.

Therefore, "acute" and "active" forms of disease should be discriminated, and not be incorporated in a single study group.

Figure 4 summarizes the controversial points in diagnosing or treating myocarditis. Two different schemes are shown. A is based on our own experience and on the Japanese multicenter study, where, in almost all cases, acute myocarditis was preceded by a flu syndrome and biopsy was performed at an early stage, i.e., within 1–2 weeks; there was a tendency to heal in many cases, albeit with some residual signs [8-11, 14, 19].

In the second, B, there was little evidence of a preceding flu syndrome; after a certain interval patients with congestive heart failure underwent a biopsy and the diagnosis of active myocarditis, not acute myocarditis, was made. In this situation, some immune reaction [38] may be suspected and immunosuppressive therapy may contribute. The results of our study suggest that in future studies the two types of disease must be discriminated.

Summary

The natural history of patients who showed evidence of viral or idiopathic myocarditis and who were treated conventionally without the aid of immunosuppressive therapy was reviewed, based on our own experience and from the literature.

In our ($n = 30$) and Kawai's experience ($n = 31$) where endomyocardial biopsies were performed at the acute stage, development into dilated cardiomyopathy occurred in only 10% of cases. Residual intraventricular conduction disturbances on the electrocardiogram were rather frequent (20%).

In a Japanese questionnaire survey of 218 patients, 40% of whom underwent biopsy or autopsy, short-term results were: complete recovery in 43%, incomplete recovery in 40%, recurrence in 3%, and death in 13%. Development into a DCM-type clinical picture occured in 15% of the cases with incomplete recovery.

Comparing the data from the literature, when immunosuppressive therapy was given the biopsies were performed long after the onset of the congestive heart failure (1–6 months), indicating that those cases were not of acute myocarditis but should be called active myocarditis. In such circumstances, immunosuppressive therapy may be indicated. However, it is still unknown whether immunosuppressive therapy is necessary in the very acute stage of myocarditis with much cellular infiltration. A randomized case analysis at both the acute and late stages of myocarditis is necessary to evaluate the efficacy of the therapy.

Acknowledgement: This study was supported by a Research Grant for the Intractable Diseases from the Ministry of Health and Welfare of Japan.

References

1. Sekiguchi M, Olsen EGJ, Goodwin JF (eds) (1985) Myocarditis and related disorders. Heart Vessels Suppl 1
2. Kawai C, Abelmann WH (eds) (1987) Pathogenesis of myocarditis and cardiomyopathy. Recent experimental and clinical studies. University of Tokyo Press, Tokyo
3. Maisch B (ed) (1987) Inflammatory heart disease. Eur Heart J 8 [Suppl J]
4. Schultheiss H-P (ed) (1988) New concepts in viral heart disease: virology, immunology and clinical management. Springer, Berlin Heidelberg New York
5. Sekiguchi M, Hiroe M, Ogasawara S, Nishikawa T (1981) Practical aspects of endomyocardial biopsy. Ann Acad Med Singapore 10 (Suppl):115–128
6. Sekiguchi M, Hiroe M, Take M, Hirosawa K (1980) Clinical and histopathological profile of sarcoidosis of the heart and acute myocarditis; II. Myocarditis. Jpn Circul J 44:264–273
7. Sekiguchi M, Hiroe M, Take M, Akamatsu T, Takahashi S (1980) Vasodilator therapy in congestive cardiomyopathy and myocarditis. In: Sekiguchi M, Olsen EGJ (eds) Cardiomyopathy, clinical, pathological and theoretical aspects. University of Tokyo Press, Tokyo and University Park Press, Baltimore, pp 257–275
8. Take M, Sekiguchi M, Hiroe M, Hirosawa K (1981) Early clinical profiles of histopathologically proven cases with acute idiopathic myocarditis and a proposal for diagnostic criteria. Jpn Circul J 45:1415–1420
9. Take M, Sekiguchi M, Hiroe M, Hirosawa K (1982) Long-term follow-up of electrocardiographic findings in patients with acute myocarditis proven by endomyocardial biopsy. Jpn Circul J 46:1127–1234
10. Hasumi M, Sekiguchi M, Morimoto S, Take M, Hirosawa K (1983) Ventriculographic findings at the convalescent stage in eleven cases with acute myocarditis. Jpn Circul J 47:1310–1316
11. Yu Z-X, Sekiguchi M, Hiroe M, Take M, Hirosawa K (1984) Histopathological findings of acute and convalescent myocarditis obtained by serial endomyocardial biopsy. Jpn Circul J 48:1368–1374

12. Hiroe M, Sekiguchi M, Take M, Matsuda M, Hirosawa K (1985) Hemodynamic studies and response to a combined therapy of nitroglycerin ointment and dopamine in patients with acute myocarditis. Heart Vessels Suppl 1:180–186

13. Hiroe M, Sekiguchi M, Take M, Kusakabe K, Shigeta A, Hirosawa K (1985) Long follow-up study in patients with prior myocarditis by radionuclide methods. Heart Vessels Suppl 1:199–203

14. Sekiguchi M, Hiroe M, Yu Z-X, Hasumi M (1987) A serial endomyocardial biopsy study on myocarditis. In: Kawai C, Abelmann WH (eds) Pathogenesis of myocarditis and cardiomyopathy. Recent experimental and clinical studies. University of Tokyo Press, Tokyo, pp 213–231

15. Sekiguchi M, Yu Z-X, Hasumi M, Hiroe M, Morimoto S, Nishikawa T (1985) Histopathologic and ultrastructural observations of acute and convalescent myocarditis. A serial endomyocardial biopsy study. Heart Vessels Suppl 1:143–153

16. Sekiguchi M, Olsen EGJ, Goodwin JF (1985) Editor's comments on the biopsy diagnosis of myocarditis. Heart Vessels Suppl 1:306–308

17. Take M, Sekiguchi M, Hiroe M, Hirosawa K (1985) A clinicopathologic study on a cause of idiopathic cardiomyopathy and arrythmia and conduction disturbance employing endomyocardial biopsy. Heart Vessels Suppl 1:159–164

18. Yu Z-X, Sekiguchi M, Hiroe M, Take M, Hirosawa K (1985) A comparative ultrastructural study on the nature of interstitial cell constituents in idiopathic myocarditis and myocardial infarction. Heart Vessels Suppl 1:154–158

19. Yu Z-X, Sekiguchi M, Hiroe M, Hasumi M, Morimoto S, Hirosawa K (1985) On the interstitial fibrotic changes in acute and convalescent myoarditis obtained by serial endomyocardial biopsy. Jpn Circul J 49:1270–1276

20. Hasumi M, Sekiguchi M, Yu Z-X, Hirosawa K, Hiroe M (1986) Analysis of histopathologic findings in cases with dilated cardiomyopathy with special reference to formulating diagnostic criteria on the possibility of postmyocarditic change. Jpn Circul J 50:1280–1287

21. Sekiguchi M, Hiroe M, Hiramitsu S, Izumi T (1988) Natural history of acute viral or idiopathic myocarditis: a clinical and endomyocardial biopsy follow-up. In: Schultheiss H-P (ed) New concepts in viral heart disease: virology, immunology and clinical management. Springer, Berlin Heidelberg New York Tokyo, pp 33–50

22. Sekiguchi M, Hiroe M, Yu Z-X, Hasumi M (1986) Observer variation study in myocarditis using ROC analysis. Presented at the XII Congress of Cardiology, Washington

23. Mason JW, Billingham ME, Ricci DR (1980) Treatment of acute inflammatory myocarditis assisted by endomyocardial biopsy. Am J Cardiol 45:1037–1044

24. Olsen EGJ (1985) Histopathologic aspects of viral myocarditis and its diagnostic criteria. Heart Vessels Suppl 1:130–132

25. Billingham ME (1985) The diagnostic criteria of myocarditis by endomyocardial biopsy. Heart Vessel Suppl 1:133–137

26. Kawai C (1988) Clinical and experimental aspects of treatment for viral myocarditis. In: Schultheiss H-P (ed) New concepts in viral heart disease: virology, immunology and clinical management. Springer, Berlin Heidelberg New York Tokyo, pp 433–437

27. Kawamura K, Kitaura Y, Morita H, Deguchi H, Kotaka M (1985) Viral and idiopathic myocarditis in Japan: a questionnaire survey. Heart Vessels Suppl 1:18–22

28. Kawamura K (1987) Report of a committee on myocarditis. Annual Report for Intractable Disease. Ministry of Health and Welfare of Japan, p 13 (in Japanese)

29. Shanes JG, Ghali J, Billingham ME, Ferrans VJ, Fenoglio JJ, Edwards WD, Tsai CC, Saffitz JE, Isner J, Furner S, Subramanian R (1987) Interobserver variability in the pathologic interpretation of endomyocardial biopsy results. Circulation 75:401–405

30. Fenoglio JJ, Ursell PC, Kelogg CF, Pil M, Drusin RE, Weiss MB (1983) Diagnosis and classification of myocarditis by endomyocardial biopsy. N Engl J Med 308:12–18

31. Edwards WD, Holmes DR Jr, Reeder GS (1982) Diagnosis of active lymphocytic myocarditis by endomyocardial biopsy: quantitative criteria for light microscopy. Mayo Clin Proc 57:419–425

32. Archard LC, Bowles NE, Freeke C, Meany B, Morgan-Capner P, Olsen EGJ, Richardson PJ (1988) Enterovirus RNA in myocarditis. Eur Heart J Suppl I:19 (abstract)

33. Kilbourne E, Wilson CB, Perrier D (1956) The induction of gross myocardial lesions by a coxsackie (pleurodynia) virus and cortisone. J Clin Invest 35:362–370
34. Tomioka N, Kishimoto C, Matsumori A, Kawai C (1986) Effects of prednisolone on acute viral myocarditis in mice. J Am Coll Cardiol 7:868–872
35. Hosenpud JD, McAnulty JH, Nlies NR (1985) Lack of objective improvement in ventricular systolic function in patients with myocarditis treated with azathioprine and predonisone. J Am Coll Cardiol 6:797–801
36. Salvi A, Hrovatin E, Dreas L, Silvestri F, Camerini F (1987) Changes in histology and left ventricular ejection fraction during immunosuppressive treatment in active myocarditis. Eur Heart J 8 (Suppl J):267–269
37. Quigley PJ, Richardson PJ, Meany BT, Olsen EGJ, Monaghan MJ, Jackson G, Jewitt DE (1987) Long-term follow-up of acute myocarditis. Correlation of ventricular function and outcome. Eur Heart J 8 (Suppl J):39–42
38. Maisch B, Deeg P, Liebau G, Kochsick K (1983) Diagnostic relevance of humoral and cytotoxic immune reactions in primary and secondary dilated cardiomyopathy. Am J Cardiol 52:1072–1078

Clinical Presentation and Evolution in Treated and Untreated Myocarditis

A. Salvi, L. Dreas, A. Di Lenarda, F. Silvestri, E. Della Grazia, B. Pinamonti,
R. Bussani, G. Sinagra, and F. Camerini

Introduction

Before the introduction of the endomyocardial bioptome as a diagnostic tool
[1] the diagnosis of myocarditis, although often clinically suspected, could not
be confirmed in vivo. This resulted in a poor understanding of the natural
course of the disease which as been clarified in the recent past, particularly by
Sekiguchi et al. and Kaway [2, 3] in Japan, where the technique of endomyocardial biopsy was initially developed, as well as by other authors [4].

Our interest in the study of myocardial diseases led to the referral of several
patients from different italian regions, in whom myocarditis was diagnosed with
endomyocardial biopsy or at postmortem. In this study we will analyze the
clinical presentation and the evolution of 40 of these patients observed in the
past 10 years.

Patients and Methods

From January 1978 to May 1989, endomyocardial biopsy was performed in 435
patients with suspected myocardial disease. According to the Dallas criteria [5],
myocarditis was diagnosed in 41 patients. In two additional patients, who died
of refractory heart failure shortly after admission, the histologic diagnosis of
myocarditis was made at postmortem.

The clinical presentation, the initial histologic aspects, and the evolution
were analyzed in 40 of these patients (15 women and 25 men with an age range
at presentation of 5–69 years, mean 38 years), while two patients with eosinophilic myocarditis and one patient with rheumatic carditis were excluded.

At the time of admission, a complete clinical evaluation was made with
particular interest to the presence of preceding viral illnesses and to the onset
of the first symptom, and included: ECG, chest X-ray, 24-h ECG recording,
M-mode and/or two-dimensional echocardiography [6], standard laboratory
investigations and Coxsackie B virus-neutralizing antibodies (in 16 patients),
and cardiac catheterization (in 39 patients). Selective coronary arteriography,
in order to exclude coronary artery disease, was performed in all patients over
25 years of age, except in two women aged 34 years who presented with
congestive heart failure, and in four patients with atrioventricular block. The

status of the coronary arteries was assessed in the youngest patients by aortography or at postmortem in the two patients who died shortly after admission.

At the end of follow-up, all patients were examined clinically and underwent ECG and M-mode and two-dimensional echocardiography; in patients with atrial tachycardia or atrioventricular block who were not treated with a permanent pacemaker, a 24-h continuous ECG was recorded.

Histologic data during follow-up were obtained in 35 out of the 38 patients in whom myocarditis was initially diagnosed by endomyocardial biopsy. In addition, all the initial histologic slides were reviewed and the amount of inflammatory cells, necrosis, and their distribution were semiquantitatively assessed by one investigator unaware of the clinical presentation and of the name of the patient.

Results

Several clinical presentations were observed (Table 1).

Table 1. Myocarditis – clinical presentation

	Fulminant heart failure	Chest pain	A–V block	Persistent atrial tachycardia	Congestive heart failure
	($n = 2$)	($n = 5$)	($n = 6$)	($n = 2$)	($n = 25$)
Influenza syndrome (< 3 months)	All	None	1/6	None	13/25
Illness duration	< 8 days	≤ 8 days	< 20 days	1–3 months	> 1 month–3 years (mean: 5 months)
Multiorgan failure	All	None	None	None	None
Abnormal ECG	All	All	All	All	All
CK	All	4/5	None	None	None
EF	19%–23%	All > 50%	All > 50%	40%–51%	7%–42% 29% (mean)
Normal LV Histology	None	4/5	All	None	None
Infiltrate	++++	++	+++/++++	++	+/++
Necrosis	++++	+	+/++	+	+
Endomyocarditis	1/2	None	5/6	None	1/25

EF, ejection fraction; *LV*, left ventricle; *CK*, increased creatine kinase.

Fulminant Heart Failure

Two young patients presented shortly after an acute viral infection with severe heart and multiorgan failure and elevated cardiac enzymes. A fulminant down-hill course ending with death within 1 week was noted. Both showed histologic features of severe necrosis and inflammatory infiltration (with endomyocarditis in one) at postmortem.

Chest Pain

In five patients the initial symptomatology was characterized by anginal chest pain and the histologic diagnosis of myocarditis was always made within few days. An abnormal ECG was present in all (mainly ST elevation or ST-T changes) usually associated with a slight elevation of CPK.

Four out of five patients showed a preserved ventricular function at echo-cardiography and/or angiography. The histologic features were characterized by mild degrees of inflammation and necrosis and none showed signs of endo-myocarditis. Two patients were treated with immunosuppressives [7], and all were followed up for 36–75 months (mean 48.6).

Endomyocardial biopsy after a mean of 5 months in four patients showed a

Table 2. Myocarditis – outcome

	Fulminant heart failure	Chest pain	A–V block	Persistent atrial tachy-cardia	Congestive heart failure
	(n = 2)	(n = 5)	(n = 6)	(n = 2)	(n = 25)
Treatment					
Immunosuppressive	1/2	2/5	3/6	2/2	20/25
Permanent PM	None	None	3/6	None	None
Follow-up (mean)	4 days	48.6 months	69 months	45 months	33.8 months
NYHA	–	Complete recovery in all	Complete recovery (3/6) I (3/6)	I	I–II (16/25)
Death	All	None	None	None	9/25
CHF	2/2	–	–	–	5/9
Arrhythmia	–	–	–	–	3/9
Noncardiac	–	–	–	–	1/9
EF	–	Normal	Normal	Normal	37% (mean)
Normal LV	–	4/5	All	All	4/22

PM, pacemaker; *NYHA,* functional class; *CHF,* congestive heart failure; *EF,* ejection fraction; *LV,* left ventricle.

healing or healed myocarditis. No recurrences of chest pain were observed, and all patients were alive and completely asymptomatic. Left ventricular ejection fraction at two-dimensional echocardiography was normal in all. One patient showed at long term (Table 2) a mild left ventricular dilatation (echo-LVEDVI $= 60 \, \mathrm{ml/m^2}$) with a normal ejection fraction (54%).

Advanced Atrioventricular Block

Advanced atrioventricular block was present in six patients who were biopsied after a relatively short history of syncope, presyncope, or fatigue.

A history of influenza-like illness was present in one, and three had a recent (< 20 days) sting (in two) or tick bite (in one). In one patient rickettsial myocarditis was diagnosed [8] and in another it was strongly suspected. Left ventricular function (at echocardiography) was normal in all. The site of the atrioventricular block (studied by electrophysiology in five out of six patients) was suprahisian in two, infrahisian in two, and both hisian and suprahisian in another patient.

Five out of six of the patients showed moderate to severe inflammatory infiltration (Fig. 1) and endomyocarditis which completely disappeared in four out of five at a control biopsy performed after 45 days of treatment with prednisone or tetracycline (in two patients). Permanent pacemaker implantation for persistent atrioventricular block was, however, required in three patients.

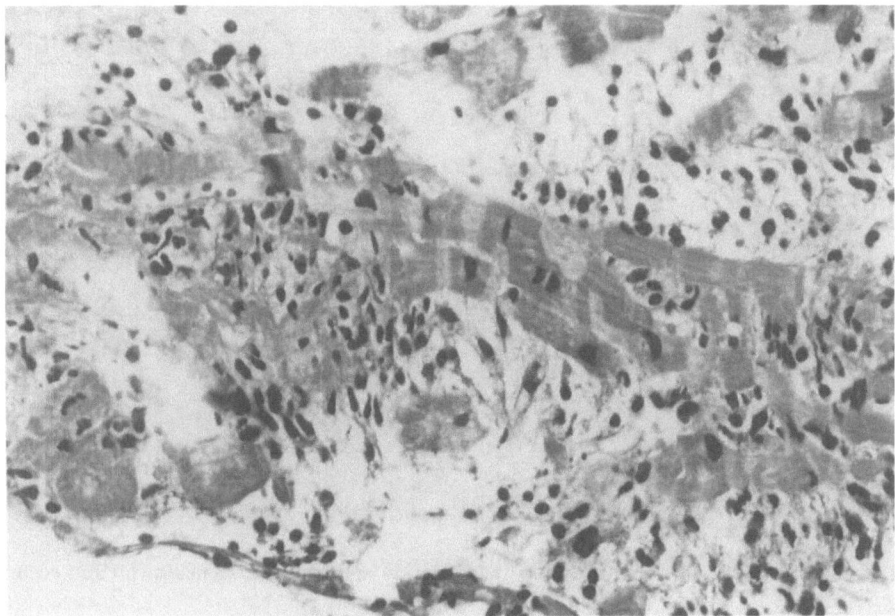

Fig. 1. Severe myocarditis. Hematoxylin and eosin; × 100

After a mean follow-up of 69 months (range 44–97 months) (Table 2), all patients were alive, asymptomatic, and normal left ventricular function and volumes were present in five. Normal sinus rhythm with normal atrioventricular conduction was present in the three patients who were not treated with permanent pacing while persistent atrioventricular block was present in the other three.

Persistent Atrial Tachycardia

Two patients underwent endomyocardial biopsy after a 1–3-month history of atrial tachycardia. The left ventricle was of normal volume but with a slight to moderate reduction of the ejection fraction. Histologic findings characterized by a mild degree of inflammatory cell infiltration were present (Fig. 2). Both were treated with immunosuppression with improvement of the histologic findings and of the left ventricular ejection fraction [7].

After a mean follow-up (Table 2) of 4 years, and 2 years at least after withdrawal of the immunosuppression, both patients were asymptomatic. The left ventricular function and volumes were normal, and the arrhythmia was absent in 24-h ECG recording during treatment with amiodarone 200 mg every 2nd day in one and digoxin 0.125 mg/day in the other.

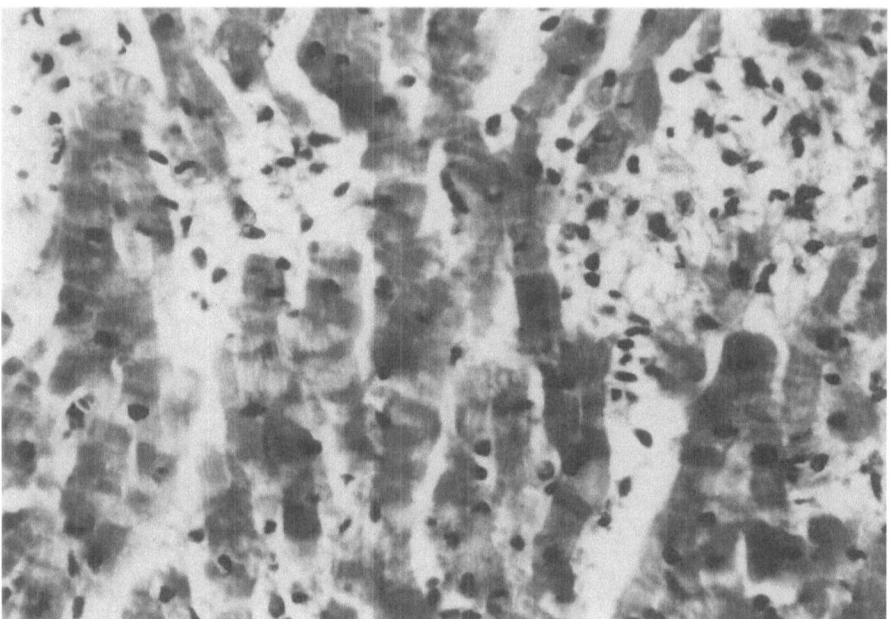

Fig. 2. Myocarditis with mild and focal inflammation and necrosis. Hematoxylin and eosin; × 100

Congestive Heart Failure

Myocarditis was histologically diagnosed in 25 patients among the 255 observed in the past 10 years, who presented with idiopathic heart failure and who were investigated with endomyocardial biopsy after exclusion of coronary artery disease. They had a relatively long (mean 5 months) history of dyspnea on exertion or at rest and at echocardiography the left ventricle appeared mildy or severely ($> 74 \, ml/m^2$) dilated, with a depressed ejection fraction (mean 29%, range 7%–42%).

An influenza-like illness in the preceding 3 months was present in more than 50% of them, and in one patient serial rising neutralizing Ab titers for Coxsackie B virus were found.

The clinical history was very long in three patients, already investigated for idiopathic heart failure 2 or 3 years before, and in whom myocarditis had been excluded at that time by examination of endomyocardial samples.

The longest clinical histories before histologic diagnosis and the slightest degrees of inflammation were observed in this group of patients.

The usual measures for the treatment of heart failure were undertaken in all patients. Immunosuppression with prednisone alone (three patients), prednisone plus azathioprine (16 patients) [8] and cyclosporine (one patient with associated polymyositis) was also employed in 20 patients.

During a follow-up of 33.8 months (range 5–89 months) nine patients died (Table 2). Postmortem examination was possible in three who died 4, 21, and 39 months after the diagnosis and showed a healed myocarditis with fibrosis. Endomyocardial biopsy during follow-up was performed in 21 patients a mean of 11 months (range 2–27) after the initial diagnostic biopsy and showed either a healed (in 19 patients) or a healing myocarditis (in two patients who eventually died and in whom postmortem examination was not obtained).

All patients underwent M-mode and two-dimensional echocardiography during follow-up, but the recordings were considered adequate for the measurements of left ventricular dimensions in 21 only. An overall increase of ejection fraction, from 29% to 37%, was observed, and two subgroups of patients were identified. Thirteen patients showed an increase of ejection fraction of more than 5%, and among them a mortality rate of 15.3% was observed (one patient suffered an out-of-hospital cardiac arrest and another had a cerebral hemorrhage during anticoagulant treatment). In other eight patients, ejection fraction decreased or remained practically unchanged. Among them five died (four due to refractory heart failure and one due to out-of-hospital cardiac arrest). Among the four patients in whom follow-up echocardiography was not adequate, two were alive and two died (one for progressive heart failure and one several days after being resuscitated from his second out-of-hospital cardiac arrest).

In four out of 13 patients (Fig. 3) who presented with severely dilated (Echo LVEDVI $> 73 \, ml/m^2$ vs. normal value of $37 \pm 7 \, ml/m^2$) and hypokinetic (Echo EF $< 40\%$) left ventricle, a complete normalization of ejection fraction and a marked reduction of volumes were observed, but the other nine remained unchanged or deteriorated. Limited information is available about the evolu-

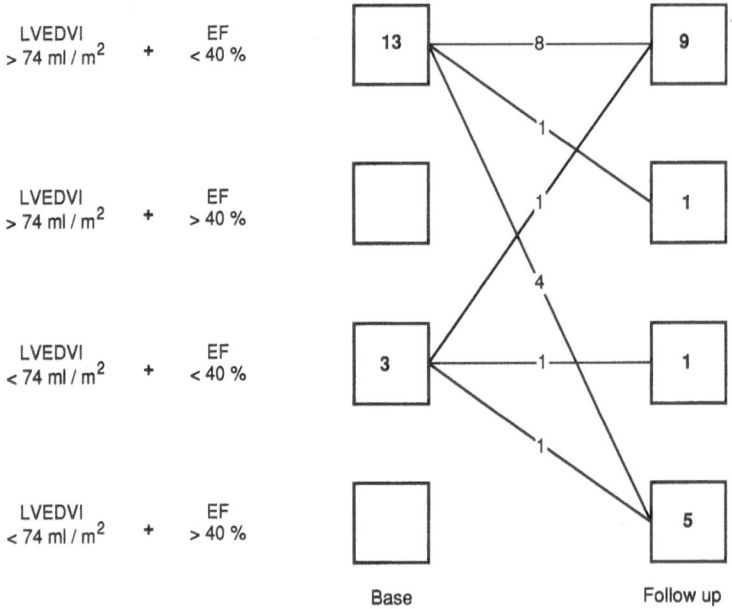

Fig. 3. Left ventricle volume (*LVEDVI*) and ejection fraction (*EF*) changes in patients with myocarditis and congestive heart failure

tion of patients with a severely hypokinetic but only mildly dilated left ventricle at the time of diagnosis. In three of these patients we observed three different behaviours: progressive ventricular dilatation, complete normalization, or persistence of severe hypokinesia and minimal dilatation.

Discussion

In this series of patients with myocarditis diagnosed by histology different clinical presentations were observed. Patients with advanced atrioventricular block or chest pain usually had a short time interval (few days → 3 weeks) between the onset of the first symptom (syncope, presyncope, or pain) and the histologic diagnosis.

A similar short clinical history was observed in two young patients who died of fulminant refractory heart and multiorgan failure. It may be of interest that most patients with these clinical findings (fulminant heart failure, advanced atrioventricular block, chest pain) showed severe degrees of inflammatory cell infiltration with marked necrosis, and endomyocarditis was present in more than half of them. On the contrary, patients with the clinical presentation of congestive heart failure had a longer history (although usually limited to few months) and the histologic picture was less remarkable.

Most cases with biopsy-proven myocarditis described in the literature are characterized by the presence of congestive heart failure of relatively recent, but not abrupt, onset [9–14]. Only a few cases with very recent onset and clinical presentation other than heart failure have been described [8, 15, 16].

In the present study, all the cases included were uniformly considered, but the difference between the two main groups appeared both in the clinical presentation and in the histologic picture and even more in the long-term follow-up.

Patients with chest pain or advanced atrioventricular block of recent onset demonstrated a very good prognosis at long term and none showed an evolution towards dilated cardiomyopathy. On the contrary, mortality was high in the group of patients with heart failure, particularly in those who demonstrated a worsened or an unchanged ejection fraction during follow-up, as already reported by Quigley et al. [4]. The higher mortality rate in this group might reflect the persistence of virus within the myocardium of these patients [17] and preliminary data seem to confirm this hypothesis. However, a complete recovery of ventricular function at rest was possible in some cases who presented with heart failure. It is still undetermined whether this evolution was secondary to the immunosuppressive treatment (employed in all of them) or spontaneous [12, 18]. The ongoing trial on myocarditis [19] will perhaps solve this dilemma.

References

1. Sakakibara S, Konno S (1962) Endomyocardial biopsy. Jpn Heart J 3:537–543
2. Sekiguchi M, Hiroe M, Hiramitusu S, Izumi T (1988) Natural history of acute viral or idiopathic myocarditis: a clinical and endomyocardial biopsy follow up. In: Schultheiss HP (ed) New concepts in viral heart disease. Springer, Berlin Heidelberg New York, pp 33–50
3. Kaway C (1988) Clinical and experimental aspects of treatment for viral myocarditis. In: Schultheiss HP (ed) New concepts in viral heart disease. Springer, Berlin Heidelberg New York Tokyo, pp 433–437
4. Quigley PJ, Richardson PJ, Meany BT, Olsen EGJ, Monaghan MJ, Jackson G, Jewitt DE (1987) Long term follow up of acute myocarditis. Correlation of ventricular function and outcome. Eur Heart J 8 [Suppl J]:39–42
5. Aretz HT, Billingham ME, Edwards WD, Factor SM, Fallon JT, Fenoglio JJ, Olsen EGJ, Schoen FG (1986) Myocarditis: a histopathologic definition and classification. Am J Cardiovasc Pathol 1:3–14
6. Pinamonti B, Alberti E, Cigalotto A, Dreas L, Salvi A, Silvestri F, Camerini F (1988) Echocardiographic findings in myocarditis. Am J Cardiol 62:285–291
7. Salvi A, Di Lenarda A, Dreas L, Silvestri F, Camerini F (1989) Immunosuppressive treatment in myocarditis. Int J Cardiol 22:329–338
8. Salvi A, Della Grazia E, Silvestri F, Camerini F (1985) Acute rickettsial myocarditis and advanced atrioventricular block: diagnosis and treatment aided by endomyocardial biopsy. Int J Cardiol 7:405–409
9. Mason JW, Billingham ME, Ricci DR (1980) Treatment of acute inflammatory myocarditis assisted by endomyocardial biopsy. Am J Cardiol 45:1037–1044
10. Zee-Cheng C-S, Tsai CC, Palmer DC, Codd JE, Pennington DG, Williams GA (1984) High incidence of myocarditis by endomyocardial biopsy in patients with idiopathic congestive cardiomyopathy. J Am Coll Cardiol 3:63–70
11. Daly K, Richardson PJ, Olsen EGJ, Morgan-Capner P, McSorley C, Jackson G, Jewitt DE (1984) Acute myocarditis: Role of histological and virological examination in the diagnosis and assessment of immunosuppressive treatment. Br Heart J 51:30–35

12. Dec GW, Palacios IF, Fallon JT, Aretz HT, Mills J, Lee D C-S, Johnson RA (1985) Active myocarditis in the spectrum of acute dilated cardiomyopathies: clinical features, histologic correlates, and clinical outcome. N Engl J Med 312:885–890
13. Hosenpud JD, McAnulty JH, Niles NR (1985) Lack of objective improvement in ventricular systolic function in patients with myocarditis treated with azathioprine and prednisone. J Am Coll Cardiol 6:797–801
14. Billingham ME, Mason JW (1984) Endomyocardial biopsy diagnosis of myocarditis and changes following immunosuppressive treatment. In: Bolte HD (ed) Virus heart diseases. Springer, Berlin Heidelberg New York Tokyo, pp 200–216
15. Sekiguchi M, Hiroe M, Take M, Hirosawa K (1980) Clinical and histopathologic profile of sarcoidosis of the heart and acute idiopathic myocarditis. Concepts through a study employing endomyocardial biopsy. II. Myocarditis. Jpn Circ J 44:264–273
16. Costanzo-Nordin MR, O'Connell JB, Subramanian R, Robinson JA, Scanlon PJ (1985) Myocarditis confirmed by biopsy presenting as acute myocardial infarction. Br Heart J 53:25–29
17. Bowles NE, Olsen EGJ, Richardson PJ, Archard LC (1986) Detection of coxsackie B virus specific RNA sequences in myocardial biopsy samples from patients with myocarditis and dilated cardiomyopathy. Lancet i:1120–1122
18. Kawamura K, Kitaura Y, Morita H, Deguchi H, Kotaka M (1985) Viral and idiopathic myocarditis in Japan: A questionnaire survey. In: Sekiguchi M, Olsen EGJ, Goodwin JF (eds) Myocarditis and related disorders. Springer, Berlin Heidelberg New York Tokyo, pp 18–22
19. Anderson JL, Fowles RE, Unverferth DV, Mason JW (1987) Immunosuppressive therapy of myocardial inflammatory disease. Initial experience and future trials to define indication for therapy. Eur Heart J 8 [Suppl J]:263–266

Immunosuppressive Therapy in Active Myocarditis

J. B. O'Connell

Pathogenesis of Myocarditis

The precise mechanisms leading to immune-mediated damage of the human myocardium following viral infection are unknown. In the murine model infection with Coxsackie B or encephalomyocarditis viruses result in self-limited viral replication in the myocardium [12, 16]. Following viral clearance, however, cytoxic T lymphocytes with heart-reactive specificity participate in the progressive myocyte injury. In some strains this immune-mediated injury is due to antibodies which are specific for cardiac antigens such as myosin rather than cytotoxic T lymphocytes [13, 18].

Analogous immune mechanisms have been proposed for the human disease but have not been proven. Although human cardiotropic virus infection is common [8], myocardial viral replication is generally asymptomatic; hence, subjects only rarely present to the physician during this phase. Patients, who have recovered from acute viral myocarditis diagnosed by clinical criteria, develop cardiomyopathy at a high frequency on long term follow-up [22]. The lack of noninvasive diagnostic techniques hinder the understanding of the immunopathogenesis of this disease in man. Nonetheless, most investigators agree that active myocarditis results from immune-mediated myocardial injury rather than direct damage by replicating virus.

Diagnostic Techniques

It was not possible to establish an accurate diagnosis of myocarditis during life until safe techniques of endomyocardial biopsy were developed. Mason et al. were first to report histologic proof of myocarditis by biopsy in patients with unexplained congestive heart failure [14]. In most instances this diagnosis was unsuspected. Clinicopathologic correlative studies have shown that the criteria for the clinical diagnosis of myocarditis do not accurately predict histologic activity on biopsy. Only duration of symptoms correlates active myocarditis. Radioisotopic techniques such as gallium-67 and indium-111 antimyosin antibody have been proposed as screening tools for active myocarditis [21, 30]. These techniques have only been applied to small study populations and cannot be recommended to establish the diagnosis.

Table 1. Incidence of myocarditis diagnosed by biopsy in unexplained congestive heart failure

Investigators	Year	Patients biopsied (n)	Myocarditis (%)
Mason et al. [14]	1980	400	2
Noda et al. [20]	1980	52	1
Baandrup and Olsen [2]	1981	201	4
Das et al. [5]	1981	12	8
Nippoldt et al. [19]	1982	34	12
Fenoglio et al. [9]	1983	135	25
Unverferth et al. [29]	1983	42	9
Strain et al. [28]	1983	64	26
Parillo et al. [23]	1984	74	26
Zee-Cheng et al. [31]	1984	35	63
O'Connell et al. [21]	1984	68	7
Daly et al. [4]	1984	69	17
Regitz et al. [24]	1984	290	6
Rose et al. [6]	1984	76	0
Dec et al. [6]	1985	27	67
Mortensen et al. [17]	1985	65	18
Hosenpud et al. [11]	1985	38	16
Cassling et al. [3]	1985	80	2
Salvi et al. [26]	1987	74	18

Although sampling error may reduce the sensitivity of active myocarditis, the specificity should be quite high. Careful analysis of reports of histologic myocarditis in patients with unexplained heart failure (Table 1), however, demonstrate a great variability in incidence [2–6, 9, 11, 14, 17, 19, 20, 21, 23–26, 28, 29, 31]. This wide discrepancy was in large part a result of a lack of uniform histologic criteria. The "Dallas" criteria, defining myocarditis as inflammatory infiltration with myocyte necrosis in the absence of ischemia, have been proposed as a working histologic definition [1], and reports since 1987 usually apply these criteria. Therefore, endomyocardial biopsy is an accurate diagnostic tool for identifying active myocarditis.

Immunosuppressive Therapy

In their original report of myocarditis in patients with unexplained heart failure, Mason et al. administered prednisone and azathioprine to those with positive biopsies because the histology was reminiscent of allograft rejection [14]. They noted clinical improvement in some patients. Other investigators have administered various immunosuppressants to patients with biopsy-proven myocarditis (Table 2), and 58% of these patients have responded [4, 6, 7, 9–11, 14, 17, 26, 27, 31]. Unfortunately these investigations were uncontrolled; the immunosuppression regimens lacked uniformity both within and among the studies; the histologic diagnosis was inconsistent because these assessments predated the Dallas criteria; and the criteria for improvement are variable. In addition, few patients with active myocarditis have not received immunosup-

Table 2. Immunosuppression in biopsy-proven myocarditis for unexplained heart failure: uncontrolled studies

Investigator	(n)	Improved (n)	Agent(s)
Mason et al. [14]	10	5	cs, a
Sekiguchi et al. [27]	3	2	cs
Edwards et al. [7]	4	2	cs
Fenoglio et al. [9]	19	8	cs, a
Hess et al. [10]	6	6	cs, a, ATG
Daly et al. [4]	9	7	cs, a
Zee-Cheng et al. [31]	11	5	cs, a, ATG
Dec et al. [6]	9	4	cs, a
Hosenpud et al. [11]	6	0	cs, a
Mortensen et al. [17]	12	8	cs, a, cy
Salvi et al. [26]	17	14	cs, a
	106	61 (58%)	

ATG, antithymocyte globulin; *a*, azathioprine; *cs*, corticosteroids; *cy*, cyclosporine.

pression. In the nine patients who did not receive corticosteroids reported by Sekiguchi, seven improved [27]. Edwards et al. found improvement in three of six without immunosuppressive [7]. Dec et al. reported six of 18 patients improved without immunosuppression [6]. The natural history of active myocarditis has therefore not been defined.

Myocarditis Treatment Trial

A multicenter study, sponsored by the National Institutes of Health, which randomly assigns therapy to patients with active myocarditis, has been developed [15]. This study incorporates 23 centers in the United States, Canada and Japan and is coordinated at the University of Utah. Following informed consent patients with unexplained congestive heart failure and an ejection fraction below 45% are randomized to receive either conventional therapy for congestive heart failure alone or conventional therapy plus prednisone and cyclosporine for six months. Patients are then followed for an additional six months on conventional treatment of congestive heart failure without immunosuppressive therapy and final assessment of ejection fraction and treadmill exercise performance is completed one year following randomization.

The purpose of this trial is to determine whether ejection fraction and treadmill exercise performance improve with immunosuppressive therapy. The control group who do not receive immunosuppressive therapy will define the natural history of active myocarditis. In the formal enrollment centers endomyocardial biopsy, right heart catheterization, echocardiography, and 24-h Holter monitoring are performed at baseline 12, 28, and 52 weeks. The information regarding sequential hemodynamic analysis, echocardiographic findings and histology will be invaluable in studying the mechanisms of active myocarditis.

In addition to the clinical trial, a cellular immunology study coordinated at the University of Nebraska utilizes serial serum and tissue samples from randomized patients to ascertain the phenotype and function of peripheral blood lymphocytes and identify the nature of the infiltrating cells. A humoral immunology study, coordinated by investigators at the Johns Hopkins University, is designed to determine the frequency of heart-specific antibody formation and the nature of the antigen that elicits this immune response. A serum and tissue bank with samples from randomized patients and controls with dilated cardiomyopathy is being maintained at the University of Utah for access by investigators interested in investigating the immune mechanisms of dilated cardiomyopathy and myocarditis.

To date over one-half of the required patients are randomized and preliminary observations suggest that approximately 10% of patients with unexplained congestive heart failure have active myocarditis. The results of this study will be key in directing future investigation regarding the immunopathogenesis and treatment of active myocarditis and in addition will further elucidate the necessity of endomyocardial biopsy in the clinical assessment of patients with unexplained heart failure. If efficacy with immunosuppression is proven, patients with unexplained heart failure should undergo endomyocardial biopsy and if the biopsy shows evidence of active myocarditis, immunosuppressive therapy should be administered. If the results demonstrate that immunosuppression is not efficacious in active myocarditis, endomyocardial biopsy is not warranted to rule-out myocarditis in patients with unexplained congestive heart failure because no alteration in therapy can be proposed. The study is not designed to assess the optimal duration of therapy nor optimal combination of immunosuppressive agents which may become the end-points of future clinical trials.

References

1. Aretz HT, Billingham ME, Edwards WD, Factor SM, Fallon JT, Fenoglio JJ Jr, Olsen EGJ, Schoen FJ (1987) Myocarditis: a histopathologic definition and classification. Am J Cardiovasc Pathol 1:3–14
2. Baandrup U, Olsen EGJ (1981) Critical analysis of endomyocardial biopsies from patients suspected of having cardiomyopathy I: morphologic and morphometric aspects. Br Heart J 45:476–486
3. Cassling RS, Linder J, Sears TD, Waller BF, Rogler WC, Wilson JE, Kugler JD, Kay DH, Dillon JC, Slack JD, McManus BM (1985) Quantitation of inflammation in biopsy specimens from idiopathically failing or irritable hearts: experience in 80 pediatric and adult patients. Am Heart J 110:713–720
4. Daly K, Richardson PJ, Olsen EGJ, Morgen-Capner P, McSorley C, Jackson G, Jewitt DE (1984) Acute myocarditis. Role of histologic and virological examination in the diagnosis and assessment of immunosuppressive treatment. Br Heart J 51:30–35
5. Das JP, Rath B, Das S, Sarangi A (1981) Study of endomyocardial biopsies in cardiomyopathy. Indian Heart J 33:18–26
6. Dec GW, Palacios IF, Fallon JT, Aretz HT, Mills J, Lee D C-S, Johnson RA (1985) Active myocarditis in the spectrum of acute dilated cardiomyopathies. Clinical features, histologic correlates and clinical outcome. N Engl J Med 312:885–890
7. Edwards WD, Holmes DR Jr, Reeder GS (1982) Diagnosis of active lymphocytic myocarditis by endomyocardial biopsy. Quantitative criteria for light microscopy. Mayo Clin Proc 57:419–425

8. Eggers HJ, Mertens TW (1987) Viruses and myocardium: notes of a virologist. Eur Heart J 8 (Suppl J):129–133

9. Fenoglio JJ Jr, Ursell PC, Kellogg CF, Drusin RE, Weiss MB (1983) Diagnosis and classification of myocarditis by endomyocardial biopsy. N Engl J Med 308:12–18

10. Hess ML, Hastillo A, Mohanty PK (1983) Inflammatory myocarditis: incidence and response to T-lymphocyte depletion. J Am Coll Cardiol 1:584 (abstr)

11. Hosenpud JD, McAnulty JH, Niles NR (1985) Lack of objective improvement in ventricular systolic function in patients with myocarditis treated with azathioprine and prednisone. J Am Coll Cardiol 6:797–801

12. Huber SA (1987) Viral and immune mechanisms in cardiac diseases. In: Spry CF (ed) Immunology and molecular biology of cardiovascular diseases. MTP Press, Boston, pp 143–159

13. Huber SA, Lodge PA (1986) Coxsackie B-3 myocarditis. Identification of different pathogenic mechanisms in DBA/2 and BALB/c mice. Am J Pathol 122:284–291

14. Mason JW, Billingham ME, Ricci DR (1980) Treatment of acute inflammatory myocarditis assisted by endomyocardial biopsy. Am J Cardiol 45:1037–1044

15. Mason JW, O'Connell JB (1989) Clinical merit of endomyocardial biopsy. Circulation 79:971–979

16. Matsumori A, Kawai C (1982) An animal model of congestive (dilated) cardiomyopathy: dilatation and hypertrophy of the heart in the chronic stage with DBA/2 mice with myocarditis caused by encephalomyocarditis virus. Circulation 66:355–360

17. Mortensen SA, Baandrup U, Buch J, Bendtzen K, Hvid-Jacobsen K (1985) Immunosuppressive therapy of biopsy-proven myocarditis: experiences with corticosteroids and cyclosporine. Int J Immunother 1:35–45

18. Neu N, Rose NR, Beisel KW, Herskowitz A, Gurri-Glass G, Craig SW (1987) Cardiac myosin induces myocarditis in genetically predisposed mice. J Immunol 139:3630–3636

19. Nippoldt TB, Edwards WD, Holmes DR Jr, Reeder GS, Hartzler GO, Smith HC (1982) Right ventricular endomyocardial biopsy: clinicopathologic correlates in 100 consecutive patients. Mayo Clin Proc 57:407–418

20. Noda S (1980) Histopathology of endomyocardial biopsies from patients with idiopathic cardiomyopathy: quantitative evaluation based on multivariate statistical analysis. Jpn Circ J 44:95–116

21. O'Connell JB, Henkin RE, Robinson JA, Subramanian R, Scanlon PJ, Gunnar RM (1984) 67 Gallium imaging in dilated cardiomyopathy with biopsy-proven myocarditis. Circulation 70:58–62

22. O'Connell JB, Mason JW (1989) Therapeutic implications of immune mechanisms in myocarditis. Springer Sem in Immunopathol 11:43–49

23. Parillo JE, Aretz HT, Palacios IF, Fallon JT, Block PC (1984) The results of transvenous endomyocardial biopsy can frequently be used to diagnose myocardial diseases in patients with idiopathic heart failure. Endomyocardial biopsies in 100 consecutive patients revealed a substantial incidence of myocarditis. Circulation 69:93–101

24. Regitz V, Knoll P, Rudolph W (1984) Clinical and hemodynamic findings in patients with histologically documented myocarditis (abst). Eur Heart J 5 (Suppl I):65

25. Rose AG, Fraser RC, Beck W (1984) Absence of evidence of myocarditis in endomyocardial biopsy specimens from patients with dilated (congestive) cardiomyopathy. S Afr Med J 66:871–874

26. Salvi A, Hrovatin E, Dreas L, Silvestri F, Camerini F (1987) Changes in histology and left ventricular ejection fraction during immunosuppressive treatment in active myocarditis. Eur Heart J 8 (Suppl J):267–269

27. Sekiguchi M, Hiroe M, Take M, Hirosawa K (1980) Clinical and histopathological profile of sarcoidosis of the heart and acute idiopathic myocarditis. Concepts through a study employing endomyocardial biopsy II myocarditis. Jpn Circ J 44:264–273

28. Strain JE, Grose RM, Hirsch CL, Kramer DC, Cho S, Factor SM (1983) Atypical presentations of myocarditis (abst). Circulation 68 (Suppl III):III-27

29. Unverferth DV, Fetters DK, Unverferth BJ, Leier CV, Magorien RD, Arn AR, Baker PB (1983) Human myocardial histologic characteristics in congestive heart failure. Circulation 68:1194–1200

30. Yasuda T, Palacios IF, Dec GW, Fallon JT, Gold HK, Leinbach RC, Strauss HW, Khaw BA, Haber E (1987) Indium-111 monoclonal antimyosin imaging in the diagnosis of myocarditis. Circulation 76:306–311
31. Zee-Cheng C-S, Tsai CC, Palmer DC, Codd JE, Pennington G, Williams GA (1984) High incidence of myocarditis by endomyocardial biopsy in patients with idiopathic congestive cardiomyopathy. J Am Coll Cardiol 4:812–819

Immunosuppressive Therapy
in Myocarditis – 24-Month Follow-up

W. Ruzyllo and Z. T. Bilinska

Introduction

Few reports are available on the fate of patients with idiopathic heart failure
and biopsy-proven myocarditis who have been treated by immunosuppression.
Quigley et al. [8] showed that an improvement in ventricular function within
6–8 months of immunosuppression for myocarditis was predictive of an excellent long-term prognosis. The aim of this study was to evaluate results of 6-
month immunosuppression therapy in a group of patients with new-onset idiopathic heart failure and biopsy-proven myocarditis at 24 months' follow-up.

Patients and Methods

From a review of the medical records of 400 patients who had undergone
endomyocardial biopsy between November 1983 and December 1986, we identified 20 consecutive patients who met the following criteria:

– New-onset unexplained heart failure ($<$ 12 months' duration);
– A left ventricular ejection fraction (LVEF) $\leq$ 45%;
– Histological confirmation of myocarditis on initial biopsy;
– Assessment of left ventricular function during at least 24 months' follow-up.

The patients underwent full evaluation including endomyocardial biopsy, heart
catheterization, and radionuclide ventriculography both at presentation and 6
months after immunosuppressive treatment. Coronary angiography was performed in adults to exclude occult coronary heart disease.

Left ventricular, right ventricular, or biventricular endomyocardial biopsy
was performed using the Cordis bioptome [9]. A minimum of three to five
samples, measuring 1–2 mm in diameter, were obtained at each procedure. The
samples were examined by light microscopy. Myocarditis was defined as the
presence of a lymphocytic infiltrate in connection with an injury of adjacent
myocytes (degeneration, necrosis). All repeat biopsy specimens were then
classified according to the Dallas criteria [2].

All patients were treated with standard medical therapy consisting of digoxin
and diuretics. Most patients were also receiving vasodilators (nifedipine or
captopril). Antiarrhythmics were used as deemed necessary. Immunosuppres-

sive treatment (oral prednisone and azathioprine) was started after 2–4 weeks of optimal conventional treatment for heart failure. Prednisone was administered at an initial dose of 1.5 mg/kg/day for the first 2 weeks, tapered to 0.75 mg/kg/day by 4 weeks, maintained until 24 weeks, and tapered off by 28 weeks. Azathioprine was given at a dose of 2.0 mg/kg/day for the entire 24 weeks but reduced if leukopenia (white blood cell count < 4000 mm^3) developed.

Long-term follow-up included routine clinical examination, chest X-ray to determine relative heart volume and radionuclide ventriculography performed after 6 months of immunosuppressive treatment and at final evaluation (24 months after initial biopsy). Left ventricular function was considered to have improved after treatment if the LVEF on the repeat ventriculogram had increased by > 5%.

Statistical Analysis

Measurements were recorded as mean ± SEM values, unless otherwise stated. Statistical analysis was performed using Student's paired t test, where appropriate. A p value of < 0.05 was regarded as statistically significant for a single set of data.

Results

The response to immunosuppressive treatment was evaluated in a total of 20 patients with unexplained heart failure and biopsy-proven myocarditis. The average age of the patients was 33.8 years (range 14–55 years). Sex distribution was 14 males and 6 females. Heart failure was < 6 months' duration in 16 patients and > 6 months' in four patients. Mean duration of the disease was 7.8 ± 10.5 months. Mean LVEF was 25.8% ± 8.9% (range 7%–45%). Inflammatory cellular infiltrates consisted predominantly of lymphocytes and were

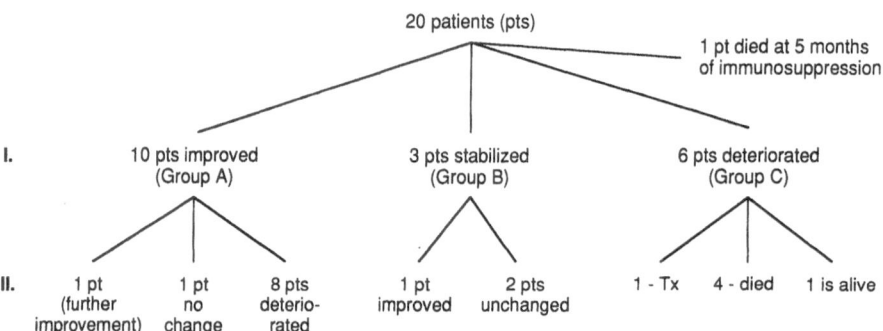

Fig. 1. Early and late results of immunosuppressive therapy. *I*, at 6 months of immunosuppression; *II*, at 24-month follow-up; *Tx*, heart transplantation

judged to be mild in nine, moderate in seven, and severe in four cases. One patient died of progressive heart failure 5 months after initial biopsy.

The individual response to immunosuppressive treatment was variable. Of the 19 patients who completed immunosuppressive treatment, left ventricular function improved in ten (50%) (group A), remained unchanged in three (15%) (group B) and deteriorated in six (30%) (group C) (Fig. 1). The mean LVEF increased from 25.85% ± 8.9% to 35.95% ± 13.3%, $p < 0.02$.

On repeat biopsy, histological examination showed resolution of both infiltrate and myocyte injury in all patients. At 24-month follow-up, eight patients from group A failed to sustain improvement. Their mean initial LVEF was 26.6% ± 9.95%. After 6 months of immunosuppressive treatment, the mean LVEF increased to 51.0% ± 7.1% ($p < 0.01$) and declined to 32.0% ± 6.8%

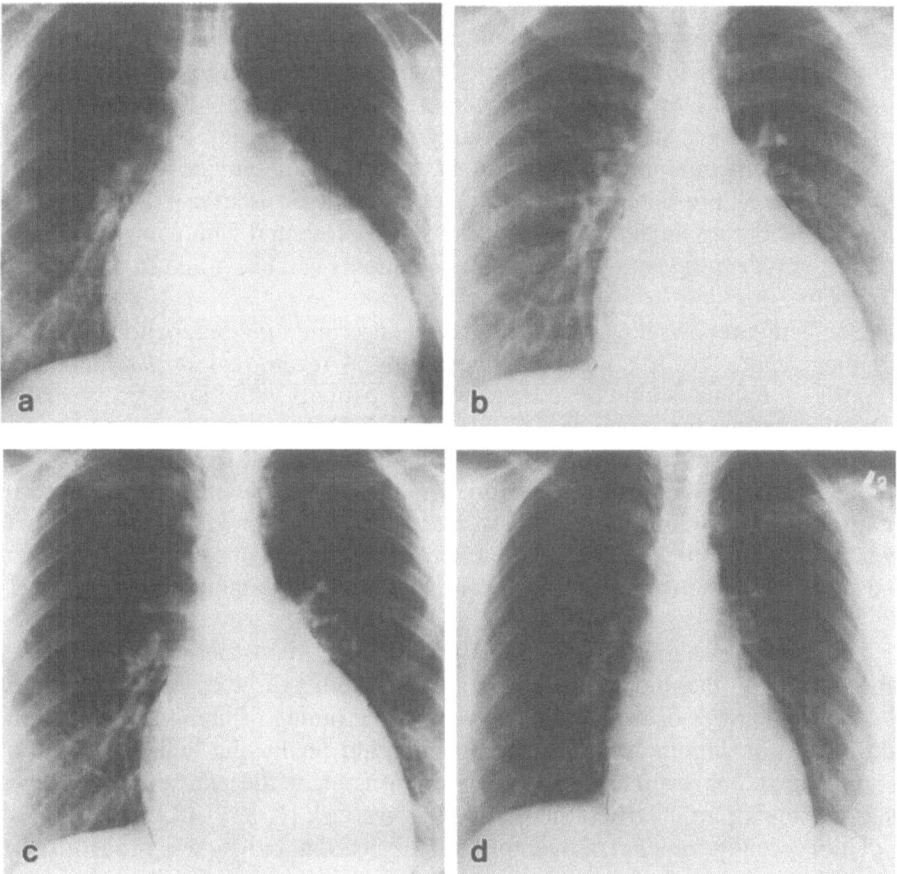

Fig. 2 a–d. Chest X-ray of a 14-year-old girl with active lymphocytic myocarditis; **a** before immunosuppressive therapy (IT), LVEF – 11%; **b** after 6 months of IT, LVEF – 17%; **c** 6 months after discontinuation of IT; **d** 18 months after discontinuation of IT, LVEF – 43%/41% (rest/exercise)

($p < 0.001$) at final evaluation. One patient, a 14-year-old girl from group A (Fig. 2) improved further. Her LVEF at the time of initial biopsy, repeat biopsy, and final determination was 11%, 17%, 43%/41% (rest/exercise), respectively. The last patient of group A remained unchanged.

Of the three patients in group B, one improved further. Her pretreatment LVEF was 22%, posttreatment LVEF 24%, and final LVEF 42%/38% (rest/exercise). The two remaining patients from group B stabilized. All patients in group C continued to deteriorate; four of them died of progressive heart failure, one underwent heart transplantation, one is alive.

Discussion

The clinical diagnosis of myocarditis is very difficult. Sudden onset of the disease and rapidly progressive heart failure do not necessarily indicate myocarditis. Some patients with such a clinical picture do not have inflammatory infiltrates on biopsy [5]. Histopathological criteria for the diagnosis of myocarditis were defined in Dallas, 1984 [2]. From a very considerable bank of biopsy data at Stanford University, it has been established that only fulminant, diffuse infiltrates, present in every biopsy fragment, lead to heart failure [3]. All except four of our patients, did not have diffuse inflammatory infiltrates on biopsy, but all presented with features of cardiomyocyte injury, and most had mild to moderate inflammatory infiltrates. All presented with congestive heart failure of recent onset (< 12 months), 16 patients had heart failure of less than 6 months' duration.

Conflicting reports have been published concerning the therapeutic benefit of immunosuppressive treatment for myocarditis. A recent review of 12 published reports on immunosuppressive therapy in 97 patients with biopsy-proven myocarditis revealed improvement in 54 (56%) [7]. Unfortunately, in these studies there were no control groups. Reports on conventional treatment in biopsy-proven myocarditis are not substantially different [7]. Of the 33 patients, 16 improved spontaneously for a 48% success rate. Thus, any improvement in left ventricular function, thought to be associated with immunosuppression, is not necessarily related to this therapy, but may represent spontaneous recovery [1, 7, 11].

Differences in patient population, sometimes insidious onset of the disease, the timing of the biopsy, interobserver variability in the interpretation of histologic features of myocarditis as well as the timing of immunosuppression, differences in immunosuppressive regimes, and finally the high incidence of spontaneous improvement make the establishment of the efficacy of immunosuppression a particularly difficult investigative task [1, 3, 7, 10, 11] .

Until recently, repeat transvenous endomyocardial biopsy was thought to be an effective method of monitoring the results of treatment [6]. Now it is well known, that histologic improvement may be present without an increase in ejection fraction, and, furthermore, clinical improvement may occur in the presence of ongoing myocarditis. Thus, the course of myocarditis is thought to be unpredictable on both histologic and clinical grounds [4, 5, 8].

Dec et al. [4] have recently reported a study of the relationship between histologic findings on early repeat right ventricular biopsy and ventricular function in patients with symptomatic heart failure, biopsy-proven myocarditis, and significantly reduced LVEF. According to them, early improvement of ejection fraction after immunosuppression was the best marker for good long-term prognosis – 83% survival for a least 3 years. In our group of 20 patients, left ventricular function worsened, accompanied by enlargement of heart silhouette in eight out of ten patients who had improved after 6-month immunosuppressive treatment. The question of defining an optimal period of immunosuppressive treatment remains.

Only two patients, one with improvement, one with no change in ejection fraction after 6 months of immunosuppression, showed late spontenous improvement at 24-month follow-up. It is noteworthy that none of these patients had dramatic clinical improvement at 3 months. The remaining two patients who stabilized at 6 months did not demonstrate deterioration at 24 months.

Weiss et al. [11] suggest that patients with myocarditis should be put on conventional therapy for at least an initial period of 6–9 months to determine whether there will be spontaneous improvement. Our patients were treated conventionally for 2–4 weeks before starting with immunosuppression.

It is well known that no conclusion about prognosis can be drawn from the degree of left ventricular dysfunction at the time of initial presentation. Our study suggests that assessment of left ventricular function after 6 months of immunosuppressive treatment cannot predict who will deteriorate and who will have further spontaneous improvement at late follow-up. It also indicates the need for careful long-term evaluation of these patients.

Until controlled, randomized studies can be completed, the role of immunosuppression for myocarditis will remain controversial.

Conclusion

Improvement of the left ventricular function after 6 months of immunosuppressive therapy does not predict long-term prognosis. Most of the patients failed to sustain improvement at 24 months follow-up.

References

1. Anderson JL, Fowles RE, Unverferth DV, Mason JW (1987) Immunosuppressive therapy of myocardial inflammatory disease. Initial experience and future trials to define indications for therapy. Eur Heart J 8 (Suppl J):263–266
2. Billingham ME (1985) The diagnostic criteria of myocarditis by endomyocardial biopsy. Heart Vessels 1 (Suppl 1):133–137
3. Billingham ME (1987) Acute myocarditis: a diagnostic dilemma. Br Heart J 58:6–8
4. Dec GW Jr, Fallon JT, Southern JF, Palacios JF (1988) Relation between histological findings on early repeat right ventricular biopsy and ventricular function in patients with myocarditis. Br Heart J 60:332–337

5. Dec GW Jr, Palacios JF, Fallon JT, Aretz HT, Mills UJ, Lee DC-S, Johnson RA (1985) Active myocarditis in the spectrum of acute dilated cardiomyopathies. Clinical features, histologic correlates and clinical outcome. N Engl J Med 312:885–890

6. Mason JW, Billingham ME, Ricci DR (1980) Treatment of acute inflammatory myocarditis assisted by endomyocardial biopsy. Am J Cardiol 45:1037–1044

7. O'Connell JB (1987) The role of myocarditis in end-stage dilated cardiomyopathy. Tex Heart Inst J 14:268–275

8. Quigley PJ, Richardson PJ, Meany BT, Olsen EGJ, Monaghan MJ, Jackcon G, Jewitt DE (1987) Long-term follow-up of acute myocarditis. Correlation of ventricular function and outcome. Eur Heart J 8 (Suppl J):39–42

9. Ruzyllo W, Purzycki Z (1981) Endomyocardial biopsy of right and left ventricle (in Polish). Kardiol Pol 24:87–99

10. Shanes JG, Ghali J, Billingham ME, Ferrans V Jr, Fenoglio JJ Jr, Edwards WD, Tsai CC, Saffitz JE, Isner J, Furner S, Subramanian R (1987) Interobserver variability in the pathologic interpretation of endomyocardial biopsy results. Circulation 75:401–405

11. Weiss MB, Marboe CC, Escala EL, Treulieb N, Fenoglio JJ Jr (1987) Natural history of untreated chronic myocarditis (active myocarditis with fibrosis). Eur Heart J 8 (Suppl J):247–250

Natural History and Prognosis of Overt Dilated Cardiomyopathy

R. E. Fowles

Heterogeneity

Dilated cardiomyopathy is by definition a syndrome of unknown causes. Many plausible etiologies have been proposed, and it is likely that the end stage of dilated cardiomyopathy results from multiple pathogenetic mechanisms. It is therefore not surprising that the course of dilated cardiomyopathy is highly variable. Indeed, the published 1-year survival of dilated cardiomyopathy ranges between 46% and 82% [1, 2]. Unfortunately, too many patients succumb during the first year despite treatment, while it is not unusual for others to survive for ten or fifteen years. In contrast, survival figures for valvular or ischemic heart disease are not so diverse. Heterogeneity in dilated cardiomyopathy is also observed with respect to functional status, quality of life, tempo of disease progression, complications, and even response to therapy.

When viewing the presentation, course and prognosis of dilated cardiomyopathy, one must take into account the heterogeneous nature of the syndrome. At this point in the study of dilated cardiomyopathy we seem to be relatively blind regarding its pathogenesis. However, clinical experience allows us to see a little more each year through new diagnostic techniques and treatment schemes.

Presentation

Overt dilated cardiomyopathy is usually manifested by a combination of functional and anatomic abnormalities. Some form of cardiac dysfunction leads to symptoms, causing the patient to present for medical attention; this reveals the anatomic hallmark of dilated cardiomyopathy, left ventricular enlargement. By definition cardiomegaly is a feature *sine qua non* for dilated cardiomyopathy, but the degree of chamber dilation is variable on presentation. Most patients are symptomatic when referred for medical evaluation, but up to 10% may have asymptomatic cardiomegaly [3].

The most common symptoms with which patients present are related to congestive heart failure, predominantly left-sided. Symptoms may be only brought on by exertion or can occur at rest, taking the form of dyspnea, fatigue, lightheadedness, etc. Right-sided congestion is rarer as an initiation to dilated cardiomyopathy. Interestingly, symptoms of heart failure tend not to correlate closely with signs or functional parameters [4]; this is often the case in dilated cardiomyopathy. It is not uncommon for dilated cardiomyopathy to present with complete cardiovascular collapse or pulmonary edema, whereas in some cases symptoms may persist for up to four years before medical consultation is sought.

Patients with dilated cardiomyopathy may present with symptoms related to arrhythmias–palpitations, lightheadedness, or even syncope and cardiopulmonary arrest. Sometimes the first symptom or sign of dilated cardiomyopathy may be a thromboembolic event, either venous/pulmonary or arterial/systemic. Occasionally, patients will present with chest pain, which may be almost anginal in nature, and can be elicited in 10%–50% of individuals with dilated cardiomyopathy.

Natural History/Course

Just as the suspected causes and the presentation of dilated cardiomyopathy, its course is on the whole quite variable. The tempo of the disease process is unpredictable. However, most studies show that the majority of deaths occur in the 2–3 years after presentation. Patients who die may suffer a relentlessly downhill course of progressive congestive heart failure, or may suddenly and unexpectedly expire. One cannot always distinguish by clinical history whether death has taken place due to heart failure or sudden lethal arrhythmia [24].

Some patients improve after presentation. Those who survive 2–3 years have a chance for stabilization or even improvement; 4-year survivors do so in 86% of cases [3] (Table 1). Of presenting patients, 20%–40% have been found to enjoy improvement or stabilization [1, 5, 6, 7]. Stevenson et al., in a dual center study [1], found that a 21% improvement rate tended to be associated with a shorter history of symptom duration (< 7 months), and with better pump function and cardiac rhythm. Gavazzi et al. [6] observed in 137 subjects followed for a mean of 4 years improvement or stabilization in 22%, which is notable because these patients presented with New York Heart Association (NYHA) class III or IV heart failure. Studies of perhaps more etiologically defineable myocardial disease have shown an improvement rate of 50% for peripartum [8] and 44% for alcoholic [9] cardiomyopathy. This raises the question of the heterogeneity of etiologies in presenting cases of idiopathic myocardial disease: perhaps much of the diversity in course is due to diversity in cause.

Table 1. Heterogeneity of prognosis: possibility of improvement

– Stabilization or improvement
　　　39%　　(Figulla) [7]
　　　22%　　(Keogh) [5]
　　　22%　　(Gavazzi) [6]
　　　21%　　(Stevenson) [1]
– Mid-course survivors have much better chance for stabilization (Diaz [3], others)

Table 2. Dilated cardiomyopathy complications: thromboembolism

Prevalence is approximately 18%–33%
Pulmonary probably equal to systemic
Anticoagulants are beneficial

The most common complications of dilated cardiomyopathy are worsening of congestive failure and arrhythmia. In a large study from Hammersmith Hospital in London, one-half of dying patients suffered deterioration of NYHA classification before death [3]. Arrhythmic symptoms are generally not highly bothersome to patients unless causing recurrent lightheadedness and presyncope. However, arrhythmias such as sustained ventricular tachycardia obviously may cause severe and dangerous disability, and the major arrhythmic complication is sudden death [10]. Arrhythmias are common in dilated cardiomyopathy. Atrial fibrillation is found in approximately 20% of patients [3–5, 10]. Although intraventricular conduction delay and left bundle branch block occur also in 20% of patients [3], heart block as a complication is rare. The most prevalent arrhythmias are ventricular. Ambulatory ECG monitoring in dilated cardiomyopathy has shown complex ventricular premature complexes (VPCs) in 93% of patients [11], multiform VPCs, pairs or runs in 87% [10], and nonsustained ventricular tachycardia (VT) in as many as 60%–80% [10–13].

Thromboembolism is a complication of the enlarged, poorly contractile chamber(s) and reduced blood flow of dilated cardiomyopathy (Table 2). Several studies have found incidences of thromboembolism between 11% and 33% [3, 5, 6, 15]. Pulmonary and systemic thromboembolism is generally evenly divided. Systemic emboli are more prevalent in atrial fibrillation [3, 6, 15]. Three studies have found anticoagulant therapy beneficial, the treated patients being spared, contrasted to approximately 20% of untreated patients suffering systemic embolic events [5, 15–17].

The response to drug therapy in dilated cardiomyopathy is generally unpredictable in the individual case. Antiarrhytmic medications are variably effective in controlling ventricular ectopy [10]. Antiarrhythmics have been shown to modify the inducibility and repetitive rate of ventricular tachycardia during electrophysiologic programmed stimulation, but without detectable effect on eventual clinical course [17].

Drug treatment of heart failure is probably most effective at improving symptomatic and functional status. The natural history of dilated cardiomyopathy is probably also altered with respect to extension of life [18]. However, many questions have yet to be answered with respect to the timing and selection of therapy in the course of dilated cardiomyopathy, whether subsets exist that may be more amenable to physiologically tailored treatment, etc.

Prognosis

The prognosis of dilated cardiomyopathy patients has been studied repeatedly and is highly variable (Table 3). In general, the overall prognosis is not good; indeed, survival is not any better and in some instances worse than that for certain neoplastic malignancies. The mortality of patients suffering congestive heart failure (CHF) from dilated cardiomyopathy may be slightly less than for patients with advanced ventricular dysfunction due to ischemic heart disease [19]. This underscores the probably heterogeneous make-up of dilated cardiomyopathy, and takes into account the subpopulations of patients who improve or stabilize, a course not so likely for extensive ischemic heart disease and CHF. Recently published studies show that in moderately sized groups of dilated cardiomyopathy patients, the actuarial 1-year survival ranges from 46% to 82% [1–3, 5, 7, 12, 15, 19]. Five-year suvival figures tend to be less diverse, centering around 50% [3, 6, 15]. This is probably due to the observed short-term demise of certain patients by 2–3 years, and the relatively more stable outlook for those remaining alive after 4–5 years [3].

Many investigators have attempted to derive clinical markers that can identify patients at higher risk for deterioration and death (Table 4). Surprisingly, features such as symptom severity at time of presentation are not strong indicators of prognosis. Duration of symptoms has a slight tendency to predict worse prognosis in some studies [1, 19] but not in others [3]. It is to be expected that older patients should have a poorer outlook; the risk of death for a 50-year-old patient can be 1.8-fold greater, and for a 70-year-old 3.4-fold greater than that for a 30-year-old patient [20]. Fuster found age 55 to be a significant cut-off for survival, older patients doing worse [15]. However, several studies

Table 3. Dilated cardiomyopathy: 1-year survival

46%	Stanford + UCLA [1]
65%	Ohio State [12]
70%	Mayo Clinic [15]
72%	Sydney [5]
72%	Hammersmith [3]
77%	Minn + Phil [19]
82%	Goettingen [2]

Table 4. Dilated cardiomyopathy: prognostic indicators

LV ejection fraction
LV conduction delay
LV complicance
Ventricular arrhythmias
Cardiac index
LV size
Symptom severity
Atrial fibrillation
Age

Table 5. Left ventricular function is a primary determinant

- Ejection fraction 0.20–0.30
- Compliance (LVEDP) (mmHg) 20
- Cardiac index (1/min/m^2) 2.5
- Stroke volume (ml/m^2) 40

have shown no statistically significant relation between age and prognosis [2, 3, 7, 19]. Other factors such as family history, ethanol use, recent pregnancy, a heralding viral illness, or viral titers have been found not to be predictive of outcome [3, 7].

The most consistently predictive factors for survival in dilated cardiomyopathy pertain to left ventricular function (Table 5). The Hammersmith group reported a tendency toward better ejection fraction at study entry in survivors (mean value of 0.33) compared to patients who died (mean 0.25) [3]. Hofmann et al. found ejection fraction (EF) to be a statistically independent determinant of prognosis, those patients with left ventricular EF greater than 0.35 enjoying twofold greater survival [2]. Stevenson et al. at Stanford and UCLA discovered that a low ejection fraction (< 0.25) was associated with unexpectedly low survival (46% at 1 year) despite subjectively limited symptoms in patients thought to be too well for transplantation [1]. Meinertz et al. showed EF to be significantly higher (mean value 0.36) in survivors than in patients dying of either pump failure or sudden death (aggregate mean EF = 0.21) [10]. Extremely low initial ejection fractions averaging 0.12 can predict likelihood of death within 6 months, compared to survivors' EF mean values of 0.23 [5], with serial deterioration of ejection fraction preceding death in all patients; an ejection fraction less than 0.10 predicts a 6-month survival of only 17% [5]. Olshausen et al. reported that left ventricular ejection fraction correlated with survival as an independent predictor, patients with EF > 0.40 showing 3-year survival 92%, but those with EF < 0.30 only 38% [21]. In the usually diffuse and homogeneous ventricular hypokinesis associated with dilated cardiomyopathy, EF correlates well with noninvasively-measured echocardiographic fractional shortening (normal range 0.30–0.50); Gavazzi et al. found fractional shortening of 0.14 to be associated with a poor prognosis [6].

The hemodynamic parameters often associated with ejection fraction, cardiac output and stroke volume, are also generally predictive of prognosis [19], although not in all studies [3]. Stroke volume less than 40 ml was associated with 100% mortality in 1 year regardless of subjective assessment in Stevenson's study [1], and predicted a hemodynamic demise as opposed to arrhythmic. Hofmann et al. found that patients with cardiac index (CI) > 2.5 l/min/m^2 were unlikey to die within 2 years, whereas those with CI < 2.5 had only 30% survival during mean follow-up of 53 months [2]. Fuster reported cardiac output as a predictor of prognosis, values less than 3.0 l/min being associated with poorer survival [2].

Left ventricular diastolic function also seems to determine prognosis. Poor hemodynamic compliance in a maximally dilated, failing chamber may be reflected by left ventricular elevated end-diastolic pressure (LVEDP) or by

Table 6. Prognosis and left ventricular size

– CT	ratio > 0.53	(Gavazzi [6], Fuster [15])
– LVEDVI	131 vs. 173 ml/m²	(Diaz [3])
	190 vs. 250 ml/m²	(Meinertz [10])
	cut-off 185 ml/m²	(Gavazzi [6])

pulmonary capillary wedge pressure. In most studies, LVEDP values greater than 20 mmHg are associated with worse prognosis [3, 10, 15], and can be an independent predictor of heart failure-related death [21]. Franciosa et al., however, make the point that in congestive heart failure, resting hemodynamics may not adequately predict outcome [19].

The degree of left ventricular enlargement in dilated cardiomyopathy tends to be connected with prognosis, but is not as strong a predictor of survival as the hemodynamic functional parameters discussed above (Table 6). A cardiothoracic ratio of greater than 0.55 was found by Fuster et al. [15] to be associated with twice the prevalence of demise, supported by findings of Gavazzi et al. [6]. Normalized left ventricular end diastolic volumes have been shown in three studies to be generally associated with survival [3, 6, 10], the cut-off of 185 ml/min/m² for favorable prognosis found by Gavazzi et al. [6] being typical.

Arrhythmias in dilated cardiomyopathy are currently the subject of extensive investigation. Most studies show a greater proportion of patients dying from sudden death than from congestive failure *per se* [2, 3, 6, 15]. Sudden death has been linked predominantly with arrhythmia as opposed to other causes such as thromboembolism or hemodynamic collapse.

The ability to predict death by analysis of rhythm disorders has been only partially successful (Table 7). As a rule, ventricular tachycardia, for example, is more prevalent in patients with worse left ventricular function, and mortality is higher overall in patients with congestive heart failure and sustained ventricular tachycardia [17]. Stevenson et al. reported a statistical association between a history of ventricular arrhythmias and mortality in general, and sudden death in particular [11]. On the other hand, other investigations have been unable to find any predictive association between ventricular arrhythmias (including ventricular tachycardia) and mortality [11]. Huang et al. [11] detected significant ventricular arrhythmias in 83% of dilated cardiomyopathy patients on ambulatory monitoring, but this prevalence was not predictive of death, sudden or otherwise. Other workers have reported similar findings [10, 11, 13]. In a

Table 7. Prognosis and ventricular arrhythmias

Majority of patients have complex VPCs or nonsustained VT
Half or more of deaths are unexpected and sudden
Correlation between arrhythmias and prognosis:
   published studies do not agree
   ECG monitoring variably predictive
   programmed stimulation not predictive
   antiarrhythmic therapy appears limited
Left ventricular function related to SD *and* rhythm

prospective, 3-year study by Olshausen et al. [21], the frequency of VPCs, pairs, and VT episodes was strongly statistically related to hemodynamic performance; indeed, more than six couplets or any VT detected over 24 h predicted death due to pump failure but not from identifiable primary arrhythmia. The number of beats in the longest VT episode was a statistically independent risk factor for congestive heart failure death, but not for sudden death. Ambulatory ECG monitoring was unable to identify patients subsequently succumbing to sudden death.

A few studies have linked ventricular arrhythmias to prognosis [10, 12, 14, 21]. Meinertz et al. [10] followed 74 patients for a mean of 11 months, detecting ventricular arrhythmias in 93%; 49% of patients even had nonsustained ventricular tachycardia. Frequency of VPCs was related to reduction in EF. Sudden death victims had on Holter monitoring significantly more ventricular arrhythmias than either survivors or patients dying of congestive failure. However, the question remains as to whether ventricular arrhythmias are a direct etiologic factor in demise, or instead a noncausal marker of the failing ventricle.

Invasive electrophysiologic procedures have been applied to dilated cardiomyopathy patients, but so far have been unable to arrive at meaningful clinical correlation with outcome. Programmed ventricular stimulation studies have shown inducibility of VT or VF in 40% [22], 89% [23], and 100% [17] of patients, but this inducibility does not predict sudden death or eventual prognosis [22]. Furthermore, treatment of such patients with specific antiarrhythmic drugs successful in the electrophysiologic study at affecting inducibility have not yet been proven protective against sudden death [17].

Intrinsic ventricular conduction delay and left bundle branch block appear to be stronger predictors of mortality than the occurrence of arrhythmias. Unverferth's study [12] ranked left bundle branch block as the number one feature associated with poor survival. Other investigators support this conclusion [2, 6, 21, 24]. Olshausen [21] found that left bundle branch block was an independent discriminatory risk factor, dying patients with conduction delay having a twofold greater likelihood of sudden death than of pump failure death.

Some studies have been able to derive statistical risk models for prognostic features in dilated cardiomyopathy. Hofmann et al. [2] reported that the risk and mode (sudden death versus pump failure) of death in 88% of their patients could be classified by a logistic regression model from multivariate analysis. Their four independent prognostic factors were ejection fraction, cardiac index, number of ventricular ectopic pairs/24h, and presence of atrial fibrillation. Unverferth et al. [12] used univariate analysis to identify statistically seven significant factors, which in descending order of prognostic importance were: left intraventricular conduction delay, pulmonary capillary wedge pressure, ventricular arrhythmias, mean right atrial pressure, left ventricular ejection fraction, presence of atrial fibrillation, and presence of S_3 gallop. In the same study, multivariate analysis revealed the three-fold combination of left conduction delay, ventricular arrhythmias, and mean right atrial pressure to be the most accurate predictor of outcome, and an equation using these factors was derived to quantify the statistical probability of 1-year survival. Meinertz et al. [10] applied linear stepwise discriminant function analysis and found that ejection fraction, cardiac index, number of ventricular pairs and runs/24 h could separate survivors from those dying of either sudden death or congestive failure. Patients with more than 20 ventricular pairs or runs per 24 h and EF less than 0.40 had an especially high risk of succumbing to sudden death.

Early attempts at prognostication by histopathologic examination of myocardium in dilated cardiomyopathy are promising. Endomyocardial biopsy, so popular in recent years, is perhaps the ultimately invasive cardiac test. Figulla et al. [7] reported that on light microscopy of biopsy samples, the specific appearance of cardiac myocyte fibers as manifested by "myofibril volume fraction" correlated with prognosis, those patients with a value of less than 0.60 having a 93% likelihood of death. Hammond et al. [25] were able to identify with a predictive accuracy of 0.70 those patients with a low (0%) versus high (37%) 18-month mortality, based on the degree of myofilament loss quantitated on electron microscopy. Certain investigative findings appear generally to support the notion that histopathology correlates with ventricular performance and prognosis [12, 26], but other studies are less conclusive [27, 28, 29].

Prognosis in congestive heart failure and dilated cardiomyopathy appears to be related to some laboratory findings, which may reflect degree of pathophysiologic deterioration or perhaps lend a clue to physiologic compensatory phenomena if not to disease mechanisms. Serum sodium concentration can be a powerful prognostic index, hyponatremia being associated with significantly shorter survival [30], and probably linked to the renin-angiotensin-aldosterone axis. Administration of angiotensin converting enzyme inhibitors tends to be more beneficial in hyponatremic patients, indicating an interaction between a risk factor, pathophysiology, treatment, and survival. Higher plasma norepinephrine levels correlate with worse prognosis in heart failure, probably indicating the role of the sympathetic nervous system in congestive heart failure [31].

Outlook

This review of the natural history and prognosis of dilated cardiomyopathy has examined studies from the past 2 decades. Dilated cardiomyopathy at this point is necessarily diverse because of our inexact understanding of its causes and disease mechanisms. Clinical, statistical studies of patient populations, however, have identified some features that help us to derive a prognostic profile. In some cases, there is hope that intervention can affect survival, as it can do for symptomatic status.

As we survey the outlook for clinical and investigative work in dilated cardiomyopathy, it appears that a few considerations are important. First, we shall perhaps benefit from earlier detection of dilated cardiomyopathy, both from the point of treatment as well as understanding of disease mechanisms. Second, improved diagnostic techniques may yet help in elucidating new information about how to approach heart failure, arrhythmias, and other complications of cardiomyopathy. Third, it is possible that subcategorization of etiologically distinct diseases within the syndrome of dilated cardiomyopathy will bring great progress in understanding and intervention. Fourth, all patients with dilated cardiomyopathy undergo treatment while being studied. The prognostic effects of treatment are now proven, so future investigations will necessarily take this into account.

References

1. Stevenson LW, Fowler MB, Schroeder JS, Stevenson WG, Dracup KA, Fond V (1987) Poor survival of patients with idiopathic dilated cardiomyopathy considered too well for transplantation. Am Heart J 83:871–876
2. Hofmann T, Meinertz T, Kasper W et al (1988) Mode of death in idiopathic dilated cardiomyopathy: a multivariate analysis of prognostic determinants. Am Heart J 116:1455–1463
3. Diaz RA, Goodwin JF, Obasohan A, Oakley CM (1987) Prediction of outcome in dilated cardiomyopathy. Br Heart J 58:393–399
4. Engler R, Ray R, Higgins CB, McNally C, Buxton WH, Bhargava V, Shabetai R (1982) Clinical assessment and follow-up of functional capacity in patients with chronic congestive cardiomyopathy. Am J Cardiol 49:1832–1837
5. Keogh AM, Freund J, Baron DW, Hickie JB (1988) Timing of cardiac transplantation in idiopathic dilated cardiomyopathy. Am J Cardiol 61:418–422
6. Gavazzi A, Lanzarini L, Cornalba C, Desperati M, Raisaro A, Angoli L, De Servi S, Specchia G (1984) Dilated (congestive) cardiomyopathy. Follow-up study of 137 patients. G Ital Cardiol 14:492–498
7. Figulla HR, Rahlf G, Nieger M, Luig H, Kreuzer H (1985) Spontaneous hemodynamic improvement or stabilization and associated biopsy findings in patients with congestive cardiomyopathy. Circulation 71:1095–1104
8. Demakis J, Rahimtoola S, Sutton G, Meadows R, Szanto P, Tobin J, Gunnar R (1971) Natural course of peri-partum cardiomyopathy. Circulation 44:1053–1060
9. Regan T (1984) Alcoholic cardiomyopathy. Prog Cardiovasc Dis 17:141–152
10. Meinertz T et al (1984) Significance of ventricular arrhythmias in idiopathic dilated cardiomyopathy. Am J Cardiol 53:902–907
11. Huang SK, Messer JV, Denes P (1983) Significance of ventricular tachycardia in idiopathic dilated cardiomyopathy: observations in 35 patients. Am J Cardiol 53:507–512
12. Unverferth DV, Magorien RD, Moeschberger ML, Baker PB, Fetters JK, Leier CV (1984) Factors influencing the one-year mortality of dilated cardiomyopathy. Am J Cardiol 54:147–152
13. Maskin CS, Siskind SJ, LeJemtel TH (1984) High prevalence of nonsustained ventricular tachycardia in severe congestive heart failure. Am Heart J 107:896
14. Holmes J, Kubo SH, Cody RJ, Kligfield P (1985) Arrhythmias in ischemic and non-ischemic dilated cardiomyopathy: prediction of mortality by ambulatory electrocardiography. Am J Cardiol 55:146–151
15. Fuster V, Gersh BJ, Giuliani ER, Tajik AJ, Brandenburg RO, Frye RL (1981) The natural history of idiopathic dilated cardiomyopathy. Am J Cardiol 47:525–531
16. Meltzer R, Visser C, Fuster V (1986) Intracardiac thrombi and systemic embolization. Ann Intern Med 104:689–698
17. Poll DS, Marchlinski FE, Buxton AE, Doherty JU, Waxman HL, Josephson ME (1984) Sustained ventricular tachycardia in patients with idiopathic dilated cardiomyopathy: electrophysiologic testing and lack of response to antiarrhythmic drug therapy. Circulation 70:451–456
18. Packer M (1988) Effect of vasodilator and inotropic drugs on clinical symptoms and long-term survival in chronic congestive heart failure. Eur Heart J 9 (Suppl H):105–108
19. Franciosa JA, Wilen M, Ziesche S, Cohn JN (1983) Survival in men with severe chronic left ventricular failure due to either coronary heart disease or idiopathic dilated cardiomyopathy. Am J Cardiol 51:831–836
20. Kinney EL (1988) Letter. Am J Med 84:797–798

21. Olshausen KV, Stienen U, Schwarz F, Kuebler W, Meyer J (1988) Long-term prognostic significance of ventricular arrhythmias in idiopathic dilated cardiomyopathy. Am J Cardiol 61:146–151
22. Das SK, Morady F, DiCarlo L Jr, Baerman J, Krol R, Be-Buitleir, Crevey B (1986) Prognostic usefulness of programmed ventricular stimulation in idiopathic dilated cardiomyopathy without symptomatic ventricular arrhythmias. Am J Cardiol 58:998–1000
23. Meinertz T et al (1985) Determinants of prognosis in idiopathic dilated cardiomyopathy as determined by programmed electrical stimulation. Am J Cardiol 56:337–341
24. Convert G et al (1980) Prognosis of primary non-obstructive cardiomyopathy. Arch Mal Coeur 227–237
25. Hammond EH, Menlove RL, Anderson JL (1987) Predictive value of immunofluorescence and electron microscopic evaluation of endomyocardial biopsies in the diagnosis and prognosis of myocarditis and idiopathic cardiomyopathy. Am Heart J 114:1055-1065
26. Schwartz F et al (1983) Quantitative morphologic findings of the myocardium in idiopathic dilated cardiomyopathy. Am J Cardiol 51:501
27. Schwartz F et al (1984) Determinants of survival in patients with congestive cardiomyopathy: quantitative morphologic findings and left ventricular hemodynamics. Circulation 70:923
28. Unverferth DV et al (1983) Human myocardial histologic characteristics in congestive heart failure. Circulation 68:1194
29. Baandrup U et al (1981) Critical analysis of endomyocardial biopsies from patients suspected of having cardiomyopathy. II. Comparison of histology and clinical/hemodynamic information. Br Heart J 45:487
30. Lee WH, Packer M (1986) Prognostic importance of serum sodium concentration and its modification by converting-enzyme inhibition in patients with severe chronic heart failure. Circulation 73:257–267
31. Rector TS et al (1987) Predicting survival for an individual with congestive heart failure using the plasma norepinephrine concentration. Am Heart J 114:148–152

Myocardial Perfusion and Metabolism in Dilated Cardiomyopathy

C. V. Leier

Introduction and Hypotheses

This report will focus on myocardial perfusion and metabolism in dilated cardiomyopathy; that is, perfusion and metabolism after the primary insult has been delivered to evoke cardiac enlargement and myocardial dysfunction. The discussion will not elaborate on the metabolic defects which may serve as the underlying etiology or as the primary insult (e.g., selenium and carnitine deficiencies). Based on several lines of evidence, this author proposes the following hypotheses. It has been my belief that these hypotheses cumulatively explain a major component of the pathophysiology and course of advanced dilated cardiomyopathy.

1) The pathophysiology of dilated cardiomyopathy includes the evolution of a state of compromised myocardial metabolism moving the clinical course into "end-stage" congestive heart failure.
2) The development of this deteriorating metabolic process has a highly variable time course and thus, can set the stage for terminal cardiac failure anytime during or after the primary insult.
3) The mechanisms for the compromised myocardial metabolism in dilated cardiomyopathy are related to:
   (a) Increased metabolic demands
   (b) Limited metabolic supply (inadequate myocardial perfusion relative to (a))
   (c) Deranged myocardial cell metabolism.
4) The final "downhill" course, the end-stage phase, for many patients with dilated cardiomyopathy is secondary to ischemia and metabolic derangements of the myocardium, particularly of the subendocardial region.

Cardiovascular Events in Dilated Cardiomyopathy Leading to the Formulation of These Hypotheses

The onset of ventricular dysfunction at a level which compromises overall cardiac and cardiovascular performance evokes a number of cardiovascular and systemic reactions. These reactions create a milieu conducive for further deterioration of ventricular and cardiovascular performance. The augmentation of sympathetic nervous system tone enhances cardiac output (via increased stroke volume and heart rate); however, excessive norepinephrine release elicits increased ventricular afterload, a detrimental event in ventricular/cardiac failure. The enhancement of renin release (followed by increased aldosterone) in cardiac failure augments cardiac-output, via the Frank-Starling mechanism, through salt-water retention. Unfortunately, the concomitantly elevated angiotensin levels and the NaCl-H_2O retention in arterial and arteriolar structures evokes additional afterload. Elevated plasma arginine vasopressin levels and blunted responsiveness to increased levels of atrial natriuretic factor may also contribute to the unfavorable milieu. These events, plus myocardial beta-receptor downregulation, are generally blamed for the progressively declining clinical course in patients who have dilated cardiomyopathy.

While the aforementioned factors are extremely important in the perpetuation of congestive heart failure, they probably do not provide the entire explanation for the progressive deterioration. Converting enzyme inhibition with resultant decreased angiotensin and aldosterone delays, but does not arrest, the clinical deterioration in heart failure. Although data are not available, it is likely that the same limitation will be seen for sympathetic blockade, with or without concomitant therapy with converting enzyme inhibition. This is particularly true once the patient has moved into the advanced stages of the disease.

Myocardial Perfusion and Metabolic Derangements in Human Dilated Cardiomyopathy

Patients with dilated cardiomyopathy and congestive heart failure typically have a reduction in the high energy phosphate levels [1–3] of their ventricular myocardium. This reduction is as apparent in acute onset ventricular dysfunction as it is in a more chronic course, and is directly related to disturbances in diastolic and systolic parameters [1, 2, 4]. Virtually all patients with dilated cardiomyopathic hearts and end-stage heart failure have severely depressed levels of high energy phosphates, the essential energy substances of the heart [3, 4].

The reduction in the myocardial content of high energy phosphates is probably both a sign and cause of the problem: the reduction results from a combination of pathophysiological events (e.g., myocardial hypoperfusion, mitochondrial dysfunction) and its depletion deprives the heart of its energy base, thereby resulting in further depression of ventricular function.

A number of mechanisms can account for the development of myocardial metabolic derangements, typified by reduced high energy phosphate content, in patients with dilated cardiomyopathy.

The major contributing mechanisms include:

(a) increased metabolic demands and requirements;
(b) myocardial hypoperfusion and/or limited metabolic supply relative to these requirements;
(c) disturbed function of the myocardial cell and subcellular structures.

Increased Metabolic Demands and Requirements

In response to cardiac dysfunction, the cardiovascular system undergoes a series of changes which increase the energy requirement and inefficiency (energy required per work output) of the cardiac myocyte and the whole heart. Increased afterload, directly related to the increase in aortic impedance, systemic vascular resistance, and ventricular systolic volume, increases ventricular wall stress, ventricular volume and myocardial oxygen consumption during systole, while further suppressing systolic performance of the ventricle. Elevated preload, secondary to salt-water retention and perhaps venoconstriction, may increase cardiac performance through the Frank-Starling effect, but also increases ventricular volume and diastolic ventricular wall stress. Enhanced sympathetic nervous system tone and nerveending release of norepinephrine with elevated circulating levels increase myocardial oxygen and energy requirements through an increase in resting and exercise heart rate and myocardial contractility (albeit still depressed).

Myocardial oxygen consumption in patients with cardiomyopathic heart failure can be normal but generally is elevated significantly [5–7]. However, when these levels are corrected for levels of cardiac systolic performance it appears that a relatively inefficient process (work output per oxygen use falls) evolves with progression of the cardiac/ventricular failure. During rapid pacing, myocardial oxygen consumption increases more for less cardiac performance in dilated cardiomyopathy than in normal controls [6].

Myocardial Hypoperfusion and/or Limited Metabolic Supply

A number of pathophysiological conditions reduce coronary blood flow and myocardial perfusion in dilated cardiomyopathy [8, 9]. Diastolic filling pressure of the left ventricle increases with unchanged or a fall in diastolic blood pressure in moderate to severe dilated cardiomyopathy; a drop in coronary perfusion pressure is a consequence of these events. The increase in heart rate in these patients reduces the time spent in diastole, compromising diastolic myocardial perfusion time [10]. The combination of reduced coronary perfusion pressure and coronary perfusion time likely accounts for a large part of the compromise of coronary blood flow and myocardial perfusion in dilated cardiomyopathy [5, 6]. When calculated or corrected for ventricular mass, coronary blood flow and oxygen delivery can become considerably reduced in hypertrophic and cardiomyopathic hearts [5, 8, 9]. Enhanced myocardial oxygen consumption and reduced myocardial blood flow and perfusion elicit a fall in coronary sinus oxygen content and an elevation in coronary sinus lactate concentration, particularly in patients with high wall stress [7]. The hypoperfusion and disturbed metabolic state is further accentuated during rapid pacing and exercise [6, 11].

The aforementioned myocardial perfusion/metabolic conditions have been demonstrated in cardiomyopathic patients without obstructive coronary artery disease [2–11] and are likely to be exacerbated by the presence of destructive coronary lesions. In the setting of dilated cardiomyopathy and congestive heart failure, *we must dispel the misconception that myocardial ischemia requires lesions of large or small arteries.* It is interesting that we have long been aware of systemic and organ hypoperfusion in heart failure, but may have ignored hypoperfusion of the heart itself.

Disturbed Cellular and Subcellular Function of the Cardiac Myocyte in Dilated Cardiomyopathy

Several lines of evidence suggest that after the primary insult the cardiac myocyte develops cellular-subcellular abnormalities during the course of dilated cardiomyopathy. Unfortunately, it becomes difficult in most human situations to determine whether the defect represents a continuum of the primary insult or an abnormality which evolves as a consequence of ventricular dysfunction and failure. The major cellular/subcellular abnormalities will be briefly presented without any intent to be comprehensive in terms of each defect or to include all the defects described.

A number of abnormalities have been described to incriminate deranged membrane function of the failing cardiac myocyte. With respect to membrane receptors, myocardial beta-receptor density is reduced, presumably secondary to chronically elevated endogenous catecholamine exposure [12]. Recent studies in an animal model [13] suggests that the available beta receptors of the failing cardiomyocyte also may not be able to effectively activate adenylate cyclase (to produce C'AMP) because of an abnormal reduction in membrane Gs protein (stimulatory guanosine triphosphate binding protein). These receptor abnormalities coupled with depleted myocardial nerve catecholamine stores and blunted production probably accounts for much of the impairment in contractile response.

Several lines of evidence suggest deranged membrane function of cardiomyocyte organelles as well. Careful ultrastructural analysis of myocardial mitochondria in patients with dilated cardiomyopathy reveals varying degrees of swelling, disrupted cristae, and structural distortion which probably contribute greatly to impaired ATP production in these hearts [13, 14]. Studies in cardiomyopathic hamsters [15] indicate that the membranous structure of sarcoplasmic reticulum also becomes dysfunctional in dilated cardiomyopathy, which when accompanied by membrane dysfunction of the sarcolemma (surface membrane of the cardiomyocyte) and other organelles leads to disturbances in calcium metabolism, movement, sequestration and release. Inadequate calcium release occurs in systole with excessive cytoplasmic levels in diastole. A state of "calcium intoxication" ensues to advance the widespread cellular and subcellular dysfunction already occurring. Systolic and diastolic dysfunction of the heart necessarily follows and progressively worsens.

As noted, depressed levels of myocardial high energy phosphates are a consistent finding in dilated cardiomyopathy with a relatively good direct relationship between these levels (e.g., ATP) and certain parameters of systolic and diastolic function [2, 3]. High energy phosphates are a necessary fuel for most cellular reactions and activity. Depression of these evokes widespread cellular and subcellular dysfunction, structural deterioration, and retardation of cellular repair.

It is likely that this reduction in high energy phosphates, generally reflecting mitochondrial dysfunction, has multiple explanations and mechanisms including those related to the primary insult. A major contributory mechanism is cellular (mitochondrial) ischemia secondary to myocardial hypoperfusion; this hypothesis is strongly supported by pharmacophysiological studies. Seventy-two hour dobutamine infusions in patients with dilated cardiomyopathy and congestive heart failure resulted in improved mitochondrial ultrastructure, normalization of myocardial ATP levels, enhanced cardiac function, and improved clinical status [3, 14, 16] via mechanisms probably related to augmented coronary blood flow, myocardial perfusion and cellular oxygenation, particularly of the subendocardium. A similar clinical response was attained with prolonged nitroglycerin infusions [17] suggesting that the beneficial metabolic effects of the dobutamine infusions were not primarily mediated by a positive inotropic effect or by beta-adrenergic stimulation.

A number of other metabolic abnormalities are now known to occur in failing dilated cardiomyopathy; the relevance of many of these has not been established for the human condition. A shift in myosin isoenzymes from the rapidly contracting high ATPase V1 myosin to the slower contracting low ATPase V3 myosin occurs in myocardial failure [18]; the (patho)physiology and impact of this finding remains to be determined in humans (and in animals for that matter).

The Self-Perpetuating, Deteriorating Course
of End-Stage Dilated Cardiomyopathy

The net effect of the aforementioned pathophysiological events is the evolution of a self-perpetuating course of biochemical, structural and functional deterioration of the cardiomyopathic myocardium. A given patient's heart arrives at a state of progressive ventricular enlargement, poor systolic function and high wall stress. Myocardial oxygen and metabolic demands increase while the supply of these tends to fall in relation to this increase. Subendocardial ischemia-infarction develops and exacerbates the entire process by further reducing systolic and diastolic function. Histologic studies indicate that the subendocardium of end-stage cardiomyopathic hearts is often replaced with fibrous tissue suggesting that the ischemia of this region may evolve into infarction [19]. Basically depressed systolic and diastolic function, high wall stress, increased metabolic demands and reduced myocardial perfusion begets the same to set the stage for a progressively deteriorating course. I firmly believe that the spiraling "downhill" course for many patients with "endstage" dilated cardiomyopathy and congestive heart failure commences with the development of a critical level of ventricular enlargement, wall stress, and coronary hypoperfusion to elicit subendocardial ischemia [19]. Cellular and subcellular physiological functions and ultrastructure become disrupted, high energy phosphates fall evoking further loss of systolic and diastolic function, failure of reparative processes, and eventual cell death. Unless an intervention can be directed at interrupting these events and reversing subendocardial ischemia, a patient will be condemned into the terminal phase of his condition.

Acknowledgement: This work has been largely supported by grants from the American Heart Association (Central Ohio Heart Chapter). Many of the concepts and data contained herein evolved out of a close 12-year association with my fellow investigator, Dr. Donald V. Unverferth. A malignancy ended his brief, but distinguished career on January 8, 1988.

References

1. Pool PE, Spann JF, Buccino RA, Sonnenblick EH, Braunwald E (1967) Myocardial high energy phosphate stores in cardiac hypertrophy and heart failure. Circ Res 1:365–373
2. Bashore TM, Magorien DJ, Letterio J, Shaffer P, Unverferth DV (1987) Histologic and biochemical correlates of left ventricular chamber dynamics in man. J Am Coll Cardiol 9:734–742
3. Unverferth DV, Magorien RD, Altschuld R, Kolibash AJ, Lewis RP, Leier CV (1983) The hemodynamic and metabolic advantages gained by a three day infusion of dobutamine. Am Heart J 106:29–34
4. Furchgott RF, Lee KS (196) High energy phosphates and the force of contraction of cardiac muscle. Circulation 24:416–428
5. Magorien RD, Unverferth DV, Brown GP, Leier CV (1983) Dobutamine and hydralazine: comparative influences of positive inotropy and vasodilation on coronary blood flow and myocardial energetics in non-ischemic congestive heart failure. J Am Coll Cardiol 1:499–505
6. Pasternac A, Noble J, Streulens Y, Elie R, Herschke C, Bourasso MG (1982) Pathophysiology of chest pain in patients with cardiomyopathies and normal coronary arteries. Circulation 65: 778–789
7. DeMarco T, Chattergee K, Rouleau JL, Parmley WW (1988) Abnormal coronary hemodynamics and myocardial energetics in patients with chronic heart failure caused by ischemic heart disease and dilated cardiomyopathy. Am Heart J 115:809–815
8. Rembert JL, Kelinman LH, Fedor JM, Wechsler AS, Greenfield JC Jr (1978) Myocardial blood flow in concentric left ventricular hypertrophy. J Clin Invest 62:379–387
9. Opherk D, Mall G, Zebe H, Schwarz F, Weihe E, Marthey J (1984) Reduction of coronary reserve: a mechanism for angina pectoris in patients with arterial hypertension and normal coronary arteries. Circulation 69:1–7
10. Meiler SEL, Boudoulas H, Unverferth DV, Leier CV (1987) Diastolic time in congestive heart failure. Am Heart J 114:1192–1198
11. Magorien RD, Frederick J, Leier CV, Unverferth DV (1987) Influence of exercise of coronary sinus flow determinations. Am J Cardiol 59:659–661
12. Bristow MR (1984) Myocardial beta-adrenergic receptor downregulation in heart failure. Int J Cardiol 5:648
13. Longabaugh JP, Vatner DE, Vatner SF, Homcy CJ (1988) Decreased stimulatory guanosine triphosphate. Binding protein in dogs with pressure-overload left ventricular failure. J Clin Invest 81:420–424
14. Unverferth DV, Leier CV, Magorien RD, Croskery R, Svirbely JR, Kolibash AJ, Dick MR, et al (1980) Improvement of human myocardial mitochondria after dobutamine: a quantitative ultrastructural study. J Pharmacol Exp Ther 215:527–532
15. Whitmer JT, Pankay K, Solaro RJ (1988) Calcium transport properties of cardiac sarcoplasmic reticulum from cardiomyopathic Syrian hamsters (BIO 53.58 and 14.6): evidence for a quantitative defect in dilated myopathic hearts not evidence in hypertrophic hearts. Circ Res 62:81–85

16. Leier CV, Webel J, Bush CA (1977) The cardiovascular effects of the continuous infusion of dobutamine in patients with severe cardiac failure. Circulation 56:468–472

17. Rouleau JL (1989) Myocardial hypoperfusion and ischemia as a complication of congestive heart failure. Congest Heart Failure Index Rev 2(1):1, 20

18. Entman ML, Michael LH (1988) Molecular and cellular basis for myocardial failure. In: Parmley WW, Chatterjee K (eds) Cardiology, vol 1. Lippincott, Philadelphia, pp 1–14

19. Unverferth DV, Magorien RD, Lewis RP, Leier CV (1983) The role of subendocardial ischemia in perpetuation myocardial failure in patients with nonischemic congestive cardiomypathy. Am Heart J 105:176–179

Complex Ventricular Arrhythmias in Dilated Cardiomyopathy: A Multicenter Italian Experience

A. Gavazzi, R. De Maria, A. Caroli, A. Di Lenarda, U. Veritti, D. Miani,
G. Sinagra, M. Luvini, R. Ometto, M. Borgia, M. Ciaccheri, C. Campana,
G. Graziano, L. Lanzarini, E. Gronda, and F. Camerini

Introduction and Review of Literature

Studies on prognosis in dilated cardiomyopathy (DCM) have generally reported a poor outcome, with almost equal prevalence of mortality due to pump failure and sudden death [1–4]. While the association between DCM and complex ventricular arrhythmias has been well recognized, a clear relationship with systolic impairment and outcome remains controversial, particularly when the issue of sudden death in these patients is addressed. In many instances of sudden death, a role played by therapeutic side effects can be assumed [5]: commonly used drugs for the treatment of congestive heart failure may cause electrolyte imbalance or have a direct arrhythmogenicc effect, whereas the

Table 1. Incidence of complex ventricular arrhythmias in DCM

Reference	Patients (n)	CVA (%)	NS-VT (%)	S-VT (%)
Huang et al. 1983 [6]	35	77	60	–
Olshausen et al. 1984 [7]	60	95	42	–
Meinertz et al. 1984 [8]	74	87	49	–
Unverferth et al. 1984 [9]	69[a]	36	16	6
Costanzo-Nordin et al. 1985 [10]	55	85	40	–
Holmes et al. 1985 [3]	31[b]	71	35	–
Haissaguerre et al. 1986 [11]	236 (76[c])	40	15	2
Neri et al. 1986 [12]	65	80	45	1.5

[a] Cases without dynamic electrocardiographic monitoring.
[b] 15 DCM and 16 ischemic heart disease patients.
[c] Cases with dynamic electrocardiographic monitoring.

NS-VT, nonsustained ventricular tachycardia; CVA, complex ventricular arrythmias; S-VT, sustained ventricular tachycardia.

proarrhythmic potential of antiarrhythmic agents is now well established. In view of the potential adverse effects of this type of treatment, a clear definition of the prognostic value of complex ventricular arrhythmias and the consequent need for their treatment is required.

A number of studies have analyzed the prevalence and role of ventricular arrhythmias as prognostic factors in DCM [6–14]. In all studies a high prevalence of complex ventricular arrhythmias was reported in DCM patients, ranging from 40% to 95%, whereas asymptomatic, nonsustained ventricular tachycardia was found in about one half of cases on average (Table 1). It is interesting to note that while symptomatic sustained ventricular tachycardia is not an unusual type of presentation for DCM in clinical practice, dynamic electrocardiographic monitoring in all studies did not show a relevant prevalence of this malignant arrhythmia.

The relationship between pump function and ventricular arrhythmias remains controversial. While some authors found significantly more depressed contractility indices in DCM patients with severe ventricular arrhythmias [7, 11–13], the analysis of other series did not yield any correlation [6, 8, 10, 14].

The prognostic role of ventricular arrhythmias is also uncertain (Table 2). In some studies [6, 7, 10, 11] no predictive value for cardiac death could be demonstrated. Other authors identified complex ventricular arrhythmias as

Table 2. Mortality and prognostic value of complex ventricular arrhythmias in DCM

Reference	Patients (n)	GM (%)	SD (%)	HF (%)	CVAev	CVA predictive
Huang et al. 1983 [6]	35	8 (34 m)	6	2	24-h HM	No
Olshausen et al. 1984 [7]	60	12 (12 m)	7	2	24-h HM	No
Meinertz et al. 1984 [8]	74	26 (11 m)	16	10	24-h HM	VE, VC, VT for SD
Unverferth et al. 1984 [9]	69	35 (12 m)	NE	NE	ECG strips	Yes
Costanzo-Nordin et al. 1985 [10]	55	20 (14 m)	20	0	24-h HM	VE for SD
Holmes et al. 1985 [3]	31[a]	45 (25 m)	39	6	24-h HM	Yes
Haissaguerre et al. 1986 [11]	236	34 (39 m)	11	23	ECG/EST/	Yes
Neri et al. 1986 [12]	65	29 (30 m)	8	21	24-h HM	Yes
Olshausen et al. 1988 [13]	73	38 (36 m)	19	18	24-h HM	VT beats for GM
Hofmann et al. 1988 [14]	110	35 (53 m)	23	12	24-h HM	VC for HF

[a] 15 DCM and 16 ischemic heart disease.

GM, global mortality; in brackets months of follow-up; *SD*, sudden death; *HF*, heart failure; *CVA*, complex ventricular arrythmias; *CVAev*, method of evaluation of CVA; *HM*, Holter monitoring; *VE*, ventricular extrasystoles; *VC*, ventricular couplets; *VT*, ventricular tachycardia; *NE*, not examined; *EST*, exercise stress test.

major risk indicators for sudden death [8, 14] or global cardiac mortality [3, 9], whereas in some series [12, 13] ventricular arrhythmias showed a prognostic value because they were related to pump function parameters, which appeared to be the strongest predictors of death.

Thus the relationship between complex ventricular arrhythmias and pump dysfunction remains a highly controversial point in the literature. Possible explanations for the contrasting findings are the small samples studied and the heterogeneous patient distribution in different series for clinical, hemodynamic, and pump function indices. The same reasons account for widely variable mortality rates in DCM patients, particularly when sudden death is considered.

In 1986 the Italian Multicenter Cardiomyopathy Study (S.P.I.C) was started. Its acknowledged main aim is the definition of natural history and identification of the most prominent prognostic factors for dilated cardiomyopathy through a prospective long-term follow-up.

The purpose of this report of a multicenter experience is:

1) To evaluate the frequency, prevalence, characteristics, and clinical significance of ventricular arrhythmias detected by dynamic electrocardiographic monitoring in a group of 178 patients with dilated cardiomyopathy,
2) To assess the prognostic significance of ventricular arrhythmias based on a long-term follow-up.

Methods

A total of 178 consecutive patients from seven centers (Florence, Milan, Naples, Pavia, Trieste, Varese, Vicenza) participating in SPIC were studied prospectively between January 1986 and January 1989. Fifty-eight of these patients had been enrolled in a pilot study undertaken prior to the beginning of SPIC. All patients underwent right and left heart catheterization, selective coronary angiography, M-mode and two-dimensional echocardiography, and right and/or left ventricular endomyocardial biopsy.

In every patient the following criteria were fulfilled:

1) Reduced left ventricular ejection fraction ($\leq 55\%$).
2) Absence of significant coronary artery disease, that is, more than 50% luminal diameter obstruction of a major coronary artery.
3) Exclusion of underlying sytemic hypertension, cor pulmonale, valvular heart disease, specific muscle disease, active myocarditis, general systemic disease.

Symptomatic status was classified according to the New York Heart Association (NYHA) criteria. According to our criteria [15], patients with end-stage cardiomyopathy and/or on the waiting list for heart transplantation were not enrolled.

Baseline dynamic electrocardiographic monitoring was performed for at least 24 h. The number of episodes of ventricular tachycardia per 24 h, the number of beats per episode, and the rate of ventricular tachycardia were evaluated.

The total number of VEs in 24 h and mean hourly frequency were calculated.

Ventricular arrhythmias were classified according to a modified Lown grading system as described by Ryan et al. [16]:

Grade 0 = No VEs in 24 h.
Grade 1 = No more than 30 VEs in any hour of monitoring.
Grade 2 = More than 30 VEs in any hour of monitoring.
Grade 3 = Multiform VEs.
Grade 4A = Two consecutive VEs (couplets).
Grade 4B = Multiform VEs and couplets.
Grade 5 = Ventricular tachycardia (three or more VEs in succession).

Sustained ventricular tachycardia was defined as an episode of tachycardia lasting more than 30 s and not self-terminating. At the time of dynamic electrocardiographic monitoring 122 patients (68.5%) were taking digitalis, 140 (78.7%) diuretics, 59 (33.1%) ACE inhibitors, 12 (6.7%) beta-blockers, 67 (37.6%) antiarrhythmics (amiodarone in 32%, other agents in 5.6%); 20 patients (11.2%) not receiving any therapy. The study began after completion of this baseline evaluation and terminated at the time of the last follow-up visit or at the patient's death. Patients underwent physical examination and 12-lead standard electrocardiography at least every 3 months. Echocardiography was performed every 6 months; chest X-ray, laboratory tests, and dynamic electrocardiography monitoring were repeated every 12 months or earlier when clinically needed. Circumstances of death were investigated by interviewing the next of kin, friends, or physician. Classification of the type of death was based on evaluation of the state of circulation immediately before death [17]. Death was considered sudden if it occurred instantaneously within minutes or during sleep and was not preceded by deteriorating cardiac failure. Death occurring during progressively impaired cardiac performance was considered secondary to heart failure.

Statistical Analysis

Continuous data are expressed as mean values ± standard deviation. Where appropriate, the t test for unpaired data or one-way analysis of variance was used to assess statistical significance. Dynamic electrocardiographic parameters were correlated to angiographic left ventricular ejection fraction by linear regression analysis. A probability value of < 0.05 was considered significant.

Survival estimates were calculated using the Kaplan-Meier life-table technique. The variables examined with univariate statistics were entered into a stepwise discriminant function analysis program to obtain the best possible discrimination between the groups of survivors and non-survivors. A single additional variable was entered into the set of discriminating variables at each step; only variables that maximized the distance between the two groups were retained.

The program also calculated two classification functions that were used to allocate each case to one of the two groups. A table was produced to compare this classification with real group. A percentage of correctly classified cases was given to allow an estimate of predictive power of the set of variables selected.

All statistical computations were performed using the Statistical Package for the Social Science Program (SPSS by SPSS Inc. Chicago, Ill.).

Results

Clinical, Electrocardiographic, Echocardiographic, and Hemodynamic Findings

The clinical, electrocardiographic, echocardiographic, and hemodynamic findings at entry into the study are summarized in Table 3. There were 136 men and 42 women, mean age 43.8 ± 13.6 years (range 8–70). The mean interval

Table 3. Clinical, electrocardiographic, echocardiographic, and hemodynamic findings in 178 patients with DCM

Presenting symptoms	(n)	(%)	Surface ECG	(n)	(%)
Heart failure	146	82	Sinus rhythm	151	84.8
Palpitations	18	10	Atrial fibrillation	27	15.2
Chest pain	17	9.5	$1_{st}/2_{nd}$ A–V block	28	15.7
Syncope	5	2.8	LVH	25	14
NYHA class I	35	19.7	RVH	1	0.5
II	39	33.1	LAH	13	7.3
III	68	38.2	LBBB	25	14
IV	16	9	RBBB	3	1.7
			RBBB + LAH	1	0.5
			Nonspecific ST-T changes	19	10.6

Echocardiography	Mean ± SD	Hemodynamics	Mean ± SD
RVEDD (mm)	22 ± 9	RAP (mmHg)	5 ± 4.7
LVEDD (mm)	70 ± 9	RVEDP (mmHg)	6.1 ± 4.9
LVESD (mm)	58 ± 12	mPAP (mmHg)	21 ± 10
LVFS (%)	17.3 ± 11	PCWP (mmHg)	15 ± 10
LVEF (%)	30 ± 11	LVEDP (mmHg)	16 ± 11
IV Th (%)	12 ± 9	CI (L/min/m²)	3.29 ± 1.2
PW Th (%)	23 ± 18	LVEF (%)	31 ± 12

1st/2nd A–V block, first and second degree atrioventricular block; *LVH,* left ventricular hypertrophy; *RVH,* right ventricular hypertrophy; *LAH,* left anterior hemiblock; *LBBB,* left bundle branch block; *RBBB,* right bundle branch block; *RVEDD,* right ventricular end-diastolic diameter; *LVEDD,* left ventricular end-diastolic diameter; *LVESD,* left ventricular end-systolic diameter; *LVFS,* left ventricular fractional shortening; *LVEF,* left ventricular ejection fraction; *IV Th,* percentage thickening of the interventricular septum; *PW Th,* percentage thickening of the posterior wall; *RAP,* right atrial pressure; *RVEDP,* right ventricular end-diastolic pressure; *mPAP,* mean pulmonary artery pressure; *PCWP,* pulmonary capillary wedge pressure; *LVEDP,* left ventricular end-diastolic pressure; *CI,* cardiac index; *LVEF,* left ventricular ejection fraction.

between the onset of symptoms and entry into the study was 811 ± 792 days (range 54-3350). Sinus rhythm was present in 151 patients (84.8%) and chronic atrial fibrillation in 27 (15.2%).

Dynamic Electrocardiographic Monitoring

Atrial arrhythmias were present in 87 patients (48.8%). Atrial extrasystoles were detected in 60 patients (33.7%) and the mean number of atrial extrasystoles in 24 h was 409 ± 1365 (range 3-8652). In one patient paroxysmal atrial fibrillation was also detected. Ventricular arrhythmias were present in 163 patients (91.6%). The mean number of VEs in 24 h was 2852 ± 6285 (range 18-44 000). VEs were rare (< 500/24 h) in 103 patients (57.8%) and frequent (> 500/24 h) in 60 (33.7%).

According to a modified Lown classification of ventricular arrhythmias [16], 15 patients (8.4%) were in grade 1, 2 (1.1%) in grade 2, 58 (33.1%) in grade 3, 9 (5%) in grade 4A, 42 (23.5%) in grade 4B, and 37 (20.5%) in grade 5. A total of 79 patients (44.3%) had couplets with a mean number of 80 ± 269 in 24 h (range 1-222). In 37 patients (20.5%), a total of 197 episodes of ventricular tachycardia were recorded (range 1-38 episodes per patient in 24 h).

Out of 37 patients with ventricular tachycardia, 14 patients (37.8%) had only one episode in 24 h, 18 patients (48.6%) had two to six episodes, and five patients (13.6%) more than 14 episodes. All episodes were nonsustained (6 ± 4 beats, range 3-24) and were noticed by the patient in 19% of cases. The mean rate of ventricular tachycardia episodes ranged from 94 to 220 beats per minute (mean 160 ± 34 beats per minute).

Ventricular Arrhythmias and Ventricular Function

Patients were grouped according to severity of ventricular arrhythmias: 90 patients (50.6%) had Lown grade 0-3 (group 1), 51 patients (28.9%) Lown grades 4A and 4B (group 2), and 37 patients (20.5%) Lown grade 5 (group 3). There were no significant differences between the groups in age, duration of illness, and NYHA functional class. Amiodarone treatment was equally distributed within the three groups (37% in group 1, 30% in group 2, 29% in group 3, p = NS). The echocardiographic and cardiac catheterization findings in these three groups are summarized in Table 4.

Weakly significant differences were found between echocardiographic right ventricular end diastolic diameter in group 2 (25.8 ± 10 mm) vs. group 1 (21 ± 8 mm) and vs. group 3 (19 ± 7 mm) with a p value < 0.02, and angiographic left ventricular ejection fraction in group 1 (33 ± 11%) vs. group 2 (28 ± 11%) and vs. group 3 (28 ± 12%), p < 0.02.

By linear regression analysis dynamic electrocardiographic parameters (total number of VEs, number of couplets, number of morphologies, number of ventricular tachycardia episodes) showed no significant relation to angiographic left ventricular ejection fraction as an index of pump dysfunction. Data are

Table 4. Echocardiographic and hemodynamic findings in 178 DCM patients according to severity of ventricular arrhythmias

	Group 1 (n = 90)	Group 2 (n = 51)	Group 3 (n = 37)	p
Echocardiography				
RVEDD (mm)	21.1 ± 8	25.8 ± 11	19 ± 7	< 0.02
LVEDD (mm)	69.5 ± 9	69.5 ± 9.5	70 ± 11	NS
LVESD (mm)	57.5 ± 10	57.5 ± 14	58.7 ± 11	NS
LVFS (%)	17.7 ± 7	18 ± 17	16 ± 8	NS
LVEF (%)	31.6 ± 12	27.9 ± 10	31 ± 11	NS
IV Th (%)	12.6 ± 10	11.3 ± 7	11.7 ± 9	NS
PW Th (%)	22.4 ± 20	22.4 ± 13	25 ± 18	NS
Cardiac catheterization				
RAP (mmHg)	4.9 ± 4	5 ± 4	5.3 ± 6	NS
RVEDP (mmHg)	6 ± 4	6.4 ± 5	6 ± 6	NS
mPAP (mmHg)	21.4 ± 10	21.4 ± 11	20.3 ± 12	NS
PCWP (mmHg)	14.2 ± 8	15.4 ± 10	15.7 ± 12	NS
LVEDP (mmHg)	16 ± 10	16.6 ± 12	17 ± 10	NS
CI (L/min/m^2)	3.36 ± 1.2	3.19 ± 1.1	3.21 ± 0.9	NS
LVEF (%)	33 ± 11	28 ± 11	28 ± 12	< 0.02

Group 1, Lown grades 0–3; Group 2, Lown grades 4A and 4B; Group 3, Lown grade 5; other abbreviations as in Table 3.

listed in Table 5. Thus, in this series, ventricular arrhythmias are apparently not related to left ventricular dysfunction.

According to the modified Lown grade (0–3 vs. 4A–5) and angiographic left ventricular ejection fraction (> 30% vs. < 30%), patients were further divided into four groups:

Group A: Lown grade 0–3 and LVEF > 30%, $n = 50$
Group B: Lown grade > 3 and LVEF > 30%, $n = 35$
Group C: Lown grade 0–3 and LVEF < 30%, $n = 37$
Group D: Lown grade > 3 and LVEF < 30%, $n = 56$.

Table 5. Relation between dynamic electrocardiographic parameters and angiographic left ventricular ejection fraction

	r [a]	p
Lown grade (n)	−0.21	NS
VEs (n)	0.13	NS
Couplets (n)	0.004	NS
PVC morphology (n)	−0.16	NS
Ventricular tachycardia	−0.2	NS

[a] Linear regression analysis.

Table 6. Dynamic electrocardiographic, echocardiographic, and hemodynamic parameters in DCM patients with different degrees of ventricular arrhythmias and ventricular dysfunction

Group	A	B	C	D	p
n	50	35	37	56	
%	28.3	19.6	20.7	31.4	
Dynamic electrocardiography					
VE/24 h	1798 ± 7564	5071 ± 7076	571 ± 2413	2785 ± 4618	< 0.05
Couplets/24 h	–	119 ± 389	–	43 ± 113	< 0.05
Morphologies	1.8 ± 0.9	2.6 ± 0.9	1.8 ± 0.9	2.9 ± 1.2	< 0.01
VT/24 h	–	2.4 ± 6.4	–	2.2 ± 6.5	< 0.05
Echocardiography					
RVEDD (mm)	17 ± 6	21 ± 8	26 ± 8	24 ± 11	< 0.05
LVEDD (mm)	67 ± 9	65 ± 9	72 ± 8	72 ± 10	< 0.01
LVESD (mm)	54 ± 9	53 ± 8	62 ± 10	61 ± 14	< 0.01
LVEFS (%)	20 ± 7	19 ± 7	15 ± 7	16 ± 17	NS
LVEF (%)	36 ± 13	36 ± 11	26 ± 10	26 ± 8	< 0.01
IV Th (%)	14 ± 10	12 ± 8	11 ± 10	11 ± 8	NS
PW Th (%)	24 ± 19	23 ± 14	21 ± 21	25 ± 17	NS
Cardiac catheterization					
RAP (mmHg)	4.0 ± 2.7	4.1 ± 2.7	6.1 ± 5.6	5.7 ± 6.1	NS
RVEDP (mmHg)	5.0 ± 3.1	4.6 ± 3.6	7.3 ± 4.2	7.0 ± 6.6	NS
mPAP (mmHg)	17 ± 8	16 ± 9	27 ± 9	23 ± 11	NS
PCWP (mmHg)	10 ± 6	11 ± 8	20 ± 8	19 ± 12	< 0.0001
LVEDP (mmHg)	14 ± 10	13 ± 9	19 ± 10	19 ± 12	< 0.01
CI (L/min/m²)	3.6 ± 1.3	3.4 ± 1.1	3.0 ± 1.1	3.0 ± 0.9	< 0.05
LVEF (%)	42 ± 7	41 ± 7	23 ± 7	21 ± 6	< 0.01

VT, ventricular tachycardia; group A, Lown grades 0–3 and LVEF > 30%; group B, lown grade > 3 and LVEF > 30%; group C, Lown grades 0–3 and LVEF < 30%; group D, Lown grade > 3 and LVEF < 30%; NS, not significant. Other abbreviations are as in Table 3. Figures are mean ± SD.

The groups were comparable by age and sex. Dynamic electrocardiographic, echocardiographic, and hemodynamic parameters in these four groups are summarized in Table 6. Groups C and D showed a significantly greater ventricular dysfunction and dilatation. The groups with a similar degree of ventricular dysfunction (A vs. B, C vs. D) were not significantly different for any parameter except presence or absence of severe ventricular arrhythmias.

Follow-up Data

The duration of follow-up ranged from 24 to 1095 days (mean 693 ± 345 days). During follow-up seven patients underwent heart transplantation, and were not included in follow-up analysis. Actuarial survival is shown in Figs. 1 and 2.

The overall survival rate at 36 months was 80%. Within 12 months nine patients died (5%), within 24 months 17 patients (9.5%), and within 36 months 23. All deaths were from cardiac causes (13.4%). Fourteen patients died of heart failure (60.8%), and nine of sudden death (39.2%).

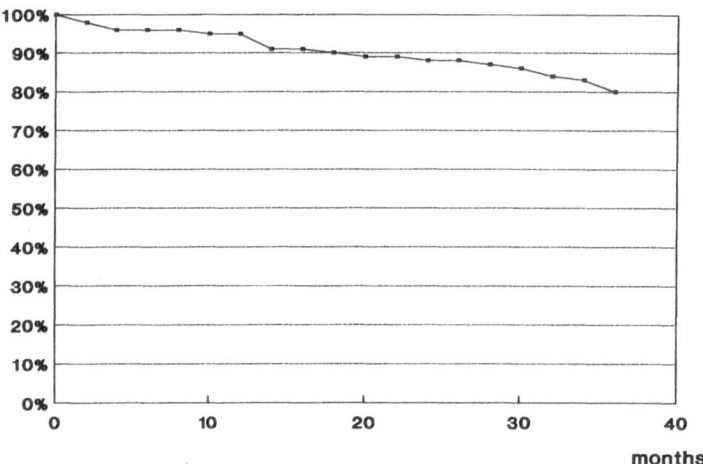

Fig. 1. Kaplan-Meier survival curve in 178 DCM patients

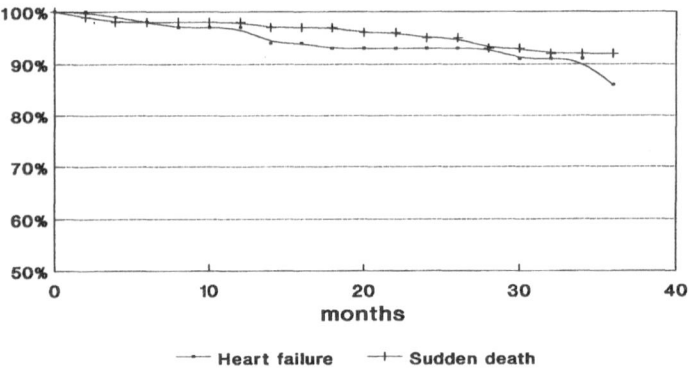

Fig. 2. Kaplan-Meier survival curve in 178 DCM patients according to cause of death

Among the variables tested in relation to prognosis, the only echocardiographic parameter showing a difference was the percentage posterior wall thickening: it was lower in nonsurvivors vs. survivors (13.5 ± 7 mm vs. 24.5 ± 17 mm, $p < 0.05$) and in patients dying from heart failure compared with survivors (12 ± 7 mm vs. 24.5 ± 17 mm, $p < 0.02$). Among the hemodynamic variables tested in relation to prognosis, the only parameter showing a difference was left ventricular ejection fraction: it was significantly lower in patients who died from heart failure compared with survivors (24% ± 11% vs. 32% ± 5%, $p < 0.05$). Although there was a trend towards a lower left ventricular ejection fraction in nonsurvivors, the difference vs. survivors was not statistically significant (27% ± 11% vs. 32% ± 11%, $p = $ NS).

Comparing mode of death in relation to severity of ventricular arrhythmias (Table 7), sudden death was found to be significantly more frequent in patients in a higher Lown grade group (9.8% in group 2 and 8.1% in group 3 vs. 1.1% in group 1, $p < 0.05$). A linear stepwise discriminant function analysis was

Table 7. DCM: mortality in Lown grade group

	(n) (%)	GM (n) (%)	HF (n) (%)	SD (n) (%)
Group 1	90 50.6	8 8.8	7 7.7	1 1.1
Group 2	51 28.7	9 17.6	4 7.8	5 9.8
Group 3	37 20.7	6 16.2	3 8.1	3 8.1
p		< 0.05	NS	< 0.05

Group 1, Lown grades 0–3; group 2, Lown grades 4A and 4B; group 3, Lown grade 5; GM, global mortality; HF, death due to heart failure; SD, sudden death.

performed using dynamic electrocardiographic, echocardiographic, and hemo-dynamic variables.

The major independent determinants of death from global mortality were percentage echocardiographic posterior wall thickening and number of ventricular tachycardia episodes (76% of the patients who died and 63% of the survivors correctly classified). The major independent determinants of death from heart failure were percentage posterior wall thickening and angiographic left ventricular ejection fraction (75% of the patients who died from heart failure and 71.3% of the survivors correctly classified). The major independent determinants of death from sudden death were Lown grade and number of ventricular tachycardia episodes (75% of the patients who died from sudden death and 71% of the survivors correctly classified).

Discussion

This study confirms a high prevalence of ventricular arrhythmias in DCM patients. In our series of 178 consecutive patients, dynamic electrocardiographic monitoring detected ventricular arrhythmias in 91.6%, a finding consistent with the results of previous studies [3, 6, 8, 12]. However, prevalence of complex ventricular arrhythmias (couplets, multiform PVCs and couplets, ventricular tachycardia) was found to be considerably lower than previously reported (49% vs. up to 95%) [3, 6–8, 10, 12].

Despite the common detection of high-grade arrhythmias, the majority of patients with DCM are asymptomatic during dynamic electrocardiographic monitoring: symptoms were present in only 19% of recorded episodes of nonsustained ventricular tachycardia in our series. Prevalence and complexity of ventricular arrhythmias in DCM seem to be higher than those reported so far in any other cardiac disease: only in hypertrophic cardiomyopathy was a similar prevalence of complex ventricular arrhythmias found [18–21], while a considerably lower prevalence was observed in ischemic heart disease after myocardial infarction [22–24].

The relationship between severity of ventricular arrhythmias and degree of ventricular dysfunction remains controversial. Some previous studies showed that complexity of ventricular arrhythmias correlated with left ventricular dysfunction [7, 11, 12, 25]. In contrast, other authors could not detect any relation between occurrence of complex ventricular arrhythmias and degree of left ventricular impairment [3, 6, 8, 10].

In the present study, the only significantly different hemodynamic parameter between patients with and without complex ventricular arrhythmias was left ventricular ejection fraction ($p < 0.02$).

However, linear regression analysis failed to demonstrate a significant relationship between any dynamic electrocardiographic monitoring variable (total number of ventricular extrasystoles, number of ventricular couplets, number of morphologies, number of ventricular tachycardia episodes), and angiographic left ventricular ejection fraction. Moreover, in our series patients with similar degrees of ventricular dysfunction (groups A and B, C and D) were not significantly different for any other variable, except presence or absence of complex ventricular arrhythmias.

Distribution of ventricular arrhythmias grade over a wide range of left ventricular ejection fraction should therefore exclude a clear-cut correlation between severity of ventricular arrhythmias and severity of ventricular dysfunction.

Our data show, by Kaplan-Meier analysis, an overall survival rate at 36 months of 80%, considerably higher than previously reported in patients with DCM [1, 2, 4, 9, 13, 14]. The low incidence of mortality during long-term follow-up might be biased by selection criteria of our study [15]: all patients with end-stage DCM and/or on the waiting list for heart transplant were not enrolled. In the present study, about 40% of patients with DCM died from sudden death and about 60% from heart failure. These rates are no different from the range of previous reports [2, 5, 12, 13].

Conflicting data on complex ventricular arrhythmias as determinants of prognosis in patients with DCM are reported: some authors found a correlation between prevalence and severity of ventricular arrhythmias and incidence of sudden death [3, 8, 14], while others did not [5, 7, 10, 12, 13]. In this study, dynamic electrocardiographic monitoring was able to identify patients with DCM prone to subsequent sudden death. There was significantly higher mortality in patients with complex ventricular arrhythmias than in patients without complex ventricular arrhythmias, because of a higher prevalence of sudden death (t test, $p < 0.05$).

Moreover, linear stepwise discriminant function analysis revealed the Lown grade and number of ventricular tachycardia episodes as major independent determinants of sudden death.

In view of the similar mortality for sudden death and congestive heart failure, it is not surprising that discriminant analysis identified a dynamic electrocardiographic variable, number of ventricular tachycardia episodes, in association with a pump function index, percentage echocardiographic posterior wall thickening, as major independent determinants of global mortality. On the contrary, no dynamic electrocardiographic monitoring variable had a prognostic impact on pump failure deaths.

These data are in partial agreement with those of Hofmann et al. [14], who found that patients who died suddenly had a significantly higher Lown grade than survivors and patients who died from heart failure. However, these authors found, by multivariate logistic regression analysis, that the presence of frequent complex ventricular arrhythmias alone was not indicative of an increased risk for sudden death. Only the combination of frequent complex ventricular arrhythmias and reduced left ventricular function identified patients at risk for sudden death. The same conclusions were reached by Costanzo-Nordin et al. with multiform VEs [10].

Limitations of the Study

It is important to note that in our prospective study, selection factors may have influenced the results. According to our criteria, patients with a low life expectancy (end-stage DCM and/or on the waiting list for heart transplantation) were excluded; therefore, the patient population was in general clinically stable and there was, not surprisingly, a low mortality. Such a low event rate may in fact impair the prognostic value of these findings.

During dynamic electrocardiographic monitoring only 11% of patients were in pharmacological wash-out; however, antiarrhythmic treatment was equally distributed among the groups with different severity of ventricular arrhythmias, thus minimizing the risk of bias.

The possibility that a specific antiarrhythmic treatment in DCM may induce a significant reduction in the incidence of ventricular arrhythmias has been suggested [26], but not confirmed [14]. On the other hand, the proarrhythmic effects of any antiarrhythmic agent should also be taken into account.

Another point of criticism may be related to the duration of dynamic electrocardiographic monitoring: while 24 h is the accepted standard, 48- or 72-h monitoring can increase the number of detected arrhythmics events.

The day to day variability of complex ventricular arrhythmics makes a correct estimate of the phenomenon difficult [27]. The large number of observations in our study probably averages this kind of variability.

In conclusion, in our study ventricular arrhythmias were frequently observed at dynamic electrocardiographic monitoring of DCM patients (91.6%). Complex ventricular arrhythmias (modified Lown grade > 3) were less frequently seen (49%). Complex ventricular arrhythmias were equally distributed in patients with different degrees of left ventricular dysfunction (angiographic left ventricular ejection fraction < or > 30%), and severity of ventricular arrhythmias was not apparently related to depression of ventricular function. There was a low global mortality in our patient population with a 40% prevalence of sudden death. Sudden death was significantly more frequent in patients with a Lown grade > 3. The Lown grade itself and number of ventricular tachycardia episodes were identified as major independent determinants of sudden death.

References

1. Fuster V, Gersh BJ, Giuliani ER, Tajik AJ, Branderburg RO, Frye RL (1981) The natural history of idiopathic dilated cardiomyopathy. Am J Cardiol 47:525
2. Gavazzi A, Lanzarini L, Cornalba C, Desperati M, Raisaro A, Angoli L, De Servi S, Specchia G (1984) Dilated cardiomyopathy. Follow up study in 137 patients. G Ital Cardiol 11:429–498
3. Holmes J, Kubo S, Cody R, Kligfield P (1985) Arrhythmias in ischemic and non-ischemic dilated cardiomyopathy: prediction of mortality by ambulatory electrocardiography. Am J Cardiol 55:146–151
4. Keogh A, Freund J, Baron D, Hickie J (1988) Timing of cardiac transplantation in idiopathic dilated cardiomyopathy. Am J Cardiol 61:418–422
5. Packer M (1985) Sudden unexpected death in patients with congestive heart failure: a second frontier. Circulation 72:681–685
6. Huang SK, Messer JV, Denes P (1983) Significance of ventricular tachycardia in idiopathic dilated cardiomyopathy: observations in 35 patients. Am J Cardiol 51:507–512
7. Olshausen KV, Schafer A, Mehmel HC, Schwarts F, Senges J, Kbler W (1984) Ventricular arrhythmias in idiopathic dilated cardiomyopathy. Br Heart J 51:195–201
8. Meinertz T, Hofmann T, Kasper W, Treese N, Bechtold H, Stienen U, Pop T, Leitner ER, Andresen D, Meyer J (1984) Significance of ventricular arrhythmias in idiopathic dilated cardiomyopathy. Am J Cardiol 53:902–907
9. Unverferth DV, Magorien RD, Moeschberger ML, Baker PB, Fetters JK, Leier CV (1984) Factors influencing the one-year mortality of dilated cardiomyopathy. Am J Cardiol 54:147–152
10. Costanzo-Nordin MR, O'Connell JB, Engelmeier RS, Moran JF, Scanlon PJ (1985) Dilated cardiomyopathy: functional status, hemodynamics, arrhythmias and prognosis. Cathet Cardiovasc Diagn 11:445–453
11. Haissaguerre M, Bonnet J, Le Goff G, Gueguen A, Broustet J, Chaussat A, Dallochio M, Besse P, Bricaud H (1986) Prévalence, signification et prognostic des troubles du rythme ventriculaire dans 236 myocardiopathies dilatées. Arch Mal Coeur 1:32–38
12. Neri R, Mestroni L, Salvi A, Camerini F (1986) Arrhythmias in dilated cardiomyopathy. Postgrad Med J 62:593–597
13. Olshausen KV, Stienen U, Schwarz F, Kbler W, Meyer J (1988) Long-term prognostic significance of ventricular arrhythmias in idiopathic dilated cardiomyopathy. Am J Cardiol 61:146–151
14. Hofmann T, Meinertz T, Kasper W, Geibel A, Zehender M, Hohnloser S, Stienen U, Treese N, Just H (1988) Mode of death in idiopathic dilated cardiomyopathy: a multivariate analysis of prognostic determinants. Am Heart J 116:1455–1463
15. Italian Multicenter Cardiomyopathy study (SPIC) (1989) In this volume
16. Ryan M, Lown B, Horn H (1975) Comparison of ventricular ectopic activity during 24-hours monitoring and exercise testing in patients with coronary heart disease. N Engl J Med 292:224
17. Hinkle L, Thaler J (1975) Clinical classification of cardiac death. Circulation 65:457–464
18. Savage DD, Seides SF, Maron BJ, Myers DJ, Epstein SE (1979) Prevalence of arrhythmias during 24-hours electrocardiographic monitoring and exercise testing in patients with obstructive and nonobstructive hypertrophic cardiomyopathy. Circulation 59:866–875
19. KcKenna WJ, Chetty S, Oakley CM, Goodwin JF (1980) Arrhythmias in hypertrophic cardiomyopathy: exercise and 48 hours ambulatory electrocardiographic assessment with and without beta adrenergic blocking therapy. Am J Cardiol 45:1–5
20. McKenna WJ, Englang D, Doi LY, Deanfield JE, Oakley CM, Goodwin JF (1981) Arrhythmias in hypertrophic cardiomyopathy. Influence on prognosis. Br Heart J 46:168–172
21. Maron BJ, Savage DD, Wolfson JK, Epstein SE (1981) Prognostic significance of 24 hours ambulatory electrocardiographic monitoring in patients with hypertrophic cardiomyopathy: a prospective study. Am J Cardiol 48:252–257

22. Bigger JT (1986) A Symposium: management of ventricular arrhythmias in patients with congestive heart failure. Am J Cardiol 57:1–41
23. Bigger JT, Coromilias J (1984) Ventricular tachyarrhythmias in the various stages of ischemic heart disease. In: Surrawicz B, Reddy CP, Pristowshy EN (eds) Tachycardias. Nijhoff, Boston, pp 355–371
24. Bigger JT, Weld FM, Coromilias J, Roinitszky LM, De Turk WE (1983) Prevalence and significance of arrhythmias in 24 hours ECG recording made within one month of acute myocardial infarction. In: Kulbertus H, Wellens HJJ (eds) The first year after a myocardial infarction. Nijhoff, Boston, pp 161–175
25. Leclercq JF, Maisonblance P, Cauchemez B, Attuel P, Coumel P (1984) Les troubles du rythme ventriculaire des myocardiopathies congestives. Arch Mal Coeur 8:937–945
26. Neri R, Mestroni L, Salvi A, Pandullo C, Camerini F (1987) Ventricular arrhythmias in dilated cardiomyopathy: efficacy of amiodarone. Am Heart J 113 3:707–715
27. Schmidt G, Ulm K, Barthel P, Goedel-Meinen L, Jahns G, Baedeker W (1988) Spontaneous variability of simple and complex ventricular premature contractions during long time intervals in patients with severe organic heart disease. Circulation 78:296–301

Essential Ventricular Arrhythmias: An Early Step Toward Cardiomyopathy?

C. Contini, D. Levorato, C. Arlotta, A. Pozzolini, M. G. Bongiorni, S. Berti, M. T. Baratto, L. Paperini, M. Piacenti, G. Kraft, and A. Biagini

Introduction

Severe ventricular arrhythmias in apparently healthy subjects have recently been shown to be associated with regional or global myocardial contractile abnormalities. In this study we have assumed, as a working hypothesis, that this association in such subjects may represent an early step toward cardiomyopathy [1–5].

This highly attractive hypothesis needs, on the one hand, to be supported by an objective marker of myocardial damage, more specific than echocardiographic abnormalities [6]. On the other hand, it also needs to be supported by the objective demonstration during follow-up that the patients will develop clinical manifestations of myocardial impairment.

Being fascinated by this hypothesis, that even implies the possibility of an early recognition of myocardial dissynergies before their overt clinical manifestation, we studied 25 patients in whom we were able to document the coexistence both of complex ventricular arrhythmias and myocardial contractility impairment. Patients were enrolled after noninvasive tests (ambulatory ECG recordings and two-dimensional echocardiography); myocardial contractility was later also assessed with radioisotopic angiography and confirmed by hemodynamic study. The presence of morphologic alterations of the myocardium was assessed by endomyocardial biopsy, at present considered the "gold standard" for this purpose [7–9]. Furthermore, patients were followed-up in our outpatients' clinic.

Material and Methods

Selection of Patients: From 1983 up today we have enrolled 25 patients in NYHA classes 1–2 who, in the absence of any apparent heart disease (ischemic, valvular, or hypertensive), presented complex ventricular arrhythmias on 24-h ambulatory ECG monitoring and regional myocardial contractile abnormalities and/or ventricular enlargement on a standard two-dimensional echocardiographic study.

Study Protocol: After the demonstration of both complex arrhythmic events and ventricular dyssynergies, patients underwent radioisotopic angiography, hemodynamic study, and right ventricle endomyocardial biopsy. All patients also underwent further biohumoral tests to exclude metabolic, rheumatologic, autoimmune, or viral disorders. During the follow-up 18/25 patients underwent ambulatory ECG monitoring and two-dimensional echocardiographic study every 6 month for 1–5 years (mean 3.3 years).

ECG Ambulatory Monitoring: Dynamic ECGs were recorded with Avionics ECG recorders model 453A and analyzed with Avionics Cardiodisplay 250. The following parameters were analyzed: total ectopic beats, mean ectopic beats and their hourly frequency, number of morphologies, pairs and bigeminy frequency, number of ventricular tachycardia episodes.

Two-Dimensional Echocardiographic Examination: Echocardiographic (Hewlett-Packard, 77020 A model) examination was obtained by left parasternal, apical, and subxifoideal approaches. Regional wall motion was evaluated by an expert echocardiographist; hypokinesia was defined as reduction in wall thickening compared with normal segments. Segments were deemed akinetic when there was no systolic thickening even though slight endocardial motion remained [10]. Ventricular enlargement was defined by an increase in end-diastolic diamenters (normal values in our laboratory $< 55\,\mathrm{mm}$ for the left ventricle and $< 26\,\mathrm{mm}$ for the right ventricle).

Radioisotopic Angiography: Blood pool scintigraphic images were performed in left anterior and oblique projections. Regional wall motion was evaluated by an experienced observer, unaware of clinical and two-dimensional echocardiographic data, with the aid of parametric images (stroke, amplitude). Biventricular global systolic function was assessed by right and left ventricular ejection fraction values computed according to previously described methods [11–13].

Hemodynamic and Angiographic Study: Intracardiac pressures were recorded at rest and cardiac output was determined by the thermodilution method. Biplane right atrioventriculography and left ventricle angiography were sequentially performed in the 30° right anterior oblique and 60° left anterior oblique projections and followed by coronary angiography.

Right Ventricular Endomyocardial Biopsy: At least three specimens, approximately 3 mm in diameter, were obtained from each patient, using 6F King's bioptome. These were immediately fixed in phosphate-buffered 10% formalin. After completion of the routine histologic procedure, the 4–5-μm thick paraffin-embedded sections were stained by hematoxylin-eosin, Masson's trichrome, and van Gieson stain. Four to five sections of each specimen were evaluated by an experienced observer, unaware of patients' data. Hypertrophy and fibrosis were diagnosed when mean cellular diameter was $> 25\,\mu m$ and the percentage of fibrous tissue per section was $> 20\%$, respectively, in two samples [7, 14, 15].

Results

Clinical Findings: Among the patients (20 males, 5 females; mean age 37.4 years, range 14–56), 16 patients were in NYHA class 1 and nine in class 2; three were completely asymptomatic; in the remaining 25 subjects symptoms included palpitations (64%), syncope (8%), chest pain (44%), fatigue (20%), and dizziness (28%). Biohumoral tests excluded in all cases rheumatologic, autoimmune, or viral disease. Physical examination disclosed a fourth heart sound in one case and a third heart sound in three patients. Seven patients showed a slightly enlarged cardiac silhouette at chest X-ray, with a cardiothoracic ratio > 0.5. No patient had pulmonary congestion.

ECG Ambulatory Monitoring: According to entry criteria, all patients had ventricular arrhythmias (Fig. 1) during the 24-h ambulatory monitoring. Particularly 13 (52%) patients had frequent premature ventricular contractions (PVCs) (> 30 PVCs per hour), 10 (40%) multiform PVCs, 16 (64%) couplets, and 13 (52%) had episodes of ventricular tachycardia (from a minimum of one episodes up to 1516 episodes in one patient). Moreover, six patients (24%) had conduction abnormalities (second to third degree atrioventricular block); atrial flutter or fibrillation was present in four patients (16%), one patient experienced episodes of sinus arrest shorter than 1.5 s, and one patient had intermittent preexcitation.

Two-Dimensional Echocardiographic Examination: The results of two-dimensional echocardiography are summarized in Fig. 2. Mono- or biventricular enlargement and dyssynergies were observed in 25 patients (right ventricle in eight patients, left ventricle in five patients, and both ventricles in 12 patients). Two patients showed only left ventricular enlargement, one patient showed isolated dyssynergies of the left ventricle.

Radioisotopic Angiography: Regional wall motion analysis demonstrated myocardial dyssynergies in all patients. Isolated right ventricle (62%), biventricular (28%) or isolated left ventricle (28%) wall motion anomalies were documented; mainly affected regions were right ventricular wall, left ventricular septum and apex; while diffuse ventricular enlargement and hypokinesia were present

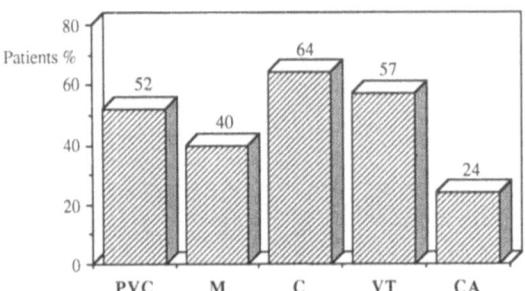

Fig. 1. Arrhythmias. *PVC*, premature ventricular contraction; *M*, multiform; *C*, couplets; *VT*, ventricular tachycardia; *CA*, conduction abnormality

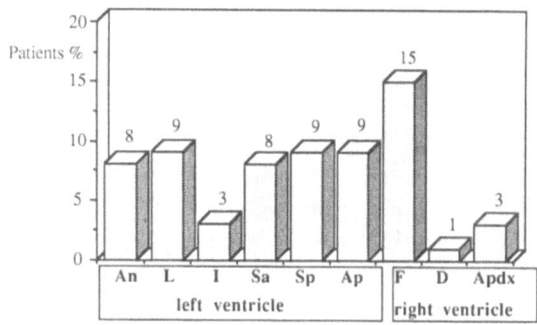

Fig. 2. Two-dimensional echocardiography. Myocardial wall: *An*, anterior; *L*, lateral; *I*, inferior; *Sa*, septum anterior; *Sp*, septum posterior; *Ap*, apex; *F*, free wall; *D*, diaphragmatic; *Apdx*, apex

in two cases. Twenty-four patients (95%) showed right and/or left ventricular ejection fraction reduction (ten right ventricle, six left ventricle, and eight both).

Follow-up: During the follow-up period, 11/18 patients showed no changes in myocardial contractility and/or chamber dimension as evaluated by two-dimensional echocardiography, while the other 7/18 patients showed some degree of worsening. In particular, five patients showed an increase of the preexisting abnormalities, while in two patients the abnormality localized to the right ventricle extended also to the left one. We did not observe any significant changes in the number and entity of ventricular arrhythmias each patient had on analysis of Holter recordings.

Discussion

In the natural history of dilated cardiomyopathy, ventricular arrhythmias are commonly found [16–19], but they are also often reported in apparently healthy subjects [1, 5] in whom some impairment in myocardial contractility and even the presence of histological alterations have been demonstrated [2, 3, 7].

Nevertheless, at present we ignore the prevalence of this association in the normal population and its clinical relevance. In this study we assumed as a working hypothesis that this association in the same subject may represent an early step toward cardiomyopathy. For this reason, we selected a group of patients with ventricular arrhythmias and some impairment in myocardial contractility and/or chamber dimension, who had not experienced any sign of myocardial failure and in whom the clinical manifestations of the disease were poor.

In this group of patients, collected over 5 years, we have carefully evaluated the extent of myocardial involvement not only with the echocardiographic technique, which could be affected by some variability in the interpretation of the results, but also with radionuclide and angiographic ventriculography, which are affected by this bias to a lesser extent [2, 20]. The accordance found in the evaluation of regional contractility by these different techniques allows us to exclude biases related to interobserver variability. Generally, our patients were characterized by a regional defect in myocardial contractility and/or dimension unrelated to an ischemic problem, as demonstrated by normal coronary angiography. The regional myocardial contraction abnormality was only seldom related to global ventricular dysfunction, as was also demonstrated by the mean ejection fraction of our population (56.2%) and by normal hemodynamic study. The alterations described were, in general, localized to both ventricles, while, when only isolated abnormalities were present, they affected mainly the right ventricle. We also consider it interesting that within the myocardial wall, the echocardiographic examination often showed, patchy areas of increased density probably related to isolated areas of fibrosis.

Regarding the arrhythmic phenomena, our population was characterized by the same ventricular arrhythmias typical of patients with overt dilated myocardiopathy [16–19]. In fact 13/25 patients showed several episodes of nonsustained and even sustained ventricular tachycardia, especially in those with right ventricular involvement, in accordance with the data in the literature which identify such patients as a subgroup at high risk of sudden death [18]. This finding demonstrates that the number and severity of ventricular arrhythmias do not seem to be correlated to the level of myocardial impairment. Therefore, it is possible to speculate that in these patients arrhythmias are not directly related to dilatation of the ventricle, but more to the intrinsic abnormality of the diseased myocytes (fibrosis, hypertrophy).

In this study we also attempted to identify which histologic alterations were present at endomyocardial biopsies. We are aware of the fact that the results obtained by endomyocardial biopsies are often nonspecific, but in this particular clinical setting we considered it interesting to have this information in order to better classify our population. Ventricular endomyocardial biopsy showed abnormal histologic findings in 14/18 patients, however, no specific diagnosis of heart disease could be reached. Combined hypertrophy and fibrosis was documented in nine cases with a similar frequency to those reported in patients with idiopathic dilated cardiomyopathy. In two cases there was an increase in the number of inflammatory cells but a diagnosis of myocarditis was not possible, for lack of myocellular necrosis. Only in one patient with isolated right ventricular dysfunction could adipose infiltrates, typical of arrhythmogenic right ventricular dysplasia, be documented. This patient showed only mild right ventricular functional abnormalities. Our and previous results demonstrate that myocardial dysfunction in arrhythmic patients may be associated with evident histologic anomalies, rarely including the specific pattern of right ventricular dysplasia, whose etiopathologic meaning is at present undefined. The assessment of biventricular histologic abnormalities and of their extent by means of endomyocardial biopsy and their morphometric evaluation would help to determine in future whether generalized myocardial damage is always associated with both electrical disturbances and ventricular dysfunction.

In conclusion, our data, obtained in a well-selected group of patients with severe ventricular arrhythmias and with myocardial contractile abnormalities, demonstrate a high correlation between the presence of these abnormalities and some evidence of myocardial damage as judged by endomyocardial biopsy. This finding enforce the hypothesis that these "alarm" ventricular arrhythmias are sometimes an isolated manifestation of heart disease.

Acknowledgements: This work was partly supported by a grant from the CNR specialized programs "Tecnologie Biomediche e Sanitarie." The authors appreciate the skillfull assistance of Miss R. Bertolini in preparing the manuscript.

References

1. Kennedy HL, Pescarmona JE, Bouchard RJ, Goldberg RJ, Carolis DG (1982) Objective evidence of occult myocardial dysfunction in patients with frequent ventricular ectopy without clinically apparent heart disease. Am Heart J 104:57–65
2. Neglia D, Levorato D, Berti S et al (1987) Diagnosi e caratterizzazione funzionale di iniziale danno miocardico in pazienti con aritmie cardiache. Cardiologia 32(8):713–718
3. Morgera T, Salvi A, Alberti E, Silvestri F, Camerini F (1985) Morphological findings in apparently idiopathic ventricular tachycardia. An echocardiographic, hemodynamic and histologic study. Eur Heart J 6:323–334
4. Bouvrain Y, Slama R, Motte' G, Waynberger M, Grevellier A (1968) Les tachycardies ventriculaires. Etiologie et évolution, à propos de 161 malades. Arch Mal Coeur 61:909–920
5. Montague TJ, Mc Pherson DD, Mac Kenzie BR, Spencer CA, Nanton MA, Horacek BM (1983) Frequent ventricular ectopic activity without underlying cardiac disease: analysis of 45 subjects. Am J Cardiol 52:980–984
6. Tajik AL, Seward JB, Hagler DJ, Mair DD, Lie JT (1978) Two-dimensional real-time ultrasonic imaging of the heart and great vessels: technique, image orientation, structure identification and validation. Mayo Clin Proc 53:271–303
7. Strain JE, Grose RM, Factor SM, Fisher JD (1983) Results of endomyocardial biopsy in patients with spontaneous ventricular tachycardia but without apparent structural heart disease. Circulation 68:1171–1181
8. Sugrue DD, Holmes DR, Gersh BJ, Edwards WD, McLaren CJ, Wood DL, Osborn MJ, Hammill SC (1984) Cardiac histologic findings in patients with life-threatening ventricular arrythmias of unknown origin. J Am Coll Cardiol 4:952–957
9. Shirey EK, Proudftit WL, Hawk WA (1980) Primary myocardial disease. Correlation with clinical findings, angiographic and biopsies diagnosis. Am Heart J 99:198–207
10. Moynihan PF, Parisi AF, Feldman CL (1981) Quantitative detection of regional left ventricular contraction abnormalities by two-dimensional echocardiography. I. Analysis of methods. Circulation 63:752–760
11. Schelbert HR, Verba JW, Johnson A, Brock GW, Alazraki NP, Ross FJ, Ashburn WL (1975) Nontraumatic determination of left ventricular ejection fraction by radionuclide angiography. Circulation 51:902–909
12. Maddahi J, Berman DS, Matsuoka T, Waxman AD, Stankus KE, Forrester JS, Swan HJC (1979) A new technique for assessing right ventricular ejection fraction using rapid multiple-gated equilibrium cardiac blood pool scintigraphy. Circulation 60:581–589
13. Neglia D, Marcassa C, Parodi O, Bellina CR, Marzullo P, Michelassi C, Berti S, Contini C, L'Abbate A (1987) Optimization of right ventricular ejection fraction measurements from first pass and gated blood pool scintigraphy. In: Guzzardi R (ed) Physics and engineering of medical imaging. Nijhoff, Dordrecht, pp 615–620

14. Kuhn H, Briethardt G, Knieren MJ, Loogen F (1978) Endomyocardial catheter biopsy in heart disease of unknown etiology. In: Kaltenbach M, Loogen F, Olsen EGJ (eds) Cardiomyopathy and myocardial biopsy. Springer, Berlin Heidelberg New York, pp 121–136
15. Baandrup U, Olsen EGJ (1981) Critical analysis of endomyocardial biopsies from patients suspected of having cardiomyopathy. I: Morphological and morphometric aspects. Br Heart J 45:475–486
16. Goodwin JF, Oakley CM (1972) The cardiomyopathies. Br Heart J 34:545–552
17. Fuster V, Gersh BJ, Giuliani ER, Tajik AJ, Brandemburg RO, Frye RL (1981) The natural history of idiopathic dilated cardiomyopathy. Am J Cardiol 47:525–531
18. Mc Kenna WJ, Krikler DM, Goodwin JF (1984) Arrhythmias in dilated and hypertrophic cardiomyopathy. Med Clin North Am 68:983–1000
19. Olshausen KV, Stienen U, Schwarz F, Kubler W, Meyer J (1988) Long-term prognostic significance of ventricular arrhythmias in idiopatic dilated cardiomyopathy. Am J Cardiol 61:146–151
20. Stamm RB, Carabello BA, Martin RP et al (1981) Comparison of regional wall motion determined by two-dimensional echocardiography, radionuclide angiography and left ventricular ventriculography. In: Rijsterborgh H (ed) Echocardiography. Nijhoff, The Hague, pp 103–110

Role of Radionuclide Angiography in the Diagnosis of Early Ventricular Dysfunction in Patients with Complex Ventricular Arrhythmias

S. Berti, D. Neglia, D. Levorato, O. Parodi, M. G. Bongiorni, M. Piacenti, M. T. Baratto, C. Arlotta, L. Paperini, G. Kraft, A. L'Abbate, A. Biagini, and C. Contini

Introduction

Dilated cardiomyopathy is defined as a heart muscle disorder of unknown etiology in which there is impaired contractile function and dilatation of one or both ventricles [1, 2]. It is known that, once clinical evidence of impaired ventricular performance is apparent, the prognosis is poor [3–5]. Hence, we should attempt to diagnose the disorder earlier in its latency period. Much evidence suggests that subjects who come to medical attention only because of ventricular arrhythmias may represent the tip of the iceberg of patients with primitive myocardial disease.

Ventricular arrhythmias are frequent in patients with dilated cardiomyopathy [6–8] and have recently been associated with predominant right ventricular dysfunction [9–11]. Moreover, occult left ventricular dysfunction [11–13] and myocardial histologic abnormalities [14–16] have been demonstrated in patients with apparently primitive ventricular tachycardia. For these reasons, patients with complex ventricular arrhythmias and without clinical evidence of heart failure may be considered as a population "at risk" of primitive myocardial disease in the early stage. At present, a complete picture of the prevalence and the extent of biventricular dysfunction in patients with complex ventricular arrhythmias is still lacking. The purpose of this study was to assess, by radionuclide angiography, the presence and the distribution of regional and/or global ventricular dysfunction in patients with apparently primitive complex ventricular arrhythmias. The reliability of this noninvasive technique in identifying subclinical functional abnormalities was evaluated by comparison with angiographic and hemodynamic data.

Methods

Study Protocol

From January 1983 to January 1988 over 400 subjects were referred to our institute because of symptomatic or asymptomatic ventricular arrhythmias. Preliminary biohumoral and clinical evaluation allowed us to exclude patients with signs or symptoms of cardiac failure (NYHA class II–IV), or documented ischemic, valvular, congenital, hypertensive heart disease, or other systemic disorders. After discontinuation of any cardiologic therapy, 24-h Holter recordings were performed in all. Twenty-seven consecutive patients (21 males, six females; mean age 30 years, range 18–62 years) with complex ventricular ectopic beats (multiform, repetitive) and/or ventricular tachycardia (more than three episodes of three beats or at least one episode of more than eight beats) were selected (group 1). In this group, radionuclide angiography (RNA) was performed, and data were compared with those of 20 normal individuals (ten males, ten females; mean age 40 years, range 14–68; group 2) studied because of palpitations and sporadic monomorphic ventricular ectopic beats ($n = 10$) or atypical chest pain and nonspecific ST-T wave abnormalities at basal electrocardiogram ($n = 10$). After the noninvasive evaluation, in 24/27 patients in group 1, who had shown regional dyssynergies, and in the ten patients in group 2 with chest pain, cardiac catheterization and coronary angiography were performed. Informed consent to enter the study protocol was obtained in all cases.

Radionuclide Angiography

Gated blood pool images were obtained by in vivo labeling of red blood cells by 0.03 mg/kg of stannous agent (Amersham) followed after 30 min by 0.93 GBq (25 mCi) of technetium-99m pertechnetate. The scintigraphic data were collected by a standard large field gamma-camera (Selo KR7, Italy) interfaced with a dedicated computer (Medusa 12 B, SEPA, Italy) or with a small field mobile camera (Apex 410m, Elscint, Israel) both equipped with a high resolution, parallel hole collimator. Acquisitions were performed in the left anterior oblique ("best septal") and anterior projections collecting a minimum of 100 000 counts/frame and stored in 24 frames of a 64×64 matrix. A narrow (10%) acceptance RR window was chosen to avoid acquisition of ectopic and postextrasystolic beats. Regional wall motion was evaluated by an experienced observer, not aware of the clinical data, with the help of parametric images (stroke, amplitude), for five left ventricular (septal, apical, anterior, lateral, and inferior) and two right ventricular regions (anterolateral and inferoapical). A score of 0–1–2 was used to indicate normal, hypokinetic or akinetic regions, while diffuse enlargement and hypokinesia of one ventricle was characterized by a global score of 5. The sum of regional scores provided right and left ventricular global wall motion abnormality indices (WMI). Ventricular dysfunction was defined by a global wall motion index score value ≥ 2. Slight volume increase with normal wall motion was not considered sufficient to identify ventricular impairment.

Right and left ventricular ejection fraction values were computed from radionuclide angiography data according to previously described methods [17, 18]. In particular, right ventricular ejection fraction measures had been previously validated in our laboratory using right ventricular ejection fraction values obtained from "first pass" analysis as a reference [19]. Scintigraphic left ventricular ejection fraction values showed a good correlation with the corresponding angiographic values obtained in the study population ($r = 0.70$, $p < 0.0001$).

Cardiac Catheterization

Intracardiac pressures were recorded at rest using fluid-filled catheters. Cardiac output was measured using the thermodilution technique. The normal range of hemodynamic values was derived from published data [20] in agreement with the standards obtained in our laboratory. Biplane right and left ventricular cineangiographies were sequentially performed injecting contrast medium into the right atrium and into the left ventricle, respectively. Coronary angiography was performed using the Judkins technique. Angiographic images were evaluated by an experienced observer for corresponding myocardial regions and with the same analysis used for radionuclide angiography. Volume increase was defined by qualitative criteria. Only sinus and not postextrasistolic beats were evaluated for wall motion analysis and pressure measurements.

Statistical Analysis

Continuous data are presented as the mean $\pm$ 1 standard deviation. Fisher's exact test was used to assess, beyond chance occurrence, agreement between noninvasive and invasive techniques. The t test for unpaired data was performed to identify differences among radionuclide angiography data obtained in different groups. Linear regression analysis was used to study the correlation between scintigraphic parameters. A probability (p) value less than 0.05 was considered significant.

Results

Clinical and Electrocardiographic Findings

Most of the patients in group 1 were symptomatic (89%) complaining of palpitations (74%), syncope (44%), and atypical chest pain (30%). Physical examination was generally normal disclosing grade I–II systolic ejection murmurs in five cases, a fourth heart sound in two cases, and a third heart sound in another case. Chest X-ray was usually normal showing a slightly enlarged cardiac silhouette with normal cardiothoracic ratio in ten cases. Biohumoral tests did not show any signs of metabolic, rheumatologic, or viral disease, while alcohol, coffee, or tea abuse or an excessive use of other pharmacologic agents were excluded. Standard ECG was generally abnormal (92%) showing ventricular ectopic beats (52%) and/or T wave abnormalities (33%) or conduction disturbances (11%). Neither maximal bicycle exercise testing nor ergonovine testing (performed in patients with chest pain) was able to evidence ischemic ECG changes.

Ventricular arrhythmias at 24-h Holter recordings were characterized as follows: complex ventricular etopic beats in 25 cases, associated with ventricular tachycardia in 19; isolated ventricular tachycardia in two cases. Prevalent left bundle branch block configuration of ventricular arrhythmias was docu-

Table 1. Main clinical data in patients with complex ventricular arrhythmias

Patient no.	Age and sex	Symptoms at admission	CS	Basal ECG	24-h Holter data (arrhythmias)		Functional data RV Dys	LV Dys
1	51 F	Palpitations, syncope	N	VEBs	CVEBs (2)[a]	VT[a]	+	–
2	43 M	Syncope	N	VEBs	CVEBs (3)[a]	VT[a]	+	–
3	36 M	Palpitations	N	N	CVEBs (2)[a]	VT[a]	+	–
4	18 M	Syncope	N	N		VT[a]	+	–
5	25 M	Palpitations, syncope	N	RBBB	CVEBs (1)[a]	VT[a]	+	–
6	19 M	Asymptomatic	N	VEBs	CVEBs (1)[a]	VT[a]	+	–
7	43 M	Palpitations, syncope, chest pain	A	NEG TW	CVEBs (1)[a]		+	–
8	25 M	Palpitations	N	NEG TW	CVEBs (3)	VT	+	–
9	62 F	Palpitations, chest pain	A	NEG TW	CVEBs (2)[a]		+	–
10	39 M	Palpitations, syncope	A	AVB I+II	CVEBs (5)	VT	+	–
11	52 M	Palpitations, syncope	N	NEG TW	CVEBs (3)	VT	+	+
12	32 M	Palpitations, syncope	A	VEBs	CVEBs (3)	VT	+	+
13	41 M	Palpitations, syncope	A	VEBs	CVEBs (3)	VT	+	+
14	51 M	Palpitations, chest pain	A	VEBs	CVEBs (3)		+	+
15	44 M	Syncope	A	VEBs	CVEBs (1)	VT	+	+
16	46 M	Palpitations	A	VEBs	CVEBs (3)[a]		+	+
17	20 M	Asymptomatic	N	VEBs	CVEBs (2)	VT	–	+
18	42 M	Palpitations, syncope	N	NEG TW	CVEBs (4)	VT	–	+
19	56 M	Asymptomatic	N	VEBs	CVEBs (3)[a]		–	+
20	43 M	Palpitations, syncope	N	NEG TW, VEBs	CVEBs (4)	VT	–	+
21	45 M	Palpitations	N	NEGTW	CVEBs (3)	VT	–	+
22	46 M	Palpitations, chest pain	A	LBBB	CVEBs (3)	VT	–	+
23	36 F	Palpitations, chest pain	N	NEG TW, VEBs	CVEBs (3)	VT	–	+
24	48 M	Chest pain	A	NEG T W	CVEBs (2)		–	+
25	26 F	Palpitations	N	N		VT[a]	–	–
26	33 F	Palpitations, chest pain	N	VEBs	CVEBs (1)[a]	VT[a]	–	–
27	30 F	Palpitations, chest pain	N	VEBs	CVEBs (1)[a]	VT[a]	–	–

[a] Prevalent LBBB configuration of ventricular arrhythmias.

CS, cardiac silhouette; *RV, LV dys*, RV, LV dysfunction at RNA wall motion analysis (WMI $\geq$ 2); *N*, normal; *A*, abnormal; *VEBs*, ventricular ectopic beats; *RBBB, LBBB*, right, left bundle branch block; *NEG TW*, negative T-waves; *AVB*, AV block; *CVEBs*, complex ventricular ectopic beats, number of morphologies in parenthesis; *VT*, ventricular tachycardia.

mented in 13 patients (48%). The main clinical and electrocardiographic data are summarized in Table 1.

In group 2, ten patients with palpitations showed sporadic ventricular ectopic beats, and ten patients with atypical chest pain showed nonspecific ST-T wave abnormalities at basal ECG and/or Holter recordings. All other clinical findings, including bicycle exercise testing and ergonovine testing performed in subjects with chest pain, were normal.

Biventricular Function: Noninvasive Results

Twenty-four out of 27 patients in group 1 (89%) showed regional wall motion abnormalities. In particular, significant ventricular dysfunction (WMI $\geq$ 2) involved the right ventricle in ten cases (37%), the left ventricle in eight cases (30%), and both ventricles in six (22%) (Tables 1 and 2). Regional dyssynergies could involve each myocardial region explored with a prevalence of the right ventricular free wall and the septal and apical walls of the left ventricle (Fig. 1).

Table 2. Noninvasive and invasive data on biventricular function in patients of group 1

Patient no.	WMI values (units)						Biventricular pressures (mmHg) Cardiac index (L/min/m^2)								
	RNA		VTG		RNA EF		RVP		PAP		LVP		AoP		CI
	RV	LV	RV	LV	RV (%)	LV (%)	S	D	S	D	S	D	S	D	
1	2	–	V	–	50	57	18	1	20	4	144	1	136	67	2.8
2	2	–	–	–	40	58	28	0	20	7	135	8	136	86	5.1
3	4	–	5	–	22^a	69	34^a	6	34^a	16^a	118	19^a	117	70	2.5^a
4	5	–	5	–	17^a	60	19	5	15	5	113	9	110	76	3.7
5	3	–	5	–	33^a	60	19	2	17	3	125	10	135	75	4.1
6	2	–	–	–	41	51	14	2	13	4	132	10	135	84	4.3
7	2	–	–	–	41	65	15	2	14	3	130	3	130	80	4.0
8	3	–	V	V	43	60	10	2	9	3	100	3	100	52	2.8
9	3	1	5	1	24^a	68	30	4	29	9	118	17^a	119	60	2.8
10	2	1	V	V	50	56	19	5	18	8	101	10	111	63	2.9
11	5	2	–	1	28^a	54	15	3	14	3	124	12	120	75	3.8
12	4	2	5	2	14^a	44^a	10	1	10	2	102	3	108	62	3.6
13	2	5	V	V	39^a	49^a	26	1	27	1	127	13^a	136	86	4.2
14	3	3	–	5	36^a	50^a	17	3	16	3	145	5	145	70	3.9
15	2	3	V	V	32^a	46^a	16	0	16	4	118	7	118	60	3.1
16	2	4	–	2	41	34^a	40^a	0	30	10	120	10	120	60	2.9
17	1	2	V	1	40	44^a	15	3	15	4	120	7	120	65	2.7
18	1	3	V	3	49	38^a	23	2	19	5	140	10	140	70	3.7
19	1	3	–	3	48	47^a	12	0	11	3	125	6	143	32	3.0
20	–	4	–	2	54	54	27	2	20	3	124	16^a	129	69	3.9
21	–	3	–	V	55	49^a	22	2	16	4	124	8	128	70	3.0
22	–	3	–	5	59	48^a	14	2	13	3	124	5	128	80	3.3
23	–	3	V	3	53	37^a	23	2	19	4	112	14^a	114	68	3.7
24	–	3	V	5	56	51	18	3	18	5	133	14^a	133	70	2.8
25	–	–	NP	NP	48	61	NP	NP	NP	NP	NP	NP	NP	NP	NP
26	–	–	NP	NP	54	62	NP	NP	NP	NP	NP	NP	NP	NP	NP
27	–	–	NP	NP	47	66	NP	NP	NP	NP	NP	NP	NP	NP	NP
Mean					41	53	20	2	18	5	123	9	125	70	3.4
SD					12	9	8	2	6	3	12	5	12	9	0.6
Normal values					$\geq$40	51	$\leq$30	8	$\leq$30	12	$\leq$150	12	$\leq$150	90	$\geq$2.6

^{a}Abnormal findings.

WMI, wall motion index; *VTG*, contrast ventriculography; *RVP*, right ventricular pressure; *PAP*, pulmonary artery pressure; *LVP*, left ventricular pressure; *AoP*, aortic pressure; *CI*, cardiac index; *S*, systolic; *D*, diastolic; *V*, volume enlargement; *NP*, not performed; –, normal findings.

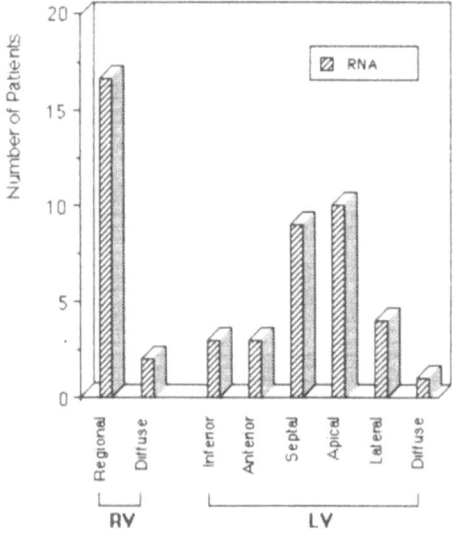

Fig. 1. Frequency distribution of regional wall motion abnormalities detected by radionuclide angiography (*RNA*) in 24 patients of group 1. *RV*, right ventricle; *LV*, left ventricle

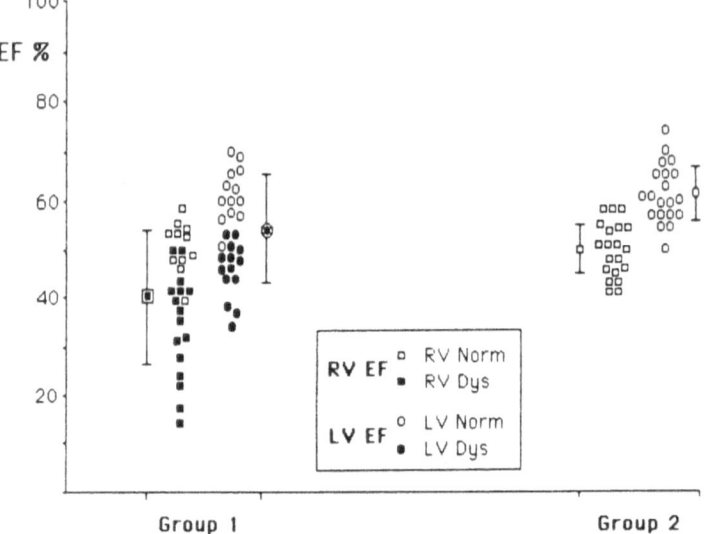

Fig. 2. Right and left ventricular ejection fraction (*EF*) values (individual and mean ± SD values) are represented in the two groups of patients. *RV, LV Norm*, normal right, left ventricular wall motion; *RV, LV Dys*, right, left ventricular dyssynergies (WMl ≥ 2). Both right ventricular and left ventricular ejection fraction values in group 1 were significantly lower than in group 2 ($p < 0.01$)

By contrast, diffuse ventricular enlargement and hypokinesia were detected in few cases.

Prevalent right ventricular origin of ventricular arrhythmias (left bundle branch block configuration) was documented in 8/10 cases with right ventricular dysfunction, in one case with left ventricular, and in one case with biventricular impairment; the same pattern was found in the three patients in group 1 with normal wall motion (Table 1).

The lower limit for normal ejection fraction was defined by mean values obtained in group 2 (right ventricular ejection fraction = 50 ± 5, left ventricular ejection fraction = 61 ± 5) minus 2 standard deviations and was in agreement with published data [17–18]. Accordingly, in group 1, 16/27 patients (59%) showed abnormal right ventricular and/or left ventricular ejection fraction values. Mean right ventricular and left ventricular ejection fraction values were significantly lower in group 1 (right ventricular ejection fraction = 41 ± 12; left ventricular ejection fraction = 53 ± 9) than in group 2 ($p < 0.01$) (Fig. 2). In particular, right ventricular ejection fraction was depressed in 9/16 cases with right ventricular dysfunction, and left ventricular ejection fraction was reduced in 11/14 cases with left ventricular dysfunction (Fig. 2). The correlation between the extent of regional dyssynergies and decrease in ejection fraction was high for the right ($r = 0.88$) and the left ($r = 0.74$) ventricle (Fig. 3).

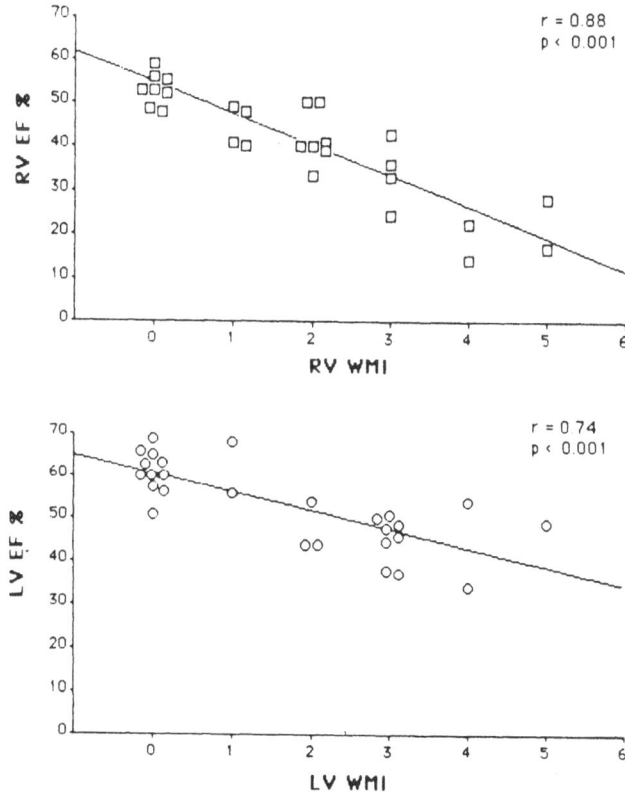

Fig. 3. Linear regression analysis of ejection fraction (*EF*) values vs. wall motion abnormality index (*WMI*) values for the right ventricle (*RV*) and the left ventricle (*LV*) in patients of group 1. Data were obtained from the analysis of radionuclide angiograms

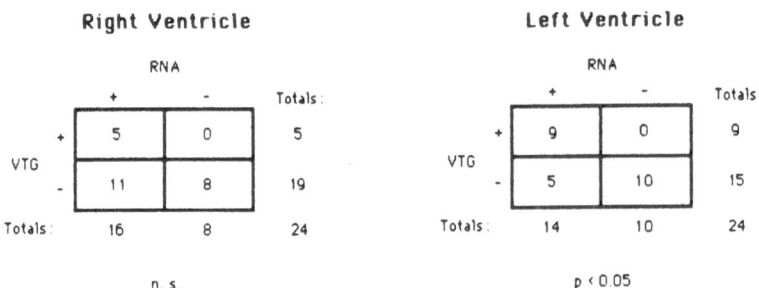

Fig. 4. Two by two contingency tables illustrate the concordance between radionuclide angiography (*RNA*) and contrast ventriculography (*VTG*) in the diagnosis of right ventricular or left ventricular dysfunction by wall motion analysis (WMl ≥ 2)

Correlation Between Noninvasive and Invasive Data

In group 1, ventricular dysfunction was demonstrated by wall motion analysis of contrast ventriculography in 13/24 cases (54%). The agreement between the noninvasive and angiographic evaluation was significant for the left ventricle ($p < 0.05$) but did not exceed chance occurrence for the right ventricle (Fig. 4). It is noteworthy that among the patients with right ventricular ($n = 11$) or left ventricular ($n = 5$) impairment, assessed by radionuclide angiography but not evident at contrast angiography, seven and five cases showed, respectively, right ventricular or left ventricular volume enlargement or minor wall motion abnormalities at angiography.

Coronary angiography documented normal coronary vessels in 24/24 cases. Hemodynamic measurements were in the normal range in 17 patients (71%), showed slight increase in left ventricular end-diastolic pressure in five, biventricular elevated pressures and depressed cardiac index in one, and elevated right ventricular systolic pressure in one other case. In group 1 as a whole, mean values of hemodynamic parameters were in the normal range (Table 2). In group 2, all ten patients studied had normal angiographic and hemodynamic findings.

Discussion

Ventricular ectopic activity generally is the result of a variety of cardiac diseases, systemic illness, and pharmacologic agents, but can also occur in apparently healthy individuals [21–23]. However, in particular subgroups of these "healthy" patients, recent reports have documented right ventricular histologic abnormalities and right ventricular or left ventricular clinically silent dysfunction [9–16]. Whether these findings are able to identify the early phase of a dilated cardiomyopathy is an open question. However, it would be interesting to know, in patients with apparently primitive complex ventricular arrhythmias, the prevalence of regional or global ventricular dysfunction and to assess which are the most reliable noninvasive tools to diagnose this disorder.

Prevalence and Extent of Myocardial Dysfunction in Patients with Apparently Primitive Ventricular Arrhythmias

In the patients selected for the present study, ventricular arrhythmias appeared clinically "primitive": in no case were signs or symptoms of cardiac failure evident at admission, and other cardiac or systemic diseases were reasonably excluded by clinical, biohumoral, and instrumental criteria. Ischemic heart disease was also excluded by means of exercise stress test, ergonovine maleate test, and coronary angiography.

This population, studied by radionuclide angiography in basal conditions, showed a high prevalence (89%) of regional myocardial dysfunction involving, with similar frequencies, the right, the left, or both ventricles. The right ventricular and/or left ventricular location of dyssynergies was somewhat correlated with the site of origin of arrhythmias as predicted from their prevalent configuration. Ventricular arrhythmias with left bundle branch block pattern were mainly associated with isolated right ventricular dysfunction while right bundle branch block or multiform patterns were present in patients with left ventricular or biventricular impairment.

Biventricular systolic function was depressed in the study population as compared with normal subjects, and the degree of ventricular global impairment was correlated with the extent of regional dyssynergies.

The combined analysis of clinical and functional data, previously described, suggests that complex ventricular arrhythmias are frequently an expression of subclinical myocardial damage which, in this early phase, is mainly regional and may involve one or both ventricles. The extent of regional impairment may determine the presence of global systolic dysfunction in each ventricle. Interestingly, the relation between increasing degrees of regional dyssynergies and lower values of ejection fraction appears steeper for the right than for the left chamber, so that only right ventricular function may be severely depressed in some of these patients (Fig. 3). Similar evidence of predominant right ventricular damage is the distinctive feature of the syndrome known as arrhythmogenic right ventricular dysplasia [9–11], and it is also documented in patients with Chagas' disease but without clinical evidence of cardiac involvement [24]. It is conceivable that all these conditions, characterized by ventricular arrhythmias without evidence of left heart failure, are different expressions of early myocardial damage which may impair right ventricular function and left ventricular regional wall motion but still spares global left ventricular performance.

Correlation Between Noninvasive and Invasive Data

Good agreement between noninvasive and angiographic diagnosis of regional impairment was demonstrated for the left ventricle but not for the right chamber. Only clearly enlarged and hypokinetic right ventricles could be recognized at angiography, even though, in our study, direct injection of the medium in the right ventricle would have probably allowed better evaluation of this chamber as shown by others [9, 10, 25].

Ventricular dysfunction demonstrated in our patients did infrequently correspond to abnormal hemodynamic measurements as expected since left ventricular dysfunction is mainly regional [13, 22, 26]. On the other hand, the right ventricle is a very compliant chamber and can probably compensate initial dysfunction by volume enlargment without pressure changes. Kennedy et al. [12] reported a higher frequency of increased left ventricular end-diastolic pressure, probably because their population also included patients with systemic hypertension.

According to our results in patients with complex ventricular arrhythmias as the only manifestation of disease, radionuclide angiography seems to be a valuable clinical tool to recognize silent myocardial dysfunction, while the invasive evaluation should be performed only when functional and/or clinical worsening is evident.

Conclusions

A high prevalence of regional myocardial dysfunction, which may involve the right and/or the left ventricle, is demonstrated in patients with apparently primitive complex ventricular arrhythmias. Global systolic dysfunction is less frequent and correlates with the extent of regional impairment while biventricular hemodynamic measurements are rarely abnormal. All these findings suggest that complex ventricular arrhythmias are associated with early myocardial damage.

Neither the causal relationship among all these aspects nor whether the progression of initial dysfunction could eventually lead to congestive heart failure can be stated at present. Nevertheless, it is now clear that complex ventricular arrhythmias are rarely an isolated manifestation of heart disease; thus, an early search for myocardial impairment and follow-up is mandatory in these patients.

Acknowledgement: This work was partially supported by a grant from the CNR specialized programs on "Tecnologie Biomediche e Sanitarie."

References

1. Goodwin JF, Oakley CM (1972) The cardiomyopathies. Br Heart J 34:545–552
2. Fitchett DH, Sugrue DD, Mac Arthur CG, Oakley CM (1984) Right ventricular dilated cardiomyopathy. Br Heart J 51:25–29
3. Hatle L, Orjavik O, Storstein O (1976) Chronic myocardial disease. I. Clinical picture related to long term prognosis. Acta Med Scand 199:399–405
4. Oakley OM (1980) Prognosis in dilated cardiomyopathy related to left ventricular function, conduction defects and arrhythmia. In: Goodwin JF, Hjalmarson A, Olsen EGJ (eds) Congestive cardiomyopathy. Hassle, Kiruna, p 249
5. Fuster V, Gersh BJ, Giuliani ER, Tajik AJ, Brandemburg RO, Frye RL (1981) The natural history of idiopathic dilated cardiomyopathy. Am J Cardiol 47:525–531
6. Huang SK, Messer JV, Denes P (1983) Significance of ventricular tachycardia in idiopathic dilated cardiomyopathy: observations in 35 patients. Am J Cardiol 51:507–512

7. Mc Kenna WJ, Krikler DM, Goodwin JF (1984) Arrhythmias in dilated and hypertrophic cardiomyopathy. Med Clin North Am 68:983–1000
8. Olshausen KV, Stienen U, Schwarz F, Kubler W, Meyer J (1988) Long-term prognostic significance of ventricular arrhythmias in idiopathic dilated cardiomyopathy. Am J Cardiol 61:146–151
9. Marcus FL, Fontaine GH, Guiraudon G, Frank R, Laurenceau JL, Malergue C, Grosgogeat Y (1982) Right ventricular dysplasia: a report of 24 adult cases. Circulation 65:384–398
10. Manyari DE, Klein GJ, Gulamhusein S, Boughner D, Guiraudon GM, Wyse G, Mitchell LB, Kostuk WJ (1983) Arrhythmogenic right ventricular dysplasia: a generalized cardiomyopathy? Circulation 68:251–257
11. Webb JG, Kerr CR, Huckell VF, Mirgala HF, Ricci DR (1986) Left ventricular abnormalities in arrhythmogenic right ventricular dysplasia. Am J Cardiol 58:568
12. Kennedy HL, Pescarmona JE, Bouchard RJ, Goldberg RJ, Carolis DG (1982) Objective evidence of occult myocardial dysfunction in patients with frequent ventricular ectopy without clinically apparent heart disease. Am Heart J 104:57–65
13. Morgera T, Salvi A, Alberti E, Silvestri F, Camerini F (1985) Morphological findings in apparently idiopathic ventricular tachycardia. An echocardiographic, hemodynamic and histologic study. Eur Heart J 6:323–334
14. Kuhn H, Briethardt G, Knieren MJ, Loogen F (1978) Endomyocardial catheter biopsy in heart disease of unknown etiology. In: Kaltenbach M, Loogen F, Olsen EGJ (eds) Cardiomyopathy and myocardial biopsy. Springer, Berlin Heidelberg New York, p 121
15. Strain JE, Grose RM, Factor SM, Fisher JD (1983) Results of endomyocardial biopsy in patients with spontaneous ventricular tachycardia but without apparent structural heart disease. Circulation 68:1171–1181
16. Sugrue DD, Holmes DR, Gersh BJ, Edwards WD, McLaran CJ, Wood DL, Osborn MJ, Hammil SC (1984) Cardiac histologic findings in patients with life-threatening ventricular arrhythmias of unknown origin. J Am Coll Cardiol 4:952–957
17. Schelbert HR, Verba JW, Johnson A, Brock GW, Alazraki NP, Ross FJ, Ashburn WL (1975) Nontraumatic determination of left ventricular ejection fraction by radionuclide angiography. Circulation 51:902–907
18. Maddahi J, Berman DS, Matsuoka T, Waxman AD, Stankus KE, Forrester JS, Swan HJC (1979) A new technique for assessing right ventricular ejection fraction using rapid multiple-gated equilibrium cardiac blood pool scintigraphy. Circulation 60:581–589
19. Neglia D, Marcassa C, Parodi O, Bellina CR, Marzullo P, Michelassi C, Berti S, Contini C, L'Abbate A (1987) Optimization of right ventricular ejection fraction measurements from first pass and gated blood pool scintigraphy. In: Guzzardi R (ed) Physics and engineering of medical imaging. Nijhoff, Dordrecht, pp 615–620
20. Grossman W (1986) Cardiac catheterization and angiography. Lea and Febiger, Philadelphia
21. Bouvrain Y, Slama R, Motte' G, Waynberger M, Grevellier A (1968) Les tachycardies ventriculaires. Etiologie et évolution, à propos de 161 malades. Arch Mal Coeur 61:909–920
22. Chapman JH, Schrank JP, Crampton RS (1975) Idiopathic ventricular tachycardia. An intracardiac electrical, hemodynamic and angiographic assessment. Am J Med 59:470–480
23. Sebastian P, Waynberger M, Beaufils P, Motte' G, Slama R, Bouvrain Y (1976) Les tachycardies ventriculaires isolées sans cardiopathie patente. Arch Mal Coeur 69:919–928
24. Marin-Neto JA, Marzullo P, Sousa ACS, Marcassa C, Maciel BC, Iazigi N, L'Abbate A (1988) Radionuclide angiographic evidence for early predominant right ventricular involvement in patients with Chagas' disease. Can J Cardiol 4:231–236
25. Robertson JH, Bardy GH, German LD, Gallagher JJ, Kisslo J (1985) Comparison of two-dimensional echocardiographic and angiographic findings in arrhythmogenic right ventricular dysplasia. Am J Cardiol 55:1506–1508
26. Pietras RJ, Lam W, Bauernfeind R, Sheikh A, Palileo E, Strasberg B, Swiryn S, Rosen KM (1983) Chronic recurrent right ventricular tachycardia in patients without ischemic heart disease: clinical, hemodynamic and angiographic findings. Am Heart J 105:357–366

Italian Multicenter Cardiomyopathy Study Group

The Italian Multicenter Cardiomyopathy Study Group (SPIC) was formed to promote knowledge on cardiomypathies in our country. Fifteen centers located all over Italy form the group (Appendix). Following a pilot study, a protocol on dilated cardiomyopathy became operative in January 1986. A protocol on hypertrophic cardiomyopathy is in the pilot study phase.

Aims of the Study

According to the WHO Expert Committee (Geneva 1984), *dilated cardiomyopathy is a heart muscle disease of unknown cause, characterized by dilation and hypertrophy of one or both ventricles with systolic pump function impairment, in the absence of other forms of heart disease or specific heart muscle disease.*

The main aims of the protocol on dilated cardiomyopathy are:

1. Identification of early clinical signs;
2. A better understanding of natural history by follow-up study;
3. Investigation of possible causal factors with particular reference to immunological and infections mechanisms.

The protocol on dilated cardiomyopathy is subdivided into two main lines (Tables 1–3): the invasive line attempts to clarify the natural history and prognosis of dilated cardiomyopathy; the noninvasive line tries to identify through long-term follow-up early signs and symptoms, which may predict development of subsequent overt dilated cardiomyopathy (Fig. 1). Patients considered candidates for heart transplantation when first seen are not included in the study.

Table 1. Entry criteria for invasive study (upper age limit 60 years)

A *One of the following criteria:*
  1. Right and/or left heart failure
  2. Severe ventricular arrhythmias
     – More than three episodes of nonsustained ventricular tachycardia
     – Sustained ventricular tachycardia
     – Multifocal ventricular ectopic beats with > 20 couplets/24 h
  3. Severe global hypokinesis: M-mode echo %FS < 20%
B *The following two associated criteria:*
  1. Cardiomegaly: cardiothoracic ratio at chest X-ray > 0.5
  2. Global hypokinesis: M-mode echo %FS 21%–25%
C *Three associated criteria of the following:*
  1. Recent onset (< 3 months) effort dyspnea in the absence of anemia, thyreotoxicosis, parenchymal lung diseases
  2. Recent onset (< 1 year) recurrent supraventricular arrhythmias
  3. Left bundle branch block
  4. Global hypokinesis: M-mode echo %FS 21%–25%
  5. Regional wall motion abnormalities at echocardiography (excluding interventricular septum in left bundle branch block)
  6. Cardiomegaly: cardiothoracic ratio at chest X-ray > 0.5
  7. Noncongenital second or third degree atrioventricular block
  8. History of systemic emboli in the absence of atrial arrhythmias
  9. More than 500/24 h ventricular ectopic beats or 10–20 couplets/24 h or one to three episodes of non-sustained ventricular tachycardia (unassociated with recurrent supraventricular arrhythmias)
  10. Severe stable ECG changes: inverted T-wave in at least three precordial leads (excluding V1)
  11. Typical chest pain not due to coronary insufficiency

Table 2. Entry criteria for noninvasive study (upper age limit 50 years)

At least one of the following criteria is required for entry;
1. Recent onset (< 1 year) recurrent supraventricular arrhythmias
2. Left bundle branch block
3. Global hypokinesis: M-mode echo %FS 21%–25%
4. Cardiomegaly: cardiothoracic ratio at chest X-ray > 0.5
5. Noncongenital second or third degree atrioventricular block
6. More than 500/24 h ventricular ectopic beats or 10–20 couplets/24h or one to three episodes of nonsustained ventricular tachycardia (unassociated with recurrent supraventricular arrhythmias)
7. Severe stable ECG changes: inverted T-wave in at least three precordial leads (excluding V1)

Characteristics of the Series

At January, 1989, 255 patients had entered the study, 176 in the invasive and 79 in the noninvasive protocol; diagnoses at entry are given in Fig. 2; 68% of patients in the invasive and 57% in the noninvasive protocol presented with symptoms. NYHA class at entry was I in 50%, II in 25%, III in 14%,

Table 3. Scheduled investigations

Noninvasive protocol
- Clinical history and physical examination
- Baseline 12-lead ECG, chest X-ray
- 24-h dynamic ECG
- M-mode and two-dimensional echocardiogram
- Exercise stress testing
- Biochemical tests and virological investigations in case of suspected myocarditis
- Radionuclide angiography (optional)

Invasive protocol
- Clinical history and physical examination
- Baseline 12-lead ECG, chest X-ray
- 24-h dynamic ECG
- M-mode and two-dimensional echocardiogram
- Exercise stress testing
- Biochemical tests and virological investigations in case of suspected myocarditis
- Radionuclide angiography (optional)
- Right and left heart catheterization
- LV cineangiography (RV cineangiography optional)
- Coronary angiography
- Right ventricular endomyocardial biopsy

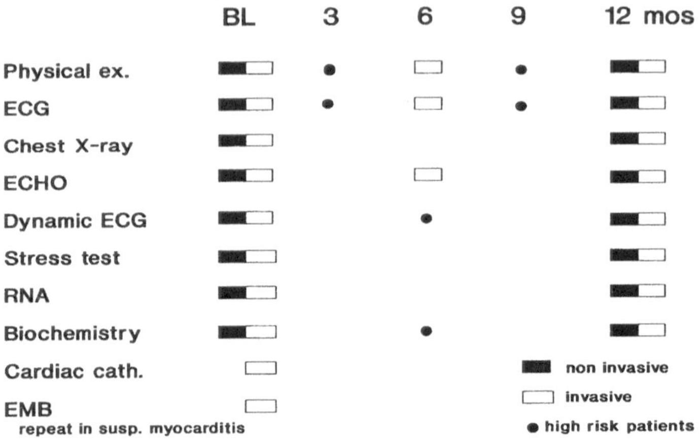

Fig. 1. Follow-up schedule (*Bl*, baseline)

and IV in 10%. Complex ventricular arrhythmias (Lown grade $> = 3$) at baseline dynamic ECG were present in a substantial proportion of patients (55% in the invasive and 38% in the noninvasive protocol (Fig. 3).

Mean echocardiographic ejection fraction was 33% ± 15% in the invasive and 55% ± 11% in the noninvasive group. Mean left ventricular end-diastolic diameter was 68 ± 11 mm in the invasive and 53 ± 8 mm in the noninvasive group. Cardiac catetherization findings in the invasive group were: mean ejection fraction 32% ± 15%; mean cardiac index 3.31 ± 1/min/m^2; mean pul-

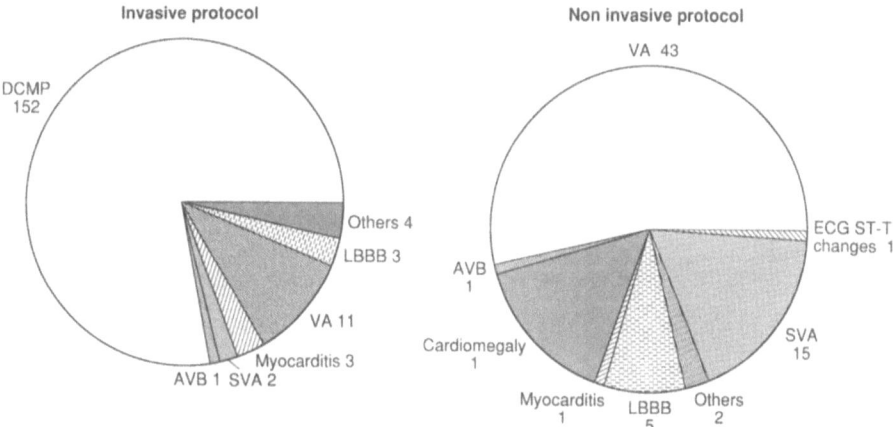

Fig. 2. Diagnosis at entry into SPIC according to protocol. *vA*, ventricular arrhythmia; *SVA*, supraventricular arrhythmias; *LBBB*, left bundle branch block; *AVB*, atrioventricular block; *DCMP*, dilated cardiomyopathy

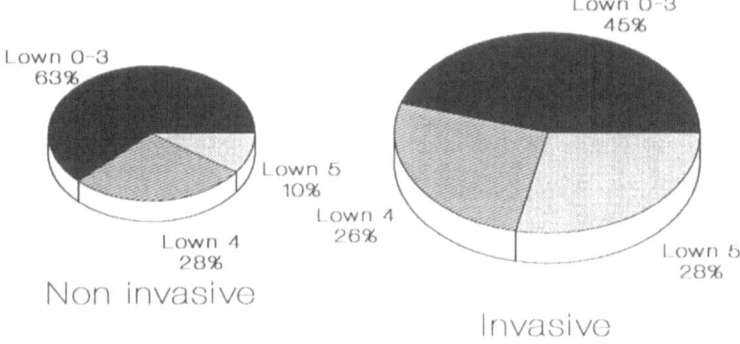

Fig. 3. Prevalence of ventricular arrhythmias at baseline dynamic ECG according to protocol

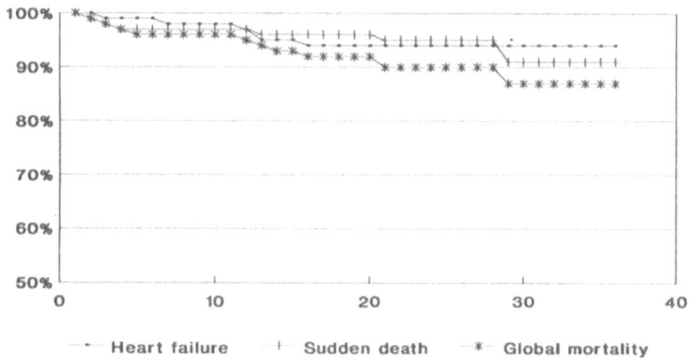

Fig. 4. Actuarial survival at 36 months of patients enrolled into SPIC. Three curves are given according to cause of death

monary artery pressure 20 ± 11 mmHg and left ventricular end-diastolic pressure 16 ± 11. At January 1989, ten patients had undergone heart transplantation, 11 had been lost to follow-up, and 15 had died (6%). The actuarial survival curve is shown in Fig. 4.

Appendix

Participating Centers in SPIC

Dipartimento di Cardiologia "A. De Gasperis," Ospedale Niguarda, Milano
  (Dr. C. De Vita)

Servizio di Cardiologia San Luca, Ospedale Careggi, Firenze
  (Dr. A. Dolara)

Divisione di Cardiologia, Ospedale San Carlo, Milano (Prof. M. Morpurgo)

Divisione di Cardiologia, Ospedale San Gerardo Monza, Milano
  (Dr. F. Valagussa)

Istituto di Patologia Medica, Universita' di Pisa, (Prof. C. Contini)

Divisione di Cardiologia, IRCCS San Matteo, Pavia (Dr. A. Gavazzi)

Divisione di Cardiologia, Ospedali Riuniti, Trieste (Prof. F. Camerini)

Divisione di Cardiologia, Ospedale di Rho, Milano (Dr. G. Parenti)

Divisione di Cardiologia, Ospedale di Circolo, Varese
  (Prof. G. Binaghi)

Divisione di Medicina, Ospedale Bassini, Cinisello Balsamo, Milano
(Prof. R. Rumolo)

Il Divisione di Cardiologia, Dipartimento di Cardiologia "A. De Gasperis,"
  Ospedale Niguarda, Milano (Prof. C. Belli)

Servizio di Cardiologia, Consorzio Provinciale Antitubercolare, Milano
  (Dr. A. Sachero)

I Divisione di Medicina, Servizio di Riabilitazione del Cardiopatico,
  Ospedale Monaldi, Napoli (Prof. M. Cafiero)

Divisione di Cardiologia, Presidio Ospedaliero, Vicenza
  (Prof. M. Vincenzi)

Divisione di Cardiologia "R. Foligno," Ospedale Civile, Treviso
  (Prof. Cuzzato)

Scientific Committee

G. Baroldi, F. Camerini, C. De Vita

Scientific Secretariat

R. De Maria, A. Gavazzi
Istituto Fisiologia Clinica del CNR, Dipartimento di Cardiologia
"A. De Gasperis", Piazza Ospedale Maggiore, 3, I-20162 Milano, Italy,
Telephone, telefax 0039-2-6473407

Dilated Cardiomyopathy in Children

C. P. Taliercio

Introduction

Dilated cardiomyopathy is a rare but serious disease in children. Clinical manifestations are primarily due to impaired systolic function of the left ventricle. Diagnostic evaluation is important to exclude masquerading cardiac abnormalities and to assess the degree of myocardial dysfunction. Treatment of dilated cardiomyopathy is not curative but directed at improving symptoms and long-term outcome.

Etiologic Considerations

Dilated cardiomyopathy is defined as a disease of unknown etiology. There are likely different etiologic mechanisms responsible for dilated cardiomyopathy both in different individual patients and different patient populations. Various diseases in childhood can result in cardiac dysfunction similar to that in dilated cardiomyopathy but may be improved by specific therapies.

Carnitine is a naturally occurring amino acid necessary for transport of long chain fatty acids into mitochondria. Carnitine deficiency can occur in myopathic or systemic forms and result in both dilated and hypertrophic cardiomyopathy [1]. Cardiac improvement has been demonstrated following treatment with oral L-carnitine. ·

Selenium is an element which helps form the biologic enzyme glutathione peroxidase. Selenium deficiency is believed to contribute to Keshan's disease, a dilated cardiomyopathy endemic to certain geographical areas in China [2]. Dietary supplementation of selenium has prevented new cases of Keshan's disease.

Various toxins can result in dilated cardiomyopathy including alcohol and anthracyclines. Anthracycline therapy is commonly utilized in a number of childhood malignancies. Although cardiotoxicity is dose-related, there is variation in the dose/toxicity relationship in individual patients. Therefore, periodic evaluation of left ventricular function is crucial for safe administration of anthracyclines.

A number of recent reports have emphasized that prolonged rapid heart rates can result in decreased left ventricular systolic function and result in a secondary dilated cardiomyopathy [3, 4]. A supraventricular tachycardia is usually the etiologic mechanism and there may be significant improvement in left ventricular function with successful treatment of the arrhythmia.

A congenital cardiac abnormality which may result in a clinical syndrome similar to dilated cardiomyopathy is abnormal origin of the left coronary artery from the pulmonary trunk [5]. Usually, the heart is perfused via an enlarged right coronary artery which has branches that ultimately anastomose to the left coronary artery by large fistulous collaterals. Flow is reversed in the left coronary artery which shunts into the pulmonary artery circulation. Left ventricular dysfunction and other manifestations of myocardial ischemia may improve with surgical correction of the anomalous left coronary origin.

Recent studies have documented that genetic factors should be considered in patients with dilated cardiomyopathy. Familial involvement was documented in approximately ten percent of patients under age 35 in a recent study of dilated cardiomyopathy from the Mayo Clinic [6]. An X-linked abnormality resulting in early dilated cardiomyopathy in males has recently been reported [7].

Myocarditis secondary to infectious (usually viral) etiologies is believed to be the initial cardiac insult in many patients with dilated cardiomyopathy in the United States and western Europe [8]. Three phases of myocardial injury have been postulated: infection, inflammation secondary to immune mechanisms, and eventual fibrosis [9]. Variability in initial symptoms and myocardial injury and difficulty in the diagnosis of current or prior myocarditis has likely contributed to the overall few cases of dilated cardiomyopathy which have unequivocally been shown to result from preceding myocarditis.

Recent reports have documented symptomatic cardiac dysfunction due to a dilated cardiomyopathy in a number of children with human immunodeficiency virus (HIV) infection [10, 11]. Abnormalities were documented in 20% of AIDS patients from one series [11]. Various etiologies (infective, immunologic, nutritional, drug toxic, etc.) may account for cardiac dysfunction in this patient population.

Clinical Manifestations

The usual mode of presentation in children with dilated cardiomyopathy is symptomatic heart failure. Symptoms may occur concurrently with or follow an upper respiratory infection. This scenario often raises the issue of a causative myocarditis. With established dilated cardiomyopathy, intervening respiratory infections commonly exacerbate symptoms of left ventricular failure. Other common clinical manifestations include symptomatic and asymptomatic arrhythmias, thromboembolism, and chest pain. Rarely, patients are asymptomatic and discovered on routine examination to have a heart murmur or cardiomegaly on chest X-ray. In children seen at the Mayo Clinic with dilated cardiomyopathy since 1973, approximately 80% presented with heart failure, 15% with arrhythmias, and 5% with asymptomatic cardiomegaly.

Laboratory Evaluation

Chest X-ray demonstrates cardiomegaly in the majority of children with dilated cardiomyopathy. Common electrocardiographic abnormalities include patterns of left ventricular hypertrophy, abnormal ventricular repolarization, conduction abnormalities, right or left atrial enlargement, and supraventricular and ventricular arrhythmias.

A complete echocardiographic examination (two-dimensional and Doppler) is a valuable test in the evaluation of children with suspected or known dilated cardiomyopathy. A variety of congenital and valvular cardiac defects can be accurately excluded by echocardiography. Short-axis views of the aortic root are able to document normal proximal coronary artery anatomy in most patients with dilated cardiomyopathy and exclude abnormal origin of the left coronary artery from the pulmonary artery. In patients with abnormal origin of the left coronary artery from the pulmonary artery, color Doppler will often show evidence of abnormal blood flow in enlarged collateral vessels in the septum.

Cardiac chamber size can be determined by echocardiography and the degree of left ventricular systolic dysfunction quantitatively assessed. Views of the left ventricular apex are important to search for left ventricular thrombus, a frequent finding in patients with significantly depressed left ventricular function. Thrombus may also form in an enlarged left atrium, especially in patients with atrial fibrillation. Standard two-dimensional echocardiography is less sensitive in documenting thrombus in this location. Doppler echocardiography is useful in assessing valvular regurgitation and diastolic filling parameters. In those children with dilated cardiomyopathy who go on to heart transplantation, Doppler techniques are becoming increasingly utilized to monitor for rejection [12, 13].

Delineation of cardiac anatomy and function by echocardiography often precludes the need for right and left heart catheterization in children with dilated cardiomyopathy. Endomyocardial biopsy is often employed to investigate myocarditis or exclude other possible etiologies. Biospy findings by light microscopy in dilated cardiomyopathy are nonspecific and include interstitial fibrosis, cellular hypertrophy, variation in myofibril size, myofibril degeneration, and hyperchromatic, enlarged nuclei. Although there has been some enthusiasm for the clinical utility regarding endomyocardial biopsy in children with dilated cardiomyopathy [14], our impression is that it does not influence clinical management in most patients. A recent editorial by two leading authorities has suggested that the proven clinical utility of current modes of endomyocardial biopsy may not justify its widespread use [15].

Arrhythmias, many asymptomatic, are common in dilated cardiomyopathy. Electrocardiographic monitoring is extremely useful in documenting cardiac arrhythmias and guiding therapy in symptomatic patients. Electrophysiology testing may be useful in selected patients. The utility of Holter monitoring and electrophysiologic testing in patients with asymptomatic arrhythmias is controversial.

Exercise testing including exercise radionuclide studies are not typically utilized in the evaluation of children with dilated cardiomyopathy. Radionuclide angiography can precisely assess left ventricular function, but this information can usually be obtained from echocardiography. A recent report suggests that indium-111 monoclonal antimyosin antibody imaging may be a reliable screening method for myocarditis [16]. This technique is still experimental.

Natural History

The natural history of children with dilated cardiomyopathy is not clearly established due to few reports in the literature and small patient numbers [17–24]. In addition, reports are generally from tertiary centers and are likely influenced by referral bias.

A recently completed follow-up of 33 children with dilated cardiomyopathy seen at the Mayo Clinic since 1973 showed a 1-year survival of 67% and 5-year survival of 47%. This survival rate was similar to a referral population of adult patients with dilated cardiomyopathy seen at the Mayo Clinic [25]. In adult patients, indices of left ventricular function are strongly correlated to prognosis [25]. This is likely true in children but has been difficult to document due to small patient numbers. In the updated Mayo Clinic series of children with dilated cardiomyopathy, several clinical parameters at initial evaluation (i.e., degree of elevation of LVEDP) tended to be more abnormal in those patients with poor outcome. However, it was not possible to predict clinical improvement or deterioration in individual patients from initial clinical parameters. Similar findings were noted in a recent report of eight children from Europe [22].

In a report from Washington University, St. Louis, children older than 2 years at presentation were noted to have an extremely poor prognosis with all 12 such patients dead on follow-up [23]. In a series from Thailand, prognosis was worse in children with dilated cardiomyopathy who were less than 2 years of age [24]. It is likely that childhood dilated cardiomyopathy represents two different diseases in the central United States and Southeast Asia. In the updated Mayo Clinic series, age at presentation was not statistically related to prognosis.

In a few children, heart size and left ventricular function will eventually return to normal. Whether this scenario results from a slowly resolving myocarditis is speculative. In the updated Mayo series, 13 of 16 survivors were asymptomatic at last follow-up (mean 7 years). Improved left ventricular function was generally documented in those patients who clinically improved and achieved asymptomatic status. However, in many of these asymptomatic patients, the left ventricular ejection fraction remained abnormal.

Treatment

Treatment is supportive and not curative in children with dilated cardiomyopathy. General measures include salt restriction and bedrest or restricted activity with exacerbation of symptomatic heart failure. Digitalis, diuretics, and vasodilators are the cornerstones of therapy for heart failure and are tailored to the individual patient. Data regarding the influence of vasodilator therapy on mortality in children with heart failure is not available. Anticoagulation with warfarin is recommended in patients with prior embolic events and pedunculated apical thrombus on echocardiography. A retrospective study in adult patients has suggested anticoagulation be considered in all patients with significant impairment of LV function [25]. However, a recent prospective study in adults with heart failure suggests no overall benefit from this approach [26]. Anticoagulation is not routinely utilized in children with dilated cardiomyopathy at the Mayo Clinic.

Antiarrhythmic therapy is utilized and individualized in symptomatic patients. There is no convincing evidence that antiarrhythmic therapy can improve outcome in patients with asymptomatic arrhythmias. Beta-blockade in dilated cardiomyopathy is controversial in adults and has not been carefully studied in children with dilated cardiomyopathy.

A major unanswered question is whether immunosuppressive therapy is helpful in patients with dilated cardiomyopathy and biopsy evidence of ongoing myocardial inflammation. Hopefully, an ongoing NIH funded trial in the United States will help answer this question.

Heart transplantation has become an established therapy for selected patients with terminal heart disease. Current 1-year survival rates are approximately 85% and 5-year survival rates 65% in adults at experienced centers [27]. Despite multiple reasons why children may not be ideal cardiac transplant candidates, several recent reports show encouraging results in children [28, 29]. Consideration of heart transplantation is appropriate in children with dilated cardiomyopathy who clinically deteriorate despite medical therapy.

References

1. Ino T, Sherwood G, Lee NB, Wilson GJ, Freedom RM, Rowe RD (1988) Cardiac manifestations in disorders of fat and carnitine metabolism in infancy. J Am Coll Cardiol 11:1301–1308
2. Su Yin, Yu Wei-Han (1979) A study on the nutritional biogeochemical relationship of selenium and Keshan disease. Chin Med J (Engl) 59:461
3. Gillette PC, Smith RT, Garson A Jr, Mullins CE, Gutgesell HP, Goh TH, Cooley DA, McNamera DG (1985) Chronic supraventricular tachycardia: a curable cause of congestive cardiomyopathy. JAMA 253:391–392
4. Rao PS, Najjar HN (1988) Congestive cardiomyopathy due to chronic tachycardia: resolution of cardiomyopathy with antiarrhythmic drugs. Int J Cardiol 17:216–220
5. Nugent EW, Plauth WH Jr, Edwards JE, Schlant RC, Williams WH (1986) Origin of the left coronary artery from the pulmonary artery. In: Hurst JW (ed) The heart. McGraw Hill, New York, pp 708–710
6. Michels VV, Driscoll DJ, Miller FA (1985) Familial aggregation of idiopathic dilated cardiomyopathy. Am J Cardiol 55:1232–1233
7. Berko BA, Swift M (1987) X-linked dilated cardiomyopathy. N Engl J Med 316:1186–1191
8. Kopecky SL, Gersh BJ (1987) Dilated cardiomyopathy and myocarditis: natural history, etiology, clinical manifestations and management. Curr Probl Cardiol 12(10):569–647
9. Stevenson LW, Perloff JK (1988) The dilated cardiomyopathies: clinical aspects. Cardiol Clin 6(2):187–218

10. Joshi VV, Gadol C, Connor E, Oleske JM, Mendelson J, Marin-Garcia J (1988) Dilated cardiomyopathy in children with Acquired Immunodeficiency Syndrome: a pathologic study of five cases. Hum Pathol 19:69–73

11. Stewart JM, Kaul A, Gromisch DS, Reyes E, Woolf PK, Gowitz MH (1989) Symptomatic cardiac dysfunction in children with human immunodeficiency virus infection. Am Heart J 117:140–144

12. Desrvennes M, Corcos T, Cabrol A, Gandjbakhch I, Pavie A, Leger P, Eugène M, Bors V, Cabrol C (1988) Doppler echocardiography for diagnosis of acute cardiac allograft rejection. J Am Coll Cardiol 12:63–70

13. Valantine HA, Appleton CP, Hatle LK, Hunt SA, Billingham ME, Shumway NE, Stinson EB, Popp RL (1989) A hemodynamic and Doppler echocardiographic study of ventricular function in long-term cardiac allograft recipients. Circulation 79:66–75

14. Leatherbury L, Chandra RS, Shapiro SR, Perry LW (1988) Value of endomyocardial biopsy in infants, children and adolescents with dilated or hypertrophic cardiomyopathy and myocarditis. J Am Coll Cardiol 12:1547–1554

15. Mason JW, O'Connell JB (1989) Clinical merit of endocardial biopsy. Circulation 79:971–979

16. Yasuda T, Palacios IF, Dec GW, Fallon JT, Gold HK, Leinbach RC, Strauss HW, Khaw BA, Haber E (1987) Indium 111-monoclonal antimyosin antibody imaging in the diagnosis of acute myocarditis. Circulation 76:306–311

17. Greenwood RD, Nadas AS, Fyler DC (1976) The clinical course of primary myocardial disease in infants and children. Am Heart J 92:549–560

18. Harris LC, Rodin AE, Nghiem QX (1968) Idiopathic nonobstructive cardiomyopathy in children. Am J Cardiol 21:153–165

19. Van Der Hauwaert LG, Boudewijn D, Dumoulin M (1983) Long-term echocardiographic assessment of dilated cardiomyopathy in children. Am J Cardiol 52:1066–1073

20. Doshi L, Lodge KV (1973) Idiopathic cardiomyopathy in infants. Arch Dis Child 48:431–435

21. Taliercio CP, Seward JB, Driscoll DJ, Fisher LD, Gersh BJ, Tajik AJ (1985) Idiopathic dilated cardiomyopathy in the young: clinical profile and natural history. J Am Cardiol 6:1126–1131

22. Schmaltz AA, Apitz J, Hort W (1987) Dilated cardiomyopathy in childhood: problems of diagnosis and long-term follow-up. Eur Heart J 8:100–105

23. Griffin ML, Hernandez A, Martin TC, Goldring D, Bolman RM, Spray TL, Strauss AW (1988) Dilated cardiomyopathy in infants and children. J Am Coll Cardiol 11:139–144

24. Pongpanich B, Isaraprasart S (1986) Congestive cardiomyopathy in infants and children: clinical features and natural history. Jpn Heart J 27(1):11–15

25. Fuster J, Gersh BJ, Giuliani ER, Tajik AJ, Brandenburg RO, Frye RL (1981) The natural history of idiopathic dilated cardiomyopathy. Am J Cardiol 47:525–531

26. Dunkman WB, Johnson GR, Cohn JR, VA Cooperative Study Group (1988) Incidence of thromboembolic events in congestive heart failure: the V-HeFT study. Circulation 78:617 (abstr)

27. Foweler MB, Schroeder JS (1986) Current status of cardiac transplantation. Mod Con Cardiovasc Dis 55:37–41

28. Starnes VA, Stinson EB, Oyer PE, Valantine H, Baldwin JC, Hunt SA, Shumway NE (1987) Cardiac transplantation in children and adolescents. Circulation 76 (Suppl V):V43–V47

29. Pahl E, Fricker EJ, Trento A, Griffith B, Hardesty R, Gold L, Lawrence K, Beerman L, Fischer D, Neches W (1988) Late follow-up of children after heart transplantation. Transplant Proc 20 (Suppl 1):743–746

Anatomoclinical Aspects of Arrhythmogenic Right Ventricular Cardiomyopathy

G. Thiene, A. Nava, A. Angelini, L. Daliento, R. Scognamiglio, and D. Corrado

Introduction

Cardiomyopathies are generally classified according to clinical and anatomic features, using an adjective to distinguish them. Thus, *dilated* (congestive) cardiomyopathy (DCM) indicates enlargement of the cardiac chambers with poor contractility and heart failure, *hypertrophic* cardiomyopathy implies hypertrophy of the ventricular septum in the setting of normal (or even increased) contractility, and *restrictive* cardiomyopathy denotes impaired compliance of the ventricles due to myocardial stiffness.

A cardiomyopathy which has been recently described has been designated as *arrhythmogenic right ventricular* (ARVC) since it is characterized by an electrical instability of the right ventricular myocardium due to fibrous-fatty replacement. This term is proposed in place of right ventricular dysplasia [1], in that the right ventricle pathologic involvement is not a congenital developmental abnormality of the right ventricular myocardium as previously held [2, 3], but an acquired, progressive atrophy of the myocardium with fibroadipose substitution. This condition should be listed with the cardiomyopathies simply because it is a primary degenerative disorder of the myocardium [4–7].

The objective of this paper is to delineate the clinicopathologic profile of this poorly known nosographic entity.

Pathologic Substrates

An involvement of the right ventricle, usually isolated, in the absence of cardiomegaly is the striking feature of ARVC. In fact, heart size and weight are usually within the upper normal limits, but the myocardium of the right ventricular free wall shows localized or diffuse atrophy with fibrous and/or fatty tissue replacement. Two distinct forms exist, lipomatous and fibrolipomatous [4].

In the *lipomatous form*, subepicardial fatty tissue infiltrates the right ventricle free wall, often so deeply as to become transmural (Fig. 1a). On histology, the myocardium is atrophic and separated, residual myocytes are scattered throughout the fatty transformation. This feature accounts for the phenomenon of intraventricular electrical dispersion of the impulse transmission, which causes late potentials and reentrant arrhythmias [8] (see below). Patchy myo-

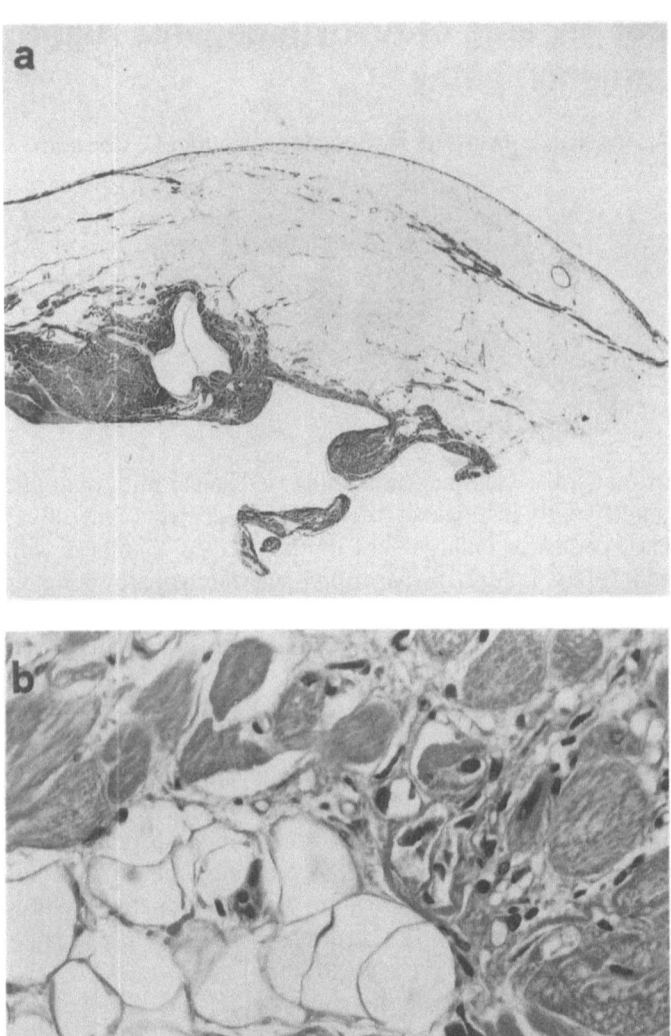

Fig. 1 a, b. ARVC lipomatous pattern, in a 16-year-old woman who died suddenly. **a** Transmural histologic section of the right ventricular free wall shows almost complete fatty transformation: note the myocardial fascicles scattered throughout the adipous tissue and the increased wall thickness. **b** Higher magnification of the residual myocardium with focal myocardial necrosis near the adipocytes. Hemotoxylin and eosin; **a** × 4; **b** × 480

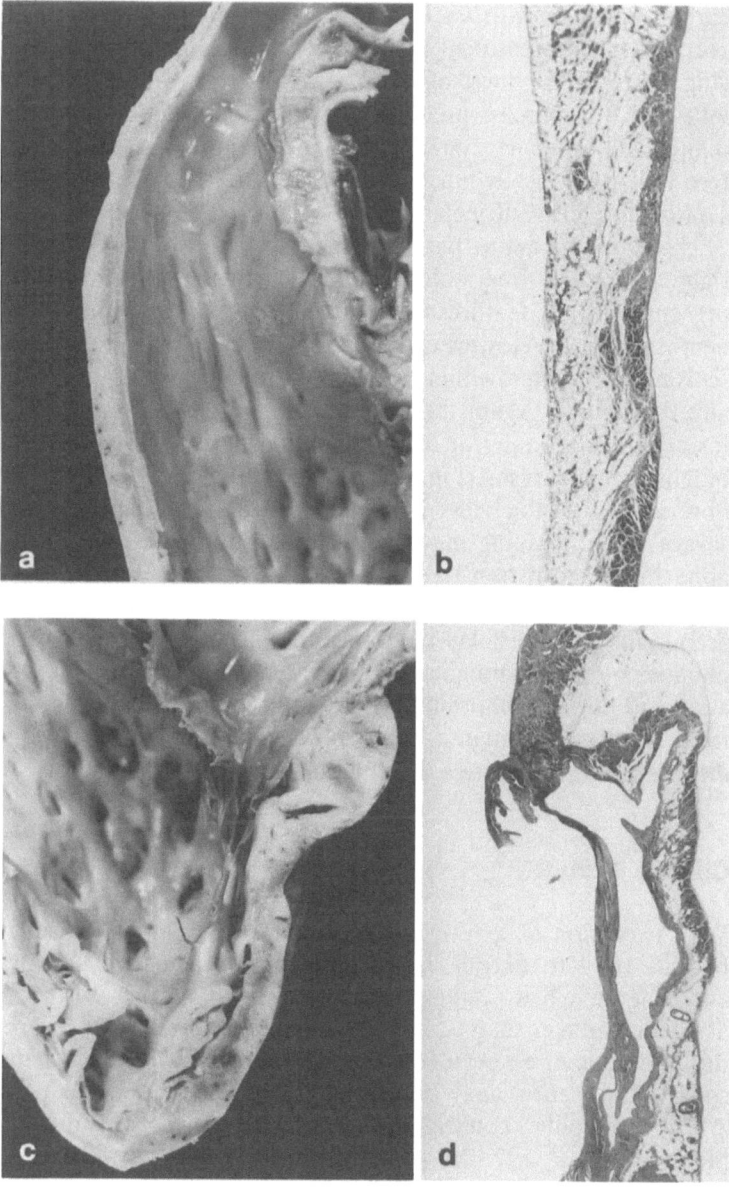

Fig. 2 a–d. ARVC, fibrolipomatous pattern, in a 19-year-old boy who died suddenly while playing soccer. **a** Dilated pulmonary infundibulum with thin, lipomatous wall and whitish endocardium. **b** Histology of **a**, showing fibrolipomatous atrophy. **c** Inferior wall of the right ventricle, below the posterior leaflet of the tricuspid valve: at postmortem,the aneurysmatic bulge appears retracted. **d** Histology of **c**, in which the subtricuspid aneurysm appears more evident. **a** Azan; ×6. **b** Weigert-van Gieson ×3

cardial damage, with vacuolization, necrosis, and macrophage inflammatory reaction, is an occasional finding and explains the progressive myocardial loss (Fig. 1b). The thickness of the free wall is preserved or even increased. When localized, the process predilects the pulmonary infundibulum, which appears dilated and even aneurysmatic. The interventricular septum and left ventricular free wall are basically normal, but spots of fatty tissue may be seen at both the septum and left ventricular apex.

The *fibrolipomatous* pattern is characterized by myocardial sclerosis of the right ventricular free wall, usually associated with fatty tissue. The fibrosis presents with the features of a scarring process suggesting repair of myocardial necrosis (Fig. 2). However, unlike the ischemic myocardial sclerosis, the fibrosis is mostly located within the subepicardial layers, even though it is occasionally transmural. Again the disease may be diffuse or localized, and the preferred site is the inferior diaphragmatic wall of the right ventricle, where wall bulging or aneurysm (Fig. 2c, d) and whitish coloured myocardium may be observed. Wall thickness is usually normal or moderately reduced; in more severe cases, thinning may be so marked that the wall has a parchment-like appearance and is translucent.

On histology, residual myocytes appear scattered within the fibrosis, again accounting for the delay in intraventricular conduction and potential reentry phenomena. The cytologic alterations typical of DCM, such as myocyte attenuation and nuclear abnormalities, are not seen in ARVC. Unlike the lipomatous form, focal involvement of the ventricular septum and left ventricular myocardium is less rare, as are scattered mononuclear inflammatory infiltrates.

Clinical Picture

With exception of a few cases, cardiac performance is usually not impaired because the left ventricle is spared [4]; in particular, dyspnea, even on effort, and congestive heart failure are absent. Chest X-ray rarely shows a cardiothoracic index greater than 0.50. Indeed, many of these patients are asymptomatic, the disease is often occult [9–11], and many subjects take part in competitive sports. Since effort may be crucial in triggering life-threatening arrhythmias, ARVC exemplifies concealed cardiac disease at risk of sudden death in athletes [4, 12].

Electrocardiography

Basal ECG displays a peculiar abnormality consisting of negative or bifid T waves on the precordial leads from V1 to V3 or even to V5–V6 [13] (Fig. 3). The explanation for this electrical *abnormality* reside in the dilation of the right ventricular cavity and in the fibrous fatty myocardial replacement, which may interfere with the repolarization wave front. An incomplete right bundle branch block is occasionally recorded (Fig. 4). The QRS complex is basically normal, although late potentials at the end of ventricular depolarization, a

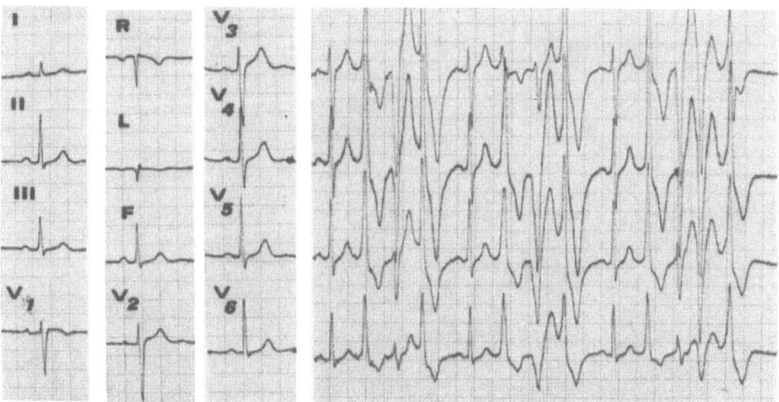

Fig. 3. ECG tracings of a 28-year-old woman who died suddenly while dancing. On the left, the basal ECG shows a negative T-wave only in V1; on the right, run of nonsustained polymorphous ventricular tachycardia on effort. At autopsy, a lipomatous variety of ARVC was found in the absence of right ventricular dilation

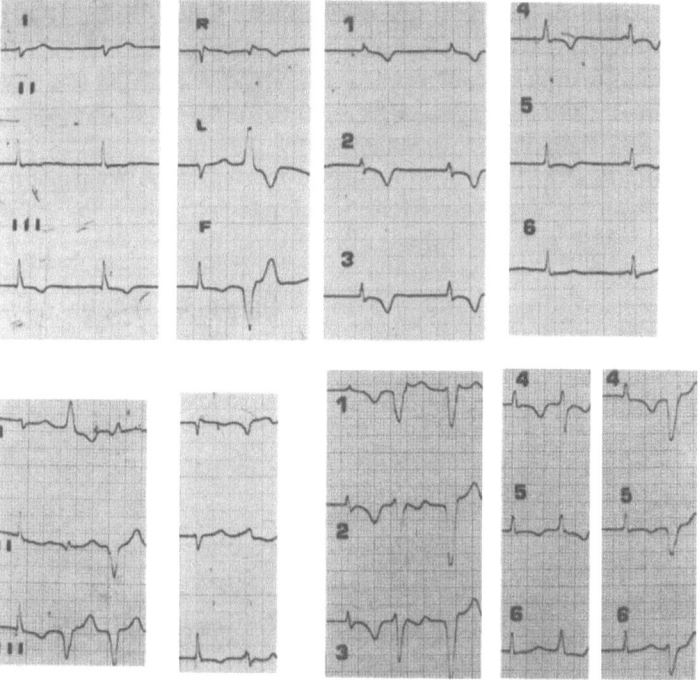

Fig. 4. Basal ECG of a cardiomegalic 22-year-old women, with symptoms of palpitation and syncope, who died suddenly during exercise: incomplete right bundle branch block and negative T-waves, from V1 to V5, are visible together with isolated, couplet, and polymorphous premature ventricular beats, with a left bundle branch block morphology

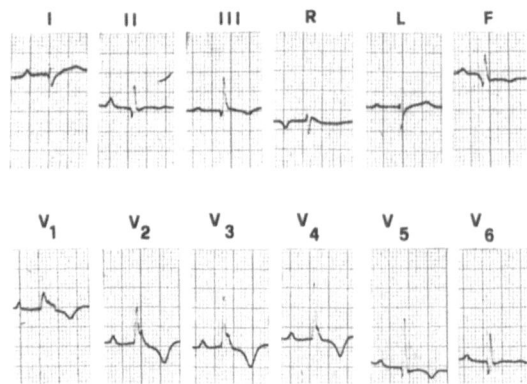

Fig. 5. Basal ECG of a 33-year-old man with ARVC, fibrolipomatous form, who died with signs of right ventricular failure: note incomplete right bundle branch block, negative T-waves from V1 to V6, and evident late potentials following the QRS complex in V1

signal of delay of the impulse transmission within the atrophic myocardium, are rarely registered (Fig. 5).

Isolated or couplet premature ventricular beats (PVB) are frequently recorded at basal ECG or at Holter monitoring and may be exacerbated by exercise testing. In our experience [9], 88% of PVB had a left bundle branch block morphology, 2% a right bundle branch block morphology, and 10% both left and right patterns. While many patients are asymptomatic, episodes of palpitation, with or without syncope, typically occur and are ascribable to sustained or nonsustained ventricular tachycardia. The pattern of ventricular tachycardia with left bundle branch block morphology is not specific, but may be considered pathognomonic of this cardiomyopathy: the same holds true for accelerated idioventricular rhythm, originating from the pulmonary infundibulum [11].

Ventricular tachycardia may transform into ventricular fibrillation [14], which is the final mechanism of cardiac arrest and sudden death in ARVC.

Echocardiographic Findings

A markedly dilated right ventricle with a depressed ejection fraction is the most common presentation of ARVC and characterizes the overt form with extensive involvement of right ventricular myocardium, when serious ventricular arrhythmias have already appeared in the natural history [15, 16]. To prevent sudden death, which is an important complication of ARVC even in asymptomatic patients, subtle echocardiographic findings must be detected to achieve an early diagnosis of the concealed form [17]. Diastolic bulge and systolic dyskinesia of the inferobasal wall just below the tricuspid valve, structural moderator band abnormalities, isolated dilation of the right ventricular outflow tract, apical dyskinesia, sacculations, and trabecular disarrangement (Fig. 6) are echocardiographic features that point to ARVC. Since, in our experience,

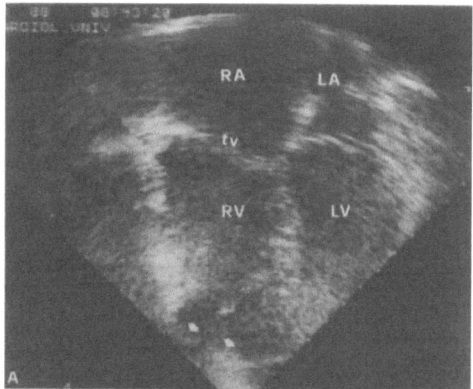

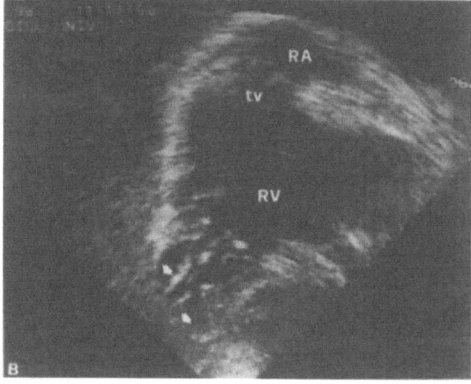

Fig. 6 A, B. Two-dimensional echocardiograms. A Apical four chamber view (systolic frame) showing saccular dilations and dyskinesia of the right ventricular apex (*arrows*). **B** Right ventricular two chamber view (systolic frame) with apical dyskinesia and disarrangements of the trabecular framework (*arrows*). *LA,* left atrium; *LV,* left ventricle; *RA,* right atrium; *RV*, right ventricle; *TV*, tricuspid valve

these criteria have a high specificity and sensitivity in the early diagnosis of ARVC in asymptomatic patients [17], cross-sectional echocardiography constitutes an effective and reliable tool in recognizing the concealed form of ARVC.

Angiocardiography and Hemodynamics

ARVC presents quantitative volumetric and hemodynamic features that clearly distinguish it from dilated cardiomyopathy and confirm its nosographic autonomy among the primary diseases of the myocardium [18, 19].

In a recently conducted study (unpublished data), we found a statistically significant difference in quantitative angiographic parameters between ARVD and DCM. Specifically, ventricular telediastolic volumes in the right ventricle were higher in DCM than in ARVC, while the ejection fraction was only moderately depressed in ARVC (mean 50%) compared to DCM (mean 30%).

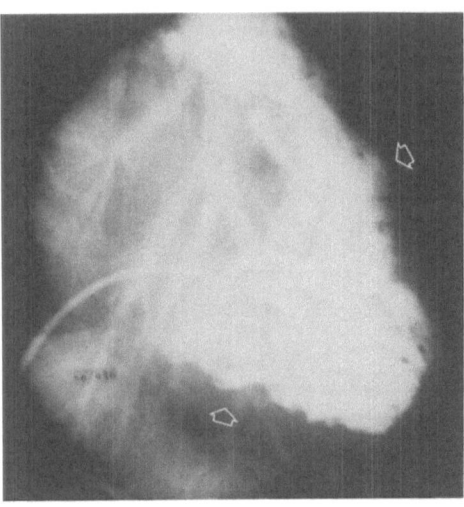

Fig. 7. Right ventricular angiography (anterior oblique view, systolic frame). The right ventricle is slightly dilated with apical dyskinesia and bulging of the inferior wall and infundibulum (*arrows*)

In the left ventricle, the mean telediastolic volume of the left ventricle was 180 ml/m^2 in DCM with severe ejection fraction impairment (mean 32%), while the mean value of telediastolic volume in ARVC was slightly increased (mean 90 ml/m^2) and the ejection fraction slightly reduced (mean 60%) ($p < 0.05$). These findings confirm that in ARVC no significant pump failure is present.

With regard to angiographic qualitative parameters, the following morphological deformations were highly sensitive and specific for diagnosis: bulging of the infundibular and/or subtricuspid inferior walls, horizontal hypertrophic trabeculae associated with deep conical images or fissuring (Fig. 7).

Endomyocardial Biopsy

Right ventricular endomyocardial biopsy [20–23] may be of great help for an in vivo morphologic confirmation of the clinical diagnosis. The efficacy of this diagnostic tool is favored by the fact that ARVC involves the right ventricle itself, so that easy transvenous access of the bioptome is feasible. Moreover, the fibroadipous replacement is frequently transmural, reaching the subendocardium, and can be detected by the endocardial approach of the biopsy. In addition, although the histopathologic substrates (fibrosis and lipomatosis) are not specific, they are readily recognized at light microscopy (Fig. 8).

Nonetheless, since the interventricular septum is mostly uninvolved, for the biopsy to be effective it should be taken on the free wall or at least on the borders between the septum and the free wall (Fig. 9). In view of myocardial atrophy, the biopsy procedure is consequently at risk of ventricular perforation and should be carried out in cardiologic units with cardiac surgery assistance for emergency thoracotomy in case of cardiac tamponade.

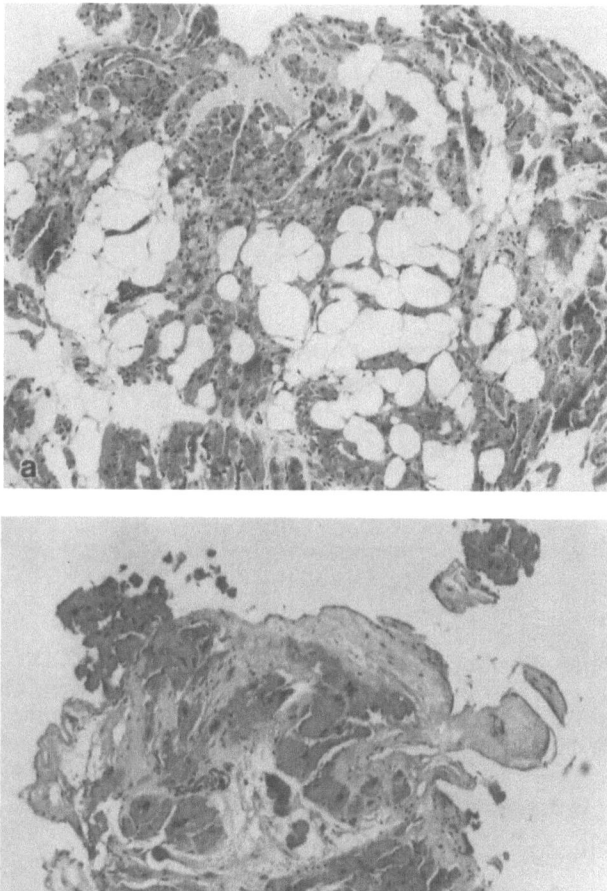

Fig. 8 a, b. Biopsy specimen in patients with ARVC. **a** Lipomatous pattern. **b** Fibrous pattern. Hematoxylin and eosin; **a** ×48, **b** ×75

To assess the diagnostic accuracy of endomyocardial biopsy in ARVC, we recently conducted a morphometric study by comparing endomyocardial biopsies from patients with ARVC with those affected by DCM (unpublished data); the first biopsy taken in patients following cardiac transplantation served as a control. Myocardial atrophy, i.e., paucity of myocardium due to fatty-fibrous replacement, was significantly pronounced in ARVC, compared to both DCM patients and controls, and had a sensitivity of 80%. Sensitivity for fibrosis was 77%, although no significant difference in the extension was found between ARVC and DCM. Lipomatosis, the true distinctive feature of the disease, had a sensitivity of only 50%, owing to the existence of the fibrous variety; it might be considered diagnostic when it constitutes more than 10% of specimen area.

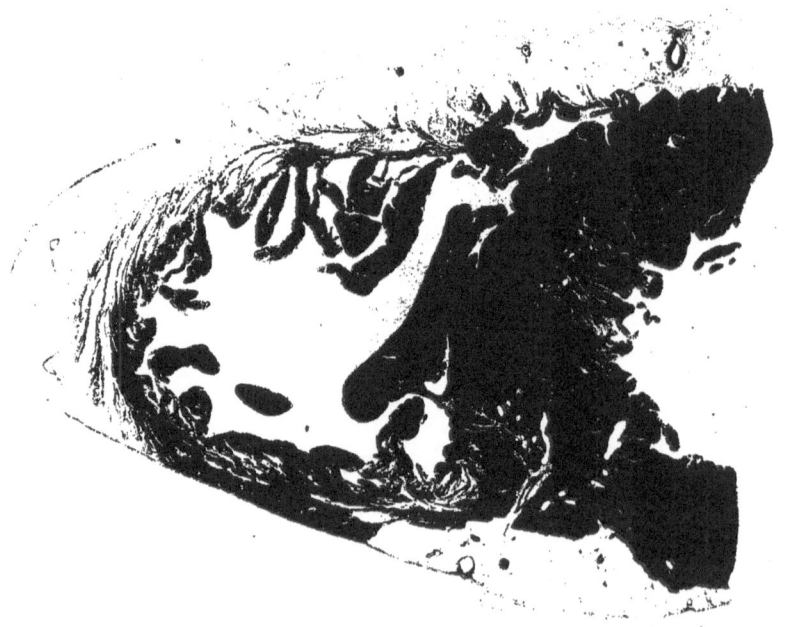

Fig. 9. Histologic cross-section of an entire heart with ARVC, lipomatous variety. Note the massive adipous transformation of the anterolateral wall, while the ventricular septum is spared by the atrophic process: for an effective biopsy, the bioptome should be directed towards the free wall. Azan × 1

Etiology and Natural History

The wide range of myocardial pathologic involvement, together with its tendency to progress [24], accounts for the polymorphism displayed by ARVC. In investigating members of nine families in which cases of juvenile sudden death had occurred [5], we found 30 living affected subjects, with a mean age of 25 years. However, because ARVC may not be clinically evident, the precise time of biologic onset is difficult to ascertain. In the above study, two patients, who did not present any abnormalities when examined at 11 years of age, were found with overt disease 4 years later. The myocardial atrophy, therefore, is not the consequence of congenital absence of the myocardium, but of acquired fatty and/or fibrous tissue substitution due to progressive myocyte degeneration and necrosis. This does not exclude the presence of the defect at birth. Although the precise cause of the disease is unknown, recent reports of familial occurrence support the idea that it might be a genetic disorder with autosomal dominance and variable expression and penetrance [5,25].

As far as its natural history is concerned, the following steps may be postulated:

1) *Concealed phase,* with or without minor arrhythmias, during which onset of myocardial atrophy brings about structural and functional alterations detect-

able by echography. Sudden death may be the first manifestation of the disease, even at this apparently benign stage, and may occur in young persons with an apparently normal heart, especially during sporting activities. Effort is the main factor precipitating cardiac arrest.

2) *Overt electrical disorder* with severe arrhythmias: the structural alterations are more prominent, with right ventricular dilation and hypokinesia; however, no signs of right ventricular pump failure are present. Sudden death is impending.

3) *Right ventricular failure* due to progression of myocardial atrophy that is so severe that right ventricular contractility is affected. Life-threatening arrhythmias and right ventricular failure may coexist at this stage.

4) *Congestive heart failure* due to biventricular depressed contractility, when the myocardial atrophy in rare long-term cases also involves the left ventricular myocardium [26]. At this stage ARVC mimics DCM, and heart transplantation represents the patient's only therapeutic option.

Acknowledgement: This work was supported by Regione Veneto, Target Project "Juvenile Sudden Death", Venice, Italy.

References

1. Marcus FI, Fontaine GH, Guiraudon G, Frank R, Laurenceau JL, Malergue C, Grosgogeat Y (1982) Right ventricular dysplasia. A report of 24 adult cases. Circulation 65:384–398
2. Virmani R, Rabinowitz M, Clark MA, Mc Allister HA (1982) Sudden death and partial absence of the right ventricular myocardium: a report of three cases and a review of the literature. Arch Pathol Lab Med 106:163–163
3. Froment R, Perrin A, Loire R, Dalloz C (1968) Ventricule droit papyrace' du jeune adulte par dystrophie congénitale. A propos de 2 cas anatomocliniques et de 3 cas paracliniques. Arch Mal Coeur 61:477–503
4. Thiene G, Nava A, Corrado D, Rossi L, Pennelli N (1988) Right ventricular cardiomyopathy and sudden death in young people. N Engl J Med 318:129–133
5. Nava A, Thiene G, Canciani B et al (1988) Familial occurrence of right ventricular dysplasia: A study involving nine families. J Am Coll Cardiol 12:1222–1228
6. Perloff J (1988) Familial occurrence of right ventricular dysplasia: a study involving nine families (editorial). J Am Coll Cardiol 12::2229–1230
7. Maron BJ (1988) Right ventricular cardiomyopathy: another cause of sudden death in the young. N Engl J Med 318:178–180
8. Fontaine G, Frank R, Tonet JL et al (1984) Arrhythmogenic right ventricular dysplasia: a clinical model for the study of chronic ventricular tachycardia. Jpn Circ J 48:515–538
9. Nava A, Martini B, Thiene G, et al (1988) La displasia aritmogena del ventricolo destro. Studio su una popolazione selezionata. G Ital Cardiol 18:2–9
10. Nava A, Scognamiglio R, Thiene G, et al (1987) A polymorphic form of familial arrhythmogenic right ventricular dysplasia. Am J Cardiol 59:1405–1409
11. Martini B, Nava A, Thiene G, et al (1988) Accelerated idioventricular rhythm of infundibular origin in patients with a concealed form of arrhythmogenic right ventricular dysplasia. Br Heart J 59:564–571
12. Thiene G, Gambino A, Corrado D, Nava A (1986) The pathological spectrum underlying sudden death in athletes. New Trends Arrhythmias 1:323–331
13. Nava A, Canciani B, Buja GF, Martini B, Daliento L, Scognamiglio R, Thiene G (1988) Electrovectorcardiographic study of negative T waves on precordial leads in arrhythmogenic right ventricular dysplasia: relationship with right ventricular volumes. J Electrocardiol 21:239–245

14. Olsson SB, Edvardsson N, Emanuelsson H, Enestrom S (1982) A case of arrhythmo-genic right ventricular dysplasia with ventricular fibrillation. Clin Cardiol 5:591–594
15. Manyari DE, Duff EJ, Kostuk WJ et al (1986) Usefulness of noninvasive studies for diagnosis of right ventricular dysplasia. Am J Cardiol 57:1147–1153
16. Scognamiglio R, Fasoli G, Nava A, Buja GF (1987) Two-dimensional echocardiographic features in patients with spontaneous right ventricular tachycardia without apparent heart disease. J Cardiovasc Ultrason 6:113–117
17. Scognamiglio R, Fasoli G, Nava A, Thiene G (1989) Relevance of subtle echocardio-graphic findings in the early diagnosis of the concealed form of right ventricular dyspla-sia. Eur Heart J 10:59–64
18. Daubert C, Descaves C, Fulgoc JL, Bourdonnec C, Laurent M, Gouffault J (1988) Critical analysis of cineangiographic criteria for diagnosis of arrhythmogenic right ven-tricular dysplasia. Am Heart J 115:448–459
19. Daliento L, Stritoni P, Isabella GB et al (1986) Malattia aritmogena primitiva del ventricolo destro: studio angiografico. Rev Lat Cardiol 7:453–460
20. Thiene G, Angelini A, Valente M (1988) Biopsia endomiocardica nella cardiomiopatia aritmogena del ventricolo, destro. Cardiologia 33 (Suppl I) 313–315
21. Sugrue DD, Holmes DR, Gersh BJ et al (1984) Cardiac histologic findings in patients with life-threatening ventricular arrhythmias of unknown origin. J Am Coll Cardiol 4:952–957
22. Morgera, Salvi A, Alberti E, Silvestri F, Camerini F (1985) Morphological findings in apparently idiopathic ventricular tachycardia. An echocardiographic, haemodynamic and histologic findings. Eur Heart J 6:323–334
23. Hasumi M, Sekiguki M, Hiroe M, Kasanuki H, Hirosawa K (1987) Endocardial biopsy approach to patients with ventricular tachycardia with special reference to arrhythmo-genic right ventricular dysplasia. Jpn Circ J 5:242–249
24. Blomstrom-Lundquist C, Sabel KG, Olsson SB 24 (1987) The long-term follow-up of 15 patients with arrhythmogenic right ventricular dysplasia. Br Heart J 58:477–488
25. Marshall WH, Furey M, Larsen B et al (1988) Right ventricular cardiomyopathy and sudden death in young people. N Engl J Med 319:174 (Letter)
26. Waller BF, Smith ER, Blackbourne BD et al (1980) Congenital hypoplasia of portions of both right and left ventricular myocardial walls. Clinical and necropsy observations in two patients with parchment heart syndrome. Am J Cardiol 46:885–891

Right Ventricular Arrhythmogenic Cardiomyopathy: The Clinical Point of View

S. Dalla-Volta

Introduction

Identification of a peculiar variant of cardiomyopathy, limited to the right ventricle and caused by a fibrolipomatous transformation of the muscular mass, either scattered or more rarely diffuse, is a recent conquest of cardiology [1].

Abnormal presence of fibrotic and/or adipose tissue was recognized in the last three centuries in various conditions:

- Fatty heart (cor adiposum), involving the subepicardium of the right ventricle [2]: the muscle is usually totally replaced by adipose tissue, whose content is increased in absolute terms
- Cardiac lipoma, a tumor presenting in infiltrative forms as well as a pedunculated mass [3]
- Right ventricular fibrolipomatous cardiomyopathy, where the walls of the right ventricle are replaced by lipomatous or fibrolipomatous tissue, but without an absolute increase in the mass of fatty tissue. Uhl's disease [4] and parchment-like heart can be considered the extreme variant of the disease.

However, only in the past 40 years has the exact meaning of the fibroadipous replacement of the right ventricular muscular mass been better appreciated.

In 1961 Dalla Volta et al. [5, 6] reported the first clinical and hemodynamic study of the disease, in four cases, stressing:

- The localization of the disease in the right ventricular wall;
- the absence of involvement of the left ventricle;
- the normality of the coronary tree;
- the frequency of ventricular arrhythmias.

In their cases the right ventricle was almost totally replaced by fibrotic and adipose tissue, with loss of the contractile power of the right ventricle, the pulmonary circulation being supported by a strong right atrial contraction ("auricularization" of the right ventricle). Negative T waves were observed in one or more right precordial leads.

In the 1970s Fontaine et al. [7, 8] studied the disease extensively: the role of the ventricular arrhythmias (premature beats and ventricular tachycardia) and the left bundle branch block pattern were recognized and therefore the name "right ventricular arrhythmogenic dysplasia" proposed. In the 24 cases of the French authors, cardiomegaly did not always occur, many cases having normal ventricular volume. Fontaine showed that the fibrolipomatous changes were mainly distributed in particular areas of the right ventricle, creating the basis for a reentry circuit, the cause of the arrhythmias and of death in some patients [8].

More recently Thiene et al. [9] observed 12 instances of right ventricular cardiomyopathy in 60 cases of sudden juvenile death in the Venetian region (northeast Italy), stressing the importance of the disease in apparently normal young people as a cause of unexpected death. Again in Padova, Nava, Martini and coworkers [10, 11] extensively reviewed a number of patients and their relatives and, by means of a carefully planned study protocol, were able to identify 196 cases presenting the clinical, electrocardiographic, and hemodynamic features characteristic of the disease. In the same period, the possibility of echocardiographic diagnosis in the various phases during progression of the cardiomyopathy was recognized by Scognamiglio and Fasoli [12]. Finally, Nava et al. [13] between 1985 and 1988 were able to show the high incidence, of familial forms of the disease in cases of different degrees of severity, but similarly potentially dangerous to life: in seven families 57 cases were recorded, the authors suggested an autosomal dominant inheritance with incomplete penetrance and variable expression: at present, in at least 30% of the 196 cases familial dependency has been shown.

It is therefore possible to say that right ventricular arrhythmogenic cardiomyopathy can be diagnosed "intra vitam" with a reasonable degree of accuracy [14]. The clinical cardiologist is now confronted with the task of suspecting and recognizing a disease which is a potential cause of sudden death in young persons.

The following review summarizes current clinical and diagnostic aspects.

Clinical Aspects

About 60% of patients are male. The age distribution shows that most cases occur in the age range of 10–35 years; no patient younger than 3 years has been observed and there is no difference in age distribution between living and deceased subjects.

The history can be indicative [14] as over 90% of cases are young people with normal exercise tolerance but complaining of arrhythmias, sometimes of many years' duration. The arrhythmias may disappear during exercise. In at least two-thirds of cases, juvenile sudden death among relatives is recorded; however, sudden death can be the first clinical manifestation, without previous arrhythmic events. Neverthless, totally asymptomatic cases are very rare.

The physical examination is usually negative and exercise tolerance is normal.

Electrocardiogram

The *resting ECG* provides useful information, through the recording of a negative T wave in one or more right precordial leads. Extension of the negative T wave on the precordium is well correlated with the degree of cardiomegaly. In the absence of cardiomegaly the T wave has counterclockwise rotation, is deviated slightly to the left, and is negative in V_1 and V_2, while in patients with enlargement of the right ventricle the rotation is clockwise, the T axis deviated posteriorly, and negative T waves can be recorded in V_3 and V_4. The QRS was for a long time considered of little value, but does give data of interest; the QRS duration is prolonged and the intracavitary recording shows that the increase in duration is due to after-potentials, which can be recorded in 15% of cases in the surface ECG. The lack of organized late potentials may explain the absence of a right bundle branch block pattern.

Very important data are obtained during Holter recording, due to the presence of the arrhythmias: premature ventricular beats and ventricular tachycardias show a left bundle branch block pattern in 90% of cases, suggesting that the origin of the conduction disturbance is inside the right ventricle.

Careful vector-cardiographic studies by Martini et al. [15] have demonstrated that there are several arrhythmogenic areas inside the right ventricle. In 60% of cases the origin of the arrhythmia is the right ventricular infundibulum, in 15% the basal interventricular septum, in 12% the apex, in 8% the middle septum, and in 8% the subtricuspid areas, giving a total of five different arrhythmogenic areas.

Different types of ventricular arrhythmias [16] have been described, all having as the most common feature the pattern of left bundle branch block (LBBB). Ventricular tachycardias (VT) presented the following clinical patterns:

– Non sustained VT in 18 cases (14 with LBBB pattern);
– Sustained VT in 9 patients (all had LBBB pattern);
– Slow VT in 8 cases (all with LBBB pattern);
– Repetitive VT in 3 cases.

During the stress test the ventricular arrhythmias presented discordant behavior. In 41% of cases arrhythmias disappeared during the test; in 20% arrhythmias appeared during the test, and in 20% during the recovery phase.

Radiology and Echocardiography

Radiology has not proved a useful method of study. However, *echocardiography* has recently proved useful, even in the early phase of the disease. A slight increase of right ventricular end-diastolic volume was observed, with a mean value of 54 ml, against 46 ml for normal persons, and the pulmonary infundibulum was slighty enlarged (32 mm against 24 mm in normal subjects); ejection fraction was normal [12].

Signs considered suggestive of the disease are the following:

- A "bald" appearance of the right ventricle, due to the reduction of the trabeculae;
- Disarray of the trabeculae with increase of echogenicity;
- Increased echogenic reflection from the "Trabecula septo-marginalis";
- Apical dyskinesia.

Usually no more than two morphological changes were present simultaneously in the same patient.

Evolution of echocardiographic findings were observed in 77% of our patients [12] within a 4-year period: increase of right ventricular dimensions and reduction of the previously normal ejection fraction occurred. These finding correlated well with an increase in frequency of arrhythmias.

All these data enable consistent identification of possible right ventricular cardiomyopathy, when the patient's history, the electrocardiogram (including the Holter recording for the detection of arrhythmias) and the echocardiogram are carefully examined.

Angiography and Biopsy

Because of the polymorphic nature of the disease and the limited number of cases recorded, angiography of the right ventricle combined with endomyocardial biopsy seems mandatory for diagnosis. Pressure in the right heart cavities and in the pulmonary circulation is normal, except in a rather small number of cases with massive involvement of the right ventricle and congestive heart failure. Occasionally the pulmonary circulation is supported by a strong atrial contraction, while the right ventricle has lost its propulsive force. Quantitative angiography of the right ventricle [17] provides the most significant data. Increases in the right end-systolic and end-diastolic volumes occur, together with dilatation of the right pulmonary infundibulum and a small reduction of the ejection fraction. The vertical axis of the right ventricle is doubled in length in comparison to the norm. Pertinent data are summarized in Table 1.

Several anomalies of the right ventricular trabeculae are observed: while the vertical and horizontal patterns are very similar to those of normal hearts, a peculiar disposition of hypertrophic horizontal trabeculae separated by deep

Table 1. Angiographic data (from [18])

Parameter	Normal	RVAC
EDV RV (ml/m^2)	94	131
ESV RV (ml/m^2)	37	62
EF RV (%)	60	53
Infundibulum diameter (mm)	2.45	5.06
Vertical axis length (mm)	5.22	12.3

RVAC, right ventricular arrhythmogenic cardiomyopathy; *EDV,* end-diastolic volume; *ESV,* end-systolic volume; *EF,* ejection fraction; *RV,* right ventricle.

fissures is specific ("aspect en pile d'assiettes" according to the French authors).

The *regional kinetics* of the right ventricle are not normal: a dyskinesia of the apex is present in 50% of cases, but the most important morphometric feature is *end-diastolic bulging* both in the infundibular area (75% of our cases) and in the subtricuspid region (90% of cases). The left ventricle is normal or presents very mild changes with hypokinetic areas in 3%–12% of cases. Finally, tricuspid prolapse was observed in 40% of cases and mitral prolapse in 18%.

These various anomalies have, when submitted to logistic discriminant analysis, shown a specificity of 95.9% and a sensitivity of 87.5%.

Biopsy of the right ventricle is a very important step in the diagnosis of the disease. In only one of 29 cases [19] studied the histological findings were normal (3.3%). In 10 cases (33%) fibrosis was the predominant feature; in 6 cases adiposis was observed (20%), and in 13 cases mixed adiposis and fibrosis (43%). In 53% of cases there were changes of myocytes (hypertrophy or nuclear changes). After calculating the percentage areas of myocytes, fibrosis, and adiposis in the normal heart, in dilated cardiomyopathy, and in right ventricular arrhythmogenic cardiomopathy, the amounts of normal myocytes found were 74%, 65%, and 47%, respectively. For the same three groups the fibrotic tissue increased from 8% to 21% and 25%; by contrast, adipose tissue was observed only in right ventricular arrhythmogenic disease. If one consideres both increase in adipose and fibrotic tissue and the reduction of myocytes, the sensitivity of the biopsy is 70% and the specificity 95%.

Clinical Course

Progression of the disease, mainly shown by the increasing number and severity of the ventricular arrhythmias as well as by the morphological changes in the right ventricle, was observed in one-fifth of our cases during an 8-year observation period.

Treatment with antiarrhythmic drugs of class one or beta-blockers seems to offer good protection against dangerous arrhythmias [20]. Of the 23 deceased cases we observed in this period, only one treated patient died, one month after he decided to interrupt the treatment; two cases presented short episodes of sustained ventricular tachycardias, easily controlled by the drugs. Patients with premature beats of Lown's class less than 3 or in whom the ventricular arrhythmias disappeared during the stress test were not treated.

Unsolved Problems

Unsolved questions are several and have recently been discussed [21]. The real incidence of the disease is not known and we are not sure that the large number of cases observed in our region depends on local genetic factors and is not related to our investigations protocol. The disease appears after 3 years of age and affects mainly young people: it is impossible to say whether it is present at birth and has a period of latency or is a progressive form which could eventually also affect the left ventricle. The relationship between sporadically occurring cases and the familial form is not clear. The localization in well-defined areas of the right ventricle may suggest intrauterine damage, such as hypoxia or infections, possibly acting through an immunogenetic mechanism.

The future of patients given antiarrhythmic treatment is unknown and it is possible that in subjects who do not die of ventricular arrhythmias cardiac failure may later develop.

Only thorough analysis of patients collected in a carefully planned study protocol followed-up over a long period will provide answers to the many unsolved questions.

References

1. Puggioni A, Martini B, Nava A (1989) La miocardiopatia aritmogena del ventricolo destro: note storiche e risultati di una ricerca epidemiologica su una popolazione selezionata. Thesis, University of Padova
2. Leyden E (1882) Über Fettherz. Ztschr Klin Med 1 5:1–25
3. Estevez J, Thompson D, Levinson J (1964) Lipoma of the heart. Arch Path 77:638–642
4. Uhl HSM (1952) A previously undescribed congenital malformation of the myocardium of the right ventricle. Bull Johns Hopkins Hosp 91:197–205
5. Dalla Volta S, Battaglia G, Zerbini E (1961) Auricularization of right ventricular pressure curve. Am Heart J 1:25–33
6. Dalla Volta S, Fameli O, Maschio G (1965) Le syndrome clinique et hémodynamique de l'auricularisation du ventricule droit. Arch Mal Coeur 58:1129–1143
7. Fontaine GH, Guiraudon G, Frank R, Cabrol C, Grosgogeat Y (1979) Arrhythmogenic right ventricular dysplasia. A previously unrecognized syndrome (14 cases). Circulation 60 (Suppl II):A65
8. Markus FI, Fontaine GH, Guiraudon G, Frank R, Laurenceau JL, Malergue C, Grosgogeat Y (1982) Right ventricular dysplasia: a report of 24 cases. Circulation 65:384–398
9. Thiene G, Gambino A, Corrado D, Nava A (1985) Sudden death in youth: postmortem study in 28 cases. Eur Heart J 6:8
10. Nava A, Canciani B, Scognamiglio R et al (1986) La tachicardia e la fibrillazione ventricolare nel ventricolo destro aritmogeno (displasia aritmogena del ventricolo destro). Spettro clinico ed elettrocardiografico. G Ital Cardiol 16:741–749
11. Nava A, Martini B, Thiene G, et al (1988) La displasia aritmogena del ventricolo destro. Studio su una popolazione selezionata. G Ital Cardiol 18:2–9
12. Scognamiglio R, Fasoli G (1985) Aspetti ecocardiografici in pazienti con aritmie ventricolari tipo BBSn senza apparente cardiopatia. In: Proceedings of international symposium of clinical electro-vectorcardiography. Bortolazzi-Stei, Padova, p 13
13. Nava A, Bottero M, Fasoli G, Scognamiglio R, Thiene G (1985) Arrhythmogenic right ventricular dysplasia: a familial form. Pace Abstract 8-A 32
14. Dalla Volta S (1989) Arrhythmogenic cardiomyopathy of the right ventricle; thoughts on aetiology. Eur Heart J 10 Supplement (in press)
15. Martini B, Canciani B, Buja GF, Bellotto F, Maddalena F, Nava (1986) L'analisi vettorcardiografica dei postpotenziali. G Ital Cardiol 16:565–572
16. Nava A, Canciani B, Daliento L et al (1988) Juvenile sudden death and effort ventricular tachicardias in a family with right ventricular cardiomyopathy. Int J Cardiol 21:111–123
17. Fontaine G, Fontaliran F, Chomette G (1986) Il ventricolo destro aritmogeno. G Ital Cardiol 16:1–3

18. Daliento L, Stritoni P, Isabella GB, Nava R, Razzolini R, Chioin R, Dalla-Volta S (1986) Malattia aritmogena primitiva del ventricolo destro: studio angiografico. Rev Lat Cardiol 7:453–460
19. Thiene G, Angelini A, Valente M (1988) Biopsia endomiocardica nella cardiomiopatia aritmogena del ventricolo destro. Cardiologia 33:313–315
20. Martini B, Nava A, Thiene G et al (1988) Right ventricular outflow tract (RVOT) tachycardias in 27 patients without apparent heart disease. New Trends Arrhyth 4:31–34
21. Dalla-Volta S (1988) La miocardiopatia fibro-adiposa del ventricolo destro. Inquadramento nosografico. Cardiologia 33:287–289

Arrhythmologic Study in Arrhythmogenic Right Ventricular Dysplasia: Prognostic Implications in Fifty Patients

R. Bettini, F. Furlanello, G. Vergara, G. B. Durante, L. Visonă, P. Dal Forno, A. Bertoldi, C. Burelli, G. L. Nicolosi, and D. Zanuttini

Introduction

In 1979 Fontaine et al. described "arrhythmogenic right ventricular dysplasia" (ARVD) [1]. This disease was characterized by hypoplasia of the right ventricular myocardium and considered similar to the disease described by Uhl in 1972 [2]. In recent literature, great attention has been paid to a wide spectrum of anatomoclinical situations which are all grouped under the still widely used term "dysplasia" [3–8]. These forms, which are often clinically nonhomogeneous, owing to the progressive degenerative tendency of the myocardium, may be considered "right ventricular cardiomyopathy" [9]. In symptomatic cases, these forms are characterized essentially by marked electrical instability, with hyperkinetic ventricular arrhythmias (HVA) which originate in the right ventricle and have a left bundle branch block morphology (LBBB). Hence the term "arrhythmogenic right ventricular disease" is justified [10, 11]. On the other hand, the existence of familiar forms [12] and the high incidence of life-threatening arrhythmias and sudden death even in young asymptomatic patients, make it necessary to identify possible risk markers in these patients.

The aim of this work is to contribute to the knowledge of prognosis in patients with ARVD by correlating the arrhythmias with the clinical course in a selected group of patients.

Materials and Method

Fifty patients [39 males and 11 females; average age 30.6 years (minimum 11, maximum 75)] affected by ARVD were studied between January 1977 and January 1988 at the Arrhythmologic Centre in Trento. The study protocol included: clinical history (50/50 patients), physical examination (50/50 patients), standard electrocardiogram (ECG) (50/50 patients), Holter monitoring (HM) (50/50 patients), ergometric test (ET) (50/50 patients), two-dimensional echocardiography with color Doppler (2D Echo) (50/50 patients), cardiac angiography (CA) (38/50 patients), electrophysiologic endocavitary study (EES) (35/50 patients), late potentials with signal averaging technique (LP) (only for patients seen in the last year) (17/50 patients), histological examination (HE) (4/50 patients).

Rigorous diagnostic echocardiographic, angiographic, and arrhythmologic criteria were applied by independent groups of observers [13–16]. A distinction was made between "localized" forms (with right ventricular segmentary involvement) and "diffuse" forms with a more extensive right ventricular disease, sometimes associated to a left ventricular involvement (LVI).

The elements drawn from the study protocol were correlated with the arrhythmic events, with sudden death (SD) and with aborted sudden death (ASD). The statistical significance was calculated with the chi-square method for $p < 0.05$.

Results

Ventricular Findings: Localized ARVD was documented in 42/50 patients (84%), and diffuse ARVD in 8/50 patients (16%). There was LVI in 30/50 patients (60%): 25 patients had wall motion abnormalities and five had mitral valve prolapse (MVP) and/or hypertrophic cardiomyopathy.

The histological reports available in 4/50 patients (8%) showed fibroadiposis of the right ventricle in 4/4 patients. In 1/4 patient the fibroadiposis was found also in the left ventricle.

Surface Electrocardiographic Study: Right bundle branch block (RBBB) was documented in 10/50 patients (20%), negative T wave in the right precordial leads (up to and beyond V_2) in 19/50 patients (38%). HVA, exclusively or mainly of LBBB morphology, were found in 50/50 patients (100%). A sinus rhythm was present in 49/50 patients, while only 2% had an atrial fibrillation. Late potentials of the signal-averaged QRS (performed in 17/50 patients) were found in 4/17 patients (23.5%).

Electrophysiological Endocavitary Study: EES was performed in 35/50 patients (70%). There were no repetitive intraventricular responses (RIVR) in 2/35 patients (5.7%), RIVR < 3 QRS complexes in 7/35 patients (20%), nonsustained ventricular tachycardia (VT) in 8/35 patients (22.8%), multiform VT[1] ≥ 10 QRS complexes in 5/8 patients, sustained VT in 18/35 patients (51.4%), multiform VT in 3/18 patients and pleomorphic VT[2] in 7/18 patients. Resuscitation was required in 5/35 patients during EES study because of the severity of the induced HVA.

Ventricular Tachycardia: Clinical VT was documented in 41/50 patients (82%): slow VT in 1/50 patient (2%), nonsustained VT in 10/50 patients (20%), sustained VT in 30/50 patients (60%) (Fig. 1); 35/50 patients underwent EES,

---

[1] Multiform VT: ventricular tachycardia with variation of the QRS morphology and/or electrical axis during the same episode without long QT.

[2] Pleomorphic VT: different morphological types of sustained ventricular tachycardia in the same patient (bundle branch block and/or variations ≥ 90° of the electrical axis and/or multiform appearance).

SYNCOPE

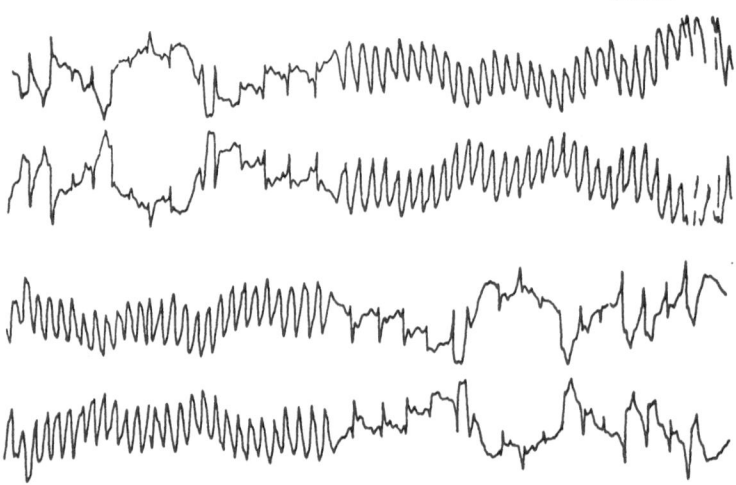

Fig. 1. A 19-year-old female diabetic patient with anamnestic syncope which was thought to be due to hypoglycemia. During a long period of dynamic electrocardiographic monitoring, this sustained ventricular tachycardia episode (250 bpm) was documented, which terminated spontaneously. The subsequent cardioarrhythmological study permitted the diagnosis of ARVD

and VT was induced in 26/35 (74.2%). Nonsustained VT was induced in 2 patients without clinical VT, in one patient with clinical nonsustained VT, in one patient with slow clinical VT, and in four patients with clinical sustained VT. Sustained VT was induced in 18 patients, all with clinical sustained VT. Altogether, multiform VT ≥ 10 QRS complexes (either clinical or induced) (Fig. 2) were documented in 12/50 patients (24%) (3/12 patients with diffuse ARVD and 11/12 with LVI). In 1/50 patient (2%), with diffuse ARVD and with LVI, nonsustained VT with acceleration (R-R cycle shortening) was documented. In 9/30 patients (30%) sustained pleomorphic VT was documented (2/9 with diffuse ARVD and 8/9 with LVI).

Antiarrhythmic Treatment: In 41/50 patients (82%), antiarrhythmic pharmacological treatment was carried out at the end of the study. In 4/41 patients, fulguration, nonautomatic antitachycardia pacemaker, crioablation, automatic implantable cardioverter defibrillator and surgical ventriculotomy, respectively, were also employed.

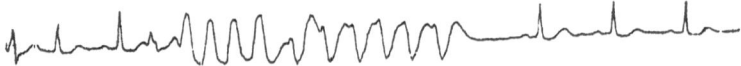

Fig. 2. A 51-year-old male amateur cyclist of a good level who died 3 months after the diagnosis of ARVD while on antiarrhythmic pharmacological treatment associated with automatic implantable cardioverter defibrillator after crioablation operation. During monitoring in intensive care unit, this multiform ventricular tachycardia run was documented: in the absence of increase of duration of the electric systole, the variation of the QRS axis is evident during the episode of only 11 QRS complexes

Clinical Course: In 50 patients the average global observation time (from the first symptom to the last control) was 8.7 years (minimum 1 year, maximum 30 years); 49/50 patients (98%) were in NYHA class I in the interval between the arrhythmic episodes. The most serious symptom occurred at an average age of 27.7 years (minimum 9, maximum 74). Life-threatening symptoms (LTS), always caused by life-threatening arrhythmias, were found in one or more episodes in 20/50 patients (40%); and more precisely these were syncope in 15/50 patients (30%) and angina and/or shock in 5/50 patients (10%). There was aborted sudden death in 5/50 patients (10%), 3/50 patients (6%) died suddenly. 4/50 patients (8%) dropped out.

Statistical Analysis of the Results: The EES induced sustained VT in only 18/24 patients with sustained clinical VT and showed a sensitivity of 75%, a specificity of 100%, and overall accuracy of 82.2%. Sustained VT was significantly correlated to the negative T wave in the right precordial leads ($p < 0.01$), while pleomorphic and multiform VT were significantly correlated to LVI ($p < 0.05$) (Table 1). The LTS were significantly correlated to sustained and pleomorphic VT ($p < 0.01$) (Table 2). Sudden death and aborted sudden death were significantly correlated to LVI and to sustained VT ($p < 0.05$) as well as to multiform and pleomorphic VT ($p < 0.01$) (Table 2).

Discussion

Our study concerns 50 consecutive patients affected by localized and diffuse forms of ARVD who underwent an arrhythmologic study at our centre because they had hyperkinetic ventricular arrhythmias. This characteristic makes our

Table 1. Statistical correlation

	Sustained VT	Pleomorphic VT	Multiform VT[a]
Negative T wave in the right precordial leads	$p < 0.01$	NS	NS
Left ventricle involvement	NS	$p < 0.05$	$p < 0.05$

[a] And/or R-R shortening including nonsustained forms.

Table 2. Statistical correlation

	Life-threatening symptoms	Sudden death and/or aborted
Left ventricle involvement	NS	$p < 0.05$
Clinical sustained VT	$p < 0.01$	$p < 0.05$
Pleomorphic VT	$p < 0.01$	$p < 0.01$
Multiform VT[a]	NS	$p < 0.01$

[a] And/or R-R shortening including nonsustained forms.

case study group (which included only patients who were symptomatic for arrhythmias) different from those in the literature [8–10, 12]. Also the duration of the clinical course (average 8.7 years), is one of the longest reported in the literature, and it is suitable for prognostic considerations [17–20]. The prevalence of the male sex (78%) is undoubtedly important, as has already been pointed out in the literature [3, 20], as is the slight functional compromission apart from the arrhythmias episodes [10, 21, 22]. The clinical course of our patients was complicated by severe clinical symptoms which were secondary to serious hyperkinetic ventricular arrhythmias. The incidence of life-threatening symptoms was high, they occurred in 40% of the patients and often during the first arrhythmic episode (18%). Finally, the incidence of hyperkinetic cardiac arrest was high (16%) with 12 episodes of resuscitation in six patients (12%) and with three sudden deaths (6%) (1/3 was resuscitated). Within the framework of the whole case study, the critical age for the most serious clinical symptoms was the third decade of life, in agreement with the literature [3, 17, 20].

In view of the stratification of risk in patients with ARVD which was the main aim of our study, interesting data emerged which correlated the arrhythmological elements with the characteristics of the anatomofunctional dysfunction and with the main events of the individual clinical course. In our cases, a significant statistical correlation with sustained VT could only be observed for negative T wave up to and beyond V_2 in the right precordial leads. This could lead to consider the alteration of the ventricular repolarization as a trustworthy index of the right ventricle, and hence of the electrical instability. Pleomorphic and multiform VT could be correlated with the presence of the LVI.

Sustained VT observed in 60% of cases, was of unfavorable prognostic significance and correlated to LTS ($p < 0.01$) and to SD ($p < 0.05$). Pleomorphic (18%) and multiform (26%) VT, even though less frequently observed, also had a negative prognostic value, since they were correlated to the most serious events of the natural history of the patients ($p < 0.01$, Table 2).

Conclusions

The data collected in our study of 50 patients with symptomatic ARVD enable us to draw some important conclusions for a prognostic stratification of these patients. In this disease the male sex prevails, the risk is not correlated to ventricular impairment, the critical age for life-threatening symptoms is between 20 and 30 years. The electrophysiological endocavitary study shows a high predictive value as regards sustained VT.

Markers of risk in patients with ARVD are:

(a) Negative T wave in the right precordial leads (statistically related to sustained VT).
(b) Left ventricular involvement, sustained VT, pleomorphic VT, multiform VT (including nonsustained forms) (statistically related to life-threatening symptoms and sudden death).

References

1. Fontaine G, Guiraudon G, Frank R, Cabrol C, Grosgogeat Y (1979) Arrhythmogenic right ventricular dysplasia: a previously unrecognized syndrome. Circulation 11: [Suppl] 11–65
2. Uhl HS (1972) A previously undescribed congenital malformation of the heart: almost total absence of the myocardium of the right ventricle. Bull Johns Hopkins Hosp 91:197–205
3. Markus FI, Fontaine G, Guiraudon G, Frank R, Laurenceau JL, Malergue C, Grosgogeat Y (1982) Right ventricular dysplasia: a report of 24 adult cases. Circulation 65:384
4. Fontaine G, Fontaliran F, Chomett G (1986) Il ventricolo destro aritmogeno. G Ital Cardiol 16/9:1–3
5. Naccarella F, Bracchetti D (1986) Il ventricolo destro aritmogeno: una displasia destra isolata o una miocardioptia diffusa? G Ital Cardiol 16:750–754
6. Rowland E, McKenna WJ, Sugrue D, Barclay R, Foale RA, Krikler DM (1984) Ventricular tachycardia of left bundle branch block configuration in patients with isolated right ventricular dilatation. Clinical and electrophysiological features. Br Heart J 51:15–24
7. Manyari DE, Klein GJ, Gulamhusein S, Boughner D, Guiraudon GM, Wyse G, Mitchell B, Kostuk W (1983) Arrhythmogenic right ventricular dysplasia: a generalized cardiomyopathy? Circulation 68 (2):251–257
8. Nava A, Martini B, Thiene G, Buja GF, Canciani B, Scognamiglio R, Miraglia G, Corrado D, Boffa GM, Daliento L, Scattolini G, Fasoli G, Stritoni P, Dalla Volta S (1988) La displasia aritmogena del ventricolo destro. G Ital Cardiol 18:2–9
9. Thiene G, Nava A, Corrado D, Rossi L, Pennelli N (1988) Right ventricular cardiomyopathy and sudden death in young people. N Engl J Med 318:129–133
10. Furlanello F, Bettini R, Vergara G, Cozzi F, Visonà L, Disertori M, Thiene G (1984) Problematica delle cardiopatie aritmogene a rischio dello sportivo con particolare riguardo alla preeccitazione cardiaca. G Ital Cardiol 14 (II):1062
11. Bettini R, Durante GB, Vergara G, Visonà L, Bertoldi A, Zardo F, Del Greco M, Furlanello F (1988) Arrhythmogenic right ventricular disease: natural history and prognostic implications in a case study of 39 patients. New Trends. Arrhythmias 4:397–401
12. Nava A, Scognamiglio R, Thiene G, Canciani B, Daliento L, Buja G, Stritoni P, Fasoli G, Dalla Volta S (1987) A polymorphic form of familial arrhythmogenic right ventricular dysplasia. Am J Cardiol 57:1405–1409
13. Moro E, Pignoni P, Nicolosi GL, Zardo F, Burelli C, Vergara G, Furlanello F, Zanuttini D (1987) Valore e limiti dell'ecocardiografia bidimensionale nell'identificazione della "displasia ventricolare destra aritmogena". G Ital Cardiol 17:661–666
14. Daubert C, Descaves C, Foulgoc JL, Bourdonnec C, Laurent M, Gauffault J (1988) Critical analysis of cineangiographic criteria for diagnosis of arrhythmias right ventricular dysplasia. Am Heart J 115:448–459
15. Josephson ME, Horowitz LN, Farshidi A, Spear JF, Kastor JA, Moore EN (1978) Recurrent sustained ventricular tachycardia. 2: Endocardial mapping. Circulation 57:440
16. Vergara G, Disertori M, Inama G, Guarnerio M, Bettini R, Durante GB, Stirpe E, Furlanello F (1984) Tachicardia ventricolare sostenuta. polimorfismo indotto. G Ital Cardiol 14:972–981
17. Baran A, Nanda NC, Falkoff M, Barold SS, Gallagher JJ (1982) Two-dimensional echocardiographic detection of arrhythmogenic right ventricular dysplasia. Am Heart J 103:1066–1067
18. Higuchi S, Caglar NM, Shimada R, Yamada A, Takeshita A, Nakamura M (1984) Sixteen year follow up of arrhythmogenic right ventricular dysplasia. Am Heart J 108:1383–1385
19. Kasanuki H, Ohnishi S (1987) Progression of arrhythmogenic right ventricular dysplasia. Abstracts of the 60th scientific session of the Am Heart Assoc. Circulation 76 [Suppl 4]:413
20. Blomstrom-Lundquist C, Sahel KG, Olsson SB (1987) A longterm follow-up of 15 patients with arrhythmogenic right ventricular dysplasia. Br Heart J 58:477–488

21. Furlanello F, Bettini R, Cozzi F, Del Favero A, Disertori M, Vergara G, Durante GB, Guarnerio M, Inama G, Thiene G (1984) Ventricular arrhythmias and sudden death in athletes. Ann NY Acad Sci 427:253
22. Furlanello F, Bettini R, Vergara G, Bertoldi A, Del Greco M, Durante GB, Frisanco L (1989) Marker and trigger mechanisms of sudden cardiac death. Excercise and sports activity. In: Bayes de Luna A (ed) Proceedings of sudden death. Barcelona (in press)

Positive Inotropic Therapy for Chronic Dilated Cardiomyopathy and Congestive Failure

C. V. Leier

Introduction

This report represents a brief overview of the current status of chronic positive inotropic therapy in dilated cardiomyopathy with heart failure. New issues about the old, namely digitalis, as well as data on the newer inotropic compounds will be presented. In the United States, the newer inotropic agents are all still investigational, but data will be discussed relevant to their current clinical status. At the onset, it is important to clearly define the term "positive inotropic drugs" as used in this text. Positive inotropic drugs are agents which increase the velocity and extent of myocardial contraction independent of loading conditions. Drugs which improve overall ventricular performance primarily through changes in afterload and preload will not be addressed.

Digitalis

With respect to digitalis we must raise the question, "what is new about the old?" We have learned over the last 3 decades, particularly over the last decade, that digitalis is a very complex drug. While digitalis does have some positive inotropic properties, these properties are relatively weak compared to those elicited with parenterally-administered inotropes (e.g., dobutamine, dopamine). Data are accruing to suggest that digitalis evokes a favorable clinical response in heart failure secondary to a number of other properties [1–4]. Some of these include sympatholytic effects (patients with congestive heart failure are generally believed to have an overabundance of sympathetic nervous system activity), normalization of baroreceptor function in heart failure, blunting the renin-angiotensin-aldosterone excess in heart failure (known to be overstimulated in many patients with congestive heart failure), a possible natriuretic effect at the renal tubular level, and a number of other properties. So it is likely that much of the clinical and laboratory improvement noted with digitalis in heart failure is, in fact, related to these noninotropic properties.

Over the past several years a number of multicenter trials have come to fruition showing that chronic digitalis therapy is more effective than chronic placebo administration. A blinded captopril versus placebo versus digoxin trial [5] and a milrinone versus placebo versus digoxin trial [6] have shown that digitalis is clearly superior to placebo in terms of improvement in ejection fraction, clinical status, and exercise performance. The results of these trials suggest that the 200-year clinical experience in the use of digitalis in heart failure has merit and credibility.

With respect to the role of digitalis in the clinical management of dilated cardiomyopathy/congestive heart failure, one can say that digitalis is the drug of choice in controlling the ventricular rate in atrial flutter/fibrillation and that for patients sinus rhythm, digitalis can be expected to improve clinical status and exercise capacity in a considerable number of patients. Digitalis therapy still has its caveats, the most noteworthy of which is tendency to cause arrhythmias in certain patients, particularly those who tend to be troubled with hypokalemia and hypomagnesemia.

Orally Administered Beta-Adrenergic Agonists

Beta-agonists act via $beta_1$-adrenergic stimulation (e.g., butopamine, prenalterol) and/or $beta_2$-adrenergic stimulation (e.g. pirbuterol, terbutaline). The latter group also elicits a considerable amount of peripheral vasodilatation through the stimulation of vascular $beta_2$-adrenergic receptors. While most of these substances clearly evoke hemodynamic changes after administration, namely an augmentation of stroke volume and cardiac output accompanied by a reduction in right and left ventricular filling pressures and pulmonary and systemic vascular resistances, the chronic administration of these compounds has been marred by several major problems [7]. First, the substances have substantial undesirable effects including tendency to cause arrhythmias, positive chronotropy, and neurological and gastrointestinal side effects. The results of chronic trials of these compounds have been relatively unimpressive, perhaps related to the proclivity for these substances to elicit pharmacodynamic tolerance. The development of pharmacodynamic tolerance and lack of clinical effectiveness with chronic administration are likely to be related to beta receptor down-regulation. With respect to the treatment of congestive heart failure, the role of adrenergic agonists is very limited and for most patients, none.

It is important to note that these comments may not apply to the group of drugs known as "partial agonists." It is possible that the partial agonists, which also have beta-blockade properties, may be more effective in the therapy of heart failure. The limited data available are not sufficient to make a statement regarding the effectiveness of the chronic administration of this special group of compounds.

Phosphodiesterase Inhibitors

The major phosphodiesterase inhibitors undergoing current clinical investigation in the United States are enoximone and milrinone. These agents act by inhibiting phosphodiesterase, resulting in an increase in intracellular cyclic AMP. The increase in cyclic AMP in the ventricle increases contractility and in the peripheral vasculature evokes relaxation of smooth muscle. Therefore, these compounds generally have positive inotropic and vasodilatory properties. The administration of these compounds to patients with heart failure generally result in a favorable hemodynamic response in the form of an increase in stroke volume and cardiac output and a reduction in systemic vascular resistance [8, 9]. In spite of these favorable hemodynamic effects, these agents have met some difficulty in their application in the chronic management of heart failure. These compounds have a relatively narrow ratio of clinical effectiveness to toxicity or side effects; in other words, the doses required to elicit convincingly favorable hemodynamic and clinical effects have a high incidence of side effects and the doses with fewer side effects are questionably effective. The results of multicenter trials have not been particularly impressive [6, 10]. Chronically administered milrinone was not superior to digitalis in improving clinical or exercise parameters, while eliciting far more undesirable effects [6]. It is not likely that the current phosphodiesterase inhibitors will replace any of the current therapies including digitalis, diuretics, vasodilators and converting enzyme inhibitors. If approved by our federal regulatory agency, these agents would only serve a supplementary role in some patients with heart failure.

Dopaminergic Agents

Examples of these drugs include levodopa, fenoldopam, and ibopamine. Commentary on these compounds will be very brief, primarily because these agents elicit a predominant vasodilatory response. They are often mistakenly placed under the category of positive inotropic drugs.

Intermittent Dobutamine Infusions

In 1977, the phenomenon of sustained clinical effectiveness after a 72-h dobutamine infusion in patients with severe congestive heart failure was reported out of our laboratories [11]. This clinical improvement lasted somewhere between 1 and 12 weeks after the infusion period [12]. These observations were confirmed by Liang et al. [13] in a blinded, controlled trial. Our laboratory published a number of reports examining mechanism of the sustained improvement and the most likely candidates include an increase in subendocardial blood flow during the infusion to generate an improvement of cellular histology, metabolism, and high energy phosphate content and a peripheral (skeletal muscle and vasculature) conditioning effect [14–17]. It is unlikely that the mechanisms are directly related to intermittent positive inotropy and for this reason, the use of the term "pulse inotropic therapy" for this intervention is not appropriate.

This form of therapy is far from being approved for use in the United States, but it is nevertheless used in many centers to elicit clinical improvement of patients with *end-stage* dilated cardiomyopathy/congestive heart failure, who are refractory to other therapies and who are not eligible for or are awaiting cardiac transplantation. Well-designed, blinded, and controlled trials are needed to examine this form of therapy and its potential mechanisms.

Is Positive Inotropic Therapy Alone a Reasonable Approach to the Chronic Management of Congestive Heart Failure?

There are a number of indications now that positive inotropic therapy alone will not turn out to be a reasonable therapeutic choice in the management of congestive heart failure. Binkley et al. [18] in our laboratories, have shown that positive inotropic drugs require proper impedance matching or the positive inotropy will not improve overall cardiac performance. It would probably be important that the positive inotropic drug maintain an adequate myocardial oxygen supply to demand ratio and thus maintain an adequate myocardial metabolic milieu. At this particular time we do not know the essential hemodynamic changes required for chronic clinical improvement in heart failure, but unless the positive inotropic agent favorably affects these parameters, the agent will probably be ineffective as a chronic treatment modality.

References

1. Covit AB, Schaar GL, Sealey JE, Laragh JH, Cody RJ (1983) Suppression of the renin-angiotensin system by intravenous digoxin in congestive heart failure. Am J Med 75:445–447
2. Fergus DW, Abboud FM, Mark AL (1984) Selective impairment of baroreflex-mediated vasoconstrictor responses in patients with ventricular dysfunction. Circulation 69:451–460
3. Strickley JC, Kessler RH (1961) Direct renal action of some digitalis steroids. J Clin Invest 40:311–315
4. Lewis RP (1986) Digitalis. In: Leier CV (ed) Cardiotonic drugs. Dekker, New York, pp 85–150
5. The Captopril-Digoxin Multicenter Research Group (1988) Comparative effects of therapy with captopril and digoxin in patients with mild to moderate heart failure. JAMA 259:539–544
6. DiBianco R, Shabetai R, Kostuk W, Moran J, Schlant RC, Wright R (1989) A comparison of oral milrinone, digoxin, and their combination in the treatment of patients with chronic heart failure. N Engl J Med 320:677–683
7. Kirlin PC (1986) Nonparenteral sympathomimetics. In: Leier CV (ed) Cardiotonic drugs. Dekker, New York, pp 151–181
8. Uretsky BF (1986) Phosphodiesterase inhibition. In: Leier CV (ed) Cardiotonic drugs. Dekker, New York, pp 183–198
9. DiBianco R (1986) The bipyridine derivatives. amrinone and milrinone. In: Leier CV (ed) Cardiotonic drugs. Dekker, New York, pp 199–242
10. Leier CV, Binkley PF, Starling RC, Huss-Randolph P (1989) Disparity between improvement in left ventricular function and changes in clinical status and exercise capacity during chronic enoximone therapy. Am Heart J 117:1092–1098
11. Leier CV, Webel J, Bush CA (1977) The cardiovascular effects of the continuous infusion of dobutamine in patients with severe cardiac failure. Circulation 56:468–472
12. Unverferth DV, Magorien RD, Altschuld R, Kolibash AJ, Lewis RP, Leier CV (1983) The hemodynamic and metabolic advantages gained by a three-day infusion of dobutamine in patients with congestive cardiomyopathy. Am Heart J 106:29–34

13. Liang CS, Sherman LG, Doherty JU, Wellington K, Lee VW, Hood WB (1984) Sustained improvement in cardiac function in patients with congestive heart failure after short-term infusion of dobutamine. Circulation 69:113–119
14. Leier CV, Huss P, Lewis RP, Unverferth DV (1982) Drug-induced conditioning in congestive heart failure. Circulation 65:1382–1387
15. Sullivan MJ, Binkley PF, Unverferth DV, Ren JH, Boudoulas H, Bashore TM, Merola AJ, Leier CV (1985) Prevention of bedrest-induced physical deconditioning by daily dobutamine infusions. J Clin Invest 76:1632–1642
16. Unverferth DV, Leier CV, Magorien RD, Croskery R, Svirebely JR, Kilibash AJ, Dick MR, Meacham JA, Baba N (1980) Improvement of human myocardial mitochondria after dobutamine: a quantitative ultrastructural study. J Pharmacol Exp Ther 215:527–532
17. Magorien RD, Unverferth DV, Brown GP, Leier CV (1983) Dobutamine and hydralazine: comparative influences of positive inotropy and vasodilation on coronary blood flow and myocardial energetics in nonischemic congestive heart failure. J Am Coll Cardiol 1:499–505
18. Binkley PF, van Fossen DB, Leier CV (1988) Contrasting effects of dopamine and dobutamine on pulsatile hydraulic load. Circulation 78:II–104

Vasodilator Therapy for Cardiomyopathy

J. N. Cohn

Introduction

The primary goals in the treatment of cardiomyopathy are improvement in the quality of life, if it is impaired by the disease, and prolongation of life by preventing progression of the disease and its complications. Although emphasis in the past was on the myocardium itself and an effort to reverse the etiologic factors and stimulate cardiac performance, in recent years it has become apparent that the peripheral vasculature may play an important role in the genesis of symptoms from cardiomyopathy and in the progression and prognosis of the heart failure syndrome. Vasodilator therapy, therefore, now has a clear place in the therapeutic armamentarium for cardiomyopathy.

Physiologic Rationale

The myopathic ventricle loses its normal capacity to maintain a constant output despite physiologic variations in impedance to left ventricular ejection [11]. This impairment may reflect a failure in part of the Frank-Starling mechanism that provides for an increase in force of contraction in response to small increments in end-diastolic fiber length. One factor in the abnormal Frank-Starling mechanism may be a reduction in dynamic diastolic compliance so that increases in end-diastolic pressure may not be accompanied by an appropriate increase in fiber length [2]. Another contribution to the impaired adjustment to impedance is probably a loss of an intrinsic autoregulatory mechanism in the myocardium [3].

The impaired ability of the ventricle to cope with an afterload stress is often accompanied by vasoconstriction in the peripheral vasculature that increases impedance to left ventricular ejection. This vasoconstriction appears to be in part related to activation of endogenous vasoconstrictor neurohormonal systems. In patients with symptoms of heart failure, plasma norepinephrine, plasma renin activity and plasma arginine vasopressin levels often are increased and this increase appears to reflect increased activity of the sympathetic nervous system, the renin-angiotensin system and the antidiuretic hormone–vasopressin system [4, 5]. The correlation between this neurohormonal activation and the severity of vasoconstriction is at best modest, however, and it is therefore likely that other mechanisms also play an important role in the systemic vasoconstriction [6].

Since most previous studies of neurohormonal mechanisms have been confined to patients with the clinical syndrome of heart failure, a possible role of neurohormonally mediated vasoconstriction in patients with cardiomyopathy in the absence of heart failure could not be assessed. In recent studies from the NIH-sponsored SOLVD study group, hormone measurements were made in patients with dilated, poorly function ventricles but without symptoms of heart failure [7]. These preliminary studies indicate that in this relatively asymptomatic population plasma norepinephrine and plasma arginine vasopressin levels are elevated although plasma renin activity is normal. Thus, it is possible that even at the asymptomatic phase of left ventricular dysfunction neurohormonal mechanisms may contribute to a heightened impedance that could have an adverse effect on left ventricular function.

Vasoconstriction has traditionally been assessed by calculation of systemic vascular resistance as the ratio of mean arterial pressure to cardiac output. This calculation, however, disregards the pulsatile component of impedance that may importantly influence left ventricular performance. We have recently been employing a pulse-wave analysis technique to study arterial vascular compliance [8]. By modelling the circulation as a modified Windkessel with a proximal and distal compliance in parallel with the resistance, computer analysis of the diastolic decay of an arterial pulse wave can provide a quantitation of both the proximal (C_1) and the distal (C_2) compliances. Since the C_1 resides predominantly in the aorta and great vessels and the C_2 in the more distal muscular arteries, these two compliances may be independently altered in various disease states.

We have previously reported that distal vascular compliance is strikingly reduced in patients with heart failure [8]. Since both norepinephrine and angiotensin when infused in dogs produce a fall in C_2 [9], it is possible that neurohormonal activation may contribute to this reduction in compliance. The quantitative importance of this compliance alteration in the total impedance load imposed on the dilated left ventricle is not yet clear, but it now is mandatory to consider both compliance and resistance in assessing the effect of disease on the vasculature and in studying the response of the vasculature to vasodilating drugs.

Clinical Response to Vasodilators

The hemodynamic effect of vasodilator drugs in patients with left ventricular failure is now well known. Drugs that relax arteries and increase venous capacitance produce an increase in cardiac output and a reduction in the elevated left ventricular filling pressure [10]. We have recently been able to show that the favorable hemodynamic effect of nitroprusside and converting enzyme inhibitors is accompanied by an increase in arterial compliance as well as a reduction in vascular resistance [11, 12].

The effect of chronic vasodilator therapy on the quality of life in patients with heart failure has been difficult to assess. Exercise tolerance testing often is used as a surrogate for quality of life, but most tests evaluate maximal exercise capacity which may not be an appropriate surrogate for the comfort with which a person may be able to carry out a more modest exercise stress. Despite this caveat, however, several sizeable trials have demonstrated that adding vasodilator drugs to background therapy with digitalis and diuretic or with diuretic alone can result in an improvement in peak exercise capacity [13–15]. In some of these studies "quality of life" has been more directly assessed by a questionnaire and these have demonstrated an improvement in response to vasodilator drug therapy. Most reported trials have utilized nitrates, nitrates plus hydralazine or angiotensin converting enzyme inhibitors as the vasodilator regimen.

Vasodilator-Heart Failure Trial

The first attempt to evaluate a possible life-prolonging effect of vasodilator therapy was the Veterans Administration vasodilator-heart failure trial (V-HeFT). In this study, 642 patient with heart failure of mild to moderate severity were randomized to receive one of three double-blind regimens in addition to digoxin and a diuretic. Forty-two percent of the patients were given a placebo and 28% were randomized to each of the vasodilator regimens, prazosin 20 mg daily or hydralazine 300 mg plus isosorbide dinitrate 160 mg daily. The study revealed a significantly prolongation of life in the group randomized to the hydralazine-isosorbide dinitrate combination vasodilator regimen [16].

V-HeFT included patients with left ventricular dysfunction and exercise intolerance of diverse etiologies. Approximately 45% of the randomized patients had heart failure presumably on the basis of coronary artery disease. Since there has been concern that the etiology of heart failure may be an important determinant of the response to therapy, the patients with coronary disease were compared to those who had heart failure in the absence of a history or findings of significant ischemic heart disease. This latter group can be classifed as idiopathic dilated cardiomyopathies (IDCM), since hypertrophic cardiomyopathy and significant obstructive valvular disease were exclusions.

Table 1 provides baseline demographic and physical findings in these two subsets of the study population. Most of the variables were similar in the two etiologic groups. However, the IDCM group was slightly younger and exhibited a slightly higher ejection fraction and slightly higher blood pressure, possibly reflecting a slightly less severe degree of left ventricular dysfunction. Exercise tolerance was similar in the two groups. The major demographic difference between the groups was in the incidence of excessive alcohol intake. More than 50% of the IDCM patients gave a history of alcohol abuse whereas this history was obtained in only 22.5% of the coronary disease group. These data provide strong support for the suggestion that alcohol is an important etiologic factor in IDCM. Since this is a male Veteran population in whom alcohol abuse may be more common than in the general population, these findings cannot necessarily be applied to the overall syndrome of IDCM. Survival was also very similar between the IDCM and ischemic groups (Fig. 1).

Table 1. Baseline variables (mean ± SD) in patients with heart failure with (CAD) and without (IDCM) coronary artery disease (V-HeFT)

	CAD	IDCM	P
Age (years)	59.2 ± 6.9	57.9 ± 8.2	0.034
Alcohol excess history (%)	22.5	54.2	< 0.00001
Hypertension history (%)	39.1	42.7	NS
Diabetes mellitus	26.4	16.2	0.002
Ejection fraction	0.27 ± 0.11	0.32 ± 0.14	0.001
Left ventricular diastolic diameter (cm/m²)	3.52 ± 0.58	3.46 ± 0.61	NS
Peak exercise VO$_2$ (ml/kg/min)	14.4 ± 3.9	14.8 ± 4.0	NS
Cardiothoracic ratio	0.53 ± 0.06	0.54 ± 0.07	0.05
Systolic blood pressure (mmHg)	116.9 ± 18.0	121.0 ± 19.0	0.006
Diastolic blood pressure (mmHg)	74.7 ± 10.0	76.4 ± 10.2	0.05
Heart rate (beats per minute)	81.3 ± 12.8	82.9 ± 13.4	NS

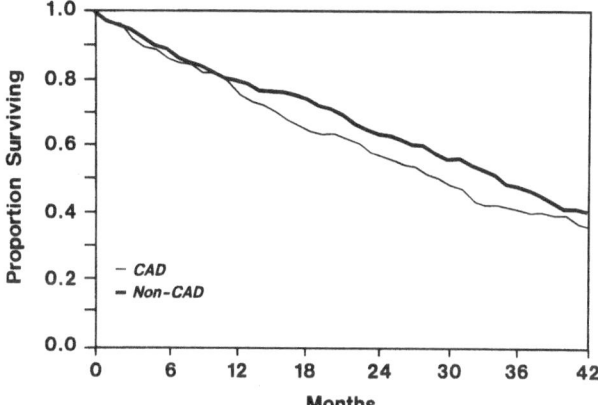

Fig. 1. Survival curves in patients with coronary artery disease (*CAD*) and with idiopathic dilated cardiomyopathy (*non-CAD*) in V-HeFT

The favorable effect of hydralazine and isosorbide dinitrate in the total heart failure population was also present in the IDCM groups. This subset analysis does not provide adequate power for a statistically significant prolongation of life in the vasodilator-treated population, but as previously reported the non-ischemic IDCM group exhibited a 27.4% reduction in adjusted mortality with hydralazine-nitrate treatment compared to placebo, whereas the ischemic group exhibited a 28.5% reduction in mortality [17] (Table 2). These data therefore provide no support for the concept that this vasodilator regimen was acting predominantly on a diseased coronary vascular bed. Rather, it would appear that muscle dysfunction, regardless of cause, is the key factor in the favorable effect of this vasodilator regimen.

An unexpected finding was that prazosin appeared to have an adverse effect in the IDCM group (Table 2). Annual mortality rate was actually higher with

Table 2. Annual mortality rate (AMR) and risk reduction (RR) in nonischemic cardiomyopathy (V-HeFT)

Placebo		Hydralazine + isosorbide dinitrate		Prazosin	
(n)	AMR (%)	(n)	AMR (%)	(n)	AMR (%)
152	15.3	104	13.3	102	21.0

	RR Unadjusted (%)	Adjusted[a] (%)	RR Unadjusted (%)	Adjusted[a] (%)
	14.1	27.4	−43.0	−15.7

[a] Adjusted for baseline variables that influenced mortality (ejection fraction, peak exercise capacity, cardiothoracic ratio, and recent antiarrhythmic therapy).

prazosin than with placebo treatment. After adjustment for baseline variables, prazosin exhibited a 15.7% increase in risk ratio which did not approach statistical significance. In the absence of a known mechanism for a specific adverse effect of prazosin in IDCM this finding must be assumed to be a chance observation.

Prevention of Progression

The unanswered question is whether early intervention with a vasodilator regimen prior to the onset of symptoms of heart failure can prevent progression of the dilated cardiomyopathy and perhaps delay or prevent entirely the development of symptomatic heart failure. Since a therapeutic trial on this population has not yet been completed, use of vasodilator drugs at this phase of the disease certainly cannot be recommended as an effective form of therapy. Nonetheless, the increase in ejection fraction observed in the hydralazine-nitrate group in V-HeFT and the prolongation of life in the same treatment group provided strong support for the idea that left ventricular dysfunction progresses in part because of the load placed on the ventricle by a high impedance to emptying. Vasodilators should counteract the adverse effects of an increase in wall stress on the progress of left ventricular dysfunction.

Vasodilator drugs should not, however, be the only therapeutic regimen to be evaluated for prevention of progression of cardiomyopathy. Agents that might block the synthesis of protein or the connective tissue matrix in the myocardium could be effective. Isozyme shifts, beta-receptor downregulation, catecholamine depletion, calcium overload and electromechanical events within the myocardium all may contribute to progressive pump failure. Interventions aimed at inhibiting any of these processes must be tested in controlled trials.

Conclusions

Vasoconstriction is a hallmark of the patient with heart failure and the load played on the ventricle by this arterial vasoconstriction appears to contribute to progression of symptoms and to a shortened life expectancy. Vasodilator drugs now should be considered an integral part of the therapeutic regimen for patients with heart failure, both because of their ability to help relieve symptoms but also because of their efficacy in prolonging life. The converting enzyme inhibitors (captopril, enalapril and lisinopril) and the combination of hydralazine with isosorbide dinitrate are the two established effective vasodilator regimens. The ACE inhibitors may, however, have important metabolic and mitogenic effects above and beyond their vasodilator property. Thus, the treatment of cardiomyopathy may eventually include the use of vasodilators plus a converting enzyme inhibitor.

Acknowledgement: This work was supported in part by the Cooperative Studies Program. Veterans Administration and by Program Project Grant POI HL 32427 from the National Heart, Lung, and Blood Institute.

References

1. Cohn JN (1973) Vasodilator therapy for heart failure: the influence of impedance on left ventricular performance. Circulation 48:5–8
2. Levine HJ, Gaasch WH (1978) Diastolic compliance of the left ventricle. Mod Concepts Cardiovasc Dis 47:95–102
3. Sarnoff SJ, Mitchell JH, Gilmore JP, Remensnyder JP (1960) Homeometic auto regulation of the heart. Circ Res 8:1077–1091
4. Levine TB, Francis GS, Goldsmith SR, Simon A, Cohn JN (1982) Activity of the sympathetic nervous system and renin-angiotensin system assessed by plasma hormone levels and their relationship to hemodynamic abnormalities in congestive heart failure. Am J Cardiol 49:1659–1666
5. Goldsmith SR, Francis GS, Cowley AW, Levine TB, Cohn JN (1983) Increased plasma arginine vasopressin in patients with congestive heart failure. J Am Coll Cardiol 1:1385–1390
6. Cohn JN (1988) Is neurohormonal activation deleterious to the long-term outcome of patients with congestive heart failure? Antagonist's view. J Am Coll Cardiol 12:554–558
7. Francis G, Benedict C, Johnston D, Kirlin P, Neuberg G, Kubo S, Hosking J, Liang C, Yusuf S (1989) Differences in neurohormonal activation in patients with left ventricular dysfunction with and without heart disease. J Am Coll Cardiol 13:264A
8. Finkelstein SM, Cohn JN, Collins RV, Carlyle PF, Shelley W (1985) Vascular hemodynamic impedance in congestive heart failure. Am J Cardiol 55:423–427
9. Mock JA, Finkelstein SM, Eaton J, Hatfield G, Cohn JN (1987) Vasoconstrictormediated reduction in vascular compliance assessed by pulse-contour-analysis. Circulation 76:IV441
10. Cohn JN, Franciosa JA (1977) Vasodilator therapy of cardiac failure. N Engl J Med 297:27–31, 254–258
11. Finkelstein SM, Collins VR, Cohn JN (1988) Arterial vascular compliance response to vasodilators by Fourier and pulse contour analysis. Hypertension 12:380–387
12. Finkelstein SM, Cohn JN, Carlyle PF, Carlyle WJ (1987) Vascular compliance response to converting enzyme inhibitors in heart failure. Circulation 76:IV179

13. Franciosa JA, Goldsmith SR, Cohn JN (1980) Contrasting immediate and long-term effects of isosorbide dinitrate on exercise capacity in congestive heart failure. Am J Med 69:559–566
14. Captopril Multicenter Research Group (1983) A placebo-controlled trial of captopril in refractory chronic congestive heart failure. J Am J Cardiol 2 (4):755–763
15. Levine TB, Olivari MT, Garberg V, Sharkey SW, Cohn JN (1984) Hemodynamic and clinical response to enalapril, a long-acting converting-enzyme inhibitor, in patients with congestive heart failure. Circulation 69:548–553
16. Cohn JN, Archibald DG, Ziesche S, Franciosa JA, Harston WE, Tristani FE, Dunkman WB, Jacobs W, Francis GS, Flohr KH, Goldman S, Cobb FR, Shah PM, Saunders R, Fletcher RD, Loeb HS, Hughes VC, Baker B (1986) Effect of vasodilator therapy on mortality in chronic congestive heart failure. Results of a Veterans Administration Cooperative Study (V-HeFT). N Engl J Med 314:1547–1552
17. Cohn JN, Archibald DG, Francis GS, Ziesche S, Franciosa JA, Harston WE, Tristani FE, Dunkman WB, Jacobs W, Flohr KH, Goldman S, Cobb FR, Shah PM, Saunders R, Fletcher RD, Loeb HS, Hughes VC, Baker B (1987) Veterans Administration Cooperative Study on vasodilator therapy of heart failure: influence of prerandomization variables on the reduction of mortality by treatment with hydralazine and isosorbide dinitrate. Circulation 75:IV49-IV54

Beta-Blockade in Dilated Cardiomyopathy

F. Waagstein

Introduction

The principle of treating severe heart failure with beta-blockade dates back to the early 1970s and was based on clinical observations in patients with three-vessel disease, acute and chronic heart failure and high resting heart rate. Almost immediate dramatic improvement was seen when practolol, a selective beta$_1$-blocker with mild intrinsic stimulatory activity (ISA) at an average dose of 20 mg was given i.v. to these patients. Table 1 describes the hypothetical pathophysiologic background of the effect of tachycardia in these patients and the possible effect of acute beta-blockade.

This observation made the basis for the use of long-term beta-blockade in patients with dilated cardiomyopathy (DCM) and resting tachycardia. The mechanism for heart failure in DCM may differ from that in ischemic heart disease with acute and chronic heart failure. In DCM we have not seen lactate production at rest and during exercise or atrial pacing indicating ischemia. Beta-blockade may, however, through reduction in heart rate and a direct effect on basal cellular metabolism, lead to reduction in myocardial energy consumption. Figure 1 illustrates the combined metabolic and hemodynamic effects of acute administration of 15 mg metoprolol i.v. in patients with DCM [1].

Evidence for the Role of the Sympathetic System in Heart Failure

There is now abundant evidence for the importance of the sympathetic system in heart failure. Table 2 lists abnormalities affecting the sympathetic system in heart failure. Serum norepinephrine is a strong predictor of death in chronic

Table 1. Effects of tachycardia which are reversed by beta-blockade

Shortening of diastole
Decrease in endocardial/epicardial flow ratio
Increase in myocardial oxygen consumption
Global ischemia
Biventricular failure

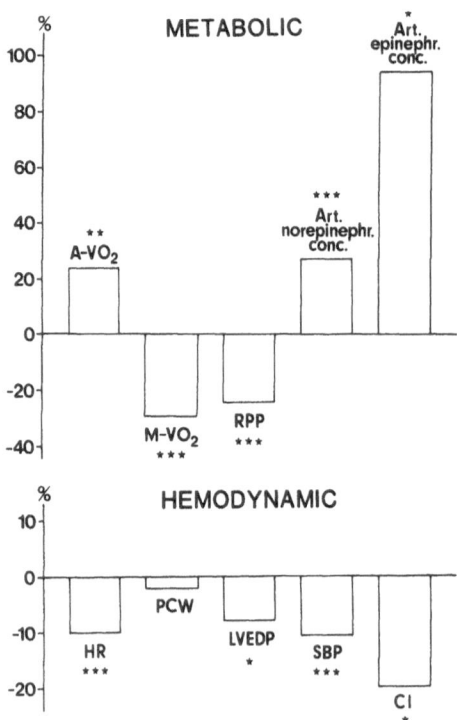

Fig. 1. Changes in metabolic and hemodynamic variables after 15 mg metoprolol i.v. in patients with DCM ($n = 18$). $A–VO_2$, arterial-venous oxygen difference; $M–VO_2$, myocardial oxygen consumption; RPP rate-pressure product; HR, heart rate; PCW, pulmonary capillary wedge; $LVEDP$, left ventricular end-diastolic pressure; SBP, systolic blood pressure; CI, cardiac index. * $p < 0.05$; ** $p < 0.01$; *** $p < 0.001$. (From [1])

Table 2. Findings in dilated cardiomyopathy

Increased serum norepinephrine
Decreased stores of myocardial norepinephrine
Down-regulation of beta$_1$-receptors
Circulating autoantibodies to beta$_1$-receptor peptide

heart failure [2], and the constant exposure to a high level of catecholamines leads to down-regulation of beta-receptors [3]. It was later shown that down-regulation is more pronounced in beta$_1$-receptor subpopulation [3]. Recently it has been shown by members of our group [4] that the activity of stimulatory G-protein is decreased [5], and by our group and others [6, 7] that circulating specific autoantibodies against the determinant peptide in the beta$_1$-receptor is significantly more common in patients with DCM compared to ischemic heart failure and controls. Whether the latter plays a pathogenic role in the development of dilated cardiomyopathy is not clear since there is no correlation between the antibody titer and the severity of the disease. Thus, it is not clear whether the sympathetic system is involved in the genesis of DCM or merely a modulating factor once the disease has arisen.

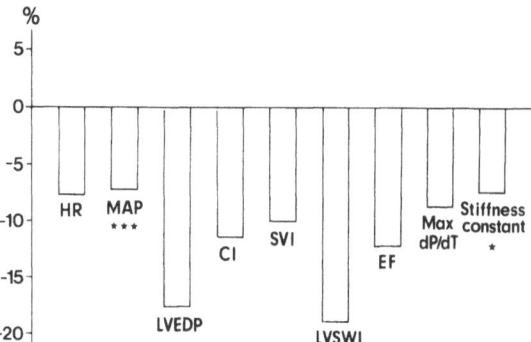

Fig. 2. Acute hemodynamic changes after 25 mg acebutalol i.v. in patients with DCM (*n* = 10). *HR*, heart rate; *MAP*, mean arterial pressure; *LVEDP*, left ventricular end-diastolic pressure; *CI*, cardiac index, *SVI*, stroke volume index; *LVSWI*, left ventricular stroke work index; *EF*, ejection fraction. (From [8])

Acute Studies of Beta-Blockade in DCM

Only a few studies have dealt with the acute effect of beta-blockade in DCM [8]. NYHA class II–IV patients who were given metoprolol or acebutalol i.v. reacted, not unexpectedly, with a drop in systolic blood pressure and cardiac index (Figs. 1, 2), whereas there was no effect on right and left ventricular filling pressure (Figs. 1, 2). We have recently shown that there is no change in ejection fraction after 10 mg metoprolol i.v. It has been suggested that the excellent tolerance for acute i.v. beta-blockade in DCM patients was due to improved compliance and decreased stiffness constant (Fig. 2) [8] observed after i.v. administration of acebutalol. We have, however, not seen any change in peak filling rate of the left ventricle when corrected for heart rate by atrial pacing after 10 mg metoprolol i.v. (unpublished observation).

Tolerance to Beta-Blockade in DCM

Although i.v. metoprolol is reasonably well tolerated in DCM, it may not be the case when metoprolol is given as a long-term oral dose. In the ongoing Metoprolol in Dilated Cardiomyopathy Trial (MDC Trial), approximately 15% of those fullfilling then inclusion criteria failed to tolerate the test dose of 5 mg b.i.d. We have not systematically studied the relation between the short-term hemodynamic response to i.v. metoprolol and an oral test dose, but it has been obvious that in some cases no signs of clinical heart failure occurred after the short-term dose compared to prolonged oral administration of a low dose of 5 mg b.i.d. or t.i.d.

When the tolerance of metoprolol was studied in an open study of 33 consecutive patients with DCM, five out of 33 did not tolerate the initial low dose, and another two patients developed intolerance to metoprolol when the dose was increased, although the initial low dose was well tolerated. The reason for the discrepancy between tolerance of i.v. beta-blockade in contrast

Table 3. Titration schema for metoprolol in DCM

Days 1– 7	5 mg b.i.d.
Days 8–14	5 mg t.i.d.
Days 15–21	10 mg t.i.d.
Days 22–28	25 mg b.i.d.
Days 29–35	25 mg t.i.d.
Days 36–42	50 mg b.i.d.
Days 43–49	50 mg t.i.d.

Table 4. Factors predicting intolerance for metoprolol in DCM

Low systolic and diastolic pressure
Low right atrial pressure
Low cardiac index
Low ejection fraction
Low LVET %

to intolerance to long-term oral administration remains obscure. One explanation may be that the acute depression of contractility from beta-blockade in itself does not induce heart failure but continued depression of contractility may do it in some instances. We therefore recommend an oral test dose instead of an i.v. test dose before it is decided whether long-term beta-blockade should be administered or not. Since most patients with severe heart failure have down-regulation of beta$_1$-receptors we recommend a very slow titration of the beta-blockade starting with 5 mg b.i.d. We suggest the titration shown in scheme Table 3. In case intolerance develops at a certain level of titration of metoprolol, it is possible to go one step back in the titration scheme or keep the patient on a certain titration level for more than 1 week. It may also be necessary to choose a final dose lower than 50 mg t.i.d.

There is no safe method for predicting whether a patient can tolerate beta-blockade or not. Certain variables, however separate those who tolerate from those who do not (Table 4). An interesting finding is that neither left ventricular diameter, left ventricular end diastolic pressure, or heart rate has any predictive value.

Short-term Studies with Beta-Blockers in DCM

The effect of short-term beta-blockade has been carefully studied using metoprolol (Figs. 3, 4) [9, 10] or acebutalol over 4 weeks in randomized placebo-controlled studies. Although these studies failed to show any improvement in invasive hemodynamics, echocardiographic findings, or exercise tolerance, it is obvious that tolerance to beta-blockers is excellent since cardiac index, left ventricular filling pressure, and ejection fraction are unchanged despite a significant decrease in heart rate indicating unchanged left ventricular performance. A considerable reduction in resting heart rate indicates a lowering of myocar-

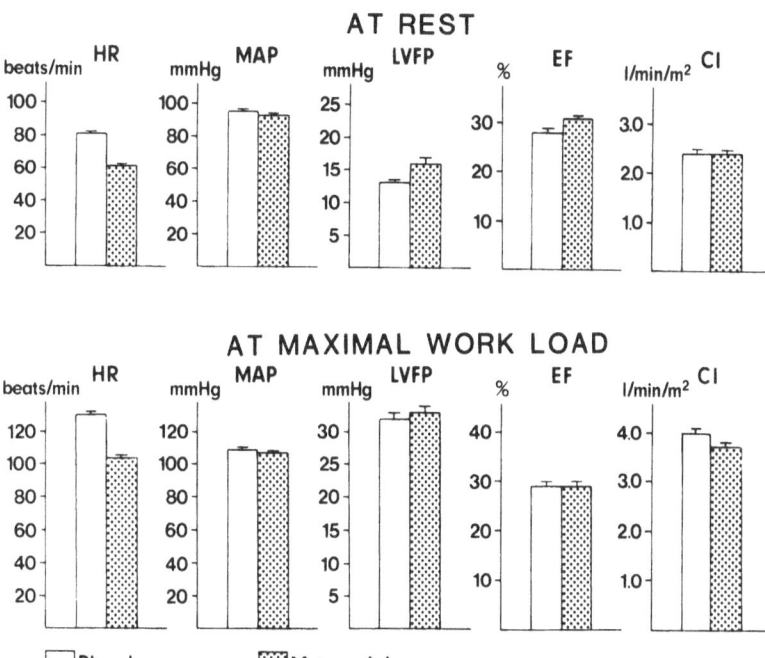

Fig. 3. Double-blind cross-over treatment with metoprolol (4 weeks) in patients with DCM ($n = 10$). *LVFP*, left ventricular filling pressure; other abbreviations as in Figs. 1 and 2. (From [9])

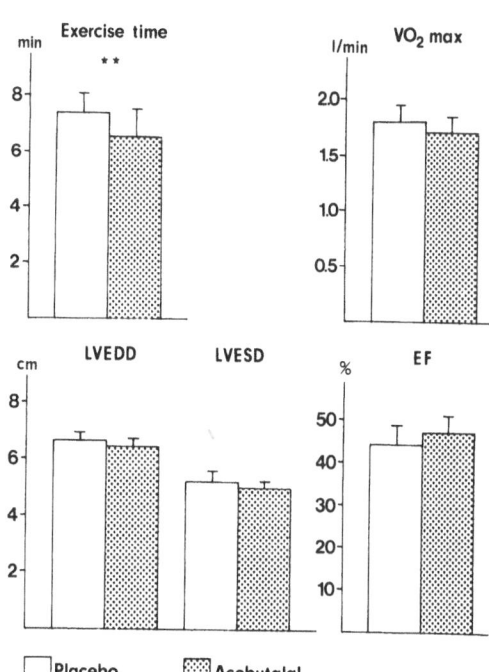

Fig. 4. Double-blind trial (1 month) with acebutalol and placebo in patients with DCM ($n = 15$). VO_2 *max*, maximal oxygen consumption; *LVEDD*, left ventricle end-diastolic dimension; *LVESD*, left ventricle end-systolic dimension; *EF*, ejection fraction. (From [10])

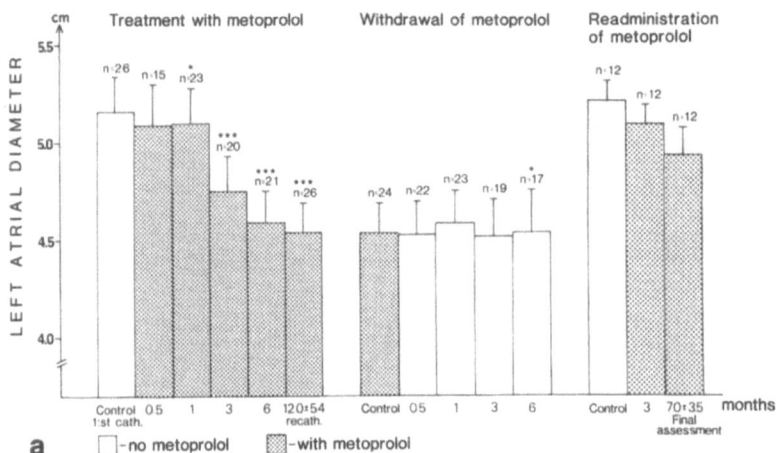

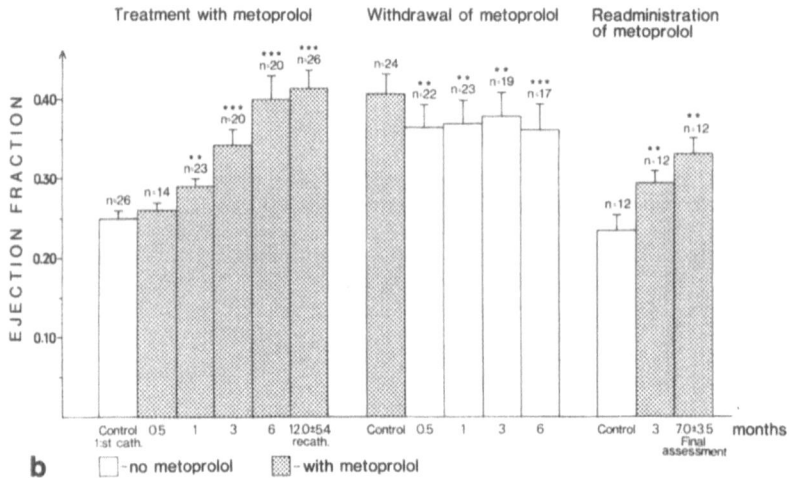

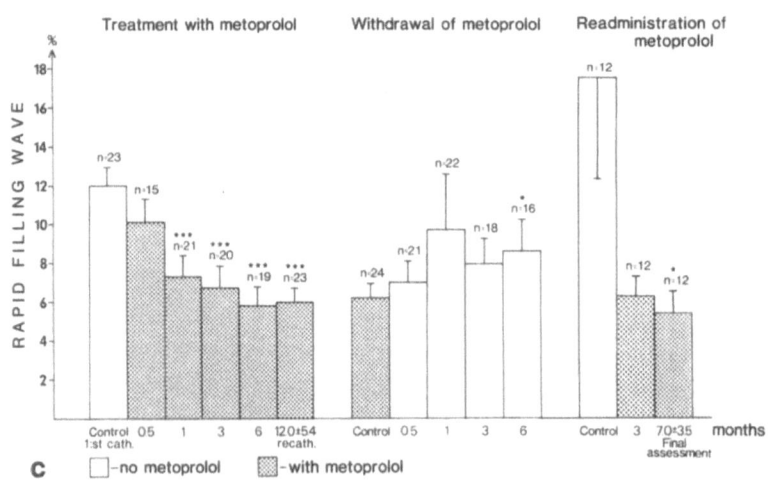

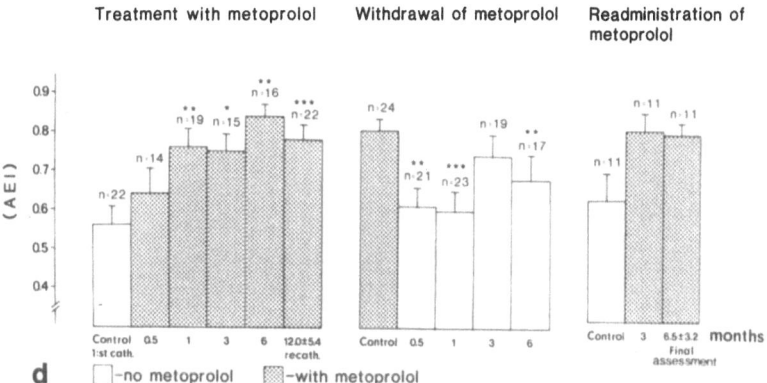

Fig. 5. a Changes in left atrial diameter in patients with DCM. **b** Changes in ejection fraction in patients with DCM. **c** Changes in rapid filling wave in patients with DCM. **d** Changes in atrial emptying index (*AEI*) in patients with DCM

dial oxygen consumption, which may be of value for long-term treatment with beta-blockers. Our own findings when using metoprolol in an open study in these patients indicate that there is no change in left atrial dimension or ejection fraction after 1 month of metoprolol treatment. Changes in these variables do not become obvious until after 3 months of treatment (Fig. 5 a, b). There are pronounced changes in rapid filling wave within 1 month (Fig. 5 c, d).

Long-term Studies with Beta-Blockers in DCM

When beta-blockers are given for 6 months or longer, it is evident from two controlled studies that there is effect on both indices of left ventricular systolic function and on exercise tolerance (Figs. 6, 7) [11, 12]. Our own data from open treatment confirm these findings. Also, invasive hemodynamic measurements at rest show that there is a significant decrease in both right and left ventricular filling pressures and increase in cardiac index (Table 5) [13]. We have not been able to correlate responsiveness or degree of improvement to initial heart rate despite the fact that, from a theoretical point of view, those with the highest heart rate should benefit more than those with a lower initial heart rate. Figure 8 shows an illustrative case of a patient with biventricular failure secondary to valvular disease. The patient had aortic and mitral valvular replacement 5 years previously and no signs of prostetic dysfunction or paravalvular leakage. The patient had a pacemaker with a constant heart rate of 70 due to third-degree atrioventricular-block. Treatment with captopril for 6 months before start of beta-blockade did not improve the patient hemodynamically. After 6 months of additional treatment with metoprolol 50 mg t.i.d., there was a marked decrease in left ventricular filling pressure and an increase in cardiac index despite an unchanged heart rate of 70 beats per minute.

Another way of demonstrating the cause relationship of observed improvement after beta-blockade treatment is to study the patients after withdrawal of

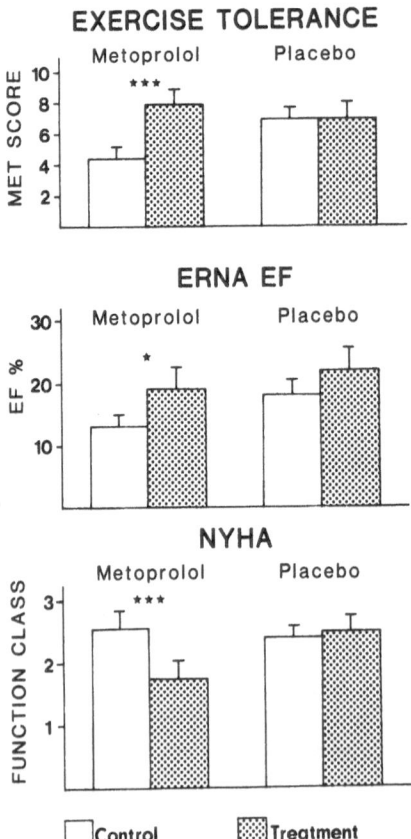

Fig. 6. Effect of long-term metoprolol treatment on exercise performance in patients with DCM. *ERNA EF*, equilibrium radionuclide angiography ejection fraction. (From [11])

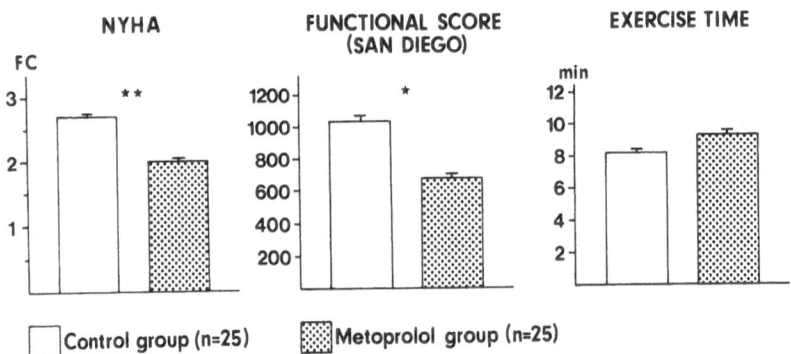

Fig. 7. Functional changes and exercise performance after long-term treatment with metoprolol in patients with DCM. (From [12])

beta-blocker treatment (Table 6) [13, 14]. In the latter study, 16/24 patients, who improved on metoprolol treatment, deteriorated within 12 months of withdrawal of metoprolol and improved again when treatment was reinstituted.

Table 5. Hemodynamic findings before and after long-term metoprolol treatment

	Baseline (n = 22)	Long-term treatment (n = 22)	p value
Heart rate (beats per minute)	93 ± 13	68 ± 12	0.0001
Systolic blood pressure (mmHg)	116 ± 20	132 ± 17	0.003
Cardiac index (l/min/m²)	2.17 ± 0.51	2.58 ± 0.43	0.005
PCW (mmHg)	23.8 ± 9.4	10.7 ± 6.2	0.0001
LVSWI (gram-meter/m²)	31.0 ± 13	64.9 ± 20.1	0.0001

All values are mean ± SD.
PCW, pulmonary capillary wedge; *LVSWI*, left ventricular stroke work index.

Table 6. Effect of withdrawal of beta-blockade

	Swedberg et al. 1980 [14] (n = 15)			Waagstein et al. 1989 [15] (n = 24)		
	C	W		C	W	
Ejection fraction	0.42	0.35	$p < 0.01$	0.41	0.32	$p < 0.0001$
Left atrial diameter	No change			4.54	4.80	$p < 0.002$
Left ventricular diastolic diameter	No change			6.44	6.81	$p < 0.0001$
Rapid filling wave ratio	Increase in 8/12 patients		$p < 0.005$	6.2	11.3	$p = 0.067$
	Follow-up time: mean 1.3 months			Follow-up time: mean 7.9 months		
Survivors	14/15			20/24		

C, control before withdrawal of chronic beta-blockade; *W*, when symptoms of dyspnea, decompensation, or sudden death occurred, or the patient had been followed for 4 months (first study) or 18 months (second study) without any signs of deterioration.

Other Findings After Long-term Treatment with Metoprolol

When patients were reinvestigated after 6 months of metoprolol treatment, it was found that there was an increase in beta-adrenergic receptor density from 39 to 80 fmol/mg protein ($p = 0.005$) [15] and an increase in peak positive dP/dt by 74% ($p < 0.05$). We had similar findings with regard to increase in beta-adrenergic receptor density. Morphometric measurements from endomyocardial biopsies before and after long-term treatment with metoprolol in patients

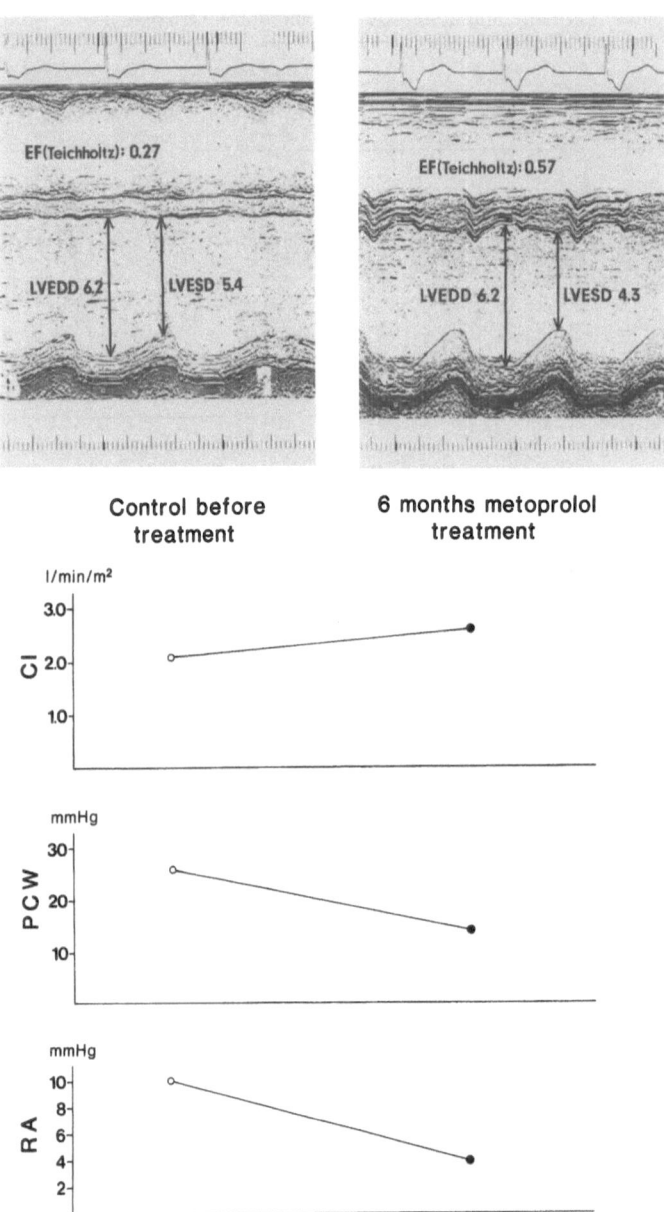

Fig. 8. Effect of long-term treatment in a patient with double valve replacement and long-term pacemaker treatment. *RA*, right atrial; other abbreviations as in Figs. 1 and 4

who improved on metoprolol and deteriorated after withdrawal of metoprolol showed an increase in both myocyte fiber diameter and myocyte nucleus diameter [13]. The latter indicates hypertrophy after metoprolol treatment which may be beneficial since a lack of compensatory hypertrophy development is an unfavorable finding predicting a poor prognosis.

Table 7. Effects on ejection fraction

	Ischemic cardiomyopathy		Other secondary cardiomyopathies	
Control	0.25 ± 0.005		0.27 ± 0.06	
		$p = 0.02$		$p = 0.05$
Metoprolol	0.31 ± 0.06		0.45 ± 0.13	

Beta-Blockade in Heart Failure Due to Ischemic Cardiomyopathy, Primary Valve Disease, and Diabetes

When a mixed group of patients with heart failure secondary to ischemic heart disease, valvular disease with permanent heart failure despite valvular replacement, heart failure secondary to diabetes, and systemic disease were given long-term treatment with metoprolol, similar findings were seen as after metoprolol treatment in patients with DCM [16], although, in patients with ischemic cardiomyopathy, the rate of improvement, as well as the absolute increase in ejection fraction, was lower than in the other secondary cardiomyopathies and DCM patients (Table 7). There was an increase in exercise duration from 431 to 522 s ($p = 0.05$) with a decrease in heart rate at maximal load from 143 to 115 ($p = 0.002$). There was a similar drop in resting left and right heart filling pressures as seen in DCM patients but no change in cardiac index. During submaximal exercise, despite a higher load, there was a tendency to a lower left ventricular filling pressure, no change in serum lactate, myocardial lactate extraction, or myocardial oxygen consumption [17].

Effect on Mortality

Until now, none of the studies has been large enough to answer the question of whether beta-blockade may affect survival in patients with severe heart failure. A comparison with historical controls in our center indicates that survival may improve after long-term treatment with beta-blockers [18]. Subgroup analysis from the postinfarction study with timolol [19] indicates that patients with big infarctions and heart failure may benefit from beta-blockade with regard to survival. To answer the question regarding the effect on survival, a multicenter trial dealing with patients with severe heart disease is in the process of studying the need for heart transplantation and survival as the primary endpoint and, in addition, heart function, exercise tolerance, and quality of life. So far (April 1989) 160 patients have been included in the trial.

Conclusion

Long-term beta-blockade seems to benefit a subset of patients with heart failure in DCM and secondary dilated cardiomyopathies with regard to heart function and exercise tolerance. There is no reliable method to choose the right patient for treatment. The mechanism for improvement remains obscure, but several mechanisms have been proposed including up-regulation of beta-receptors' and improvement of the energetic balance in the myocardium. Many problems remain to be solved, but since there is an increasing interest in this research field at present, the future seems to be promising for this new therapeutic principle.

References

1. Waagstein F, Hjalmarson A, Swedberg K, Wallentin I (1983) Beta-blockers in dilated cardiomyopathies: they work. Eur Heart J 4 [Suppl A]:17
2. Cohn JN, Levine TB, Olivari MT, Garberg V, Lura D, Francis GS, Simon AB, Rector T (1984) Plasma norepinephrine as a guide to prognosis in patients with chronic congestive heart failure. N Engl J Med 311:819–823
3. Bristow MR, Ginsburg R, Umans V, Fowler M, Minobe W, Rasmussen R, Zera P, et al (1986) Beta-1 and beta-2-adrenergic-receptor subpopulations in non-failing and failing human ventricular myocardium: Coupling of both receptor subtypes to muscle contraction and selective beta-1-receptor down-regulation in heart failure. Circ Res 59:297–309
4. Insel PA, Ransnäs LA (1988) G-proteins and cardiovascular disease. Circulation 78:1511–1513
5. Ransnäs LA, Hjalmarson A, Insel PA (1988) Dilated cardiomyopathy is associated with an impaired activation of the stimulatory G protein, G_s, by GTP in heart membranes (Abstr.) Circulation [Suppl 2] 78:II–178
6. Limas CJ, Goldenberg IF, Limas C (1989) Autoantibodies against beta-adrenoceptors in human idiopathic dilated cardiomyopathy. Circ Res 64:97–103
7. Magnusson Y, Waagstein F, Andersson A, Marullo S, Guillet J-G, Vahlne A, Hjalmarson A, Hoebeke J (1989) Auto-antibodies against the $beta_1$-adrenergic receptor in patients with idiopathic dilated cardiomyopathy (DCM). Abstract C9, New Trends in Cardiomypathies, Florence, June 1989, p 58
8. Ikram H, Chan W, Bennett SI, Bones (1979) Haemodynamic effects of acute beta-adrenergic receptor blockade in congestive cardiomyopathy. Br Heart J 42:311
9. Currie PJ, Kelly MJ, McKenzie A, Harper RW, Lim YL, Federman J, Anderson ST, Pitt A (1984) Oral beta-adrenergic blockade with metoprolol in chronic severe dilated cardiomyopathy. J Am Coll Cardiol 3:203
10. Ikram H, Fitzpatrick D (1981) Double-blind trial of chronic oral beta-blockade in congestive cardiomyopathy. Lancet 2:490
11. Engelmeier RS, O'Connell JB, Walsh R, Rad N, Scanlon PJ, Gunnar RM (1985) Improvement in symptoms and exercise tolerance by metoprolol in patients with dilated cardiomyopathy: a double-blind, randomized, placebo-controlled trial. Circulation 72:536
12. Anderson JL, Lutz JR, Gilbert EM, Sorensen SG, Yanowitz FG, Menlove RL, Bartholomew M (1985) A randomized trial of low-dose beta-blockade therapy for idiopathic dilated cardiomyopathy. Am J Cardiol 55:471
13. Waagstein F, Caidahl K, Wallentin I, Bergh C-H, Hjalmarson A (1989) Long-term beta-blockade in dilated cardiomyopathy. Effects of acute and chronic metoprolol treatment followed by withdrawal and readministration of metoprolol. Circulation 80,3:551-563
14. Swedberg K, Hjalmarson Å, Waagstein F, Wallentin J (1980) Adverse effects of beta-blockade withdrawal in patients with congestive cardiomyopathy. Br Heart J 44:134-142

15. Heilbrunn SM, Shah P, Bristow MR, Valantine HA, Ginsburg R, Fowler M (1989) Increased beta-receptor density and improved hemodynamic response to catecholamine stimulation during long-term metoprolol therapy in heart failure from dilated cardiomyopathy. Circulation 79:483–490
16. Waagstein F, Blomström-Lundquist C, Andersson B, Hjalmarson A, Wallentin I (1987) Long-term effects of metoprolol in severe heart failure due to ischemic cardiomyopathy, primary valve disease and diabetes (Abstr.) Circulation [Suppl] 76 (4):IV–358
17. Andersson B, Blomström-Lundquist C, Waagstein F (1988) Exercise hemodynamics and myocardial metabolism in severe heart failure during chronic betablockade treatment. Circulation [Suppl] 78 (4): II–575
18. Swedberg K, Waagstein F, Hjalmarson A, Wallentin I (1979) Prolongation of survival in congestive cardiomyopathy by beta-blocker blockade. Lancet 1:1374
19. Norwegian Multicenter Study Group (1981) Timolol-induced reduction in mortality and reinfarction in patients surviving acute myocardial infarction. N Engl J Med 304:801-807

Role of Antiarrhythmic Treatment in Dilated Cardiomyopathy

F. Furlanello, P. Dal Forno, G. Mosna, A. Bertoldi, R. Accardi, G. Inama,
R. Bettini, G. Vergara, and A. Valentini

Background

In recent years, there has been a growing interest in the problems of arrhythmias, particularly hyperkinetic ones, in dilated cardiomyopathy (DCM) patients, both from the point of view of incidence and of prognostic significance. In fact, DCM patients present not only a high prevalence of arrhythmias, but also a high rate of cardiac mortality.

Many studies on arrhythmias in DCM patients are concerned with Holter monitoring (HM) observation [1–11], and some study programmed electrical stimulation (PES) [12–18], or both [10, 14], or the signal-averaged electrocardiography (late potentials detection) [19]. Few studies on the role of antiarrhythmic (AA) treatment in these patients are available to date [6, 7, 15–18, 20].

Thus, the main dilemma is the real usefulness of AA treatment in the prevention of cardiac arrhythmic sudden death and of death due to congestive heart failure (CHF) in these patients, because the benefit/risk ratio is very low due to the occurrence of depressant effects of the AA drugs on the ventricular function, SA function, and atrioventricular conduction, or due to proarrhythmic effects.

There are still many questions regarding the correlation existing between cardiac arrhythmias and cardiac death in DCM patients, and the resulting role of AA treatment; for example:

- What is the incidence of arrhythmias in DCM patients, and what is their prognostic implication in the clinical course, particularly in sudden death and in cardiac mortality?
- Are the arrhythmias an independent risk factor of mortality or are they correlated to the degree of ventricular impairment, or are they both?
- What is the arrhythmogenic mechanism (reentry, increased automaticity, trigger automaticity, pause dependent, etc.), and how can it be identified or induced?
- What is the rationale of antiarrhythmic treatment, and in what type of arrhythmias is it mandatory even if there is low benefit/risk ratio?
- Are there substantial differences as regards the problem in the different stages of the disease?

Table 1. Twenty-four DCM patients with lethal VT – 23 male, one female

Mean age (years)	44.07 ± 18.3
Mean follow-up (months)	38.22
Overall mortality	9 patients (37.5%)
Cardiac mortality	8 patients (33.3%)
Sudden death	4 patients (16.6%)
CHF death	4 patients (16.6%)

We have tried to answer some of these questions by examining the DCM patients in the light of the classification of the hyperkinetic ventricular arrhythmias (HVA) based on subdivision into "benign," "potentially lethal," or "lethal" forms according to whether the risk of sudden death is absent, present but unpredictable, or very high, respectively [21].

The DCM patients can be classified into *patients with potentially lethal HVA*, normally asymptomatic (complex ectopic ventricular beats, nonsustained VT), and *patients with lethal HVA*, symptomatic for palpitations, pre-syncope, syncope, cardiac arrest: recurrent sustained ventricular tachycardia (VT) (monomorphic or pleomorphic), ventricular fibrillation (VF).

The possible overlapping of both forms of HVA which exist in the same patient can be a limitation of this subdivision, i.e., asymptomatic nonsustained VT may become sustained and symptomatic. Despite these limits, we believe the subdivision of the DCM patients into potentially lethal HVA patients and lethal HVA patients can be useful in order to clarify the role played by AA treatment.

The management of the two different forms is in fact usually different: it is based on HM and is not mandatory in the potentially lethal arrhythmic patients; it is based on PES and is mandatory in the lethal arrhythmic patients. In the discussion on DCM patients with lethal HVA, we add our personal experience of a retrospective study on a cohort of 24 patients with clinically documented sustained VT and quite long mean follow-up (38.22 months) (Table 1).

Role of AA Treatment in DCM Patients with Potentially Lethal HVA

The highest incidence of HVA appears to be in patients with DCM as opposed to other cardiac diseases [22]: ectopic ventricular beats (EVB) in 80–100 patients, with a complex form in 80% and nonsustained VT in 40%–50% of the patients [6–11]. *EVB complex forms and nonsustained VT can be typically considered as potentially lethal HVA in DCM patients, due to both electrophysiologic characteristics and presence of severe underlying disease.* The almost ubiquitous presence of potentially lethal HVA in DCM complicates the differentiation between patients at low and high risk for the purpose of the AA drug treatment. Nevertheless, although data are not conclusive and are sometimes conflicting [1, 11], potentially lethal HVA can be considered as an independent indicator of risk of sudden death in DCM patients, particularly if the NYHA class is more than 2 and ejection fraction (EF) is less than 40% [2, 7, 10, 23]. In fact, both univariate and multivariate analyses, used to determine which factor or combination of factors could most accurately predict survival and death, almost constantly include the presence of both asymptomatic HVA (particularly pairs and/or nonsustained VT) and indexes of depressed ventricular function [2–5, 7, 10, 22].

Thus, the aims of the AA treatment in DCM patients with potentially lethal HVA seem to be clear: to prevent sudden cardiac arrhythmic death, to control hemodynamic symptoms while avoiding side effects of AA drugs on ventricular functions, on atrioventricular (AV) and intraventricular (IV) conduction, and/or proarrhythmic-type effects. But the realization of this therapeutic program in a clinical setting appears to be unlikely for several reasons.

First of all, 20%–30% of the DCM patients present atrial fibrillation, with a possible predictive negative role [3, 4] and about 25% of the patients have A–V and/or IV conduction disturbances that may complicate the antiarrhythmic treatment. Secondly, if an AA treatment is particularly justified in DCM patients, particularly those at risk, with both depressed LV function and frequent pairs and/or episodes of nonsustained VT [2, 10], this is a typical situation with potentially harmful drug side effects. Finally, the hypothesis that the AA therapy might prevent sudden cardiac death in DCM patients with potentially lethal HVA is still to be tested. The recent results of the CAST study in patients with previous acute myocardial infarction (7% of sudden deaths with AA drug class 1C versus 3% with placebo at 10-months' follow-up) represent a severe warning. At present the treatment of potentially lethal arrhythmias in patients with DCM remains a clinical problem.

In the absence of important conclusive data, we advise an individualized approach to therapy based on the clinical situation of each patient. In individual patients with DCM and potentially lethal HVA, we must balance the risk of AA therapy against the potential benefits which are often unproven. We should only treat patients in whom the risk of sudden cardiac death appears to be great and/or in whom the hemodynamic consequences of HVA are intolerable in the short and long term.

It is strongly recommended that therapy be started in hospital to minimize either complications of the proarrhythmic type or depressant effects due to AA drugs on the SA function, AV conduction, and ventricular function.

Despite the long-term side effects, amiodarone remains one of the most useful agents in this type of DCM patient [6, 7]. Amiodarone could be administered with smaller maintenance doses (20 mg/kg/week) [6] than those used for lethal HVA [24].

Role of AA Treatment in DCM Patients with Lethal HVA

The majority of the studies of arrhythmias in DCM patients have been concerned with asymptomatic potentially lethal HVA with particular attention to nonsustained VT. Thus, the clinical incidence and the AA management of symptomatic sustained recurrent VT and/or VF, which is the most important lethal HVA, are not well known despite their importance as regards sudden death in DCM patients. Moreover, the role of PES is controversial in the patient with and without clinically spontaneous sustained VT/VF [10, 15, 17, 18]. The incidence of lethal HVA due to DCM is about 15% of all sustained VT for all types of cardiopathy; moreover, 10%–15% of the recipients of AICD (Automatic Implantable Cardioverter Defibrillator) devices are DCM patients. Even though the incidence of lethal HVA in DCM patients is not high, these arrhythmias are clinically relevant because of the hemodynamic consequences and the high mortality rate: their treatment is absolutely mandatory.

Personal Experience

Our study group included 24 patients with DCM and clinically recurrent sustained VT, who were admitted to the Arrhythmologic Centre of Trento over the last 6 years. The mean age was 44.07 ± 18 years; 23 patients were males (Table 1). DCM was diagnosed in patients who had diffuse left ventricular dysfunction without significant valvular or coronary artery disease or history of angina or myocardial infarction. All patients with specific disorders involving heart muscle as part of a general systemic disease were excluded.

All patients had left ventricular EF ≤ 55%, 17 patients were in NYHA functional class < 3; seven were in NYHA functional class ≥ 3. Two-dimensional Doppler color echography and 24-h HM were performed in 24/24 pa-

Table 2. DCM patients with lethal VT – treatment

Amiodarone		17
Alone	7	
+ Propafenone	1	
+ Mexiletine	2	
+ Sotalol	1	
+ Flecainide	1	
+ Tocainide	1	
Propafenone		2
Sotalol		3
Alone	1	
+ Flecainide	1	
+ Propafenone	1	
PM-AT VVI		1
PM-AT VVI or DDD AT (Symbios 7005/Spectrax SXT)		7
AICD		1

PM, Pacemaker; AICD, Automatic Implantable Cardioverter Defibrillator.

tients; coronary and ventricular angiography was performed in 19/24 patients including all patients older than 40 years of age; PES was performed in 22/24 patients.

Twenty-three patients had clinically recurrent sustained VT, and three patients had incessant ventricular VT, two of whom had also recurrent VT. Six patients (25%) had atrial fibrillation; 4/24 (16%) patients had left bundle branch block. Patients were evaluated directly or questioned by transtelephonic means or by their physicians. The actuarial survival curve at 5 years was evaluated for each patient using the Kaplan-Maier method.

Seventeen out of 24 (70.8%) of patients (Table 2) underwent a loading dose of amiodarone of 20 mg/kg body weight per day for 4–5 days and then received 30 or 40 mg/kg body weight per week according to our previous studies of plasma levels of amiodarone and desethyl-amiodarone [24, 25]. Both the loading dose and the long-term regimen allow therapeutic and safe plasma levels of the drug [26].

In each patient who took amiodarone, T_3-T_4-fT_4-TSH were performed before and every 4 months of treatment. In addition to amiodarone, 6/17 (35.3%) patients received other AA drugs (one patient – propafenone, one patient – flecainide, one patient – sotalol, two patients – mexiletine, one patient – tocainide). Five patients were treated with other AA drugs: propafenone (two patients), sotalol three patients: in one patient alone, together with flecainide in one patient, and with propafenone in one patient. Nine (37.5%) patients had implantable cardiac pacing: externally activated antitachycardia pacemakers were implanted in 7/16 (43.7%) patients (either Medtronic Spectrax SXT for ventricular pacing or Symbios 7005 for dual-chamber pacing). One patient underwent AICD implantation.

Results

The mean follow-up was 38.22 months. The overall mortality was 9/24 (37.5%). The overall cardiac mortality was 8/24 (33.3%). Four patients (16.6%) had sudden death at home (Table 3). Four patients (16.6%) had cardiac nonsudden death due to progressive CHF (Table 4), one patient had noncardiac death. The actuarial survival curve at 5 years was 81.3% for sudden death, 60% for CHF death, and 48.8% for overall cardiac mortality (Fig. 1). The four sudden deaths represented 50% of all cardiac deaths. The mean age of these patients was 46.7 years. All patients were in NYHA < 3 with a mean left ventricular ejection fraction of 42.5%. All patients were treated with amiodarone alone or in combination and a PM-AT VVI (Pacemaker Antitachycardia Ventricular Inhibited) was implanted in one patient. These four patients had short outcome and they had sudden death during a mean follow-up of 7.25 months [12, 24]. In three patients a sustained VT was inducible with PES; in the fourth patient in whom a sustained VT was not inducible, VT became incessant.

Four patients (mean age 48.25 years) had cardiac death due to CHF, all patients were in NYHA functional class ≥ 3 with a mean left ventricular EF of 25.7%; three patients were treated with amiodarone, one patient with propa-

Table 3. Sudden death in DCM patients

Pa-tient no.	Age (years)	Sex	NYHA class	ECG	PES	EF (%)	Treatment	Follow-up (months)
1	55	M	II	Af A-V block	Sustained VT inducible	35	Amiodarone PM-AT VVI	13
2	46	M	II	SR	Sustained VT inducible	35	Amiodarone	6
3	70	M	II	SR, AF	Sustained VT inducible	55	Amiodarone	1
4	16	M	I	SR Incessant VT	Sustained VT not inducible, then incessant VT	45	Amiodarone + tocainide	9

Af, atrial fibrillation; SR, sinus rhythm.

Table 4. CHF death in DCM patients

	Age (years)	Sex	NYHA class	ECG	PES	EF (%)	Treatment	Follow-up (months)
1	66	M	III	SR SSS – A-V block	Sustained VT not inducible	17	Propafenone PM VVI	12
2	39	M	III	SR A-V block	Sustained VI not inducible	26	Amiodarone PM VVI	48
3	27	M	III	SR LBBB Incessant VT	Sustained VT inducible, then incessant VT	30	AICD Amiodarone, then flecainide	4
4	61	M	III	SR SN dysfunction A-V block	Sustained VT inducible	30	Amiodarone PM-AT VVI	42

SR, sinus rhythm; SSS, sick sinus syndrome; LBBB, left bundle branch block; SN, sinus node.

fenone, three patients had implantable cardiac pacing, and one patient underwent AICD implantation. The mean follow-up was 26.5 months. All four patients had sustained VT (2/4 inducible with PES), in one patient VT became incessant.

Three patients, mean age 17.6 years, had incessant VT which was refractory to drugs (and in one to AICD) before death. One had sudden death, one death was due to CHF, and one had heart transplantation.

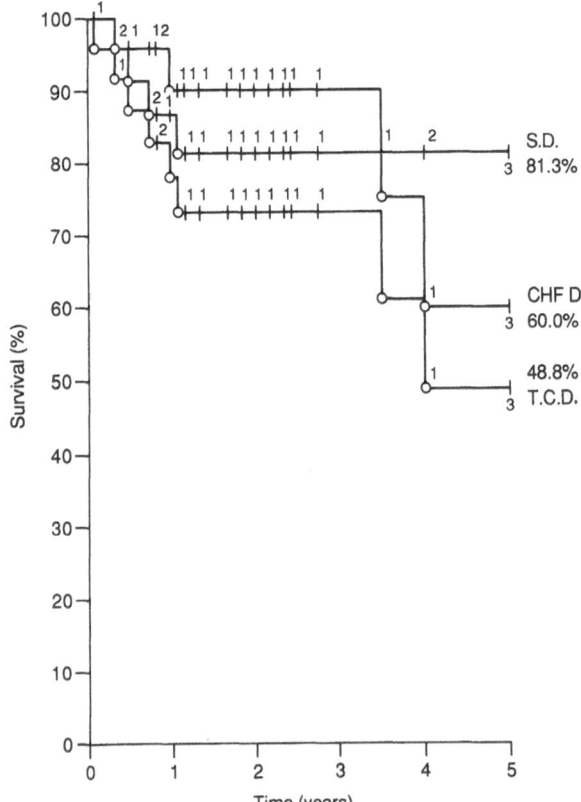

Fig. 1. Survival in dilated cardiomyopathy (24 patients)

Outcome

The actuarial survival curve at 5 years for NYHA class < III (17/24 patients) was 74.8% for sudden death, 100% for CHF death (Fig. 2). In the patients with NYHA ≥ III (7/24 patients), the actuarial survival curve for CHF death was 22.9% (Fig. 3). The actuarial survival curve for EF > 30% (18/24 patients for sudden death was 75%, for CHF death it was 94.1%, and for total cardiac death it was 70.6% (Fig. 4). The actuarial survival curves for EF ≤ 30% (6/24 patients) for sudden death was 100%, for CHF death it was 40% (Fig. 5).

In 2/17 patients (11.7%) amiodarone was withdrawn because of serious side effects due to hyperthyroidism after 10 and 12 months of treatment (Table 5).

The actuarial survival curve for total cardiac mortality at 5 years (Fig. 6). was 34.8% in patients (17/24) who were taking amiodarone; the survival curve after 2 years was 70% in patients on amiodarone and 75% in patients on other AA drugs (5/22) (not significant).

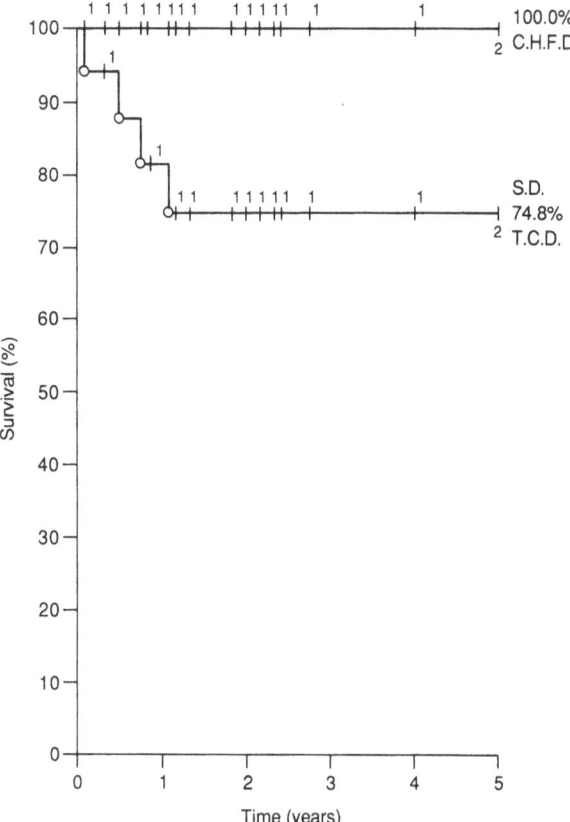

Fig. 2. NYHA class < III
(17 patients)

Comment

Our retrospective study on a cohort of 24 DCM patients with clinically recurrent sustained VT confirmed a high rate of cardiac deaths which were both sudden and due to CHF. Sudden death represented 50% of all cardiac deaths, and it occurred in the 1st year of the clinical course; conversely, cardiac death due to CHF occurred later. In addition, sudden death occurred in DCM patients in lower functional classes and with higher EF than cardiac death due to CHF.

   Our observation showed that DCM patients with sustained VT are at a high risk of sudden death in the 1st year of clinical observation, even though treatment carefully included amiodarone and electrical devices. Thus, this critical period of follow-up should be scrupulously carried out.

   Another observation is the following: in DCM patients with lethal VT and with cardiac death due to CHF (in whom device implantation helps to control SA and AV dysfunction and long-term AA treatment) the sustained ventricular arrhythmias during the clinical course lose their predictive value and clinical importance.

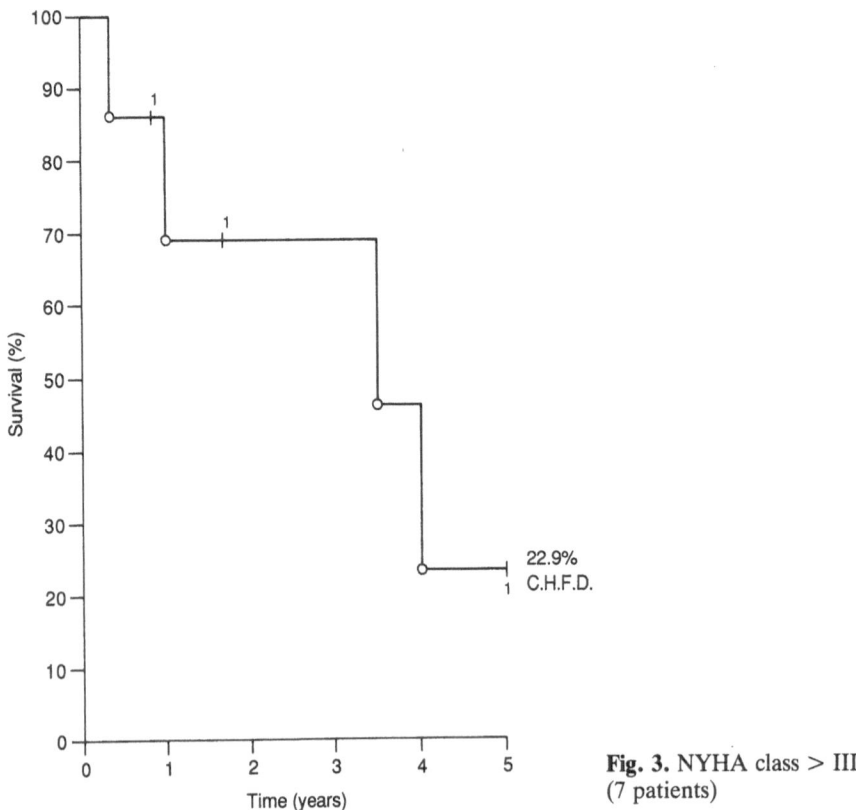

Fig. 3. NYHA class > III (7 patients)

Finally, in DCM patients with incessant sustained VT, lethal HVA can be considered as:

(a) "Secondary" to ventricular dysfunction
(b) A cause of hemodynamic cardiac deterioration
(c) An intractable arrhythmias situation for refractoriness and proarrhythmic responses to AA drugs. It may be an indication for cardiac transplantation.

Conclusions

In the patient population with DCM, the presence of lethal HVA, particularly sustained recurrent VT, represents a major clinical problem as regards sudden death. The management of these sustained VT remains arduous even though the AA armentarium available today includes PES-guided therapy. A cause of limited drug efficacy and of high rate of both sudden death and death due to CHF is related to electrophysiological substrate. First of all, many arrhythmogenic mechanisms (either alone or in combination) may be involved, e.g.,

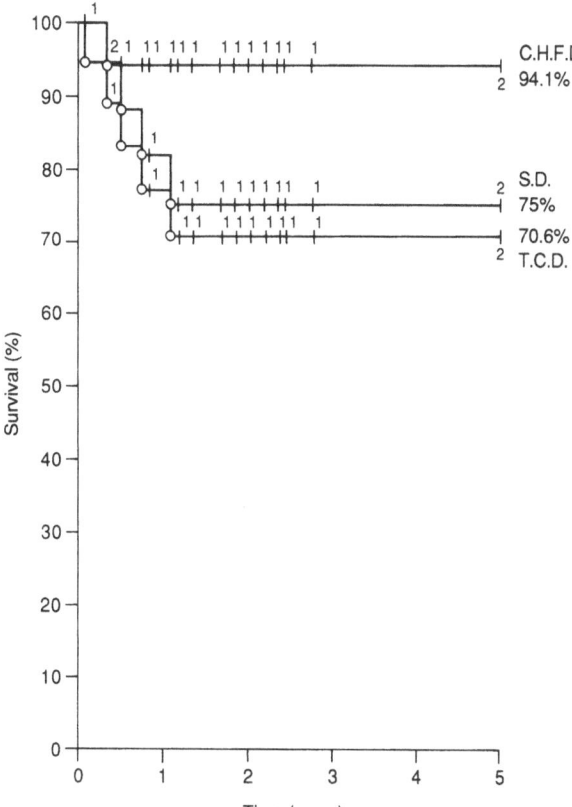

Fig. 4. Ejection fraction > 30% (18 patients)

reentry, automaticity, trigger automaticity, pause-dependent, etc. The progression and diffusion of primary myocardial compromission limit the pharmacologic test prediction and cardiac surgical options. On the contrary, the primary myocardial disease may modify the electrogenetic mechanism of VT during the clinical course to cardiac heart failure.

The patients with sustained VT and DCM are typically at risk of sudden death due to arrhythmias in the 1st year of the outcome. This is independent of both functional class and left ventricular indexes. Thus, young people with good functional class may be at risk, as can be observed in individual athletes [26, 27] with cardiac arrest and sudden death.

As a clinical implication, the initial observation period of DCM patients with sustained VT should include a careful, aggressive, diagnostic, and therapeutic approach which involves nonpharmacologic options. In the surviving patients, the deterioration of ventricular function plays a major role in the clinical course to cardiac death, and the sustained VT may lose their clinical importance. Finally, some patients, in general the younger ones, at the end stage of their clinical course of DCM, may complain of incessant refractory sustained VT which is probably secondary to ventricular dysfunction and may be an additive

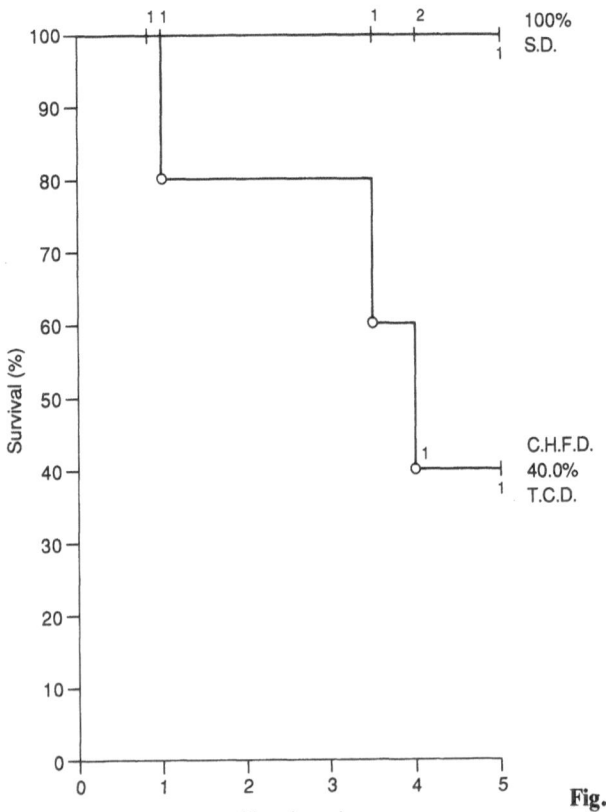

Fig. 5. Ejection fraction < 30% (6 patients)

Table 5. Amiodarone withdrawn because of major side effects: 2/17 (11.7%) DCM patients

Patient No	Sex	Age (years)	Follow-up (months)	Cause
1	M	30	10	Hyperthyroidism
2	M	66	12	Hyperthyroidism

cause of hemodynamic deterioration. In these patients, who are prone to proarrhythmic and depressant response to AA drugs, the only reliable option is cardiac transplantation.

General Conclusions

The role of antiarrhythmic treatment for the prevention of sudden death in potentially lethal HVA in DCM patients, particularly those with low EF and high functional NYHA class, is not clear. The treatment can be performed in

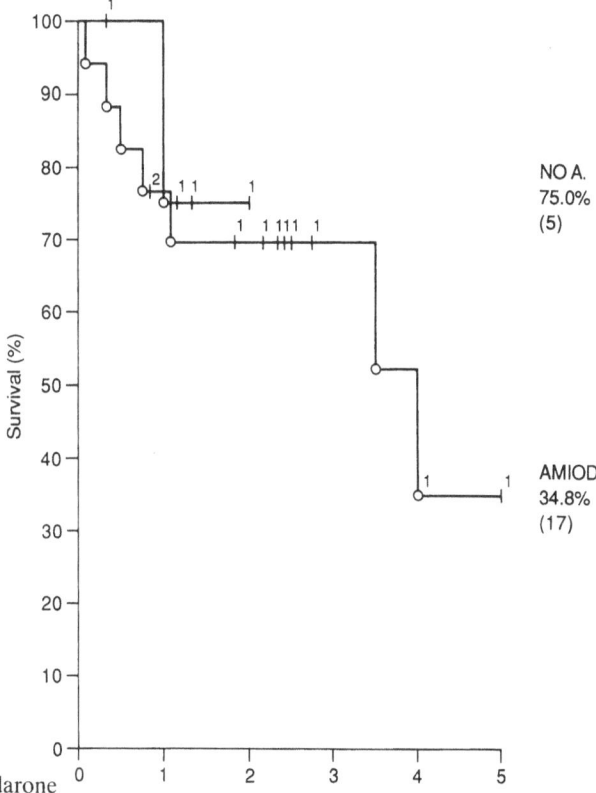

Fig. 6. Drug treatment: amiodarone vs. other drugs (22 patients)

individual patients following a careful approach in order to avoid proarrhythmic and depressant effects of AA drugs. Amiodarone is the first-choice drug.

In the DCM patients with lethal HVA, the treatment is mandatory, particularly in the 1st year of the clinical course when the risk of sudden death is higher. The therapeutic approach should be quite aggressive and based (when reliable) on PES and electropharmacologic tests to assess drug efficacy. Since the primary goal of the treatment is the prevention of sudden death, a partial result such as a partial suppression of inducible arrhythmias could be accepted, if the latter are hemodynamically well tolerated [28].

At present, amiodarone, in spite of its long-term side effects, plays an important role in the treatment of DCM patients with lethal HVA. Drug combination and implantable cardiac pacing, including antitachycardia externally activated systems or cardioverter-defibrillator units, allow the patient to be kept under quite effective, long-term treatment, even as a bridge to cardiac transplantation.

Finally, in the patients under long-term amiodarone treatment, it is necessary to use a standardized drug regimen and to perform a careful clinical surveillance during follow-up in order to individuate or prevent side effects.

References

1. Von Olshausen K, Stienen U, Schwartz F, Kübler W, Meyer J (1988) Long term prognostic significance of ventricular arrhythmias in idiopathic dilated cardiomyopathy. Am J Cardiol 61:146–151
2. Hofmann T, Meinertz T, Kaspar W, Geibel A, Zehender M, Hohnloser S, Stienen U, Tree N, Just H (1988) Mode of death in idiopathic dilated cardiomyopathy: a multivariate analysis of prognostic determinants. Am Heart J 116:1455
3. Romeo E, Pelliccia F, Cianfrocca C, Cristofani R, Reale A (1988) Identification of patients with idiopathic dilated cardiomyopathy at high risk of sudden cardiac death. Cardiostimolazione 6 (4):249
4. Unverferth DV, Magorien RD, Moeschberger ML, Baker PB, Fetters JK, Leier CV (1984) Factors influencing the one-year mortality of dilated cardiomyopathy. Am J Cardiol 54:147–152
5. Stewart RAJ, Adams K, McKenna WJ, Oakley CM (1988) Prediction of sudden death in dilated cardiomyopathy. Eur Heart J 9 [Suppl 1]:287
6. Neri R, Mestroni L, Salvi A, Pandullo C, Camerini F (1987) Ventricular arrhythmias in dilated cardiomyopathy: efficacy of amiodarone. Am Heart J 113:707
7. Meinertz T, Hofmann T, Kasper W, Treese N, Bechtold H, Stienen U, Pop R, Leitner V, Andersen D, Meyer J (1984) Significance of ventricular arrhythmias in idiopathic dilated cardiomyopathy. Am J Cardiol 53:902–907
8. Von Olshausen K, Schafer A, Meheml HC, Schwartz F, Senges J, Kübler W (1984) Ventricular arrhythmias in idiopathic dilated cardiomyopathy. Br Heart J 51:195
9. Costanzo-Nordin MR, O'Connell JB, Engelmeier RS, Moran JF, Scanlon PJ (1984) Ventricular tachycardia in dilated cardiomyopathy: a variable independent of hemodynamics, morphology and prognosis (abstr). J Am Coll Cardiol 3:594
10. Meinertz T, Hofmann T, Zehender M, Geibel A, Kasper W, Just H (1988) Arrhythmias in dilated cardiomyopathy, In: Cosin J, Bayes de Luna AJ, Garcia Civera R, Cabades (eds) Cardiac arrhythmias. Pergamon, New York, pp 431–453
11. Von Olshausen K, Schafer A, Meheml HC, Schwartz F, Senges J, Kübler W (1984) Ventricular arrhythmias in idiopathic dilated cardiomyopathy. Br Heart J 51:195–201
12. Nobile A, Spampinato A, Nava S, Montenero S, Bellocci F (1988) Usefulness of programmed ventricular stimulation in patients with idiopathic dilated cardiomyopathy and non sustained ventricular tachycardia. Cardiostimolazione 6 (4):247
13. Gössinger H, Siostrzonek P, Jung M, Grimm G, Schmoliner R, Mösslacher H (1988) Programmed ventricular stimulations in patients with dilated cardiomyopathy and nonsustained ventricular tachycardias. A follow-up study. Cardiostimolazione 6 (4):249
14. Gonska BD, Bethge KP, Kreuzer H (1989) Can electrophysiologic studies predict sudden death in patients with idiopathic dilated cardiomyopathy? In: 4th European Symposium on Cardiac Pacing, Stockholm, 28–31 May 1989, abstract book, p 122
15. Rae AP, Spielman SR, Kutalek SP, Kay HR, Horowitz LN (1987) Electrophysiologic assessment of antiarrhythmic drug efficacy for ventricular tachyarrhythmias associated with dilated cardiomyopathy. Am J Cardiol 59:291–295
16. Naccarelli GV, Prystowsky EN, Jackman WM, Heger JJ, Rahilly GT, Zipes DP (1982) Role of electrophysiologic testing in managing patients who have ventricular tachycardia unrelated to coronary artery disease. Am J Cardiol 50:165
17. Poll DS, Marchinsky FE, Bucton AE, Doherty JU, Waxman HL, Josephson ME (1984) Sustained ventricular tachycardia in patients with idiopathic dilated cardiomyopathy: electrophysiologic testing and lack of response to antiarrhythmic drug therapy. Circulation 70:451
18. Liem LB, Swerdlow CD (1988) Value of electropharmacologic testing in idiopathic dilated cardiomyopathy and sustained ventricular tachyarrhythmias. Am J Cardiol 62:611–616
19. Borggrefe M, Egloff J, Budde T, Fetsch T, Karbenn U, Breithardt G (1988) Clinical value of late potentials as a marker of electrical instability in dilative cardiomyopathy. In: Santini M, Pistolese M, Alliegro A (eds) Progress in clinical pacing. Excerpta Medica, Amsterdam, p 247

20. Almendral JM, Josephson ME (1988) An electrophysiological approach to drug therapy of ventricular arrhythmias. In: Bayes de Luna A, Betriu A, Permanyer G (eds) Therapeutics in cardiology. Kluwer, Dordrecht, pp 66–78
21. Bigger JT (1986) Relation between left ventricular dysfunction and ventricular arrhythmias after myocardial infarction. Am J Coll Cardiol 57:8B
22. Brandenburg RO (1985) Cardiomyopathies and their role in sudden death. J Am Cardiol 5:185B–189B
23. Rapaport E (1988) Sudden cardiac death. Am J Cardiol 62:31–61
24. Furlanello F, Dal Forno P, Inama G, Accardi R, Bertoldi A, Bettini R, Guarnerio M, Valentini A, Vergara G (1988) Antiarrhythmic drug therapy in the prevention of post infarction sudden death. Results with amiodarone. In: Santini M, Pistolese M, Alliegro A (eds) Progress in clinical pacing. Excerpta Medica, Amsterdam, p 393
25. Furlanello F, Inama G, Dal Forno P, Padrini R, Piovan D, Pessina AC (1983) Amiodarone in the antiarrhythmic therapy. Pharmacol Res Commun 15:881–890
26. Inama G, Padrini R, Furlanello F (1984) Amiodarone antiarrhythmic treatment and blood level: methods of administration. In: Proceedings of the 6th International Congress of Cardiology. OIC Medial Press, Florence, pp 329–335
27. Furlanello F, Bettini R, Vergara G, Bertoldi A, Del Greco M, Durante GB, Frisanco L (1989) Marker and trigger mechanisms of sudden cardiac death. Exercise and sports activity. In: Bayes de Luna A (ed) Proceedings of sudden death. Barcelona (in press)
28. Borggrefe M, Trampisch HJ, Breithardt G (1988) Reappraisal of criteria for assessing drug efficacy in patients with ventricular tachyarrhythmias: complete versus partial suppression of inducible arrhythmias. J Am Coll Cardiol 112:140–149

Cardiac Transplantation
for Dilated Cardiomyopathy

W. J. Kostuk, N. R. Singh, P. W. Pflugfelder, A. H. Menkis, and F. N. McKenzie

Introduction

In recent years, new approaches for the medical treatment for heart failure have evolved. While the use of vasodilators and specifically angiotensin converting enzyme inhibitors has improved both functional status and survival, long term prognosis unfortunately remains poor [1–4]. Since the initial human heart transplant over 20 years ago, there has been a progressive improvement in long-term survival [5]. Moreover, cardiac transplantation results in marked alleviation of symptoms and improved quality of life in patients with end stage heart failure. Indeed, patients undergoing successful cardiac transplant are capable of resuming normal physical activity which is in sharp contrast with their severe physical limitations prior to surgery. With the availability of cyclosporine [6], the cardiac transplantation program at University Hospital, London, Canada commenced in April 1981. Between then and December 1988, 186 transplants were performed in 179 patients with end-stage heart disease. Heart failure was the result of ischemic heart disease (IHD) in 86 patients and cardiomyopathy (CM) in 80 patients. In the remainder, transplantation was for end-stage valvular heart disease in eight, congenital heart disease in five, and seven patients required retransplantation. In this discussion only the patients with IHD and CM will be evaluated. Of the 80 patients with CM, one patient had amyloidosis, two hypertrophic CM, one postpartum CM, one adriamycin-induced CM, and one patient had acute myocarditis. In the remainder no identifiable cause of dilated CM was identified.

In this paper, the indications for and the results of cardiac transplantation in patients with dilated CM are compared with those in whom ventricular damage has resulted from IHD.

Indications for Transplant (Table 1)

Before committing a patient to cardiac transplantation, alternate therapies such as coronary artery bypass graft surgery, with or without aneurysmectomy, valve replacement in the setting of compromised left ventricular function and attempts to control rhythm disturbances including the use of an implantable automatic defibrillator should first be exhausted [7]. Intensive medical therapy

Table 1. Criteria for heart transplantation

Indications
1. Terminal heart disease with life expectancy of less than 12 months.
2. No possibility of benefit from conventional medical or surgical therapy.
3. No major or irreversible secondary organ dysfunction.

Contraindications
Absolute
1. Fixed elevation of pulmonary vascular resistance (> 8 Wood units).

Relative
1. Age > 60 years
2. Active sepsis
3. Unresolved pulmonary infarction
4. Insulin-dependent diabetes
5. Irreversible secondary organ dysfunction
6. Functionally limiting peripheral or cerebrovascular disease
7. Active peptic ulcer disease
8. Malignancy
9. Ongoing substance or alcohol abuse
10. Evidence of poor compliance

with vasodilator therapy as well as the use of newer inotropic agents such as milrinone has been of value in some patients with biventricular failure [4, 8]. It is important to recognize that in many cases these alternative treatments are at best a temporizing measure. Many of the individuals who benefit from alternative treatment may ultimately require transplantation.

The major criterion for selection of recipients has been and remains symptomatic terminal heart disease, that is a cardiac disorder in which survival is realistically not expected to exceed 6–12 months. A more recent indication has been intractable ventricular arrhythmias and extensive left ventricular dysfunction. These patients may not manifest severe heart failure yet there is no doubt as to the certainty of limited survival as a result of their rhythm disorder.

Among individuals with significant left ventricular dysfunction, there are several parameters statistically associated with increased mortality, including functional class and objective measures of exercise capacity, the degree of both left and right ventricular dysfunction, the presence of significant ventricular arrhythmias, the hemodynamic status of the patient and neuroendocrine abnormalities. Stability of congestive heart failure is also a significant determinant of survival. Those in whom congestive heart failure is worsening are much more likely to die within 12 months compared to those who have had a more stable course. There are conflicting reports in the literature about the independent association of ventricular arrhythmias to mortality in patients with heart failure. The suggestion is, however, that more complex ventricular arrhythmias are predictive of sudden death [9]. In general, the presence of biventricular failure with low cardiac output is associated with a poor prognosis [10].

During the past 5–8 years, there has been considerable broadening of acceptance criteria for cardiac transplantation, such that the majority of previous absolute contraindications have become relative contraindications. Elevation of

Table 2. Preoperative demographic and hemodynamic findings

	Cardiomyopathy n = 80	Ischemic heart disease n = 86
Sex: Male	63	82
Female	17	4
Age (years)	37 ± 14	50 ± 7
RAP (mmHg)	12 ± 6	11 ± 7
PAP (mmHg)	37 ± 9	38 ± 12
PAWP (mmHg)	28 ± 8	30 ± 10
CO (l/min)	3.5 ± 1.1	3.5 ± 1.1
PVR (Wood units)	3.0 ± 1.6	3.5 ± 2.2
LVEF (%)	14 ± 6	16 ± 5

Values: means ± SD. *RAP*, mean right atrial pressure; *PAP*, mean pulmonary artery pressure; *PAWP*, mean pulmonary arterial wedge pressure; *CO*, cardiac output; *PVR*, pulmonary vascular resistance; *LVEF*, left ventricular ejection fraction.

pulmonary vascular resistance (> 8 Wood units) remains the only absolute contraindication to cardiac transplantation. Patients in their sixth decade are no longer denied cardiac transplantation. In our experience, survival and rehabilitation are not adversely affected in this age group. Individuals over 60 years remain a relative contraindication. Such individuals invariably have other organ dysfunction and many lack the stamina required for good recovery during the early postoperative period. In our centre, few such individuals undergo transplantation. We have limited ourselves to patients with a short history of cardiac failure (i.e., < 1–2 years) with absolutely no other confounding systemic abnormality. Noncompliant patients as well as substance and alcohol abusers are poor candidates for transplantation.

Patient Characteristics (Table 2)

Patients with end-stage cardiac dysfunction whether due to IHD or CM were identical with regard to preoperative hemodynamics. Both groups had similar degrees of elevated filling pressures, reduced cardiac output and normal to mildly elevated pulmonary vascular resistance. Left ventricular ejection fraction was identical and invariably less than 20%. The major difference between the two groups was with regard to age and sex. The CM patients were younger (mean age 37, range 13–62 years) and 21% were females. The IHD group was older (mean age 50, range 24–64 years) and was predominantly (95%) male.

Outcome

Survival (Fig. 1): Current actuarial survival is 83%, 80%, and 77% at 1, 3, and 5 years, respectively, and for our last 100 patients is 89% in spite of operating on more critically ill patients. The majority of deaths have occurred within the first 90 days of surgery. The causes of death following transplantation were

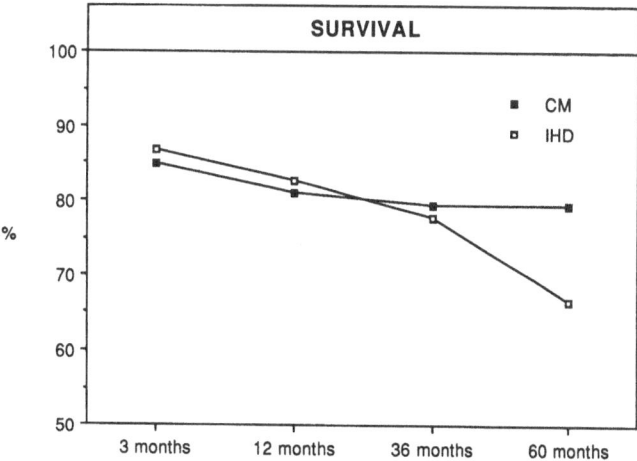

Fig. 1. Actuarial survival for 80 patients with cardiomyopathy (*CM*) and 86 patients with ischemic heart disease (*IHD*)

independent of the etiology of the heart disease that prompted the transplantation initially. Of the 21 early (< 90 days) deaths, five (24%) were the result of rejection. In five patients, the graft did not function adequately and death occurred within 24 h of surgery. The majority of immediate graft failures occurred early in our experience and were felt related to inadequate preservation. In five patients early death was related to improper patient selection. These individuals had known preexisting pulmonary infarction or infections. In the remaining six patients, early death was the result of infection in two, pulmonary embolism in two, pancreatitis in one, and intracerebral hemorrhage in one. The ten late (> 90 days) deaths (mean of 605 days, range 152–2323 days) were as a result of chronic rejection in six patients, malignancy in two patients, pulmonary embolism in one, and unknown cause in one patient.

Exercise Capacity (Table 3): By 3 months following transplantion, exercise capacity returns to normal. On follow-up, this improvement is maintained over the ensuing 36 months. In our patient population, exercise results following transplantation have been consistently better in the CM group compared to the IHD group, likely related to the age difference of the two groups.

Table 3. Exercise capacity following transplantation

Time (months)	Cardiomyopathy			Ischemic heart disease		
	3	12	36	3	12	36
Exercise duration (s)	650 ± 174[a]	663 ± 205[a]	633 ± 158[a]	516 ± 123	543 ± 131	490 ± 108
Peak workload (Mets)	12 ± 3[a]	13 ± 3[a]	12 ± 3[a]	10 ± 3	10 ± 3	9 ± 3
Peak heart rate	145 ± 18[a]	154 ± 21[a]	158 ± 19[a]	134 ± 17	146 ± 14	138 ± 16

[a] $p < 0.05$ cardiomyopathy vs. ischemic heart disease.
Means ± SD.

Table 4. Filling pressures at rest before and following cardiac transplant

| | Cardiomyopathy | | Ischemic heart disease | |
	RAP	PAWP	RAP	PAWP
Preoperatively	12 ± 6	28 ± 8	11 ± 7	30 ± 10
1 week	9 ± 6	15 ± 5	10 ± 6	16 ± 6
3 months	6 ± 2	14 ± 4	6 ± 2	14 ± 4
12 months	5 ± 2	12 ± 4	5 ± 2	12 ± 3
36 months	5 ± 2	12 ± 3	5 ± 2	12 ± 2

Values: means ± SD. *RAP,* mean right atrial pressure (mmHg); *PAWP,* mean pulmonary arterial wedge pressure (mmHg).

Left Ventricular Ejection Fraction: Resting left ventricular ejection fraction is normal by 3 months and is similar for both groups (IHD 57 ± 9% and CM 58 ± 7%). With exercise, left ventricular ejection fraction increases in a normal fashion in both groups (IHD 60 ± 9% and CM 64 ± 8%). Rest and exercise ejection fractions have remained normal on long-term follow-up in both groups.

Hemodynamics (Table 4): At 1 week following transplantation filling pressures remain mildly elevated, although they gradually decrease over the ensuing weeks to remain normal long term. There is no difference in the resting hemodynamics in patients with a pretransplant diagnosis of CM or IHD.

Cardiac output following transplantation is normal at rest and exercise and remains so long term. During supine exercise, striking increases of pulmonary artery, pulmonary arterial wedge and right atrial pressures have been seen. In a study of 20 patients following heart transplantation [11], the mean pulmonary artery pressure rose 45% during the first stage of exercise and by peak exercise increased 87% above resting values. The pulmonary arterial wedge pressure increased significantly with passive leg elevation and during the first stage of exercise rose 61% above baseline values. By peak exercise the mean pulmonary arterial wedge pressure was more than double the resting value. Similarly, the right atrial mean pressure increased significantly with passive leg elevation and nearly tripled at peak exercise. All values promptly returned to baseline after exercise. The cardiac output increased 98% during exercise, mediated primarily by an increase in stroke volume during early exercise.

Morbidity: Myocardial rejection in the setting of cyclosporine use is observed within the first 90 days of surgery in most patients (IHD 60% and CM 70%). The frequency of rejection is similar regardless of preoperative diagnosis (IHD 1.1 ± 1.2 and CM 0.9 ± 0.8 episodes).

The introduction of cyclosporine as an immunosuppressive agent has been associated with a number of adverse effects, in particular hypertension and nephrotoxicity [12]. With the passage of time, there is a gradual increase in both systolic and diastolic arterial pressure. By 1 year, 50% of individuals require treatment for hypertension and this increases to 70% by 3 years.

In our early experience, cyclosporine was given intravenously in the perioperative period; this was associated with a high incidence of nephrotoxicity. Subsequently, we have delayed oral cyclosporine administration until 3–5 days postoperatively and maintain a whole blood cyclosporine level of 300–500 ng/ml. At the same time equine antilymphocyte globulin (ALG) is administered intravenously for the first 3–5 days postoperatively.

Nevertheless, serum creatinine rises gradually following transplantation. Early postoperatively, serum creatinine is normal while by year 1, the mean values range from 150–175 mmol/L. Close monitoring of cyclosporine blood levels is essential and after 6 months levels of 150–250 ng/ml are maintained. If necessary, azathioprine is added to the long-term cyclosporine and prednisone regimen so that cyclosporine levels can be further reduced. Approximately 40% of individuals require this three-drug regimen.

The development of vascular disease has been reported to range from 5%–25% in the 1st year following surgery and 20%–44% at 3 years [13–16]. In our experience, large vessel vascular disease is an unusual phenomenon [17]. Qualitative analysis has revealed only three of 83 patients with any angiographic abnormality at follow-up, one with minimal luminal irregularities in the right coronary artery at 1 year, a second with a 50% diameter stenosis of the proximal left anterior descending artery and minimal irregularity of the proximal circumflex artery at 1 year, and a third patient who developed a new 30% diameter eccentric proximal right coronary artery stenosis at 3 years follow-up. Our cumulative incidence of graft vascular disease assessed angiographically was 2% at 1 year and 4% at 3 years. Subsequent to this reported study, one additional patient who exhibited normal coronary vasculature at 1 year following transplantation exhibited severe, diffuse triple vessel vascular disease at 2.5 years.

Quantitative analysis of these same patients, however, has showed a small but significant decrease in coronary luminal diameter over time. In addition, seven of eight hearts obtained at autopsy or retransplantation showed significant degrees of diffuse fibrointimal hyperplasia, unsuspected from angiography performed as recently as 7 days earlier. Thus, diffuse vascular disease may be insidious, progressive and often undetectable by current angiographic techniques.

Hypercholesterolemia is a common phenomenon following heart transplantation in patients who receive cyclosporine and prednisone immunosuppression. The total serum cholesterol level progressively increases such that at the end of one year follow-up 84% of patients have a serum cholesterol level higher than 5.2 mmol/L and 52% have serum levels higher than 6.2 mmol/L. Patients with a high serum cholesterol level, defined as higher than 5.2 mmol/L are more apt to be older and exhibit higher preoperative cholesterol and a greater frequency of pretransplant diagnosis of IHD. We have also found that the cumulative steroid dose is higher at one year in patients with a higher serum cholesterol. The cumulative cyclosporine dose and the frequency of rejection episodes did not differ between those with normal or high serum cholesterol. The long-term implications and optimal therapy for hyperlipidemia in heart transplant patients are unknown at the present time.

Retransplantation: In this series retransplantation was required in seven patients, five in the CM group, and two in the IHD group. In the latter, graft failure occurred within 1 week of surgery. In the CM group rejection necessitated retransplantation in three patients from 40 to 81 days. In one patient graft failure resulted in retransplantation at 16 days. In the final patient retransplantation was carried out at 488 days following her initial transplantation for acute myocarditis. This patient had no problem for the first 13 months following transplantation but began to note palpitations related to junctional tachycardia (120–140 per minute) which was associated with hypotension. Initially, myocardial biopsy and cardiac function were normal. In the ensuing weeks, however, her cardiac function became abnormal and biopsy showed evidence of giant cell myocarditis. In spite of increasing immunosuppression and antifailure medication, her cardiac function continued to deteriorate necessitating retransplantation.

Summary

During the past decade there has been a progressive improvement in survival following cardiac transplantation, irrespective of etiology. The majority of deaths tend to occur in the first 3 months following surgery. Many of these deaths are related to improper patient selection i.e., operating in the presence of known pulmonary embolism/infarct or infection, often in desperation to prevent the death of a young patient with CM. Unfortunately, we lack the ability to predict the point in time where survival with medical therapy is less than that which can be achieved with transplantation. Indeed, many deaths are sudden and have been attributed to ventricular arrhythmia. Until an ideal prognostic marker is available, we need to utilize not only symptoms and functional class but also hemodynamic and other factors such as malignant arrhythmia for selecting patients for cardiac transplantation. The appropriate timing of cardiac transplantation remains a challenge.

Following transplantation, functional status and exercise tolerance return to normal. Morbidity (hypertension, nephrotoxicity and hypercholesterolemia) associated with immunosuppressive therapy is common yet each of these adverse effects is modifiable with alterations in the cyclosporine dose. Cardiac transplantation is an effective form of therapy for patients with end-stage heart disease regardless of the etiology.

References

1. Cohn J, Archibald D, Ziesche S, Franciosa JA, Harston WE, Tristani FE, Dunkman WB, Jacobs W, Francis GS, Flohr KH, Goldman S, Cobb FR, Shah PM, Saunders R, Fletcher RD, Loeb HS, Hughes VC, Baker B (1986) Effects of vasodilator therapy on mortality in chronic congestive cardiac heart failure: results of a Veterans Administration Cooperative Study. N Engl J Med 314:1547–1552
2. The CONSENSUS Trial Study Group (1987) Effects of enalapril on mortality in severe congestive cardiac failure. Results of the cooperative North Scandinavian enalapril survival study (CONSENSUS). N Engl J Med 316:1429–1435

3. Captopril Multicenter Research Group (1983) A placebo-controlled trial of captopril in refractory chronic congestive heart failure. J Am Coll Cardiol 2:755–763

4. Stevenson LW, Dracup AK, Tillisch JH (1989) Efficacy of medical therapy tailored for severe congestive heart failure in patients transferred for urgent cardiac transplantation. Am J Cardiol 63:461–464

5. Solis E, Kaye MP (1986) Registry of the international society for heart transplantation: third official report. J Heart Trans 5:2–5

6. Borel JF, Deurer C, Magnee C, Stahelin H (1977) Effects of the new antilymphocytic peptide cyclosporine A in animals. Immunology 32:1017–1025

7. Winkle RA, Mead RH, Ruder MA, Gaudiani VA, Smith NA, Buch WS, Schmidt P, Shipman T (1989) Long-term outcome with the automatic implantable cardioverter-defibrillator. J Am Coll Cardiol 13:1353–1361

8. DiBianco R, Shabetai R, Kostuk W, Moran J, Schlant RC, Wright R (1989) A comparison of oral milrinone, digoxin and their combination in the treatment of patients with chronic heart failure. N Engl J Med 320:677–683

9. Packer M (1985) Sudden unexpected death in patients with congestive heart failure: a second frontier. Circulation 72:681–685

10. Diaz RA, Obasohan A, Oakley CM (1987) Prediction of outcome in dilated cardiomyopathy. Br Heart J 58:393–399

11. Pflugfelder PW, McKenzie FN, Kostuk WJ (1988) Hemodynamic profiles at rest and during supine exercise after orthotopic cardiac transplantation. Am J Cardiol 61:1328–1333

12. Racusen LC, Soley K (1988) Cyclosporine nephrotoxicity. Int Rev Exp Pathol 3:107–157

13. Bieber CP, Hunt SA, Schwinn DA, Jamieson SA, Reitz BA, Oyer PE, Shumway NE, Stinson EB (1981) Complications in long-term survivors of cardiac transplantation. Transplant Proc 13:207–211

14. Jamieson SW, Oyer PE, Baldwin J, Billingham M, Stinson EB, Shumway NF (1984) Heart transplant for end-stage ischemic heart disease: the Stanford experience. Heart Transplant 3:244–227

15. Gao SZ, Alderman EL, Schroeder JS, Silverman JF, Hunt SA (1988) Accelerated coronary vascular disease in the heart transplant patient: coronary arteriographic findings. J Am Coll Cardiol 12:334–340

16. Uretsky BF, Murali S, Reddy PS, Rabin B, Lee A, Griffith BP, Hardesty RL, Trento A, Bahnson HT (1987) Development of coronary artery disease in cardiac transplant patients receiving immunosuppressive therapy with cyclosporine and prednisone. Circulation 76:827–834

17. O'Neill BJ, Pflugfelder PW, Singh NR, Menkis AH, McKenzie FN, Kostuk WJ (1989) Frequency of angiographic detection and quantitative assessment of coronary arterial disease one and three years after cardiac transplantation. Am J Cardiol 63:1221–1226

Long-Term Treatment with Amiodarone for the Prevention of Sudden Death in Patients with Dilated Cardiomyopathy

M. Ciaccheri, G. Castelli, M. Nannini, V. Troiani, C. Arcangeli, P. Marconi, and A. Dolara

There is considerable controversy about the treatment of asymptomatic ventricular arrhythmias in patients with congestive heart failure [1]. Antiarrhythmic therapy has been reported either to prolong survival and decrease the incidence of sudden death (SD) [2], or only to reduce mortality [3]. Patients with dilated cardiomyopathy (DC) and complex ventricular arrhythmias have been treated successfully with amiodarone and no patient has died suddenly during therapy [4]. Others have underlined that the evidence for results is still lacking [5]. We report the results of our study on the efficacy of amiodarone for the prevention of SD in patients with DC and ventricular tachycardia (VT).

Material and Methods

One hundred and fifteen patients with DC entered the study from January 1981 to March 1989; 86 were male and 29 female. Their age ranged from 19 to 72 years with a mean of 49.6 ± 10. All were diagnosed according to the criteria proposed by Goodwin and Oakley [6], i.e., heart muscle disorder with depressed systolic function without known cause. At entry into the study all patients had one or more of the following clinical features:

1) symptoms and signs of left- or right-sided congestive heart failure or both;
2) roentgenographic evidence of cardiomegaly with cardiothoracic ratio > 0.5;
3) electrocardiogram abnormalities in the form of left ventricular conduction delay and/or left ventricular hypertrophy;
4) history of systemic emboli.

Patients were not included if there was a history of coronary artery disease or excessive alcohol intake (1 g/kg per day for 5 years). Patients with clinical evidence of systemic hypertension (> 170/90 mmHg), cor pulmonale, valvular heart disease, or systemic disease involving the heart were also excluded. All patients underwent M-mode and two-dimensional echocardiography which showed dilatation and/or hypokinesia of one or both ventricular cavities according to the Feigenbaum criteria [7]. Coronary angiography was performed in 68 patients. Patients were excluded from the study if there was an obstruction > 50% of a major coronary artery and a left ventricular ejection fraction

> 0.50 at left ventricular angiography. Endomyocardial biopsy was performed in 37 patients, none showed evidence of active myocarditis. Ventricular arrhythmias were classified according to Lown criteria.

Monitoring Procedure

All patients underwent 24-h Holter monitoring at entrance into the study. Perpendicular leads approximating V1 and V5 were recorded simultaneously. The tapes were analyzed by two of the authors (CA; PM) using an Del Mar Avionics Evaluator model 9500. Each arrhythmic event was written out in real time on standard electrocardiographic paper.

Each patient without VT was routinely controlled by serial ECG ambulatory monitoring every 6 months during the whole follow-up period. If VT was detected both at entrance into the study and during follow-up, treatment with amiodarone was started, and the examination was repeated after 1 month. If VT disappeared, Holter monitoring was again performed every 6 months; if VT persisted, Holter monitoring was performed after 3 months.

Nonsustained VT was defined as three or more ventricular ectopic beats occuring in succession at a rate > 100 per minute. Sustained VT was defined as an episode of tachycardia lasting more than 30 s and not self-terminating.

Antiarrhythmic Treatment

Sixty-one patients who had at least one episode of nonsustained or sustained VT during the follow-up period were treated with amiodarone 600 mg/day in the 1st week, 400 mg/day in the 2nd week, and 200 mg/day thereafter for 5 days a week. If episodes of VT were present in the follow-up period, the dose was again increased to 400 mg/day. The cumulative therapy period was 1881 months, equivalent to a mean of 30 months for each patient. Thyroid function tests were performed every 6 months; chest X-rays, eye examinations, and liver function tests every year.

Follow-up

The study began at the date of the first ambulatory ECG monitoring and terminated at the death of the patient or at the time of the last follow-up visit. Each patient was controlled every 3 months or earlier when clinically needed. Deaths occurring within 1 h from the onset of symptoms were defined as sudden. The mean follow-up period for the total population was 46 months. The mean follow-up period for patients treated with amiodarone was 41 months; for patients who were not treated, it was 51 months.

Results

VT was found in 61/115 patients (53%) both at the beginning of the study and during the follow-up period; the number of episodes varied from one to twelve (mean three) for each patient. The number of ectopic beats ranged from 3 to 54 with a maximum rate of 210 per minute. In 32/61 VT persisted despite treatment. Nineteen patients died during follow-up, and ten of them died suddenly. Eight out of ten were under therapy with amiodarone; in four cases VT was abolished by the drug, and in the other four it was not; in these two subgroups the numbers of patients in NYHA functional class were, respectively, as follows: class II–III, 4 and 3; class IV, 0 and 1. The other two patients who died suddenly did not take amiodarone or any other antiarrhythmic drug. Seven patients died of refractory congestive heart failure, and two of noncardiac causes (Fig. 1).

In 11 cases there were modifications of thyroid function (rise of T4 and FTI), and severe adverse side effects were observed in seven (hypothyroidism in four, hyperthyroidism in three); in these seven patients it was necessary to stop treatment. In other patients we observed gastric intolerance (one case), elevation of transaminases (one case), and corneal deposits (three cases) which needed drug withdrawal (Table 1).

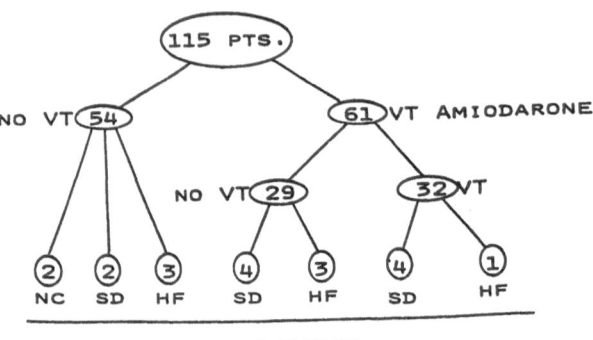

CAUSES OF DEATH

Fig. 1. Causes of death. Mean follow-up: whole group, 46 months; treated group, 41 months; nontreated group, 51 months. *VT*, ventricular tachycardia; *NC*, noncardiac; *SD*, sudden death; *HF*, heart failure

Table 1. Amiodarone side effects (16/61 patients)

Eleven cases of increased levels of T_4-FTI
    → Three cases of clinical hyperthyroidism
    → Four cases of clinical hypothyroidism
One case of gastric intolerance
One case of increased levels of SGOT, SGPT
Three cases of corneal deposits

Discussion

The percentage of VT found in the present study (53%) is similar to that reported by others in DC patients [8–11]. While some authors think that these arrhythmias are not a negative prognostic marker for SD [9, 12], others [13] have underlined that these patients are at high risk, and a therapeutic intervention is therefore mandatory.

Amiodarone has been proven to be able to abolish ventricular arrhythmias in our experience as well as in that of others [14]. Our results are nevertheless different from those observed by Neri et al. [4] who reported no SD in patients with ventricular arrhythmias treated with amiodarone. The different treatment design may have some importance. Neri et al. [4] did not use serial ECG ambulatory monitoring in patients who initially had no ventricular arrhythmias and who were used as a control group. Since detection of arrhythmias is sometimes possible only with repeated ambulatory ECG monitoring, there may be some bias in the selection of Neri et al.'s patients. We followed every patient with ambulatory ECG monitoring, and, if VT was detected at any time during the whole follow-up period, the patient was treated with amiodarone. Thus the entire group of treated and nontreated patients was evaluated only retrospectively at the end of the follow-up period.

A possible limitation of our study is the lack of serum amiodarone and desethylamiodarone concentrations. Accordingly, the doses used could not be adequate to control arrhythmias. Morady et al. [15] reported that the drug given at maintenance doses of 600 mg/day was able to abolish ventricular arrhythmias in 91% of patients who survived a cardiac arrest. It must be noted that the follow-up period for their patients was only 19 months.

In conclusion, amiodarone treatment is able to abolish ventricular arrhythmias in a large percentage of patients with DC, but in our experience it does not prevent SD. The drug has a number of side effects, and its use in every patient with ventricular arrhythmias is not justified. Other methods, such as programmed stimulation or signal averaging, may be useful to identify patients at risk.

References

1. Francis GS (1988) Should asymptomatic ventricular arrhythmias in patients with congestive heart failure be treated with antiarrhythmic drugs? J Am Coll Cardiol 12:274–283
2. Simonton CA, Daly PA, Kereiakes D, Modin G, Chatterjee K (1987) Survival in severe left ventricular failure treated with the new nonglycosidic, nonsympathomimetic oral inotropic agents. Chest 92:118–123
3. Dargie HJ, Cleland JGF, Leckie BJ, Inglis CG, East BW, Ford I (1987) Relation of arrhythmias and electrolyte abnormalities to survival in patients with severe chronic heart failure. Circulation [Suppl 4]:98–107
4. Neri R, Mestroni L, Salvi A, Pandullo C, Camerini F (1987) Ventricular arrhythmias in dilated cardiomyopathy: efficacy of amiodarone. Am Heart J 113:707–715
5. Schmitt C, Brachmann J, Waldecker B, Rizos I, Senges J, Kubler W (1987) Amiodarone in patients with recurrent sustained ventricular tachyarrhythmias: results of programmed electrical stimulation and long-term clinical outcome in chronic treatment. Am Heart J 114:279–283

6. Goodwin JF, Oakley CM (1972) The cardiomyopathies. Br Heart J 34:545
7. Feigenbaum H (1986) Echocardiography, 4th edn. Lea and Febiger, Philadelphia
8. Meinertz T, Hofmann T, Kasper W, Treese N, Bechtold H, Stienen U, Pop T, Leitner ER, Andresen D, Meyer J (1984) Significance of ventricular arrhythmias in idiopathic dilated cardiomyopathy. Am J Cardiol 51:507–512
9. Huang SK, Messer JV, Denes P (1983) Significance of ventricular tachycardia in idiopathic dilated cardiomyopathy: observations in 35 patients. Am J Cardiol 51:507–512
10. Olshausen KV, Shaper A, Mehmel HC, Schwarz F, Senges J, Kubler W (1984) Ventricular arrhythmias in idiopathic dilated cardiomyopathy. Br Heart J 51:195–201
11. Chakko CS, Gheorghiade M (1985) Ventricular arrhythmias in severe heart failure: incidence, significance and effectiveness of antiarrhythmic therapy. Am Heart J 109:497–504
12. Maskin CS, Siskind SJ, Le Jemtel TH (1984) High prevalence of sustained ventricular tachycardia in severe congestive heart failure. Am Heart J 107:896–901
13. Follansbee WP, Michelson EL, Morganroth J (1980) Non-sustained ventricular tachycardia in ambulatory patients: characteristics and association with sudden cardiac death. Ann Intern Med 92:741–747
14. Heger JJ, Prystowsky EL, Jackmann WM, Naccarelli SV, Warfel KA, Ruikenberger RL, Zipes DP (1981) Amiodarone: clinical efficacy and electrophysiology during long-term therapy for recurrent ventricular tachycardia or ventricular fibrillation. N Engl J Med 305:539–545
15. Morady F, Sauve MJ, Malone P, Shen EN, Schwartz AB, Bhandari A, Keung E, Sung RJ, Scheinmann MM (1983) Long-term efficacy and toxicity of high-dose amiodarone therapy for ventricular tachycardia or ventricular fibrillation. Am J Cardiol 52:975–979

Subject Index